Physiotherapy for Children

Edited by

Teresa Pountney PhD, MA, MCSP

Research Lead/Physiotherapist, Chailey Heritage Clinical Services, East Sussex

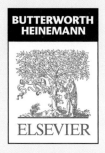

BUTTERWORTH
HEINEMANN

ELSEVIER

EDINBURGH   LONDON   NEW YORK   OXFORD   PHILADELPHIA   ST LOUIS   SYDNEY   TORONTO   2007

**BUTTERWORTH
HEINEMANN**
ELSEVIER

An imprint of Elsevier Limited

First published 2007
© 2007, Elsevier Ltd

ISBN-13: 978 0 750 68886 4

British Library Cataloguing in Publication Data
A catalogue record for this book is available from the British Library.

Library of Congress Cataloging in Publication Data
A catalog record for this book is available from the Library of Congress.

Note
Neither the Publisher nor the Authors assume any responsibility for any loss or injury and/or damage to persons or property arising out of or related to any use of the material contained in this book. It is the responsibility of the treating practitioner, relying on independent expertise and knowledge of the patient, to determine the best treatment and method of application for the patient.

Working together to grow
libraries in developing countries

www.elsevier.com | www.bookaid.org | www.sabre.org

ELSEVIER   BOOK AID
International   Sabre Foundation

ELSEVIER your source for books, journals and multimedia in the health sciences

www.elsevierhealth.com

The Publisher's policy is to use paper manufactured from sustainable forests

Printed in China

Physiotherapy for Children

For Elsevier:

Publisher: Heidi Harrison
Associate Editor: Siobhan Campbell
Project Manager: Morven Dean
Design: Andy Chapman
Illustration Buyer: Gillian Richards
Illustrator: Graham Chambers and Chartwell Illustration

Contents

Preface

This book is aimed at undergraduate students and qualified physiotherapists who are beginning a career in paediatrics. It aims to provide an understanding of a range of conditions which affect children and how these are managed. Other professionals may also find it a useful resource particularly those who see children occasionally.

Health professionals working with children need to have knowledge of the wider framework in which physiotherapy occurs and the issues pertinent to working with children. This framework includes the interventions and also the context in which they occur. Paediatric physiotherapists work with children from their arrival in the neo-natal unit until they reach adulthood and need to be aware of growth and its impact on treatment. Adolescence and other ages can be difficult for any child and will affect how a child responds to treatment interventions.

All the chapters are written by expert clinicians in their specialty, are based on research evidence and combine the theoretical and practical aspects of physiotherapy practice. Chapters include:

- Evidence based research to support clinical interventions
- A multidisciplinary approach to treatment provision with the child and family at the centre of the team
- Outcomes measures to evaluate treatment interventions
- Case studies to illustrate clinical practice

PART 1 APPROACHES TO WORKING WITH CHILDREN

These chapters set the scene for delivering physiotherapy services to children and form the background to how treatment is provided to children. The chapter on the legal and ethical framework underpins an approach to working with children to ensure that they are treated foremost as children, are safe and are included in decision making regarding their treatment. It outlines the basic principles of this framework by which paediatric physiotherapist are bound.

Paediatric physiotherapy is delivered in a wide variety of settings. This chapter will cover how physiotherapy interventions are included in different settings and what is considered to be best practice. It explores these settings and how they impact on provision, describes why working with children is different from working with adults, how policy and organizational changes affect service delivery and the changing role of the paediatric physiotherapist within this framework.

PART 2 ASSESSMENT AND OUTCOME MEASURES

The outcomes measures chapter seeks to offer advice in locating, evaluating and using outcome measurement tools that are appropriate for the paediatric patient population. It explores how decisions are made regarding which outcome measures are most appropriate based on the framework of International Classification of Functioning, Disability and Health (ICIDH). A range of commonly used outcome measures are given with detailed information to guide the reader to an appropriate measure.

The gait analysis chapter covers the use of motion analysis and how it provides a full understanding of a child's gait pattern. This information can be used to make informed decisions regarding interventions such as surgery and orthotics.

PART 3 NEUROLOGY

This series of chapters gives an insight into the most common neurological conditions encountered by paediatric physiotherapist. Motor control in developmental neurology offers an overview of paediatric neurology and explores the changing vista of motor control and views on infant development. The use of the ICIDH framework as a basis for developing a rational evidence based therapy approach is discussed alongside other aspects of therapeutic options.

Neo-natal care for physiotherapists is a combination of neurological development and respiratory care. This chapter combines these two important aspects including assessment of the nervous system and respiratory system, specific conditions and their presentation, follow-up of the high risk infant, intervention and treatment principles.

Cerebral palsy is an umbrella term for a wide spectrum of neurological impairment. The management of the motor aspect of cerebral palsy and its associated conditions such as epilepsy is covered and physiotherapy interventions are reviewed in the light of current evidence.

The mechanism of neural tube defects and the impact of spinal lesions are described. The second half of the chapter considers a child's physical management including surgery and how physiotherapy input changes through a child's life.

The historical background, terminology, differential diagnosis relating to developmental co-ordination disorder (DCD) is described in this chapter. A guide to service provision including assessment and an outline of intervention approaches is covered. Trends in current research are summarised and present a national and international picture of DCD.

Assistive technology is widely used by physiotherapists as an integral part of the management of neurological and other conditions. This chapter offers an overview of mechanical and electronic assistive technology and explores how its use can be optimized by assessment and provision as part of a multidisciplinary team. It covers the range of products which a physiotherapist is most likely to encounter when involved with families and children.

PART 4 ACQUIRED BRAIN INJURY

This section covers the acute and long-term management of acquired brain injury (ABI). Together the chapters follow the management of children with ABI from admission to hospital to reintegration. Details of incidence and causes, the different stages of recovery and the myriad of other factors which affect recovery of motor ability such as sensory and attention difficulties are explored.

PART 5 MUSCULOSKELETAL

Musculoskeletal conditions range in severity from minor injuries and problems to disabling conditions. The orthopaedic chapter covers conditions for which physiotherapists routinely provide treatment including talipes equinovarus, leg lengthening techniques and Perthes disease.

The scope of rheumatology is wide and varied and this chapter explores the gamut of conditions encountered within the field of rheumatology. It outlines the presentation and physiotherapy management and provides a detailed assessment section and description of the new group of medical therapies called the "biologics".

Duchenne muscular dystrophy is the commonest of the muscular dystrophies and this chapter provides in-depth information on the mechanism causing the condition, its presentation and management. Details of further research into this condition and how management is changing are included.

Many children engage in sport at a variety of levels and sustain injuries, and treatment of these injuries in children requires consideration of their maturity. This chapter gives an insight into the treatment of sport injuries in children, how injuries are sustained, treatment and rehabilitation to ensure a child is safe to return to sport.

PART 6 CARDIO-RESPIRATORY

The three chapters which comprise this section of the book consider the anatomy and physiology of the immature respiratory system, cardiorespiratory physiotherapy for the acutely ill, non-ventilated child and paediatric intensive care. The first chapter provides a background to how a child's anatomy and physiology differs from the adult and how it changes with growth and development and is a basis for the following chapters.

The second chapter provides an introduction to the basic concepts which impact upon assessment and treatment of respiratory illness in non-ventilated children and offers strategies for the treatment of common symptoms. The focus is on the infant and young child throughout as older children and adolescents can be assessed and treated in a similar manner to adults.

Physiotherapists now take a much more advanced role in respiratory care in the Paediatric Intensive Care Unit and this chapter explores their involvement in aspects of weaning from ventilation, the process of extubation, performing diagnostic procedures, taking blood gases and ordering investigations and prescribing. Useful sections on assessment and on-call working are included.

PART 7 ONCOLOGY AND PALLIATIVE CARE

This section covers the incidence and management of cancer in children and young people and specifically looks at the impact of these treatments on a child or young person and the role the physiotherapist can play in the treatment process. Details of some common conditions requiring physiotherapy input are described based on research, best practice and clinical experience.

PART 8 CHILD AND ADOLESCENT MENTAL HEALTH

The role of the physiotherapist in the management of young people with mental health problems is not always clear. This chapter aims to explore the physiotherapist's role as a valuable member of a multidisciplinary team working in this area to manage very real physical problems such as poor cardiovascular fitness due to inactivity, weakness associated with disuse and unusual gait patterns, and to provide advice and structure to support return to premorbid functioning.

Although this book primarily considers the physical management of children, as physiotherapists we must take a wider view of our treatment set in the context of a child's life and remember that above all childhood should not be compromised.

Paediatric physiotherapy has an evolving evidence base on which we can base our clinical practice to ensure that we use effective treatments and interventions to optimise a child's health. We have the tools to measure some of these outcomes and need to use these to build on our clinical practice and research to continue the advances seen in paediatric physiotherapy. To do this most effectively we need to involve children and families in this process.

Children and young people need to have an active role in their treatment and have their views listened to and acted upon. The National Service Framework for Children and Young People (2004) advocates actively involving children and young people in decisions affecting them. Engaging children and families as partners in physiotherapy treatment adds an additional dimension to how we work and helps ensure that the children and young people reach their potential within the limitations of their conditions.

Acknowledgements

This book is the result of many individuals' dedication and support. Thanks are therefore owed:

To all the authors who have shared their knowledge and expertise to bring together the publication of this book. They have all given precious time from their busy professional and home lives to contribute to the book and produce a resource for paediatric physiotherapists and other health professionals to use in their clinical practice. Their commitment to the book is much appreciated.

To Chailey Heritage Clinical Service who have supported me in this venture, and to the clinicians who have contributed chapters. Their willingness to discuss and advise on decisions regarding text and illustrations and their encouragement to carry on has been invaluable. I would like to thank Donna Cowan, Alice Wintergold and Pat Wilcox individually for their support.

To the Association of Paediatric Chartered Physiotherapists whose members have provided the mainstay of authors of this books. This book is a recognition of the work of the association and the depth and breadth of work in which it is involved. Their suggestions and advice on the content of the book have shaped it to hopefully meet the needs of paediatric physiotherapists. Many thanks to all those colleagues, of whom there are too many to mention individually, who have helped, encouraged and supported me.

To Professor Ann Moore for suggesting my name to Elsevier as a potential editor and encouraging me to undertake the project.

To Siobhan Campbell and Morven Dean who have patiently supported me through the project as a novice editor.

And finally, special thanks go to my family, Richard, Lizzie and William, and friends who have kept me sane and happy throughout the production of the book.

Terry Pountney

Contributors

Rebecca Biggs MSc, Grad Dip Phys, MSCP
Clinical Specialist Paediatric Physiotherapist,
St Mary's NHS Trust, London, UK

Jill Brownson JP, MSCP, Grad Dip Phys
Paediatric Physiotherapy Manager,
St Mary's NHS Trust, London, UK

Donna Cowan PhD, BSc, MIET, MIPEN CSci
Consultant Clinical Scientist and Head of
Rehabilitation Engineering Service, Chailey Heritage
Clinical Services, East Sussex, UK

Sarah Crombie MSc, MCSP
Superintendent Paediatric Physiotherapist, Royal West
Sussex NHS Trust, Chichester, UK

Jan Davies MCSP, Grad Dip Phys
Paediatric Macmillan Clinical Specialist, Royal
Manchester Children's Hospital, Manchester, UK

Helen Dewdney BSc (Hons), MCSP
Acute Paediatric Physiotherapy Team Leader,
St Mary's NHS Trust, London, UK

Michelle Eagle PhD, MSc, MCSP
Consultant Physiotherapist, Newcastle Muscle Clinic,
Institute of Genetics, Newcastle, UK

Julia Graham MSc, MCSP
Clinical Specialist, Paediatric Physiotherapy, and
Therapy Services Manager, Maternal and Child Health
Division, Basingstoke and North Hampshire
Foundation NHS Trust, Hampshire, UK

Liz Hardy BSc (Hons), MCSP
Team Leader, Acute Paediatric Physiotherapy,
Newcastle-upon-Tyne Hospitals NHS Foundation
Trust, Newcastle-upon-Tyne, UK

Jeanne Hartley MSc, MCSP
Clinical Specialist Physiotherapist, Paediatric
Orthopaedics, Great Ormond Street Hospital for
Children NHS Trust, London, UK

Robyn M. Hudson BSc, BSc App Physio
Clinical Specialist Physiotherapist, Paediatrics and
Adolescents, Physiotherapy Department, University
College Hospital London, London UK

Adele Leake MCSP, MSc
Senior Lecturer, Sheffield Hallam University, Faculty of
Health and Well Being, Sheffield. UK

Susan Maillard MSc, SRP, MCSP, Dip Physiotherapy
Clinical Specialist Physiotherapist in Paediatric
Rheumatology, Great Ormond Street Hospital,
London, UK

Ann Markee MCSP
Senior Community Physiotherapist for Children,
Rugby, UK

Anna Mayhew PhD, M Med Sci, MCSP
Research Physiotherapist, Imperial College, London, UK

Margaret Mayston PhD, MSc, BAppSc, MCSP
Senior Lecturer, Department of Physiology, University
College London, London, UK

Gillian McCarthy FRCP, FRCPCH
Honorary Consultant Neuropaediatrician, Chailey
Heritage Clinical Services, East Sussex, UK

Victoria Mitchinson MSc, BSc (Hons), MCSP
Senior Paediatric Physiotherapist, Children's and
Teenage Oncology, Newcastle-upon-Tyne Hospitals
NHS Trust, Newcastle-upon-Tyne, UK

Lesley Nutton MCSP, Grad Dip Phys
Senior Paediatric Physiotherapist, Bobath Scotland,
Glasgow, UK

Judith M. Peters PhD, MSc, BA, MCSP
Honorary Clinical Specialist Physiotherapist, Great
Ormond Street Hospital for Children NHS Trust,
London, UK

Teresa Pountney PhD, MA, MCSP
Research Lead Physiotherapist, Chailey Heritage
Clinical Services, East Sussex, UK

Fiona Price BSc, MCSP
Senior Physiotherapist, Sheffield Children's NHS
Foundation Trust/North Trent Regional Neonatal
Unit, Sheffield Teaching Hospitals NHS Foundation
Trust, Sheffield, UK

Julie Sparrow MSc, Grad Dip Phys, MCSP
Senior Lecturer, University of Teeside, Middlesborough,
UK

Nicky Thompson MSc, MCSP
Clinical Specialist in Gait Analysis, Oxford Gait
Laboratory, Nuffield Orthopaedic Centre, Oxford, UK

Patricia Wilcox MCSP
Physiotherapist, Children's Head Injury Service, Chailey
Heritage Clinical Services, East Sussex, UK

Alice Wintergold BEng, MSc, MIPEM, CEng, CSci
Clinical Engineer, Chailey Heritage Clinical Services,
East Sussex, UK

Approaches to working with children

1

Ethical and legal framework of paediatric physiotherapy practice

Julia Graham

INTRODUCTION

Paediatric physiotherapists are bound by, and practise within, a legal and ethical framework. The basic principles of this framework are outlined below but inevitably there are exceptions to most rules and this should not be relied upon as the ultimate definitive guide but rather a starting point for further investigation.

Readers must also be aware that the legislation discussed applies to England and Wales and to some extent Northern Ireland. The system within Scotland and elsewhere in Europe may be entirely different. Physiotherapists should therefore familiarize themselves with the relevant legislation relating to children for the country in which they practise.

> Physiotherapists need to have sufficient familiarity with the basic principles of the law so that when faced with a difficult situation they know immediately the laws which apply and the point at which they need to seek expert advice (Dimond 1999, p. 2).

Understanding the relevant legislation related to the field in which they work is an important factor of a physiotherapist's competency to practise. An awareness of patients'

rights, issues of consent, professional governance, professional liability and duty of care, to name but a few, are all issues within this framework that arise regularly in day-to-day practice.

THE LEGAL SYSTEM

The legislative framework and the law set out a *minimum* standard of what you should or should not do – what is legal and illegal, but be aware that what was legal one day may well be illegal the next. The law can change and be amended at any time.

There are predominantly two fields to the legal system: criminal law and civil law.

Criminal law deals with acts that are regarded by the state as 'wrongs' – a criminal offence has taken place. Criminal law is usually investigated by the police in conjunction with the Crown Prosecution Service. The law seeks to deter and punish those who are guilty of committing the crime, through prosecution.

- For a person to be guilty of a crime the court must be satisfied *beyond reasonable doubt* that a person did the wrong. This is known as the *standard of proof*
- In most cases there must have been an *intention* to do the wrong
- There are strict rules of *evidence* in criminal cases.

The law in this case has to arrive at a single determinate conclusion – guilty or not guilty.

Civil law regulates wrongs and disputes between individuals, companies and some public bodies such as local authorities. Unlike criminal law, there is no primary intention to punish. Civil law can be used to:

- Compensate for harm done (injury due to road traffic accident)
- Prevent harm occurring (injunction in domestic abuse)
- Adjudicate on conflicting claims (who should look after a child following divorce of the parents).

For someone to succeed in a civil action, the standard of proof is the *balance of probabilities*.

There are however some instances when the same action may result in proceedings under criminal and civil law. For example, a mother who seriously injures her child through ill treatment may be prosecuted under criminal law for child cruelty and the local authority, under civil law, may apply for a care order to remove the child from the home.

Statute law is written law, made by legislation of the European Community and Acts of Parliament of the UK government. The process by which Acts of Parliament are made is a recognized procedure. A bill introduced into the House of Lords or House of Commons follows a set pathway which includes hearings, committee and report stages. Once accepted by both houses and given royal assent by the signature of the Queen, it becomes an Act of Parliament.

Acts of Parliament are often supplemented by rules and regulations. Statute law includes employment law and contract issues. It is statute law that empowers our professional bodies such as the Health Professions Council.

The courts interpret statutes and in some instances create new law – judge-made common law, or case law.

Primary legislation is passed by an Act of Parliament, e.g. The Children Act 1989. It can only be changed by Parliament. Secondary legislation sets out how the primary legislation should be applied in practice and is as binding as primary legislation, although may be more easily changed. In addition to primary and secondary legislation, the government produces a large number of circulars and guidance, e.g. *Working Together to Safeguard Children* (Department of Health, Home Office, Department for Education and Employment 1999), the *Framework for the Assessment of Children in Need and their Families* (Department of Health, Department for Education and Employment, Home Office 2000), *National Service Framework for Children, Young People and Maternity Services* (Department of Health 2004). Although these are not binding in the same way as legislation, they do have strong persuasive force in legal proceedings and failure to follow them is likely to prejudice a case, unless there is good reason for not doing so.

RIGHTS OF THE CHILD AND YOUNG PERSON

It is important as practising paediatric physiotherapists to promote the rights of children. The possession of rights is an expression of value because those who lack rights are clearly valued less (Kurtz 1994). Recognition and respect are basic human rights for a child or young person; they are what children and young people want; they help children and young people to stay safe and promotion of the rights of children and young people is stated in law. Examples given below demonstrate some of the guidance, legislation and governance that have particular relevance to children.

United Nations Convention on the Rights of the Child (1989)

Although not enacted into English law to give children the same legal rights as adults, the UK government ratified the United Nations (UN) Convention on the Rights of the Child in 1991, accepting responsibility for the development of rights-based, child-centred health care. The UN Convention includes 45 articles, the guiding principles of which are summarized below:

- All of the rights in the convention apply equally to *all* children
- The best interests of the child shall be a primary consideration in all actions and decisions concerning that child
- Every child has a basic and unequivocal right to life and to survival and development
- All children have the right to express and have their views given due weight in all matters that affect them.

The UN Convention imposes responsibilities on the state, parents/carers and guardians to ensure all children are properly looked after, educated and provided with good-quality health care. The state must ensure that the rights set out in the UN Convention are put into practice.

The Children Act 1989

The principles of the UN Convention are reflected within the Children Act 1989 (England and Wales). This Act set up a new framework for the protection and care of children and established clear principles to guide decision-making in relation to their care. The overriding principle is that the child's welfare shall be the court's paramount consideration in any proceedings affecting the child.

The main principles of the Children Act 1989 are listed below:

- Welfare of the child is paramount: safeguarding and promoting it are priorities
- Children should be brought up and cared for in their own families
- Delay in the resolution of court proceedings and provision of service must be avoided
- Children should be kept informed about what happens to them and should participate in decisions about their future
- Parents continue to have responsibility even if the child is not living with them
- Parents with children in need should be helped to bring up their children themselves
- Help should be provided as a service to the family with minimal intrusion into family life
- Service providers must listen to and work in partnership with children and parents
- Needs arising from race, culture, religion and language must be taken into account by service providers.

The Children Act 2004

The Children Act 2004 (England and Wales) followed publication of the government's formal response to the Victoria Climbie inquiry and the Green Paper *Every Child Matters* in September 2003 (HM government 2003). *Every Child Matters* proposed changes in policy and law to maximize opportunities and minimize risks for all children, focusing services more effectively around their needs and those of the family. The initial Green Paper was followed by two others: *Every Child Matters: Next Steps* (March 2004), which set out a programme of change to promote the well-being of all children, and *Every Child Matters: Change for Children* (December 2004), setting out a national framework for local change programmes.

The overall aim of the Act is to create transparent accountability for children's services, promote better joint working and provide a voice for children through the establishment of a Children's Commissioner.

The second part of the Act focuses on integrated planning, commissioning and delivery of children's services. One of the outcomes of the Act is a requirement of local authorities to appoint a Director of Children's Services to be accountable for the local authority's education and social services relating to children.

The Human Rights Act 1998

The Human Rights Act 1998 came into force in October 2000 and ensures that all UK laws, policy and practice are compatible with the European Convention on Human Rights (1950). Previous to this Act the primary legal question for health care staff was whether their proposed intervention was lawful – now an assessment must be made as to whether the proposed actions in any way involve a person's human rights and whether they can be legitimately interfered with. Children also have rights under the Act, although they are not the primary focus of the legislation. In cases involving children the rights and authority of the parents are also likely to be taken into consideration.

Some of the rights and freedoms expressed in the Human Rights Act 1989 that are pertinent to children and young people include:

- The right to life
- Prohibition of torture
- Prohibition of slavery and forced labour
- Right to liberty and security
- Right to respect for private and family life
- Freedom of thought, conscience and religion
- Freedom of expression
- Prohibition of discrimination
- Protection of property
- Right to education.

Disability Discrimination Act 1995

The Disability Discrimination Act 1995 (DDA 1995) makes treating disabled people less favourably than other people, without justification, unlawful in areas such as buying goods, using services, finding somewhere to live and getting a job. The definition of a disabled person within the Act is 'someone who has a physical or mental impairment that has a substantial and long-term adverse effect on his or her ability to carry out normal day to day activities'. This includes children and young people.

Since October 2004 the DDA 1995 has required businesses and other organizations to take 'reasonable steps' to tackle physical barriers to disabled people who want to access their services. This may involve putting in a ramp for those with level access needs, providing larger signs for people with visual impairment and improving access to toileting and washroom facilities.

The Disability Discrimination Act 2005

The Disability Discrimination Act 2005 (DDA 2005) extends the provisions in the DDA 1995, including amongst others:

- Making it unlawful for operators of transport vehicles to discriminate against disabled people
- Ensuring that discrimination law covers all the activities of the public sector
- Requiring public bodies to promote equality of opportunity for disabled people.

CONSENT

In current health care ethics there is great value set upon respect for patient choice. With the changing and evolving rights of the child and young person this is becoming much more of an issue in the paediatric specialities.

> It is a fundamental ethical principle that every person has the right to determine what happens to his/her own body (Chartered Society of Physiotherapy 2005a).

As has been discussed above, the child and young person, if deemed to be cognitively able, regardless of age, should be properly informed and consulted throughout their health care intervention episode. Gaining a child's or young person's consent prior to assessment or intervention is not only a legal requirement but also a matter of common courtesy and part of the patient–physiotherapist relationship.

In England, Wales and Northern Ireland the age of majority is 18 and the young person becomes an adult as far as the law is concerned (Smith 2005). In Scotland this is 16.

For individuals to give valid consent they must be mentally competent. Competency is function-specific – the level of understanding should be assessed in relation to the task in hand. A young person of 16 or 17 has a statutory right to give consent, as may a child of younger than 16 if 'Gillick-competent' (Dimond 1999). The consent must be given without coercion, force, deceit or duress.

The term 'Gillick competency' stems from the case Gillick *v* W. Norfolk and Wisbech Area HA 1986 and a House of Lords ruling in which children under 16 years of age who are deemed to have sufficient understanding and intelligence to be capable of making up their own minds can give valid consent to treatment (Brook 2000, Hedley 2002). A Gillick-competent child is entitled to confidentiality in all aspects of information imparted to professionals during health care intervention unless it is in the best interests of the child to pass this on to the appropriate authorities, e.g. in suspected child abuse cases. If possible the physiotherapist working with a child in this situation should discuss the need for disclosure and gain the child's or young person's consent before doing so.

A child or young person may have the capacity to consent to some interventions but not others; for example, in some emergency situations. Capacity to consent will depend on the complexity and implication of treatment or, in some instances, the consequence of not giving treatment. If a child is deemed competent to consent it is not necessary to seek additional consent from parents or guardians (those with parental responsibility). It is, however, usually seen as good practice as the family is a vital source of support throughout the intervention period and often for a long time afterwards and their involvement may be crucial to the best outcome for the child.

It is worthy of note that a young person of 16 does not have the right to refuse treatment and he/she cannot override the consent given by those with parental responsibility or by a court. This power to overrule the child's views is exercised on the basis of the 'welfare principle', which holds that the best interests of the child, both physical and psychological, are paramount (Chartered Society of Physiotherapy 2005a).

Where there is dispute between parents (for example, where parents are divorced) over the course of action with regard to decisions about treatment for their child, either party can go to court for a specific issue or prohibited steps order to be made (Dimond 1999).

Valid consent

There are four identified components to valid consent (Vernon & Welbury 2002):

1. The child or young person must have the capacity, i.e. be mentally competent, to consent
2. The child or young person must be able to receive information, weigh up and understand that information and communicate his or her decision regarding that information
3. The consent must be given freely, i.e. the child or young person must not be under duress at the time
4. The child or young person must have been given sufficient information to make a decision about the treatment, including any possible side-effects and the consequences of not receiving the treatment proposed and any alternative available. The consent must not be obtained fraudulently.

If any one of these requirements is not met then the intervention may be deemed unlawful and lead to a claim for trespass or battery.

Documentation must show the process of how consent has been obtained. Refusal or withdrawal of consent is also important to note and the physiotherapist must then discuss with the child or young person and/or family the implications of this and the possible alternatives that could be offered (see case studies 1.1 and 1.2).

HEALTH CARE ETHICS AND THE ETHICAL PRINCIPLES OF THERAPY PRACTICE

Health care decision-making is now frequently questioned by the children and families with whom we work. Justification of our actions and demonstration of our clinical reasoning are essential skills in day-to day practice. More often than not a clinical decision will bring with it the issues of ethical analysis and implicit moral judgements (Kurtz 1994).

Ethical values change over time and across cultures and there are therefore no absolute right and wrong answers. Ethical decisions must be justified in terms of ethical reasoning and in the light of each particular case.

There are five basic ethical principles of which paediatric physiotherapists should be aware in their day-to-day practice (Sim 1997):

1. *Beneficence*. One should strive to promote the interests of others by conferring benefits upon them, that is, to produce a positive good for the person and to remove harm from a person. This demonstrates a positive requirement to act on the part of the physiotherapist so that the individual – the patient – will be better off for that action.
2. *Non-maleficence*. One should seek to avoid inflicting harm on others, that is, to refrain from doing that which would make another person – the patient – worse off (a negative requirement).
3. *Respect for autonomy*. Autonomy is defined as the 'capacity to think, decide and act on the basis of such thought and decision freely and independently'.
4. *Respect for persons*. Deal with others with due consideration for their dignity as individuals. Value the inherent worth and uniqueness of each person.

5. *Justice*. Deal with others in a way that is fair and in accordance with their individual merit. Everybody should be treated in the same way unless there are relevant differences between individuals which justify their being treated differently.

With regard to the ethical principles of paediatric physiotherapy practice, a child should be:

- Regarded as a child first
- Valued as an individual
- Treated with dignity
- Treated with respect
- Safe.

The fundamental ethical consideration should always be the best interests of the child or young person (the welfare of the child or young person is paramount). Factors to be considered prior to any physiotherapeutic intervention should include:

- The child's or young person's own ascertainable wishes, feelings and values (religious and cultural)
- The child's or young person's ability to understand what is proposed and weigh up the alternatives presented
- The child's or young person's potential to participate more in the decision if provided with additional support or explanations − pre-admission visits, assistance and communication, picture stories
- The child's or young person's physical and emotional needs
- The risk of harm or suffering
- The views of the parents and family
- The implications for the child and family for treatment or non-treatment
- Evidence of the effectiveness of the proposed treatment particularly in relation to other alternatives and options
- Prioritization of options that maximize the child and young person's future opportunities and choices
- Evidence of the likelihood of improvement with treatment
- Evidence about the anticipated extent of improvement
- Risks arising from delayed or non-treatment

(List adapted from British Medical Association 2001.)

Physiotherapists in paediatric practice must be aware of the power − knowledge imbalance that exists in their professional relationship with the child and family and take conscious steps to prevent this leading to exploitation in the unequal relationship.

CODE OF PROFESSIONAL CONDUCT

Physiotherapists work to a code of professional conduct. This means that they have a duty of care − a moral and legal duty − to those with whom they work.

A duty of care can be found to exist at common law wherever it is reasonable to contemplate that another person might be affected by one's acts or omissions (Donoghue *v.* Stevenson HL 1932 in Chartered Society of Physiotherapy 2005b).

A duty of care arises when an individual can reasonably foresee that his/her actions or omissions could result in harm. In the physiotherapist–patient relationship the physiotherapist is providing a service to that patient and there is an expectation that the physiotherapist will have a certain level of skill, expertise and knowledge and be competent to practise.

The professional code of conduct has a twofold purpose: public protection and professional protection.

The professional code sets standards by which physiotherapists are accountable for all their professional activity. In practice, the duty of care can be identified at three levels: the individual physiotherapist, the employing agency and the professional body, i.e. the Chartered Society of Physiotherapy and Health Professions Council.

Individual physiotherapists are personally accountable for their acts (what they do) or omissions (what they fail to do) and what they say, in a professional context, e.g. advice given to a child or young person or the carers of that child. Physiotherapists must justify the child's and family's trust and confidence in them.

Individual physiotherapists are rarely sued because their employer is indirectly responsible for their actions while they are carrying out the duty for which they have been employed. This is known as vicarious liability. However, if physiotherapists take action which is outside their scope of practice, the employer may argue that the employer is not responsible as those actions were not deemed to be within the scope of the role the physiotherapist was employed to undertake.

Physiotherapists also have a duty of care to those to whom they delegate tasks. Delegation is commonplace in paediatric physiotherapy − in particular in the community setting. Learning support assistants are often trained to undertake school programmes in the education setting. The delegating physiotherapist must ensure the assistant is competent to undertake the responsibility for the care of the child with regard to the therapy activity.

Documentation in this instance is of the utmost importance. It is essential that there is evidence of a clear assessment process, clinical reasoning for the intervention chosen, accurate information of who has been trained and what exactly they have been trained to do with a named child in a specified situation. Those undertaking these tasks must be aware that they should not transfer these skills to any other child in their care. The training is for a specific child in a specific situation undertaking a specific task.

SUMMARY

As practising paediatric physiotherapists we should all advocate for the rights of the child and young people. We need to respect children and young people – they often know things that adults do not – and remember they see the world from a different perspective. It is part of antidiscriminatory practice and equal opportunities to approach our health care intervention this way. Respecting children will help them respect others. Involving children and young people as service users in the planning of services will improve the efficiency and effectiveness of those services. Involving children and young people will promote their social inclusion and place in society.

The basic health rights of children and young people can be summarized as follows:

- To receive child-centred health care
- To be looked after without discrimination
- To be encouraged to develop their full potential
- To take opportunities to be involved and choose not to be involved in decision-making

- To receive clear information and the right to decline information
- To be able to express opinions
- To receive support and encouragement in decision-making
- To ask someone else to decide
- To receive explanations when their preferences cannot be met
- To confidentiality
- To redress where appropriate (complaints)

(British Medical Association 2001, p. 14.)

Many of these principles are evident in much of the legislative framework described above and policy guidance such as the *National Service Framework for Children, Young People and Maternity Services* (Department of Health 2004); therefore, as paediatric physiotherapists it is not only a moral duty to uphold them but our legal responsibility.

CASE STUDY 1.1

When working with a child, irrespective of the age or cognitive ability of the child, it is good practice to explain what you, as a physiotherapist, intend to do during your contact and why (demonstrating your clinical reasoning), always including the parent and carer in the discussion.

The physiotherapist must always ask the child if he or she is happy to be handled – for example, if the physiotherapist has to assess the range of movement

available in the ankle, permission must be asked of the child (and the parent) before removing or asking the child to remove the shoe and sock and handling the foot.

Once assessment is complete the ongoing treatment plan and goals of intervention should be established in collaboration with the child and carer. In this way agreement about the physiotherapy programme can be reached by all parties concerned.

CASE STUDY 1.2

A physiotherapist working with a child who has complex cerebral palsy but is cognitively able, who is aware that the child has an appointment with an orthopaedic consultant to discuss possible surgery, could in collaboration with colleagues in the speech and language therapy department ensure that the child (if unable to use verbal communication) has the appropriate language in an augmentative communication device, or pictures in a communication book to enable the child to ask the appropriate questions of the doctor about the proposed surgery.

Prior to this appointment the physiotherapist may be able to spend some time with the child talking about the surgery and implications of rehabilitation following the surgery to allow the child to be more fully informed

when he or she meets with the doctor. The physiotherapist could attend the appointment to act as an advocate for the child.

The physiotherapist could ensure that the doctor offers enough time during the appointment to allow the child to express his/her views and ask questions. This may involve early contact with the clinic organizer to adjust appointment schedules as this may demand more time than a routine appointment slot.

If the child is not cognitively able the physiotherapist must act as an advocate for the child and family in situations such as this and ensure that the family is fully informed of the implications of any proposed surgery and the expected outcomes for the child.

REFERENCES

British Medical Association 2001 *Consent, Rights and Choices in Health Care for Children and Young People.* London: BMJ Books.

Brook G 2000 Children's competency to consent; a framework for practice. *Paediatric Nursing* 12: 31–35.

Chartered Society of Physiotherapy 2005a *Consent PA60*. London: Chartered Society of Physiotherapy.

Chartered Society of Physiotherapy 2005b *Legal Work Pack*. London: Chartered Society of Physiotherapy.

Department of Health 2004 *National Service Framework for Children, Young People and Maternity Services*. London: DH Publications.

Department of Health, Department for Education and Employment, Home Office 2000 *Framework for the Assessment of Children in Need and their Families*. London: Stationery Office.

Department of Health, Home Office, Department for Education and Employment 1999 *Working Together to Safeguard Children*. London: Stationery Office.

Dimond B 1999 *Legal Aspects of Physiotherapy*. Oxford: Blackwell Science.

Hedley M 2002 Treating children: whose consent counts? *Current Paediatrics* 12: 463–464.

HM government 2003 *Every Child Matters*. London: Stationery Office.

Kurtz Z 1994 Children's rights and health care. *Children and Society* 8: 114–131.

Sim J 1997 *Ethical Decision Making in Therapy Practice*. Oxford: Butterworth Heinemann.

Smith F 2005 *The Children Act 2004 Personal Guide*. Croydon: Children Act Enterprises.

Vernon B, Welbury J 2002 Consent for the examination or treatment of teenagers. *Current Paediatrics* 12: 458–462.

FURTHER READING

Chartered Society of Physiotherapy 2000 *Law Briefing: The Human Rights Act 1998*. London: Chartered Society of Physiotherapy.

Smith F 2005 *How Old do I Have to be...? Personal Guide*. Croydon: Children Act Enterprises.

Smith F, Lyon T 2004 *The Children Act 1989 Personal Guide*, 4th edn. Croydon: Children Act Enterprises.

WEBSITES

inclusion.ngfl.gov.uk: a website giving advice on special educational needs and inclusion issues.

www.caeuk.org: Children Act Enterprises – offer useful publications about family and criminal law.

www.dfes.gov.uk: Department for Education and Skills website – useful for information and resources.

www.dh.gov.uk: Department of Health website providing health and social care policy guidance and publications.

www.direct.gov.uk: government website containing useful information and links about a range of issues, both local and national.

www.drc.org.uk: a useful website containing information and links on disability issues. The Disability Rights Commission has one key goal: 'a society where all disabled people can participate fully as equal citizens'.

www.everychildmatters.gov.uk: Every Child Matters Change for Children website containing information and access to publications related to children and families.

www.gmc-uk.org: General Medical Council website containing medical information and access to helpful publications.

www.humanrights.gov.uk: Department for Constitutional Affairs website containing information on human rights.

www.opsi.gov.uk/acts/acts2005: Office of Public Sector Information website offering access to government acts.

www.teachernet.gov.uk/publications: useful website for information and publications.

www.unhchr.ch: Office of the United Nations High Commissioner for Human Rights – information and access to publications on human rights.

2 Delivering physiotherapy services to children and young people

Sarah Crombie

INTRODUCTION

Children's services, in their approach, design and delivery, are continually undergoing constant change, with health services rethinking their models of delivery, priorities for provision and direction of future developments. Physiotherapy services, alongside other children's health services, need to take a more holistic approach to a child's management, ensuring that not only are the health needs considered, but also family, social, emotional and educational needs. The role of the paediatric physiotherapist is thus not only the delivery of therapy, but also extends into a consultancy, educational and training role. A paediatric physiotherapist needs to develop highly specialist clinical skills alongside those of communication and teaching in order to meet the needs of the child within a multiprofessional and multiagency framework. Over the past decade, government recommendations for working with children and subsequent legislation in health, education and social care have reflected these changes and are determining the necessary direction of future service development. This chapter aims to describe:

1. Why working with children is different from working with adults

2. How policy and organizational changes affect service delivery

3. The changing role of the paediatric physiotherapist within this framework.

WHY SHOULD CHILDREN'S SERVICES BE DIFFERENT?

The approach to the philosophy of the care of children, whether in health, education or social care, has undergone a radical review over the past decade. Children are beginning to take on a new priority in both legislation and practice and there is wide acknowledgement that children have very differing needs from those of adults (Department of Health 2001b, 2004b, World Health Organization 2005). Children present with different medical conditions, have vulnerabilities of dependence and age and are very much developing individuals with social, emotional and educational needs (Audit Commission 1993). Children's services and those who work within them must reflect this in their approach and delivery of services.

Involving children and families in their care

Involving children, young people and their families in decision-making around their care is fundamental to successful health interventions (Carter et al 1994) and is one of the key messages from *The National Service Framework for Children* (Department of Health 2004b). Family-centred services involving the principles of effective information exchange, respectful supportive care towards all members of the family, partnership and enablement have been shown to improve the outcome for children with long-term difficulties and their families (King et al 2004). Parents have been found to be more satisfied with services and care provided, adhere to the advice given and suffer less stress.

Children should be viewed as having rights of their own at whatever age (United Nations 1989) and be encouraged to demonstrate choice and consent to treatment. How children and young people's views are sought, however, needs careful consideration before treatment or management interventions can be decided. Information given to children needs to be age-appropriate, taking into account a child's cognitive ability, communication skills and cultural background (World Health Organization 2005). This is often a challenge when children are perceived to be too young to decide on intervention, not cognitively aware enough or unable to communicate their needs easily. Strategies may need to be used such as demonstration, pictures, toys or signing systems in order to convey ideas to a non-verbal child. There has been more research in recent years, regarding the ability of young children to make important decisions about their care (Alderson 1993) and children should always be asked for their consent wherever possible (Department of Health 2001a). Older children and teenagers often have different communication styles, peer support and an increasing need for independence and privacy. Although parents have the right to be the child's parents and make decisions on their behalf, some parents may need encouragement to 'take a back seat' in order that a young person's views may be aired. With this in mind, the physiotherapist must make great efforts to ensure that information is communicated to both a child and young person in as appropriate and understandable a manner as possible and that his or her views are sought and valued.

Effective communication of information is the first vital step for an informed decision around intervention to be made and the basis on which consent may be given. The issue of consent is an important and sometimes difficult issue when working with children, and needs to be fully considered when any intervention is proposed. Parents have the right to consent for very young children, but as children mature and are more able to make decisions for themselves, the issue of consent becomes less clear. How this is obtained and the issues around consent are more fully discussed in Chapter 1.

Decision-making regarding possible physiotherapy intervention thus needs to be a joint venture between a child, family and physiotherapist with considerations made for others involved with the child (Carter et al 1994). These decisions can often not be made in a clinical setting without taking into account the child's family life, educational, social, cultural and emotional needs. A child or young person is part of a family and this needs to be considered in order that any intervention is tailored to meet their specific needs. Following assessment, the physiotherapist will have made decisions about where he/she feels intervention would be most effective. This needs to be fully discussed with the child and family so that they are able to make decisions not only about the possible effectiveness of interventions, but the practical implications for their child and family. They may want to ask themselves questions such as: are they able to bring the child for treatment on a regular enough basis? Will the child comply with an orthotic appliance? Do they have enough space for equipment at home? (see case study 2.1)

Collaborative goal-setting

Collaborative goal-setting is another key approach to successful physiotherapy intervention. Involving a child and family in goal-setting contributes to improved working relationships, adherence and thus effectiveness of interventions (Carter et al 1994, King et al 2004). As with the decision-making process prior to intervention, collaborative goal-setting involves placing a child and family in the forefront, ensuring that they have sufficient information to decide jointly with their physiotherapist what might be realistic goals. Physiotherapists are important facilitators in this, and need to help families to take account of factors which may influence this decision. The more complex a child's difficulties or social and family situation, the more difficult it may be to set realistic and achievable goals. This may be accomplished by breaking down wider, more far-reaching goals into smaller goals that are achievable in the short term. If a child, young person or the parents are either not clear about goals of treatment or not in agreement with goals which have been set, engagement with any intervention process may not be effective. Goals must be meaningful to the child or young person, and the physiotherapist needs to discover what might motivate each individual. An example of this might be a young teenager with intermittent back pain who is not compliant with her home exercises. Unless the physiotherapist is able to discover what motivates this particular young woman, and find out what her goal of coming to therapy might be, any intervention may not be effective.

Working as a team

Collaboration in goal-setting and in a child's management often extends beyond the child and family to include others involved in their care. Working with children is often a multiprofessional and multiagency practice (Carter et al 1994, Department of Health 2004b). The Team Around the Child model (Department of Health 2004a) advocates that children's needs are central to their management and that a range of different professionals from various agencies may need to work collaboratively to meet a child's needs. This may be a virtual team in that the professionals may come from various organizations and not necessarily be co-located.

When working with children, the paediatric physiotherapist may need to liaise with a wide range of health professionals within the immediate environment, with tertiary centres or with outside agencies. This requires communication skills not only to communicate effectively with the child and family, but with all those involved with the child's management. Within the acute hospital environment, the physiotherapist will need to work closely with others involved with the child's daily treatment and management. This may include liaison

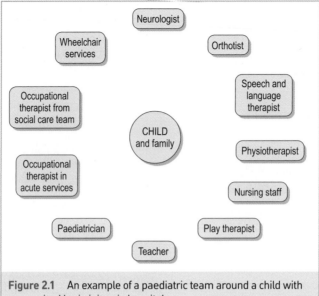

Figure 2.1 An example of a paediatric team around a child with an acquired brain injury in hospital.

with paediatricians, nursing staff, play therapists, hospital teachers, speech and language and occupational therapists (Figure 2.1). When the child is discharged and ongoing care is necessary, information may need to be shared with community or local acute services and management plans jointly agreed. A team approach is essential for the holistic management of those children requiring intervention at a number of centres.

For a child with ongoing physiotherapy needs in the community, the physiotherapist will be required to liaise not only with health professionals, but also with other agencies such as education and social care. A boy with complex developmental difficulties may, for example, have physiotherapy intervention at a child development centre where he is also seen by the occupational and speech and language therapists. He may also go to a nursery where he has a key worker who is responsible for his management during the day. He may need equipment at home which is provided by the occupational therapist from social care and the family may have a social worker. A child with a physical disability will need appropriate handling and positioning throughout the day and therefore the physiotherapist will need to liaise with all those responsible for his care.

The National Service Framework for Children (Department of Health 2004b) highlights the need for a key worker system for such children who have contacts with a multitude of professionals. This key worker model aims to provide a more holistic and joined-up approach to the child's management. This person would be chosen by the family to be responsible for coordinating their child's care

and may be one of the professionals who has the most contact with them.

Communication and confidentiality

When liaising with a wide range of people involved in a child's care, the issue of confidentiality of information is an important one. To whom can you talk about a child's difficulties and what consent do you need for this? Sharing of information is vital for collaborative working (World Health Organization 2005), and there is currently a government drive to promote this further and more formally with the use of the Common Assessment Framework (Department of Health 2004a). This aims to develop a system where important information can be shared among appropriate professionals, act as a lever for multiagency working and ensure equality of services. Other important documents to consider regarding confidentiality of information are the United Nations Convention on the Rights of the Child (United Nations 1989), Caldicott Report (Department of Health 1997), Data Protection Act (1998) and the *NHS Code of Practice* (Department of Health 2003a). Children have the same rights to confidentiality as adults, but these may not always be respected, especially where there are difficulties with communication due to their age or cognitive ability and their parents are not present. When discussing a child's problems with others, especially in a situation such as in a school, where the parent is absent, it is important to ensure that children's problems are not discussed in front of them without their permission and that others not involved with the child's care, including other children, are not able to overhear conversations. A child's rights to confidentiality should only be breached in exceptional circumstances, such as when there are concerns regarding child protection, and then only to appropriate professionals in line with local policies (see Ch. 1).

KEY POINTS

- A child has a right to confidentiality of information
- A child and young person's privacy must be respected; only necessary information should be shared
- Ask for a child and family's consent to share personal information
- Local child protection policy should be adhered to
- Sharing of information is vital for effective team-working

ORGANIZATIONAL CHANGES AFFECTING SERVICE DELIVERY

Historically, services to children in the National Health Service have been hospital-based with the primary emphasis on the child's health and clinical need. Physiotherapy services have followed this medical model, providing treatment or rehabilitation within a therapeutic setting such as a hospital or child development centre, and working in liaison with other health care providers. Over the past two decades this emphasis has shifted to spread services, wherever possible, out of the hospital environment into community, educational and social care settings (Audit Commission 1993). Currently, paediatric physiotherapists work in a range of health care settings, such as acute hospital wards, outpatient clinics and child development centres (Association of Paediatric Chartered Physiotherapists 2002). Tertiary centres provide additional specialist clinics or services such as gait assessment, orthopaedic and wheelchair clinics (Department of Health 2003b). Physiotherapists commonly extend their practice out into special and mainstream schools, nurseries, children's homes and respite homes. They work in collaboration with a range of health professionals as well as staff in education and social services. Nationwide, there is a wide diversity of provision in child health services in both the acute and community settings (Department of Health 2004b), with service delivery models developing according to how services are organized locally. With regard to childhood disability, for example, some areas provide a comprehensive family-centred service encompassing all disabling conditions throughout childhood and adolescence. Other areas, however, provide clinics only catering for under-5s with severe disorders such as cerebral palsy, and then only in a fragmentary fashion (British Association

for Community Child Health 2000). Although service delivery models for physiotherapy need to be variable to meet the needs of the local or hospital population, physiotherapists must strive to develop care pathways and guidelines for practice in order to ensure common standards for the physiotherapy management of children.

Children's services have undergone rapid changes over the last decade, with government inquiries leading to the Victoria Climbie Report (Department of Health 2003c) and Bristol Royal Infirmary Inquiry (Department of Health 2001b) which have highlighted problems in the care of children across all services, including the National Health Service. This has resulted in the need to improve standards of care for children, and for all children's services to work more collaboratively, in order that the child's needs are not viewed separately by different agencies and to develop a more holistic approach to their care. The government's *Change for Children: Every Child Matters* implementation programme (Department of Health 2004a) follows the Children Act in 2004. This Act laid down the legislative framework on which this programme is now being implemented. Its aim is to align closely *The National Service Framework for Children* (Department of Health 2004b), which has been produced to effect change in the health sector, with wide-ranging changes in education and social care. The development of children's trusts, children's centres and extended schools will not only affect how services are delivered to children in education and social care, but also how some health services are commissioned and delivered in order to provide more collaborative multiagency working.

The *National Service Framework for Children* (Department of Health 2004b) advocates a fundamental change in children's services so that they are designed and delivered around the needs of the child. It proposes that children's services should be more child-centred and encompass all aspects of the child's health and well-being. Some of the key messages from the framework affecting physiotherapy services are as follows:

- A child should be at the centre of services
- A holistic approach to a child's welfare should be taken
- Children, young people and their families should be given increased information, power and choice, and encouraged to take a more active part in decisions around their care
- Health professionals working with children need specialist training so that they are aware of the important issues surrounding the management of children, such as child protection and child-centred care
- Interventions should be needs-led, rather than service-led
- There should be improved access to services, with more co-located, multidisciplinary services
- Partnerships are vital with all agencies involved in the care of children
- Healthy lifestyles should be promoted for all children

- There should be a focus on early intervention
- Evidence-based practice is needed.

Many of these recommendations are already part of good practice in current physiotherapy services. Many services, for example, deliver therapy to the child over a number of sites such as children's homes, nurseries, health centres and schools; focus on early intervention; have developed multiagency working practices; and encourage self-management of chronic disease and illness. Over the next decade, however, the impact of this framework should ensure that these recommendations continue to improve practice, with children spending less time in hospital, having more choice and say in their treatment and management and paving the way for the development of standards of working practice with children. A national mapping programme of children's services is currently being undertaken to audit levels of service delivery across England as a first step to benchmarking standards (Department of Health 2004b). How physiotherapy services continue to deliver therapy to children will need to develop with this framework in mind. An example of this is increased multisite working, such as in extended schools and in the new children's centres.

The development of children's trusts will move physiotherapy services, which have historically been based primarily on health service sites, increasingly to other community bases such as schools and nurseries. Children's trusts aim to integrate key services for children within a single organizational focus (Department of Health 2004a). The aim of the trusts is to connect local education authorities, children's social services and community health services and thus improve multiagency working for the benefit of the child and family. Their remit will be eventually to commission services, and either provide them directly or contract out to other existing services. How physiotherapy services will ultimately work within the framework of these trusts is as yet unclear.

With a strong focus on early intervention in the *Every Child Matters* implementation programme, Sure Start children's centres are designed to promote the physical, intellectual and social development of preschool children by bringing together health, social services and early education, as well as voluntary, private and community organizations and parents themselves, to provide integrated services for young children and their families. Paediatric physiotherapists have either been seconded or are fully employed to work in these children's centres. This can be viewed as an important move from health-based multidisciplinary working, such as in a child development centre, to more closely aligned multiagency working involving social and educational aspects of the child. Services may be delivered on one site, linked together with other service providers for a more integrated approach to the child's care.

Involving children, young people and parents in planning service delivery is part of government policy (Department of Health 2000). Children and young people need to be involved in service planning and development as users in their own right (Fajerman & Tresecter 2000, Kirby et al 2003). The report on the Bristol Royal Infirmary Inquiry (2001) commented that health services are often not designed to meet the needs of children and that if services are to be improved, consultation with this group of users is vital. With Department of Education and Skills funding, Contact a Family and the Council for Disabled Children have produced a guide, *Parent Participation*, on how professionals can involve parents in planning and developing services (Contact a Family 2004). Physiotherapy services therefore need to consider how service planning takes into account these views, especially for children with communication difficulties and for those for whom English is not their first language.

PHYSIOTHERAPY IN HOSPITAL SETTINGS

Many paediatric physiotherapists are employed in hospital settings to treat children on paediatric wards, in outpatient settings or in hospital clinics. There has been a gradual move in hospital children's services to manage children's conditions away from the traditional acute setting to one that is more community-based (Audit Commission 1993, Department of Health 2004b). An example of this is the management of children with cystic fibrosis. Children may come to a hospital outpatient department for monitoring and review and may be admitted on to the paediatric ward during acute episodes. At other times, and often whilst recovering from acute episodes, the child may be treated and managed at home. *The National Service Framework for Children* (Department of Health 2004b) and *The National Service Framework for Long-Term Conditions* (Department of Health 2005) endorses this move to community services wherever possible, and this is likely to have an impact on the delivery of services for many children with long-term chronic conditions.

Some children, however, do need the specialist resources required for their acute condition which necessitates admission to a hospital ward. The role of the paediatric physiotherapist will vary depending on the range of conditions with which children present, regional hospitals admitting more acutely ill children and with conditions requiring specialist provision such as paediatric intensive care. Physiotherapists have traditionally been required to treat children with respiratory, orthopaedic, neurological, oncological and developmental conditions, and for postsurgical care, but now their caseloads may often include children with psychological and mental health disorders and a wider range of acute and chronic paediatric conditions.

A physiotherapist working in a local district hospital with one or two general paediatric wards will need to be competent to treat children with a wide range of conditions, but may not be responsible for extremely sick children or those with rare conditions, who will be sent to larger more specialist units. These children, however, will often be transferred back to the original hospital for longer-term rehabilitation or management. Physiotherapists in these positions have the benefit of a local paediatric team, with easier access to liaison with community staff. They may, however, need to liaise closely with tertiary centres when local children are treated or managed for specialist care. Physiotherapists working in larger regional hospitals may be required to work on specialist wards such as for children with orthopaedic, respiratory, oncological or surgical conditions. They may then develop highly specialist skills in the treatment and management of children with these conditions and work alongside a dedicated multiprofessional team.

When treating a child in hospital, the physiotherapist faces different challenges from treating a child in more familiar surroundings. There is often much anxiety when a child is admitted to hospital, not only from the parents, but also from the child or young person (Audit Commission 1993). Effective communication skills are vital in order to develop a relationship with the child and family, involving open sharing of information and clear explanations of interventions at an age-appropriate level to enable the child to be involved in decisions wherever possible. It may be difficult to gain cooperation from young children when they are in a strange environment and feeling unwell. The physiotherapist must consider how to gain informed consent in these circumstances and gain the cooperation of the child. This is often more time-consuming than when treating adults with similar conditions as the child may take some time to develop trust in a strange adult. Parents are often anxious themselves and need to feel actively involved in treatment decisions and interventions. Parents may be taught physiotherapy techniques such as percussion in order to treat their child, who would otherwise not allow a physiotherapist to treat them, or to continue treatment in between the therapist's sessions or postdischarge. Play specialists are often employed on paediatric wards (Audit Commission 1993) and are usually someone with whom the child may have already developed a good relationship. They may be vital colleagues who can encourage children to continue with their exercises or encourage mobility, at times when the therapist is not there.

If ongoing physiotherapy is necessary following discharge from hospital, the physiotherapist has a role to liaise closely with services in the community. This may be a simple referral to a physiotherapy department for a child with an orthopaedic condition, or for a more complex referral such as the discharge of a child following a head injury. There needs to be a planned discharge programme. This will involve close liaison with not just the physiotherapy and other health services, to ensure ongoing treatment, but with a range of other agencies. The child may need the wheelchair service to provide mobility or specialist seating, or social services to provide equipment at home or at school.

Physiotherapists treat children as outpatients either in the hospital setting or as part of community services, sometimes as part of the child development centre. Children and young people with musculoskeletal problems, orthopaedic or gait difficulties are often seen in the physiotherapy outpatient department. This may be part of adult services, or more commonly as part of specialized children's services. If children are seen in adult departments within the hospital, it is important that the facilities provide for the needs of the child and young person, such as ensuring specialist staff, play facilities and a suitable environment (Department of Health 2004b). Many physiotherapists work in conjunction with other health professions to provide specialist hospital clinics such as for the assessment and provision of orthotics, rheumatology, respiratory or follow-up baby clinics. These joint clinics are important to ensure effective use of time and multiprofessional working for children with complex conditions (see case study 2.2).

PHYSIOTHERAPY IN COMMUNITY SETTINGS

Child development centres

Physiotherapists working with children with long-term conditions are often part of a child development team, based in a child development centre. These centres have been in operation since the 1960s and usually comprise a multidisciplinary team of community paediatricians, speech and language therapists, physiotherapists and occupational therapists, and may include community nursing staff and clinical psychologists (British Association for Community Child Health 2000). Staff at the child development centre usually work in close liaison with other health service workers such as general practitioners, health visitors, podiatrists, orthotists, audiologists and paediatric dietitians. Physiotherapists working in a child development team would be responsible for meeting the physical needs of children aged 0–19 years with a wide range of disabilities. They may see children at the child development centre, but a main part of their work would be to visit children in special and mainstream schools, nurseries, in community clinics and in the child's home. Physiotherapists therefore need to work collaboratively not only with the child and family, but also with health service staff and those in education and social services. The *National Service Frameworks for Children* (Department of Health 2004b) and for *Long-Term Conditions* (Department of Health 2005) advocate the use of the key worker or case manager system to enable families to have a focal person who can coordinate services and ensure that they work collaboratively to meet the child's or young person's needs. It may be that physiotherapists are well placed to function in this role. Case study 2.3 demonstrates the physiotherapy role with a young child with a chronic disability.

Working in mainstream schools

The government strategy of enabling children with special educational needs (SEN), such as those with physical disabilities, to become part of an inclusive mainstream system has had a major impact on the working practice of paediatric physiotherapists (Audit Commission 2002). Prior to the Education Act in 1981, children with specific physical difficulties were educated and their health needs managed within a special school environment with designated trained staff. Physiotherapists worked in these schools treating or managing a number of children with physical disabilities on one site. There was little involvement with other school-aged children outside the hospital outpatient environment.

The Special Educational Needs and Disability Act (2001) and the Special Educational Needs Code of Practice (Department of Education and Skills 2001) have moved inclusion forwards so that now most children with SEN are in mainstream education. The impact of this strategy on service delivery has been huge, with organizational changes involving the necessity to provide therapy over numerous sites (Audit Commission 2002). Physiotherapists managing school children with physical difficulties, who need help with physical access, mobility in school or in accessing the national curriculum, will need to be involved to some extent with the child's school.

The role of the physiotherapist has now moved from a primarily therapeutic model to a more complex role, including teaching, consultation and advice. The school may need advice on access for the child and adaptations to the school environment. They need to understand the nature of the child's condition and how it will affect his or her functioning in school. This may include understanding the child's ability to move around the classroom and school, join in with classroom activities and facilitating socialization. Some schools may prefer to develop a whole-school approach to disability and involve all staff members in this education process. Others may choose to train up only those who are specifically involved with the child or young person.

In lieu of national guidelines or standards of practice for delivering therapy to school-age children, various models of working have emerged. These are dependent on variables such as the child and family needs, individual school practice and physiotherapy resources. Schools with more than one child requiring therapy may have more frequent access to a therapist and develop greater expertise in the management of physical disability compared to a school with only one disabled child. Some mainstream schools have specialist units within them to ensure that the child has sufficiently experienced school staff to manage those with complex disabilities.

Therapists, along with the child, family and school, need to make joint decisions regarding the delivery of therapy, where this should occur and by whom. Teaching assistants in school are often trained by physiotherapists to carry out aspects of a child's physical programme and to facilitate inclusion in the school environment. At present, this is dependent on the child having time allocated in their statement of SEN or the school allocating specific teaching assistant time. Although physiotherapy services to schools are variable, it is now advocated that therapists should be extending current support to disabled children, minimizing their disruption to education, and educating and supporting school staff so that therapy may be built into the child's daily routine (Department of Health 2004b).

Legislation and government guidelines for working with children have given physiotherapists some benchmarks for expected working practice (Department of Education and Skills 2001, Special Educational Needs and Disability Act 2001). Key points for physiotherapists to consider when working with children in mainstream schools are as follows:

- Parents have a right to express a preference for mainstream schooling for their child
- Children with SEN are expected to be fully included in all aspects of school life
- Children should be consulted over the management of their SEN in school
- Partnerships with parents are essential
- Interventions for each child should be regularly reviewed to assess their impact, the child's progress and the views of the child, teachers and parents
- Multiagency working is essential for effective information-sharing and collaborative practice
- Those required to participate in a child's statutory assessment must do so within a specified timescale. Statements should be clear and detailed to specify monitoring arrangements and review
- Liaison with the child's school is essential and this should be with the teacher and the SEN coordinator, and in consultation with parents (see case study 2.4).

Working in special schools

Although the government thrust is to encourage mainstream schooling wherever possible, special schools do exist in most areas. Physiotherapists working in special schools would be treating and managing children with a range of long-term conditions such as cerebral palsy, muscular dystrophy and other physical disabilities associated with learning difficulties. Some children will have more complex disabilities, including communication, visual or sensory difficulties requiring the specialist staff and facilities a special school can provide. Staff in these schools will be more experienced in the management of children with physical difficulties, often carrying out therapy programmes on a regular basis and supporting the child during the school day. These children often require postural management and the use of specialist equipment, which the staff will need to use with the child throughout the day. The principles for therapists working in these schools, however, are similar to those of working in mainstream schools (see case study 2.5).

SUMMARY

Children and young people require specialist service provision. They have different requirements to those of adults: they need child-centred services appropriate for their age, cognitive ability, cultural background and family circumstances. Physiotherapy services require appropriately trained staff who can meet the needs of children and young people across a range of hospital and community settings. In the light of recent government legislation there is now a strong drive towards improving the quality and standard of all services for children. For physiotherapy services, this will mean a shift in how services are organized and delivered. The focus will be on child-centred services, breaking down traditional organizational barriers in order to promote improved multiagency planning of services and collaborative working. There are already examples of this in the early-years setting. Physiotherapists have an established role to play in the treatment and management of children, but should not miss important opportunities ahead to extend and develop their role.

CASE STUDY 2.1

Alicia is a 7-year-old girl with lower-limb shortening. She was assessed by the orthopaedic surgeon for a leg-lengthening operation. She will have to wear an Illizarov frame for 6 months, requiring regular, frequent physiotherapy sessions and a home exercise programme. She will become more dependent on her parents during this time due to her reduced mobility and need for assistance with self-care. There will also be considerable discomfort or pain following this operation.

Alicia and her parents need to consider not just the final outcome of the operation, but how this will practically affect the family over the next few months. There are two younger siblings to take into account, her father is unable to bring her regularly for appointments and her mother is still waiting to take her driving test and is therefore reliant on buses. The physiotherapist has an important role to play in helping the family make their decision, by discussing the implications of this operation on Alicia herself, the family commitment necessary and the amount of therapy needed over the course of the next few months, whether as an outpatient or at home.

CASE STUDY 2.2

Sam is 3 years old and has been admitted to the ward with a chest infection. The physiotherapist has found it difficult to engage him in physiotherapy, as he is nervous of being touched by strange adults and is feeling very anxious about being in hospital. Sam's mother has been shown postural drainage and percussion techniques and is assisting the physiotherapist in Sam's physiotherapy. Sam enjoys going to the playroom as he finds this a non-threatening environment and the play therapist is able to encourage him to practise deep-breathing techniques using bubbles and blowing games as part of his play. Physiotherapy is therefore conducted in conjunction with Sam's mother, the play therapist and the physiotherapist.

CASE STUDY 2.3

Sasha is 3 years old and has cerebral palsy. She attends a playgroup at the specialist child development centre where she receives regular physiotherapy, occupational therapy and speech and language therapy. The physiotherapist works collaboratively with all the therapists and medical staff to ensure that there is collaboration of practice. As well as her therapy sessions, Sasha goes to a mainstream nursery and the physiotherapist visits her there to ensure that the staff are confident and competent in managing her needs whilst at nursery. She has specialist equipment at nursery such as a chair and a standing frame which the

continued

physiotherapist needs to adjust periodically and ensure correct usage. The physiotherapist sees Sasha's parents regularly at the child development centre to work on activities together and set joint goals. Sometimes the physiotherapist needs to go home to check Sasha's postural management equipment there or to discuss issues in the home environment. Here she will work with the occupational therapist from social services in order to provide appropriate adaptive equipment for home. Sasha wears splints on her feet and needs to go to see the orthotist and physiotherapist together to review her orthotic provision. The physiotherapist is now referring Sasha to a tertiary centre to be assessed for a suitable wheelchair and is investigating the possibility of a tricycle for her.

CASE STUDY 2.4

William is a 5-year-old boy with hemiplegia and has just started at his local mainstream school. The school has never had a pupil with a physical disability before and is keen to learn how they can ensure that he is included in everyday school activities. The physiotherapist met with the school special needs coordinator, William's new teacher and his parents before the summer holidays to discuss his abilities and potential difficulties at school. William will need extra support for dressing and undressing, will not be able to play safely on the outdoor apparatus without supervision, needs support in PE and general encouragement throughout the day to use the affected side of his body. He wears an orthosis on his ankle and a Lycra arm splint. These will need to be taken off for some activities and staff at school will need to be competent to help William reapply these. The physiotherapist works alongside the occupational therapist to ensure that school staff who are involved with William understand the nature of his condition and the difficulties he may have in school. They need to be advised on how best to support him in order to maintain and further develop his physical skills within the school environment and to be included in all school activities.

CASE STUDY 2.5

Olivia is 10 years old and attends a school for children with severe learning difficulties. She has a severe physical disability as well as visual and learning impairments. The teaching assistants in her class all know her well and have been taught by the physiotherapist correct positioning in her specialist equipment. She stands in her standing support daily and sits in her special chair for individualized activities. The staff carry out an integrated therapy programme with her as well as assisting her to join in class activities. The physiotherapist's role is that of continued management of Olivia's physical status, aiming to minimize contractures and deformities and optimize her physical ability in order to facilitate learning and promote function, communication and inclusion.

REFERENCES

Alderson P 1993 *Children's Consent to Surgery*. Buckingham: Open University Press.

Association of Paediatric Chartered Physiotherapists 2002 *Paediatric Physiotherapy Guidance for Good Practice*.

Audit Commission 1993 *Children First: A Study of Hospital Services*. London: HMSO.

Audit Commission 2002 Special educational needs: a mainstream issue. Available online at: www.audit-commission. gov.uk.

British Association for Community Child Health, Child Development and Disability Group 2000 *Standards for Child Development Centres*. London: Royal College of Paediatrics and Child Health.

Carter B, Corby B, Cooper L et al 1994 *Appreciating the Best: Multi-Agency Working Practice Project*. Executive report. Preston: University of Central Lancashire.

Children Act 2004 London: HMSO.

Contact a Family 2004 Parent participation: improving services for disabled children. Available online at: www.cafamily.org.uk.

Data Protection Act 1998 London: Stationery Office.

Department of Education and Skills 2001 *Special Educational Needs Code of Practice*. Nottingham: DfES Publications.

Department of Health 1997 *The Caldicott Committee: Report on the Review of Patient-Identifiable Information*. London: HMSO.

Department of Health 2000 *NHS Plan: A Plan for Investment, A Plan for Reform*. London: HMSO.

Department of Health 2001a *Seeking Consent: Working with Children*. London: DH Publications.

Department of Health 2001b *The Report of the Public Inquiry into Children's Heart Surgery at the Bristol Royal Infirmary, 1984–95: Learning from Bristol*. London: Stationery Office.

Department of Health 2003a *Confidentiality: NHS Code of Practice*. London: DH Publications.

Department of Health 2003b *Specialised Services National Definition Set: 23 Specialised Services for Children*. London: HMSO.

Department of Health 2003c *The Victoria Climbie Report*. London: HMSO.

Department of Health 2004a *Change for Children: Every Child Matters*. London: HMSO.

Department of Health 2004b *The National Service Framework for Children, Young People and Maternity Services*. London: HMSO.

Department of Health 2005 *National Service Framework for Long-Term Conditions*. London: HMSO.

Education Act 1981 London: HMSO.

Fajerman L, Tresecter P 2000 *Children are Service Users Too: A Guide to Consulting Children and Young People*. London: Save the Children.

King S, Teplicky R, King G 2004 Family-centered services for children with cerebral palsy: a review of the literature. *Seminars in Pediatric Neurology* 11: 78–86.

Kirby P, Lanyon C, Cronin K, Sinclair R 2003 *Building a Culture of Participation: Involving Children and Young People in Policy, Service Planning, Delivery and Evaluation*. Nottingham: DfEs publications.

Special Educational Needs and Disability Act 2001 London: HMSO.

United Nations 1989 *The UN Convention on the Rights of the Child*. London: UNICEF.

World Health Organization 2005 *European Strategy for Child and Adolescent Health and Development*. WHO Regional Office for Europe.

FURTHER READING

Care Co-ordination Network UK 2004 New standards for key working. Available online at: www.york.ac.uk/inst/spm/ccnukstandards.htm.

Department of Education and Skills 2002 *Removing Barriers to Achievement: the Government's Strategy for SEN*. Nottingham: DfES Publications.

Department of Health 2005 *National Service Framework for Long-Term Conditions*. London: HMSO.

Department of Health 2005 The development of a profile of children's health services in England. Available online at: www. dh.gov.uk.

Sloper P 2004 Facilitators and barriers for co-ordinated multi-agency services. *Child Care, Health and Development* 30: 571–580.

Assessment and outcome measures

3 Outcome measurement in paediatric physiotherapy

Adele Leake

INTRODUCTION

The value of precise and timely outcome measurement has become more widely recognized within the last 15 years. Major government initiatives, including *The Patients' Charter* (Department of Health 1991), *The Health of the Nation* (Department of Health 1992), *Clinical Governance in the New NHS* (Department of Health 1999), *The NHS Plan* (Department of Health 2000) and more recently the White Paper *Choosing Health: Making Healthier Choices Easier* (Department of Health 2004), have added to the emphasis placed on evidence-based practice (EBP) and the evaluation of clinical effectiveness. Sackett et al (1997), in their work on evidence-based medicine, suggested that EBP should include critical evaluation of current work to see if it could be improved. These drivers have led many professions within the health service to examine areas of traditional practice more closely. The use of physiotherapy time, the nature of intervention and the longer-term effects of practice have become increasingly important in the cost – benefit analysis within the National Health Service. These and other external pressures have added impetus to the use of outcome measurement within routine physiotherapy clinical practice and in physiotherapy research. The value placed upon accurate, appropriate and timely outcome measurement is demonstrated in the professional body standards and is expected to be a key attribute of professional practice. The Chartered Society of Physiotherapy's *Core Standards of Physiotherapy Practice* (2005) support that physiotherapists should select and use outcome measures appropriate to the patient and that are of high quality. The physiotherapist is advised to ensure that the measure used can evaluate change in the patient's health status and that the

physiotherapist should apply the measure in a timely manner.

Within these recommendations, it is essential that physiotherapists working in paediatrics understand the key features of good practice in outcome measurement. This chapter seeks to offer advice in locating, evaluating and using outcome measurement tools that are appropriate for the paediatric population. Finding and using an appropriate measurement tool is often a challenge to physiotherapists, particularly when ensuring the process remains child and family-centred. The whole process of assessment, goal-setting, management and evaluation must be focused on ongoing collaboration with children and their families, other professional groups and service providers. Therefore, decisions regarding use of measurement tools cannot be taken in isolation but must form part of this continuous process toward meeting the requirements of these key participants. Ditmarr & Gresham (1997) suggest that the use of assessment and measurement tools will help to improve the relationship between the clinician and the patient/family by improving communication, demonstrating the link between provision and outcome, improving the outcome by continuous evaluation and identifying any changes in provision required.

SELECTION AND EVALUATION OF MEASUREMENT TOOLS

The selection and evaluation of measurement tools from a wide range of available measures can be overwhelming and it would be impossible to consider within this chapter the whole range of measures available or to appraise each one. Therefore a selection of high-quality clinical and research measures are evaluated and their relative strengths and weaknesses discussed. The range of measures included here illustrates good practice in measurement of a range of different constructs in paediatric physiotherapy practice. However, it should be noted that other measures are available and it is recommended that the clinician consider a range of measurement tools prior to implementing one particular tool in practice.

In order to make rational, informed decisions on the use of an outcome measurement tool it is essential to consider carefully the purpose and requirements of the measure.

Many factors need investigation, including the reason for measurement (research or clinical purposes), the construct to be measured, the reliability and validity of the measure, the cost of implementing the measure and the value of the information gained. It would be inappropriate to suggest that one particular measurement tool could meet a multitude of different measurement needs and it may be that physiotherapists need to use several measures to gain the range of information they need to inform their clinical practice. In selecting and using the right measurement tool physiotherapists should use their clinical experience to help justify their choice. Consideration of prior experience and proficiency must be applied to inform clinical decision-making (Sackett et al 1997), therefore measures and management programmes should be appraised in the light of clinical experience. Measurement cannot be the sole determinant of sound clinical decision-making.

Phillips et al (1994) suggest that in order to measure outcomes effectively several key points must be considered, most importantly: what do you want to achieve? Without this clear aim, explicitly stated, it is unlikely that the end-result will be productive and indeed a great deal of time and effort, by both physiotherapist and patient, might be wasted. A measurement tool suited to a research setting may be far too extensive to use in normal clinical practice, therefore the most appropriate measure may be a clinically relevant one.

In addition to its primary purpose, a measure may have four key functions:

1. to discriminate from the norm, across subjects
2. to predict future status
3. to evaluate change over time, across time
4. to describe the status of the subject at a particular point in time (Jackowski & Guyatt 2003).

Discriminative measure

The discriminative measure is based on norm-referenced data so that one can compare the child with the norm. For example, a child is referred for assessment to see if he or she has a significant developmental delay and whether this requires intervention.

Predictive measure

The predictive measure looks forward to attempt to predict what might happen to the child over time. For example, a child with poorly controlled asthma charts his or her peak flow on a daily basis to predict a worsening of the condition prior to a significant attack.

Evaluative measure

The evaluative measure shows how a child is different from the last time the measure was used and therefore shows change in specific measured criteria over time. For

Table 3.1 International Classification of Functioning, Disability and Health (ICIDH-2) definitions of the dimensions and related outcome measurement tools

Dimension	Definition	Example of typical outcome measures
Body function and structure	Body functions are physiological functions of the body systems Body structures are the anatomical parts of the body, such as organs, limbs and their components	Balance scales Range of movement Muscle strength Motor tasks Movement and force analysis of gait Sensory awareness, e.g. functional reach test, goniometery
Activity	The performance of a task or action by an individual	Motor development tests Walking tests Self-care evaluations Play skills, e.g. 6-minute walking test, Gross Motor Function Measure (GMFM), Alberta Infant Motor Scales (AIMS)
Participation	An individual's involvement in life situations in relation to health conditions, body functions and structures, activities and contextual factors	Integration into school Fulfilment of roles and perceived needs Parental care indices Attitudinal scales of ability and disability, e.g. School Functional Assessment, Canadian Occupational Performance Measure (COPM), Juvenile Arthritis Self-Report Index (JASI)

example, a child with arthritis is repeatedly measured with the same measurement tool to determine the rate and nature of change in function and joint range following physiotherapy intervention for a 6-week period. In contrast, a descriptive measure gives a snapshot in time of the child measured against agreed criteria. For example, a child about to change from paediatric to adult-based physiotherapy services is reviewed with an agreed measurement tool that both services understand, to offer information describing the patient's condition at transfer of care.

The way in which you decide to measure will depend upon the reason for the use of measurement, but also upon what construct you wish to measure. For example, a different approach to measurement may be used when seeking to measure a child's interactions in school compared with measuring range of movement. It is important to determine the measurement construct. It is often helpful to look to the World Health Organization's (2001) *International Classification of Functioning* (ICF) model which uses the categories of 'body functions and structure', 'activity' and 'participation' to assist health professionals to ensure consideration of the whole nature of health and well-being (Table 3.1).

Which type of measurement tool is suitable will depend upon the answer to some important questions.

Finally, the physiotherapist must consider the quality of the measurement tool.

A measurement tool must measure the particular attributes and be trustworthy. Several considerations must be made when trying to determine the usefulness of a particular measure. These are *reliability* and *validity*.

A reliable measure will give the same result if a tester repeated the measure over a short period on the same

---

CRITICAL QUESTIONS

1. **What do you want to achieve?**

2. **What construct do you want to measure?**
    Having established the construct and the reason for measurement, it is vital that practical constraints are considered. Often these practical issues override what can be done (Ditmarr & Gresham 1997). For the measurement tool to be successful the person administering the tool is a vital component, so consideration should be given to training and the time available for familiarization with a tool. Similarly, if investing time in using a new measurement tool, consider whether the tool can be used on numerous occasions to ensure that the operator becomes proficient and skilful in its administration. It may be that the tool requires a significant amount of time to administer and the child and family may be unable or unwilling to participate for an extended period purely for measurement purposes, so consider the needs of the family and their priorities. The cultural context

should not be overlooked: a family may find elements of a measurement tool inappropriate or offensive. It is particularly important to consider the cultural differences that may occur when questioning families within the participation dimension. Families from different cultural backgrounds may have different attitudes and beliefs with regard to family roles and the concept of childhood.

The use of a particular method of measurement may be important to physiotherapy practice. Physical testing may be the only appropriate way to measure the dimension of body functions and structure and may be part of the ongoing clinical assessment of a management programme. Measurement tools that require extended periods of observation and interaction with families and children are costly in terms of staff time, but may be vital to ensure accurate measurement within a research programme. In contrast, a self-reported questionnaire, which can be completed and then returned to the physiotherapist, may be quick and easy to complete and offer an insight into the child and family's perceptions of their abilities and needs. Alternatively, a combination of methods may be useful to maximize the results obtained, allowing the physiotherapist to see the link between body systems, activity and participation, thus demonstrating their impact on participation and life skills.

3. **What practical considerations are there?**
    For example, training, time, location, cost, availability of measure, family circumstances and cultural sensitivities.

4. **What method will be appropriate for the measurement tool?**
    Such methods include observation, self-report or facilitated questionnaire and physical testing.

---

subject, but also gives the same result if several testers were to apply the test to the same subject. A standardized measure is often more reliable. It offers a clear rationale for testing, usually in a tester manual. It seeks to ensure that each tester applies the test in the same way and therefore their results will be comparable.

A valid measure is one that measures what it truly intends to measure. Measures should be rigorously tested to demonstrate validity. Part of the concept of validity is sensitivity and specificity. A tool that is sensitive and specific will be responsive to real difference either between patients or in a single or group of patients over time.

CRITICAL QUESTION

5. **Is there a good-quality measurement tool?**
    Reliability and standardization, validity, sensitivity and specificity are important factors to consider.

Reliability

Reliability is the test of a measure's repeatability and accuracy. A reliable measure gives results that are reproducible and consistent. Reliability is often tested by repeating the measure on a stable population over a period of time. The results are then examined for consistency, to show whether the results correlate on each occasion of measurement. The statistical testing of correlation is usually done using a Pearson correlation calculation. A good result from a very close correlation should give a Pearson correlation coefficient very close to 1. A result of 1 demonstrates an exact correlation, exactly the same result being produced on each occasion. Obviously when dealing with people and children in particular, this is unlikely; therefore a correlation coefficient between 0.7 and 0.9 is usually accepted as being of a good standard. This statistical test can be used to examine several elements of reliability, including reproducibility (test – retest correlation), intrarater reliability (correlation between repeated measures by one tester), interrater reliability (correlation between different testers) and population reliability (correlation within a particular sample group).

Reproducibility

A measure needs to be reliable in reproducing the same results on several occasions when no change could have occurred. This is often assessed by repeating the measure on several occasions over a short period (test – retest reliability). The results for the test and retests are compared using a correlation statistic (Bland & Altman 1986). If the measure is reliable and has good reproducibility the test and retest measures should be very similar, therefore they should correlate strongly. The researchers who introduce new tests will work extremely hard to ensure that a test is reproducible by all those who might use it. This might involve:

- production and testing of standardized instruction manuals and training courses to ensure that each tester applies the test in the same way
- repeated and selective testing of each component within a test to ensure that it is truly valuable and reproducible and refinement of the test components.

Intrarater reliability considers the consistency of the result if the same person applied the measure on repeated occasions and is often considered alongside reproducibility. This considers how reliable you are in the way you apply the measure and interpret the findings. This is often closely linked to the clarity of standardization of a measure. If the instructions for application and interpretation of results are very clear and minimize subjectivity then you are likely to repeat the testing and the scoring in a very similar way each time. This will then enable a very close correlation between results each time you apply the test when no real change has occurred.

Interrater reliability considers the effect of several different people applying the same measure when no change should have occurred. The population is stable and there are no true changes. The results from a measure with good interrater reliability will be very similar even if several people apply the measure. This aspect is very important if you wish to compare your results to those of other people. It is also important for research where more than one tester is involved, e.g. multicentre trials. To be able to integrate your findings with those published or collected by other people, the measure must have good interrater reliability. Interrater reliability is often improved by training, updating and discussion between testers.

Population reliability is tested with a specific population in a specific environment. It is important to consider if the reliability-testing population is similar to the one with which you are intending to use the measure. Reliability of a measure may change when applied to different client groups in different settings.

It is easy to see how results of testing might be different in these examples:

1. A group of 10-year-old children with Down's syndrome versus a group of 10-year-old children with cerebral palsy
2. A group of 13-year-old children with cystic fibrosis versus a group of 5-year-olds, even if their disease is similar
3. A group of dyspraxic children in school versus the same group tested in a quiet child development centre setting.

Validity

This is the extent to which a measure records what it intends to record or 'the degree of correspondence between the concept being measured and the variable used to represent the concept' (Law 2002). Validity has several components and ideally a high-quality measurement tool should be able to show a high level of validity in each one.

Content or construct validity is often considered by examining the findings in different aspects of a measure when it is constructed to see if they are truly responding to changes occurring in the population or if they are testing something less relevant. During initial development statistical testing of the new tool components enables the developers to add and subtract components until only those with high validity remain. Each component forms a useful and valid part of the complete tool.

Concurrent validity is often measured by comparing a new tool to a well-established high-quality tool. If both tools demonstrate similar responses under the same testing conditions then the tools can be said to have a high level of concurrent validity. In the field of paediatric measurement it can be difficult to establish concurrent validity due to the small number of high-quality tools currently available.

However some tools, e.g. Functional Independence Measure for Children (WeeFIM), Peabody Developmental Motor Scales (PDMS-2) and the Gross Motor Function Measure (GMFM) have been developed with concurrent validity testing (Campbell et al 1988, Palisano 1993).

Sensitivity

Some measures are sensitive to change throughout a population; however, because the abilities and disabilities of the children we see vary due to pathology, age and environment, it is particularly important that we try to consider the sensitivity of a measure.

Some measures have an upper limit for effectiveness. For example, it would be ineffective to measure balance in a very able 7-year-old using a measure which gives a maximum score when completing five successive steps. These measures would be insensitive to any improvement due to a 'ceiling effect'. The child has already scored a maximum or very nearly maximum and so any improvement could only give a very slight change in test result. The test will therefore lack sensitivity to change in upper range.

Some measures are insensitive in their lower range; they are unable to reflect smaller changes in progress at the lower end of the scale. This is often due to the scoring levels being too wide apart for less able children to gain increased scores. For example, a child with low tidal lung volumes might not reach the next point on an incentive spirometer with 50-ml intervals. These children would come up against a 'floor effect' preventing them from demonstrating any progression on this measurement scale.

The ceiling and floor effects can also prevent a measure from giving accurate information regarding deterioration. If the steps between scores are too large, too small or inappropriately weighted then the measure may not demonstrate a deterioration which is functionally important.

In addition, some measurement tools must show good levels of sensitivity and specificity. This is particularly relevant for diagnostic or screening tools. Sensitivity is the extent to which the measurement tool detects a disorder when it is truly present. A sensitive tool has few false-positive findings. Specificity is the extent to which the measurement tool rules to a disorder of dysfunction when it is actually present, commonly called a false-negative finding (Ditmarr & Gresham 1997).

General utility

Each physiotherapist must decide upon the utility of a measure, based upon many competing factors, e.g. the client group, their age, the time available, the clinical or research requirements, the environment, the key components considered to be most important and the child's range of ability. It is not always possible to ensure that all factors are equally considered; however a measurement tool must be chosen based on best fit.

The following sections aim to review some of the most frequently used, good-quality outcome measurement tools in paediatric practice at the present time. These tools are a selection of parent/carer/child questionnaires, physical measures and observational measures of task performance. By reviewing a range of different types of measurement tool, physiotherapists can gain an understanding of the variety of tools available. Each review describes the subject group for which the measure was designed and the main purpose of the tool. The review also suggests the level of validity, reliability and sensitivity to assist the reader in choosing a high-quality measurement tool. The list is not exclusive – other measurement tools are available – but these reviews aim to demonstrate the range of tools available and offer a starting point for physiotherapists seeking to evaluate and analyse their impact on patient care. Reviews of other tools which could be suitable can be found in Law et al (2001) and Finch et al (2002).

1. Canadian Occupational Performance Measure (COPM)
2. School Function Assessment
3. Functional Independence Measure for Children (WeeFIM)
4. Child Health Questionnaire
5. Cystic Fibrosis Questionnaire
6. Pediatric Evaluation of Disability Inventory (PEDI)
7. Gross Motor Function Measure (GMFM)
8. Peabody Developmental Motor Scales (PDMS-2)
9. Functional Reach
10. Walk test (6-minute) (6MWT)
11. Alberta Infant Motor Scale (AIMS)
12. Chailey Levels of Ability
13. Movement Assessment Battery for Children Scale (M-ABC test)
14. Paediatric Pain Profile (PPP)

CANADIAN OCCUPATIONAL PERFORMANCE MEASURE (COPM)

Source:	Law M, Baptiste S, Carswell A et al 1998 *The Canadian Occupational Performance Measure*, 3rd edn. Toronto: CAOT. Available online at: www.caot.ca/copm/.
Purpose:	To detect change in self-perceived performance and satisfaction in self-care, productivity and leisure occupations.
Groups tested:	Children with disabilities: the parents completed the COPM.
Description:	Semistructured interview that takes 30 minutes to administer. Tasks are rated in terms of importance 1–10 (not important – extremely important). The five highest-ranking tasks are then rated on perception of performance (not able to do it – able to do it extremely well) and satisfaction with performance (not satisfied – extremely satisfied). Can be used to determine performance goals based on the client's perceptions of self-care, productivity and leisure.
Standardization:	Standardized by specific administration method and scoring; instruction manual available. No normative data are available.
	Reliability: Test – retest good = 0.7–0.9.
	Validity: Good.
Strengths:	A useful measure of interactions between the child and environment, measuring real and meaningful experiences for the child/parent. Fosters a client-centred approach to measurement and management.
Weaknesses:	Cannot help to determine the underlying problem within the perceived problem areas defined by the child/parent. Parent-reported difficulties may not truly reflect the opinions of the child.
Clinical utility:	Most therapists found it easy to administer and score, helpful in defining clinical goals, but somewhat dependent upon the ability of the child/parent and the interviewer to elicit reasoned answers.

SCHOOL FUNCTION ASSESSMENT

Source:	Harcourt Assessment, Halley Court, Jordan Hill, Oxford, OX2 8EJ. www.harcourt-uk.com.
Purpose:	To measure a student's performance of functional tasks that support the student's participation in school. Includes both study and social tasks within an elementary school setting.
Description:	Ordinal measure of 317 items. Scaled either 1–4 or 1–6, dependent on the item. Can be used in sections or as a whole:
	• Equipment, technology, appliances, tools
	• Educational services
	• Personal care
	• Social relations
	• School
	• Play
	• Transportation.
	Rating scale completed by respondents who are familiar with the student's typical performance, e.g. teachers, physiotherapist, occupational therapist, non-teaching support staff.
Standardization:	Based on items required for successful school performance; manual is clear and easy to read.
	Reliability: High = >0.9.
	Validity: High.
Strengths:	Robust and easily administered scale corresponds to current exclusivity policies.
Weaknesses:	Perceptions may need to be gathered from a number of individuals to complete the whole assessment. Individual opinions may differ
Clinical utility:	A very useful tool in establishing areas of strength and of concern in school integration.

FUNCTIONAL INDEPENDENCE MEASURE FOR CHILDREN (WEEFIM)

Source:	Centre for Functional Assessment Research and Uniform Data Systems. www.udsmr.org.
Purpose:	To measure the severity of disability and changes in functional ability of children. To 'weigh the burden of care', i.e. physical, technological and financial resources.
Groups tested:	Children between 6 months and 8 years with neurodevelopmental disabilities.
Description:	An 18-item observational measure. Items are gathered into six domains and in two scales: the cognitive and the motor scale. Items are scored from 1 to 7 on the amount of assistance required to complete the item task. Completed by direct observation or by interview of primary care-giver. Takes approximately 20 minutes to complete.
Standardization:	Validated on typically developing children.
	Reliability: High = >0.9.
	Validity: Good = 0.7–0.9.

Strengths	• Suitable for various disciplines • Clear instructions • Easily administered interview format to seek carers' and/or professionals' perspective • Can be administered at home, school or in the community setting • Requires no special equipment.
Weaknesses	• Complex scoring and interpretation • Reported attributes are at risk of subjective bias.

CHILD HEALTH QUESTIONNAIRE

Source:	Landgraf JM 1996 *The Child Health Questionnaire (CHQ) Users' Manual.* Boston, MA: The Health Institute. New England Medical Centre, 750 Washington St, Boston MA 02111, USA.
Purpose:	To measure the physical and psychosocial well-being of children over the age of 5.
Groups tested:	Parents of children with asthma, attention-deficit hyperactivity disorder, epilepsy, psychiatric diagnoses and juvenile rheumatoid arthritis.
Description:	A questionnaire format administered to children as a self-report or to their parents as the parental report. Can be self-administered or used in an interview format. Questions are answered on a 4-week recall basis and answered on a four-point ordinal scale. There are multiple forms of the parent report questionnaire and it can take between 15 and 45 minutes to complete depending on the form used.
Standardization:	The scale is norm-referenced and clinical profiles are available for the groups stated above.
	Reliability: Not reported.
	Validity: Not reported.
Strengths:	Useful tool to gain the perspective of the child or parent on the child's physical and psychosocial health.
Weaknesses:	This measure is primarily a research tool and so it takes some time to become accustomed to its application. It has complex scoring system and the manual is extensive. Further testing of validity and reliability in the clinical setting is required.
Clinical utility:	May be appropriate for research physiotherapists wishing to seek clarification of the child's or parent's perspective on health and well-being. Clinical physiotherapists would tend to ask pertinent questions from a family and child rather than use this weighty measurement tool.

CYSTIC FIBROSIS QUESTIONNAIRE

Source:	Quittner AL, Buu A, Watrous M, Davis M 2000 *CFQ Cystic Fibrosis Questionnaire; A Health-Related Quality of Life Measure.* User manual. English version 1.0 (2000).
Purpose:	Designed to measure the physical, emotional and social impact of cystic fibrosis on individuals and their families.
Groups tested:	Children with cystic fibrosis between the ages of 6 and 13 and their parents, adolescents and adults with cystic fibrosis (14 years and older).
Description:	There are three versions of the CFQ: a teen adult version (CFQ 14+), a parent version (CFQ-PT) and a child version (CFQ-C). Each version is developmentally appropriate and can be self-administered or used in an interview format. A range of items are rated on a four-point scale of frequency (always – never) difficulty (a lot – no difficulty) and true – false ratings (very true – very false) or weighted statements on a four- or five-point scale. Each version takes an average of 20 minutes to complete. At least two-thirds of the items must be completed to enable scoring.
	Reliability: Internal consistency good = 0.7–0.9, test – retest not reported.
	Validity: Good.
Strengths:	A valuable tool in seeking the perception of children, adults and carers with regard to the complex health and well-being issue of patients with cystic fibrosis.
Weaknesses:	Validity and reliability require further investigation. Children and adults with lower levels of English may find the self-administered questionnaire difficult to complete.
Clinical utility:	A relatively quick and comprehensive measurement tool, able to be given to respondents prior to clinical assessment to complete the larger picture of their quality of life.

PEDIATRIC EVALUATION OF DISABILITY INVENTORY (PEDI)

Source:	Harcourt Assessment, Halley Court, Jordan Hill, Oxford. OX2 8EJ. www.harcourt-uk.com.
Purpose:	Evaluative measure of ability and activities of daily living via interview.
Groups tested:	Children with physical or physical and cognitive disabilities. Test has been used in studies of children with orthopaedic and neurological problems. Applicable to children from 6 months to 7½ years, although it can be used for older children who are functionally delayed.
Description:	A standardized structured interview for use with parents or professionals working with young children who are asked to give their impression of the child's typical performance. Divided into scales of functional skills, care-giver assistance and modifications. Scales can be collectively or independently administered. Each scale considers abilities in self-care, mobility and social function. Administration takes between 20 minutes and 1 hour depending upon the child's level of ability.
Standardization:	Standardized scores from a normal population of children can be used for norm-referencing. Manual and scoring information gives clear guidance for standardizing administration.
	Reliability: Internal reliability and test – retest reliability is high: = >0.9. Interrater reliability ranges from poor to high, with particularly low intra-class correlation (ICC) scores reported between some parent and professional impressions.
	Validity: Good.
Strengths:	Measures important constructs of life skills via interview. Can be used in any setting. Easy to administer with clear instructions.
Weaknesses:	Complex to interpret. Reported involvement may give opportunity for bias or disagreement of perceptions.
Clinical utility:	Clinically appropriate tool for investigation of the amount of assistance a child may need in functional activity and social interactions.

GROSS MOTOR FUNCTION MEASURE (GMFM)

Source:	Cambridge University Press: www.cup.org.
Purpose:	To assess change in gross motor function for children with disabilities.
Groups tested:	Children with cerebral palsy, Down's syndrome, osteogenesis imperfecta, developmental delay. The GMFM-66 has been specifically weighted for use with children with cerebral palsy.
Description:	A criterion-referenced measure. The original GMFM-88 has 88 items arranged into five dimensions. The newer GMFM 66 has 66 items in one dimension. The items consist of observation of the performance of a standardized physical task. Each item is assigned a score on a four-point scale (0–3).
Standardization:	Each item is clearly described and standardized performance outcome descriptors assist with scoring. An extensive manual supports the assessor.
	Reliability: High to good.
	Validity: High to good.
Strengths:	A commonly used measurement tool for children with cerebral palsy. The GMFM-66 is quicker to administer due to having fewer items and allows for interval scale measures rather than ordinal scale measure, thereby enabling a higher level of statistical analysis.
Weaknesses:	Some indication of ceiling and floor effects leading to a higher level of error near the upper and lower limits of the measure. Standardized equipment is required, which may make this measure unsuitable for the community environment.
Clinical utility:	A well-respected and well-used measurement tool.

PEABODY DEVELOPMENTAL MOTOR SCALES (PDMS-2)

Source:	DLM Teaching Resources, One DLM Park, Allen TX75002, USA.
Purpose:	Evaluative, discriminative and descriptive task performance measure of gross and fine motor development of children.
Groups tested:	Children aged between 0 and 83 months.
Description:	Takes on average 20–30 minutes to complete one subtest, 45–60 minutes to complete the entire test. Observer-scored test of 282 items in six subtests: reflexes, stationary control, locomotion, object manipulation, grasping and visual – motor integration.
	Gross motor and fine motor scales can be performed in isolation or together.
Standardization:	Standardized scores enable comparison with age-expected levels of ability. There is a manual and some equipment is available with the testing kit to assist standardization of administration.
	Reliability: High = >0.9.
	Validity: Good.
Strengths:	Easy to administer, administered in school or rehab setting. Gives ordinal and interval measure, norm-referenced.
Weaknesses:	Should not be used to discriminate between normal and delayed between 0 and 5 months. Gross motor scale between 48 and 59 months should be reported as ranges with caution. Unclear scoring in children with hemiplegia. A large amount of equipment is required to complete the testing.
Clinical utility:	Useful for sharing age-equivalence scores with parents and at multidisciplinary team meetings. May also provide useful information for statement reports.

FUNCTIONAL REACH

Source:	Duncan PW, Weiner DK, Chandler J, Studenski S *Graduate Program in Physical Therapy and Centre for the Study on Aging and Human Development.* Durham, NC: Duke University, Veterans Administration Medical Center.
Purpose:	To assess postural performance during voluntary movements required in everyday life. A test of functional forward reach in standing.
Groups tested:	Healthy children, children with balance dysfunction, children with lower-limb spasticity.
Description:	A level tape or stick is secured to the wall at the height of the acromion. From a relaxed standing position the child raises the arm until it is parallel with the stick. The placement of the third metacarpophalangeal joint (hand in a fist) is noted; the subject then reaches as far as possible without taking a step or touching the wall. Two practice trials and three measurement trials are completed. The mean distance over the three measurement trials is calculated to give the functional reach length.
	Reliability: High = >0.9.
	Validity: High.
Sensitivity:	Good.
Strengths:	A quick and clinically relevant measure of balance ability in standing. Can be modified to suit individuals in a seated position.
Weaknesses:	Children with lower ability may refuse to reach out of the base and therefore there is a significant floor effect.
Clinical utility:	Extremely useful measure suited to clinical practice.

WALK TEST (6-MINUTE) (6MWT)

Source:	Butland RJA, Pang J, Gross ER, Woodcock AA, Geddes DM 1982 Two-, six- and twelve-minute walking tests in respiratory disease. *British Medical Journal* 284: 1607–1608.
Purpose:	To assess exercise tolerance.
Groups tested:	Originally designed for those with respiratory conditions, but also used with those with cystic fibrosis, arthroplasty, transplant candidates, children with end-stage heart and lung disease.
Description:	The distance walked in 6 minutes is measured. A greater distance indicates better exercise tolerance. Patients are instructed to walk from end to end of a quiet enclosed corridor. They must cover as much ground as possible but may rest if they become too short of breath or tired to continue. They should resume walking as soon as they are able. The distance walked, number and duration of rests are measured. Can be combined with measurements of pulse rate, perceived effort, oxygen saturations, pain numerical scoring, if required.
	Reliability: Good = 0.7–0.9.
	Validity: Good.
Strengths:	An easily interpreted clinical tool, with good standards of reliability and validity which have been extensively tested in a variety of patient populations.
Weaknesses:	Requires the subject to apply maximal physical effort to represent a true measure of physiological exercise tolerance. More recently, 6MWT has been appropriately used as a measure of ability to undertake physically demanding activities of daily living.
Clinical utility:	A good clinical measurement tool which can be suitable for many levels of ability, including the patient who is able to run, converting the walk to a running test. Can be used for many patient groups, including those with neurological and orthopaedic conditions.

ALBERTA INFANT MOTOR SCALE (AIMS)

Source:	Piper MC, Darrah J *Motor Assessment of the Developing Infant* 1994. Philadelphia, PA: WB Saunders.
Purpose:	To measure the motor development of infants aged 0–18 months to identify children who are delayed or deviant in their development or maturation and evaluation of development and maturation over time.
Groups tested:	Children aged between 0 and 18 months.
Description:	Takes on average 30 minutes to complete. It is an observational scale requiring minimal handling by the assessor and aims to identify the positive aspects of a child's motor development. A user-friendly measure, assessing the child in four main postures: prone, supine, sitting and standing. The measure scores the child on the achievement of key postures and transitions.
Standardization:	Standardized scores enable comparison with age-expected levels of ability. There is a manual available and some equipment is available with the testing kit to assist standardization of administration.
	Reliability: High = >0.9 for single occasions and over time.
	Validity (concurrent): High: 0.98.
Strengths	• Easy to administer. Children often cooperate with this test as it is quick and easy. Any appropriate toys can be used to stimulate movement and postures during the test
	• Administered in school or rehab setting
	• Gives ordinal and interval measure, norm-referenced.
Weaknesses:	Can be problematic in scoring and you need to keep an eye on the quality of movements as well as the accomplishment of developmental milestones. The measure will not recognize asymmetry or poor-quality movement. The scoring system identifies a window for investigation and assumes the child can accomplish all the skills in the lower developmental levels.
Clinical utility:	Useful for sharing age-equivalence scores with parents and at multidisciplinary team meetings. May also provide useful information for statement reports.

CHAILEY LEVELS OF ABILITY

Source:	Pountney TE, Mulcahy CM, Clarke S, Green EM 2004 *Chailey Approach to Postural Management*. East Sussex: Chailey Heritage Clinical Services.
Purpose:	To record levels of physical ability in children with moderate to severe disability. It identifies components of posture that are limiting function. Can be used in and out of equipment to determine effects of provision of postural management equipment.
Groups tested:	Children and young people with cerebral palsy.
	This ability offers a method of postural analysis capable of identifying components of ability which are limiting postural control. It can be used as a guide for treatment interventions and is widely used in the provision of postural management equipment. Children can be reassessed within their equipment to determine if the equipment has improved their postural ability and also to identify the potential for functional activity once positioned, e.g. ability to control posture within or outside base.
Description:	It is an observational assessment for use with children and adults to assess an individual's consistent posture and ability in lying, sitting and standing. It is based on developmental biomechanics. The measure takes approximately 30 minutes and a child is encouraged to move using appropriate toys and instructions with the minimal amount of handling.
	Reliability: Reliability has been established for the lying and sitting scales. Interrater reliability of 0.94, intrarater reliability of 0.92 were established for standing; 0.65 for supine lying, and 0.73 for prone lying.
	Validity: Concurrent and content validity has been established on all scales.
Strengths:	This scale is easy to administer and requires no special equipment. Being largely observational, the test is not contaminated by handling. Based on a normal developmental model, the test identifies how function can be altered by changed biomechanics of posture.
Weaknesses:	The ceiling of the scale is independent standing so cannot assess more advanced skills in standing.

MOVEMENT ASSESSMENT BATTERY FOR CHILDREN TEST (M-ABC TEST)

Source:	Harcourt Assessment: http://www.harcourt-uk.com/index.aspx
Purpose of test:	To identify and evaluate movement problems in children with specific motor learning difficulties.
Description:	The M-ABC test has a total of eight items for each age band for children aged 4–12 years with minimal motor dysfunctions that may include children with developmental coordination disorder. These are divided into three sections to assess manual dexterity, ball skills and balance skills. The tests and scores are graded according to age.

Scores are recorded on a quantitative scale with a complementary qualitative description to provide more information regarding performance aspects of the task.

The quantitative scores are based either on time taken to perform the task or number of accurate attempts. The raw scores are converted to normative scores from which percentile rankings can be taken. Suggestions are made as to which scores would indicate cause for concern.

Qualitative descriptions include phrases such as 'misaligns pegs,' during peg board task or 'lands with straight legs' during the jumping activity. Together these two scores provide an accurate picture of the child's performance. Takes 20–40 minutes.

Reliability:	Strong test – retest interrater reliability.
Validity:	Criterion validity has been established with other perceptuomotor tests.

PAEDIATRIC PAIN PROFILE (PPP)

Source:	http://www.ppprofile.org.uk/index.htm.
Purpose:	The Paediatric Pain Profile is designed to help in assessing pain in children with severe neurological impairments, especially those whose impairments restrict their ability to communicate through speech. These children are dependent on their carers to interpret their signs of pain. It aims to identify behaviours which have been found to be the most important indicators of pain.
Description:	The PPP is a 20-item behaviour-rating scale, with each item being rated on a four-point scale, from 'not at all' to 'a great deal.' Completed scores will range from 0 to 60. Scores of 14 were generally indicative of severe to moderate pain. The profile will provide a pain history, baseline and ongoing assessments and actions and outcomes.

Reliability:	Summated scale very good (0.73–0.87).
Validity:	Face, concurrent and construct validity established.

REFERENCES

Bland JM, Altman DG 1986 Statistical methods for assessing agreement between two methods of clinical measurement. *Lancet* 1: 307–310.

Campbell SK, Wilhelm IJ, Phillips W, Slaton DS 1988 Comparative performance of infants on three tests of gross motor development. *Physical Therapy* 68: 818.

Chartered Society of Physiotherapy 2005 *Core Standards of Physiotherapy Practice*. London: Chartered Society of Physiotherapy.

Department of Health 1991 *The Patients' Charter for England*. London: HMSO.

Department of Health 1992 *The Health of the Nation*. London: HMSO.

Department of Health 1999 *Clinical Governance in the New NHS*. London: HMSO.

Department of Health 2000 *The NHS Plan*. London: HMSO.

Department of Health 2004 *Choosing Health: Making Healthier Choices Easier*. London: HMSO.

Ditmarr S, Gresham G 1997 *Functional Assessment and Outcome Measures for the Rehabilitation Health Professional*. Aspen Publications.

Finch E, Brooks D, Stratford P et al 2002 *Physical Rehabilitation Outcome Measures: A Guide to Enhanced Clinical Decision Making*, 2nd edn. Lippincott/Williams & Wilkins.

Jackowski D, Guyatt G 2003 A guide to health measurement. *Clinical Orthopaedics and Related Research* 413: 80–89.

Law M (ed.) 2002 *Evidence Based Rehabilitation: A Guide to Practice.* Slack: New Jersey.

Law M, Baum C, Dunn W 2001 *Measuring Occupational Performance: Supporting Best Practice in Occupational Therapy.* Slack: New Jersey.

Palisano RJ 1993 Neuro-motor and developmental assessment. In: Wilhelm IJ (ed.) *Physical Assessment in Early Infancy.* New York: Churchill Livingstone, pp. 173–224.

Phillips C, Palfrey C, Thomas P 1994 *Evaluating Health and Social Care.* McMillan Press.

Sackett D, Richardson W, Rosenberg W et al 1997 *Evidence Based Medicine; How to Practice and the EBM.* New York: Churchill Livingston.

World Health Organization 2001 International classification of functioning, disability and health. Available online at: http://www.who.int/classifications/icf/en/index.html.

FURTHER READING

Chartered Society of Physiotherapy 2005 Outcome measurement. Available online at: http://www.csp.org.uk/effectivepractice/outcomemeasures.cfm.

Law M (ed.) 2002 *Evidence Based Rehabilitation.* Slack: New Jersey.

Roberts AR, Yeager KR 2004 *Evidence-Based Practice Manual: Research and Outcome Measures in Health and Human Services.* Oxford University Press.

Canadian Occupational Performance Measure

Law M, Baptiste S, McColl MA et al 1990 The Canadian Occupational Performance Measure: an outcome measurement protocol for occupational therapy. *Canadian Journal of Occupational Therapy* 57: 82–87.

School Function Assessment

Davies PL, Soon PL, Young M et al 2004 Validity and reliability of the School Function Assessment in elementary school students with disabilities. *Physical and Occupational Therapy in Pediatrics* 24: 23–43.

Hwang J, Davies PL, Taylor MP et al 2002 Validation of School Function Assessment with elementary school children. *OTJR: Occupation Participation and Health* 22: 48–58.

McEwen IR, Arnold SH, Hansen LH et al 2003 Interrater reliability and content validity of a minimal data set to measure outcomes of students receiving school-based occupational therapy and physical therapy. *Physical and Occupational Therapy in Pediatrics* 23: 77–95.

Gross Motor Function Measure

Bjornson KF, Fraubert CS, McLaughlin JF et al 1998 Test – retest reliability of the gross motor function measure in children with cerebral palsy. *Physical and Occupational Therapy in Pediatrics* 18: 51–61.

Ruck-Gibis J, Plotkin H, Hanley J et al 2001 Reliability of the Gross Motor Function Measure for children with osteogenesis imperfecta. *Pediatric Physical Therapy* 13: 10–17.

Russell DJ, Avery LM, Rosenbaum PL et al 2000 Improved scaling of the gross motor function measure for children with cerebral palsy; evidence of reliability and validity. *Physical Therapy* 80: 873–885.

Russell D, Rosenbaum P, Gowland C et al 2002 *Gross Motor Function Measure (GMFM-66 and GMFM-88) User's Manual.* Clinics in Developmental Medicine no. 159. London: Mackeith Press.

Functional Independence measure (WeeFIM)

Braun S 1998 Featured instrument. The Functional Independence Measure for children (Wee FIM instrument); gateway to the WeeFIM system. *Journal of Rehabilitation Outcomes Measurement* 2: 63–68.

Braun SL, Granger CV 1991 A practical approach to functional assessment in paediatrics. *Occupational Therapy Practice* 2: 46–51.

McAuliffe CA, Wenger RE, Schneider JW et al 1998 Usefulness of the Wee-Functional Independence Measure to detect functional change in children with cerebral palsy. *Pediatric Physical Therapy* 10: 23–28.

Ottenbacher K, Msall ME, Lyon N et al 1999 Measuring developmental and functional status in children with disabilities. *Developmental Medicine and Child Neurology* 41: 186–194.

Peabody Developmental Motor Scales

Gebhard AR, Ottenbacher KJ, Lane SJ 1994 Interrater reliability of the Peabody Developmental Motor Scales: fine motor scale. *American Journal of Occupational Therapy* 48: 976–981.

Hinderer KA, Richardson PK, Atwater SW 1989 Clinical implications of the Peabody Developmental Motor Scales; a constructive review. *Physical and Occupational Therapy in Pediatrics* 9: 81.

Palisano RJ 1986 Concurrent and predictive validities of the Bayley motor scale and the Peabody Development Motor Scales. *Physical Therapy* 66: 1714.

Russell DJ, Ward M, Law M 1994 Test – retest reliability of the fine motor scale of the Peabody Developmental

Motor Scales in children with cerebral palsy. *Occupational Therapy Journal of Research* 14: 178–182.

Schmidt LS, Westcott SL, Crowe TK 1993 Interrater reliability of the gross motor scale of the Peabody Developmental Motor Scales with 4- and 5-year-old children. *Pediatric Physical Therapy* 5: 169–175.

Pediatric Evaluation of Disability Inventory

Berg M, Jahnsen R, Froslie KF et al 2004 Reliability of the Pediatric Evaluation of Disability Inventory (PEDI). *Physical and Occupational Therapy in Pediatrics* 24: 61–77.

Haley SM 1997 The Pediatric Evaluation of Disability Inventory (PEDI). *Journal of Rehabilitation Outcomes Measurement* 1: 61–69.

Hayley SM, Coster WJ, Fass RM 1991 A content validity study of the pediatric evaluation of disability inventory. *Pediatric Physical Therapy* 3: 177–184.

Child Health Questionnaire

Langgraf JM, Maunsell E, Speechhley KN et al 1998 Canadian – French, German and UK versions of the Child Health Questionnaire; methodology and preliminary item scaling results. *Quality of Life Research* 7: 433–445.

Cystic Fibrosis Questionnaire

Henry B, Aussage P, Grosskopf C et al 1998 Evaluating quality of life in children with cystic fibrosis; should we believe the child or the parent? *Pediatric Pulmonology* 26 (suppl.).

Quittner AL, Sweeny S, Watrous M et al 2000 Translation and linguistic validation of a disease specific quality of life measure for cystic fibrosis. *Journal of Pediatric Psychology* 25: 403–414.

Functional Reach

Donahoe B, Turner D, Worrell T 1994 The use of Functional Reach as a measurement of balance in boys and girls without disabilities; ages 5–15. *Pediatric Physical Therapy* 6: 189–193.

Duncan PW, Weiner DK, Chandler J, Studenski S 1990 Functional Reach: a new clinical measure of balance. *Journal of Gerontology* 45: M192–M197.

Ninik TM, Turner D, Worrell TW 1995 Functional reach as a measurement of balance for children with lower extremity spasticity. *Physical and Occupational Therapy in Pediatrics* 15: 1–15.

Wheeler A, Shall M, Lewis A, Sheperd J 1996 The reliability of measurements obtained using Functional Reach in children with cerebral palsy aged 3–16 years. *Pediatric Physical Therapy* 8: 182–183.

6-Minute Walk Test

Gultmans VAM, van Veldhoven NHMJ, de Meer K et al 1998 The six-minute walking test in children with cystic fibrosis; reliability and validity. *Pediatric Pulmonology* 22: 85–89.

Guyatt GH, Sullivan MJ, Thompson PJ et al 1985 The 6-minute walk; a new measure of exercise capacity in patients with chronic heart failure. *Canadian Medical Association Journal* 132: 919–923.

Nixon OA, Joswaik MK, Fricker FJ 1996 A six-minute walk test for assessing exercise tolerance in severely ill children. *Journal of Pediatrics* 129: 362–366.

Solway S, Brooks D, Lacasse Y, Thomas S 2001 A qualitative systematic overview of the measurement properties of functional walk tests used in the cardiorespiratory domain. *Chest* 119: 256–270.

Law M, Baptiste S, Carswell A et al 1998 *The Canadian Occupational Performance Measure*, 3rd edn. Toronto: CAOT.

Alberta Infant Motor Scale (AIMS)

Darrah J, Piper M, Watt MJ 1998 Assessment of gross motor skills of at-risk infants; predictive validity of the Alberta Infant Motor Scale. *Developmental Medicine and Child Neurology* 40: 485–491.

Piper MC, Darrah J 1994 *Motor Assessment of the Developing Infant*. Philadelphia, PA: WB Saunders.

4 Clinical gait analysis

Nicky Thompson

INTRODUCTION

Clinical gait analysis is a process in which an individual's gait pattern is measured, abnormalities are identified, causes are proposed and treatment recommendations are developed. This may be in a routine clinic setting using visual observation or video recording but increasingly a gait or motion analysis laboratory is now the clinical setting that facilitates this process using dedicated motion capture systems and a specialized multidisciplinary team. Although clinicians have highly developed visual observation skills when assessing an individual, the complex nature of some gait pathologies often defies simple visual analysis and provides no insight into the cause of the gait abnormality or any quantitative basis for treatment. In recent years advances in computer technology have led to routine instrumented gait analysis and the ability to measure a variety of gait parameters precisely and dynamically. This has not only helped progress our understanding of the biomechanics of normal and pathological locomotion but has also led to advances in the treatment of complex gait disorders.

Gait analysis has been found to be of great value in many pathologies, but is currently most highly developed clinically in neurological conditions. In paediatrics the most common condition likely to be referred for clinical gait analysis is a child with cerebral palsy, where complex gait deviations occur simultaneously in three planes of motion. Primary deviations are often confounded by compensatory strategies and increasing height and weight. A referral for gait analysis is now routine prior to consideration of surgery in children with spastic diplegia and most children with hemiplegia.

NORMAL GAIT

In order to understand pathological or abnormal gait it is necessary to have a detailed understanding of normal human walking as a reference frame (Perry 1992, Rose & Gamble 2005). Gait is defined as a repetitive sequence of limb movements to advance the body forwards safely with minimum energy expenditure. It is this repetitive or cyclical nature of walking, which is remarkably consistent between individuals (Whittle 2001), that lends itself to objective measurement. Figure 4.1 shows a complete gait cycle, i.e. one stride from foot strike to foot strike again on the same leg. It serves as a reminder of the complexities of human bipedal motion which is uniquely functional and efficient. Muscle activity and joint motion occur at various lower-limb joints and in three planes simultaneously, and the speed at which these motions occur is much faster than the ability of the human eye to process it. Even a minor gait deviation or abnormality will clearly have an effect on such gait efficiency. When several deviations occur simultaneously, as commonly seen in children with cerebral palsy, for example, then the effect can be profound (Figure 4.2).

The gait cycle can be subdivided into periods, tasks and phases (Figure 4.3). The two major periods of the gait cycle are stance and swing. Stance can be further broken down into five separate phases: (1) initial contact (IC); (2) loading response (LR); (3) mid-stance (MSt); (4) terminal stance (TSt); and (5) pre-swing (PSw). Swing phase can be broken down into three phases: (1) initial swing (ISw); (2) mid-swing (MSw); and (3) terminal swing (TSw). Generic terminology has developed to describe these phases in order to apply to children with a wide variety of pathologies. Thus 'heel strike' is more widely applicable as 'initial contact' or 'foot strike', and 'push-off' as 'terminal stance'. Overall the tasks that must be accomplished during a single cycle include weight acceptance, single-limb support and limb advancement. Weight acceptance occurs during the first two phases of IC and LR, single-limb support during the second two phases of MSt and TSt, and limb advancement during the last four phases of PSw, ISw, MSw and TSw. It is helpful to understand the mechanism by which these tasks occur.

A single gait cycle or stride begins when one foot strikes the ground and ends when it strikes the ground again.

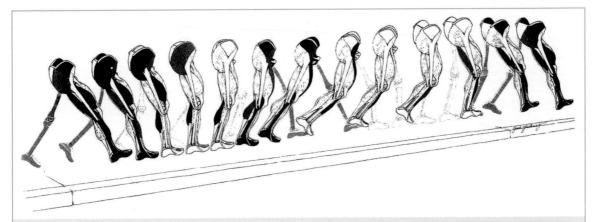

Figure 4.1 A complete gait cycle, with phasic muscle action denoted by intensity of grey shading. This figure illustrates the complex nature of gait, with motion occurring at several joints simultaneously in three planes. Reproduced from Rose & Gamble (2005) with permission.

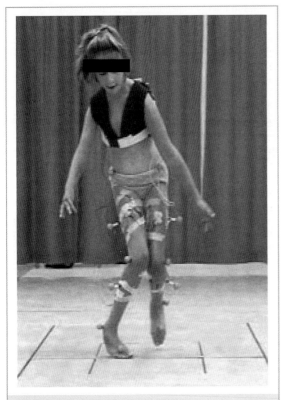

Figure 4.2 Complex nature of gait deviations in a child with spastic diplegic cerebral palsy.

Events in the gait cycle are defined sequentially as occurring at specific percentages of the gait cycle. Heel strike occurs at 0% and 100% of the cycle. During normal walking toe-off occurs at approximately 60% of the gait cycle. Therefore stance accounts for approximately 60% of the

gait cycle (Figure 4.4a) and swing 40% (Figure 4.4b). Opposite toe-off and opposite heel strike occur at 10% and 50% of the cycle respectively. Double support periods occur twice during the gait cycle and each phase of double support lasts about 10% of the cycle. The length of the double support is directly related to walking speed: as speed increases, the period of double support decreases and the absence of double support indicates a person is running rather than walking. The percentage of the gait cycle spent in single- or double-limb support is a reflection of the strength and stability of the musculoskeletal system and the coordination and maturation of the central nervous system. So in ambulant children at the more severe end of the spectrum of cerebral palsy, excessively long periods of double support would be indicative of poor overall gait function.

Normal walking has five major prerequisites, which are often lost in pathological gait. Treatment principles are based on restoring these attributes, as defined by Gage (2004):

1. Restoration of stance phase stability
2. Improvement of swing phase clearance
3. Appropriate pre-positioning of the foot in terminal swing
4. Enablement of an adequate step length
5. The reduction of energy expenditure.

GAIT MATURATION

It is not usually possible to undertake formal three-dimensional (3D) gait analysis in very young children. In typically developing children, collecting gait data from toddlers, i.e. children who have achieved independent ambulation but do not have a mature gait pattern, is a very difficult task. Their attention span and cooperation are limited and their gait pattern is characterized by inconsistency as the central nervous system matures. Shortly after learning to walk children learn to run,

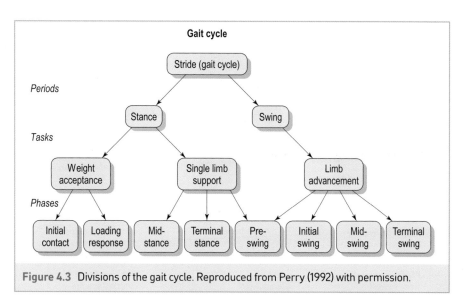

Figure 4.3 Divisions of the gait cycle. Reproduced from Perry (1992) with permission.

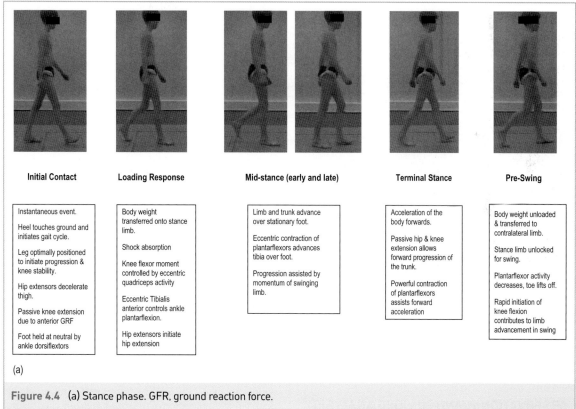

Initial Contact	Loading Response	Mid-stance (early and late)	Terminal Stance	Pre-Swing
Instantaneous event. Heel touches ground and initiates gait cycle. Leg optimally positioned to initiate progression & knee stability. Hip extensors decelerate thigh. Passive knee extension due to anterior GRF Foot held at neutral by ankle dorsiflextors	Body weight transferred onto stance limb. Shock absorption Knee flexor moment controlled by eccentric quadriceps activity Eccentric Tibialis anterior controls ankle plantarflexion. Hip extensors initiate hip extension	Limb and trunk advance over stationary foot. Eccentric contraction of plantarflexors advances tibia over foot. Progression assisted by momentum of swinging limb.	Acceleration of the body forwards. Passive hip & knee extension allows forward progression of the trunk. Powerful contraction of plantarflexors assists forward acceleration	Body weight unloaded & transferred to contralateral limb. Stance limb unlocked for swing. Plantarflexor activity decreases, toe lifts off. Rapid initiation of knee flexion contributes to limb advancement in swing

(a)

Figure 4.4 (a) Stance phase. GFR, ground reaction force.

which can be their preferred method of locomotion and difficult to slow down. Variability in joint motions, temporal parameters and the timing of muscle activity during the gait cycle occur as the gait is maturing. The immature gait is characterized by a wide base of support with absence of reciprocal arm swing (Figure 4.5a), flat foot contact, absence of knee flexion during loading response and excessive hip and knee flexion during swing. As a child gets older the variability of gait measurements decreases and adult joint motions or kinematics are mostly achieved by the age of 3 years (Figure 4.5b), whereas temporal parameters take longer to mature and adult temporal parameters are mostly achieved by age 7 years (Table 4.1) (Sutherland et al 1988).

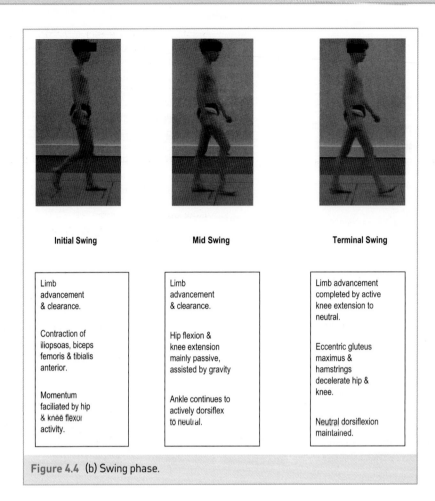

Initial Swing

Limb
advancement
& clearance.

Contraction of
iliopsoas, biceps
femoris & tibialis
anterior.

Momentum
faciliated by hip
& knee flexor
activity.

Mid Swing

Limb
advancement
& clearance.

Hip flexion &
knee extension
mainly passive,
assisted by gravity

Ankle continues to
actively dorsiflex
to neutral.

Terminal Swing

Limb advancement
completed by active
knee extension to
neutral.

Eccentric gluteus
maximus &
hamstrings
decelerate hip &
knee.

Neutral dorsiflexion
maintained.

Figure 4.4 (b) Swing phase.

It is important to appreciate the clinical relevance of the normal variability of the maturing gait pattern. It is not normally possible to undertake formal 3D gait analysis much before the age of 5 years. Video analysis can be undertaken at an earlier age but in order to interpret any gait data reliably it must be consistent, or the inconsistencies must be taken into account. All gait laboratories should have their own normal adult and child databases for comparison with pathological gait, and intertrial consistency of an individual's gait pattern is evaluated prior to interpretation of data. In the young child it is advisable to age-match temporal parameters between the ages of 5 and 7 years.

OBSERVATIONAL AND 2D VIDEO ANALYSIS

In clinical practice, visual gait observation is often necessary to determine problems and decide on treatment. This may consist purely of visual observation without the use of any equipment or 2D video recording may be employed. Visual observation is subjective, dependent on the skill of the clinician, and provides no permanent record of the gait pattern. Rapid, complex or subtle events in the gait cycle are likely to be missed since the speed at which an observer is able to process what is seen is much slower than the speed at which the events actually take place as someone walks. Video recording provides a permanent qualitative description of the subject's walking ability. The slow-motion facility allows analysis of events that are occurring simultaneously at several joints during the gait cycle, which is not possible by visual observation alone. Krebs et al (1985) reported that observational gait analysis is more reliable with a single observer and least reliable between multiple observers. Furthermore, viewing a video tape of someone walking with both single and multiple observers is more reliable than visual observation alone, and reliability is further improved when slow-motion videotaping is employed.

Standardized techniques of video recording will also improve reliability. In order to analyse the data accurately it is important to record true sagittal and coronal views, rather than oblique views which will distort the images. So, for example, to judge whether hip extension in terminal stance is complete or limited, it is necessary to obtain a true

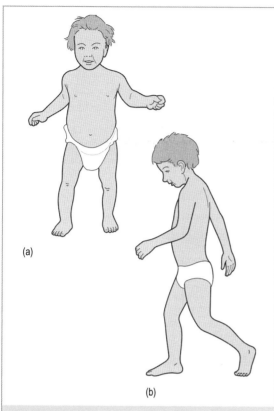

(a)

(b)

Figure 4.5 (a) Walking pattern of a 15-month-old boy. Note the broad base of support and the absence of reciprocal arm swing. (b) Maturation of kinematic parameters mostly occurs by 3 years. Note the development of reciprocal arm swing and knee-loading response in early stance.

sagittal view with the subject walking at right angles to the camera. To make a judgement on pelvic obliquity, for example, the camera needs to be positioned so the subject is walking directly towards and away from the camera to obtain a true coronal view. It is therefore advisable to fix the cameras in these planes, using tripods if possible, rather than follow the child with a hand-held camera. If standardized positions are adopted this will also facilitate more accurate comparisons where changes in the gait pattern are monitored over time. In addition to sagittal and coronal views it may be useful to record a panned sagittal view to form an overall impression of the gait pattern, standing views to compare static versus dynamic postures, as well as close-up views of the feet, both static and dynamic, particularly if foot deformity is an issue.

A child needs to be appropriately dressed to facilitate visual analysis, so shorts that maximally expose the legs and cropped top or rolled-up T-shirt to expose the lower back and upper pelvis are helpful. Observational analysis is generally more difficult at the proximal joints. The mass of the trunk and soft tissue at the hips and pelvis obscures bony landmarks and some of the motion occurring at these joints.

A systematic approach to viewing gait is recommended. Various forms have been developed to assist the clinician in taking a more organized, sequential approach to analysing gait patterns; this may include both subtle and obvious gait deviations and primary problems and compensatory strategies. The observational gait analysis form from Ranchos Los Amigos Medical Center (Figure 4.6) (Perry 1992) was developed by identifying commonly observed gait deviations and their phasic occurrence in patients with neurological disorders. The Edinburgh Visual Gait Score (Read et al 2003) was developed specifically for use in children with cerebral palsy. The authors report that the score correlates well with measurements obtained from instrumented gait analysis in the same patients and can also detect postoperative change.

Table 4.1 Maturation of temporal parameters					
	Age (years)				
	1	**2**	**3**	**7**	**Adult**
Single support (%)	32.1	33.5	34.8	36.7	36.7
Toe-off (%)	67.1	67.1	65.5	62.4	63.6
Speed (cm/s)	63.7	71.8	85.5	114.3	121.6
Cadence (steps/min)	176.7	168.8	163.5	143.5	114
Step length (cm)	21.6	27.6	32.9	47.9	65.5
Stride length (cm)	43	54.9	67.7	96.6	129.4
Modified from Sutherland et al (1988).					

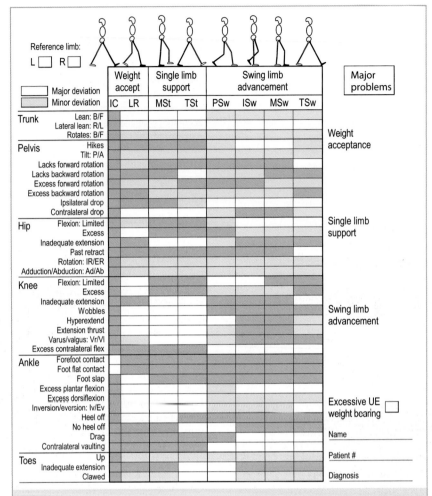

Figure 4.6 Observational gait analysis form from Ranchos Los Amigos Medical Center. Reproduced from Perry (1992) with permission. IC, initial contact; MSt, mid-stance; TSt, terminal stance; PSw, pre-swing; ISw, initial swing; MSw, mid-swing; TSw, terminal swing; UE, P/A, IR/ER.

The process of analysis requires a clear understanding of what motions occur at each joint in each plane (Table 4.2) and the ability to describe deviations from normal. One can then systematically observe pathological gait moving from proximal to distal through each plane. By adopting such a sequential approach one can more easily begin the problem-solving process.

Both visual and video analysis are limited in that they are descriptive rather than quantitative, and provide 2D rather than 3D information. The latter is particularly important in growing children with neurological problems where torsional abnormalities are common, e.g. femoral anteversion. Many gait abnormalities in the transverse plane cannot be seen without the aid of 3D analysis. So, for example, in Figure 4.2, it would not be possible using 2D video analysis to ascertain whether the right thigh is adducted or internally rotated or both, and whether any internal thigh rotation is a primary problem or secondary to pelvic retraction. Obviously the treatment will vary depending on the problem.

3D GAIT ANALYSIS

The primary contribution of the gait analysis laboratory to the clinical assessment of a child's walking ability is quantitative gait data. The clinical assessment of a child, data collection and interpretation, and treatment recommendations are undertaken by a specialist multidisciplinary team, usually consisting of both clinical and technical staff. Typically this may include an orthopaedic surgeon, physiotherapist and bioengineer, orthotist and technician.

Table 4.2	Joint motions occurring in the three planes		
	Sagittal	**Coronal**	**Transverse**
Trunk	Upper-body tilt	Side flexion	Rotation
Pelvis	Pelvic tilt	Pelvic obliquity	Rotation
Hip	Flexion/extension	Abduction/adduction	Rotation
Knee	Flexion/extension	Varus/valgus	
Ankle	Dorsi-/plantarflexion		Foot progression angle

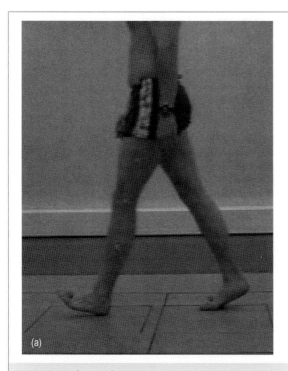
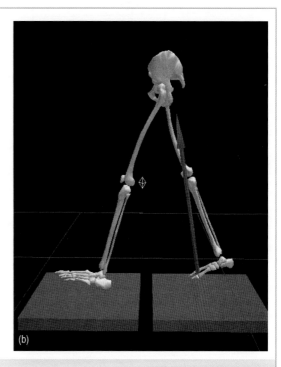

(a) (b)

Figures 4.7 (a and b) As the patient walks along the walkway, the three-dimensional position of reflective markers is tracked by specialized cameras and computer software provides three-dimensional animation of the skeleton during walking. The ground reaction force is measured by force plates in the floor.

Although each professional will have a different area of expertise, it is important all team members have an overall appreciation of the clinical picture as well as the applications and limitations of the technology, in order to facilitate the gait analysis process.

The parameters that are routinely measured in a laboratory are joint motions (kinematics) using a motion capture system, forces through the joints (kinetics) using force plates and dynamic muscle activity using electromyography (EMG). This data can usually be recorded simultaneously – a child is instrumented with reflective markers (Figure 4.7a)

and EMG electrodes and walks at a self-selected speed along a level walkway over force plates in the floor. The current software provides 3D animation of the skeleton during walking (Figure 4.7b), synchronized with movie capture and simultaneous display of kinematic and kinetic data. This allows an interactive approach to analysing data and also provides an exciting teaching tool.

Additionally pressure distribution under the foot can be measured using a pressure mat or pedobarograph, as well as energy expenditure by recording oxygen uptake or carbon dioxide output to compute a variety of metabolic indices.

Kinematics

Kinematics is the measurement of the position of a child's body segments and joints. To achieve this, small retro-reflective markers are aligned with specific bony landmarks and joint axes on a child's skin using a standard biomechanical gait model (Davies & Deluca 1996). As a child walks along the walkway the 3D position of these markers is tracked by several specialized cameras which are

floor- or wall-mounted around the walkway and interfaced to a central computer. The cameras strobe the markers with infrared or visible light, and the light reflected from the markers back to the cameras is processed by computer programs to establish highly accurate 3D trajectories. From these marker position data, the 3D angular motion of particular body segments and the motion between the segments, i.e. joint motion, are calculated mathematically (Figure 4.8). Temporal parameters such as walking speed,

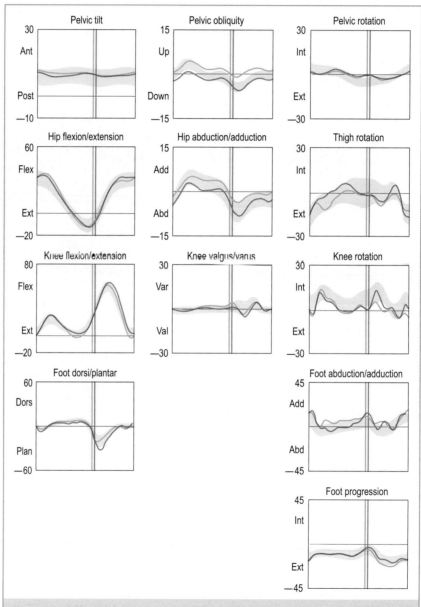

Figure 4.8 Kinematic graphs of a healthy subject (grey line = (R) leg, blue line = (L) leg) +/− one standard deviation (pale blue band). Gait cycle is on the x axis and degrees of motion on the y axis. (L) hand column displays sagittal plane, middle column coronal plane and (R) hand column transverse plane kinematics.

stride length, step length and cadence can also be calculated.

Kinematics measures joint motion, without regard to its causes, but significantly contributes to clinical problem-solving in its own right. The ability to measure 3D motion makes it possible to distinguish the plane in which the motion is occurring, and at what joint or level within the plane (Table 4.2), so treatment can be focused more accurately to the individual. For example, a common gait abnormality seen in children with cerebral palsy is an internally rotated gait pattern, often characterized by internal foot progression and in-turning of the knees. This abnormal transverse plane motion can occur at various different levels, e.g. pelvic rotation (i.e. retraction or protraction), internal hip rotation, knee rotation and/or forefoot adduction. By using clinical estimates of bony torsions together with transverse-plane kinematics, the cause of abnormal foot progression can be isolated. Kinematics also gives us the ability to measure dynamic activity versus the information collected during a clinical examination which is based on static examination. So, although clinical examination is important in guiding the interpretation of the gait data, clinicians treating gait abnormalities are interested in the dynamic aspects of walking ability. For example, muscle tone may change significantly with the position of a child and whether he or she is moving or at rest.

The use of kinematic analysis has led to the ability to classify gait patterns in both hemiplegic and diplegic cerebral palsy. As certain patterns are representative of specific pathology, this is helpful in understanding the associated set of possible causes and treatment options. Sutherland & Davids (1993) classified knee patterns in diplegic cerebral palsy. The most common gait abnormalities of the knee in children with cerebral palsy occur in the sagittal plane. Based on their experience of performing gait analysis on more than 588 children with cerebral palsy, four primary gait abnormalities of the knee were identified: jump knee, crouch knee, stiff knee, and recurvatum knee (Figure 4.9). Jump, recurvatum and crouch are stance-phase problems whilst a stiff knee pattern is a swing-phase problem. Any of the stance phase problems may be accompanied, and usually are, by pathology of the knee in swing (Figure 4.9a). In addition to assessing the child's pathology prior to treatment, kinematics also aids assessment of the outcome of treatment. Crouch is often associated with fixed contractures requiring surgical correction of deformities (Figure 4.10). Case study 4.2 further discusses the treatment of crouch gait.

Winters et al (1987) defined four main gait patterns in hemiplegia (types I–IV), with type I being the least involved and type IV the most severely involved, with increasing proximal involvement of the lower limb reflecting greater severity (Figure 4.11). These types can be differentiated by gait analysis and then treatment can be tailored to the specific pattern type.

The interpretation of kinematic and kinetic patterns requires some skill. For a more detailed understanding of patterns associated with neurological disorders, the reader is referred to Gage (2004).

Kinetics

Kinetics are the internal and external forces that cause and control movement and the ability to measure them gives us a more comprehensive understanding of a child's gait pattern. In walking, the internal forces are generated from muscle activity and stabilizing ligaments whereas the external forces are due to gravity and the reaction of the ground on the foot. The ground reaction force (GRF) can be measured by a force platform and is equal in magnitude and opposite in direction to the force exerted by the weight-bearing limb (Newton's third law).

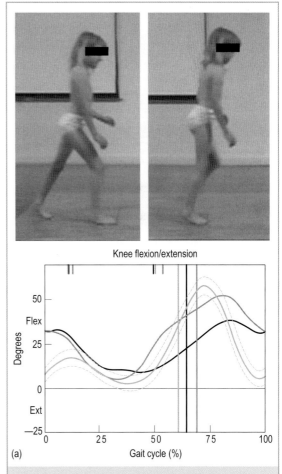

Knee flexion/extension

Figure 4.9a Jump knee pattern showing increased knee flexion at initial contact which corrects to normal or near normal knee extension in mid-stance. Often due to overactive hamstrings +/− rectus femoris spasticity. Sagittal kinematics also reveal stiff knees in swing (L) leg (grey line) > (R) leg (black line).

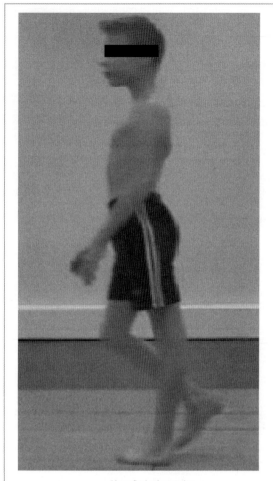

Knee flexion/extension

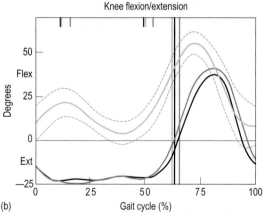

(b)

Figure 4.9 (b) Recurvatum knee pattern. Sagittal plane kinematics confirm severe knee hyperextension throughout the stance phase. Often caused by overactivity of the gastrocnemius, which prevents forward progression of the tibia, known as the plantarflexion–knee hyperextension couple.

If a force is applied at a distance from the centre of an axis of rotation, or a joint centre, this creates a moment that must be balanced by an equal and opposite moment at that joint. The result is a force couple (two parallel forces acting in opposite directions, which combine to produce a moment) which will cause angular acceleration of the limb segment unless resisted by an opposing moment at the joint. In walking the external moments about a joint in the weight-bearing limb can be estimated from the product of the GRF and the perpendicular distance to a joint centre (Figure 4.12). This allows the relative magnitudes of the moments about joints to be readily appreciated but has limitations in that it does not account for gravitational or inertial forces of the limb segments. In order to account for all components of force, modern 3D gait analysis systems utilize inverse dynamics to calculate the net internal joint moments.

Unlike kinematics, which describe visually observable quantities, such as the angle of knee flexion, kinetic quantities cannot be directly observed. The computed internal moments at each joint can be displayed graphically at each joint in three planes in the same format as kinematics. By superimposing a real-time ground reaction vector on to a video screen it is also possible to have a visual representation of the external joint moments throughout stance. In normal gait it can be seen that the GRF acts close to hip, knee and ankle joint centres, so minimizing the moments about these joints in the interests of energy efficiency (Figure 4.13).

Kinetics are important in planning and evaluating the outcome of a variety of treatments, and particularly orthopaedic surgery, in children with cerebral palsy. Kinetic data should be interpreted along with the corresponding kinematic and EMG data to provide more information about the cause of a gait deviation and help distinguish between primary and secondary problems and coping or compensatory mechanisms. Primary gait abnormalities result directly from the brain injury in cerebral palsy and are attributable to abnormal muscle tone, loss of selective motor control and impaired balance. The secondary abnormalities, i.e. muscle contracture and abnormal bone growth, arise as a result of the abnormal forces imposed on the skeleton over time by the primary abnormalities. Gage (2004) has coined the phrase 'lever arm dysfunction' to describe the distortions of bones that regularly occur in a child with cerebral palsy. Bones constitute the levers upon which muscles act and become distorted due to alteration in the leverage imposed on them by the abnormalities in muscle tone. Kinetics can evaluate the resulting abnormal moments, e.g. a reduced hip abductor moment associated with increased femoral anteversion and their correction following surgical correction.

Kinetics are also a useful tool for prescribing orthoses, evaluating their effectiveness, as well as 'tuning' orthoses (Butler et al 1992).

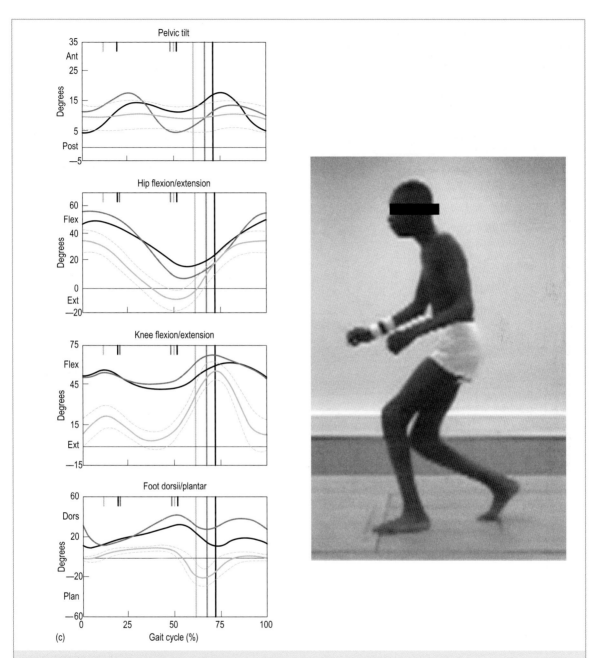

Figure 4.9 (c) Crouch-knee pattern. Defined as persistent knee flexion of 30° or more throughout stance. Often combined with excessive hip flexion and ankle dorsiflexion, as shown on the kinematics.

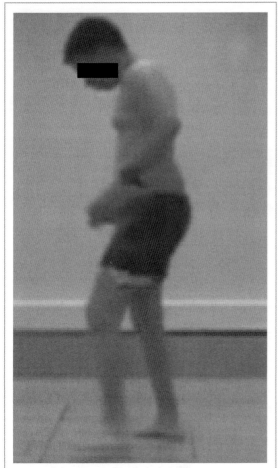

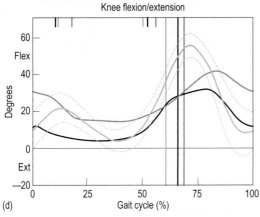

Figure 4.9 (d) Stiff-knee pattern. This is a swing-phase problem characterized by delayed and reduced peak knee flexion on kinematics, often due to overactivity of rectus femoris. Note compensatory trunk side flexion to aid clearance in swing.

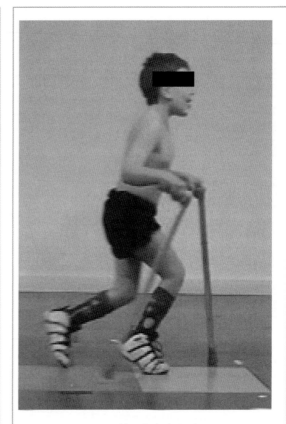

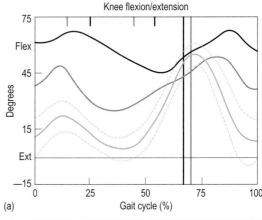

Figure 4.10 Crouch-knee pattern (a) preoperatively and (b) near-normal knee kinematics after multilevel surgery (which included psoas, hamstrings and gastrocnemius lengthenings plus rectus femoris transfers and derotation femoral osteotomies bilaterally). The child was unable to walk barefoot preoperatively, so graphs show comparison kinematics in orthoses.

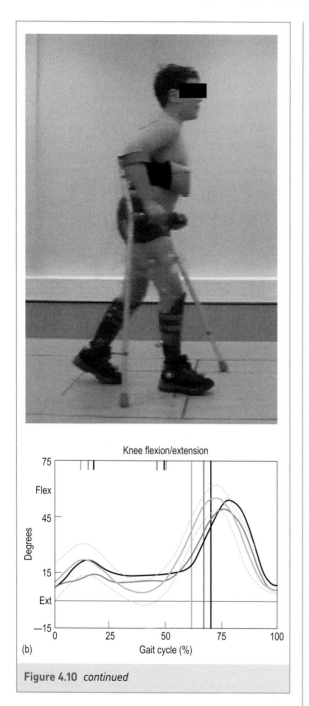

Knee flexion/extension

(b)

Figure 4.10   *continued*

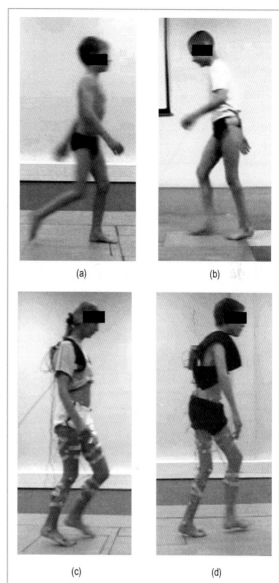

(a)   (b)

(c)   (d)

Figure 4.11 (a) Type I hemiplegia: equinus in swing. (b) Type II equinus in stance and swing (left leg) ± knee recurvatum. (c) Type III foot and knee involvement. (d) Type IV foot, knee and hip involvement.

Dynamic electromyogram

Muscle activation during walking can be measured by dynamic EMG recording. Although it may be inferred from observing a child walk, it is often difficult to determine accurately which muscles are active or inactive during a particular phase of gait and this difficulty may be compounded by lower-limb deformity or impaired motor control. The timing and action of muscles are important components of gait and contribute to our understanding of the cause of a problem, particularly if a muscle lengthening or transfer is being considered as a treatment option.

The net EMG signal is a summation of the motor unit action potentials that are generated as the muscle contracts.

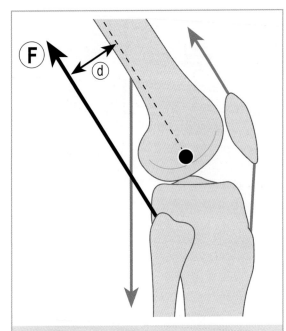

Figure 4.12 Moment (M) = force (F) $\times$ distance (d) from the joint centre. Muscles/tendons cross joints at a distance from the joint centre, producing moments. The internal joint moment represents the body's response to the external loads associated with gait.

EMG recording can be obtained from either surface or fine-wire electrodes and the type is decided by the muscle of interest. Surface electrodes are suitable for large muscles close to the surface of the skin. They detect motor unit action potentials from a large surface area of muscle, which also increases the possibility of measuring 'cross-talk' from adjacent muscles. They cause no discomfort to a child and cross-talk can be minimized by careful positioning of electrodes and verification of the signal. If a muscle is small or deeply situated it can only be measured using fine-wire electrodes – a fine wire is introduced into the muscle via a needle and its placement verified by electrical stimulation. This requires a skilled clinician and is associated with some discomfort so is unsuitable for young children.

The normal EMG patterns of the lower extremity during gait for both children and adults are well documented (Perry 1992) and a gait laboratory will have its own normal database for reference purposes. An EMG signal is mainly interpreted in terms of timing and the relative intensity of muscular action, and reported in relation to the stance and swing phases of the gait cycle (Figure 4.14). One of the primary gait abnormalities in cerebral palsy, described earlier, is the stiff-knee gait pattern (Sutherland et al 1990) which is characterized by foot clearance problems during swing. A cause of this may be abnormal activity of the rectus femoris

during the swing phase of gait when the muscle would normally be quiescent, and this can be confirmed by EMG recording. This abnormal muscle activity results in delayed and reduced peak knee flexion in swing, which can be seen on the sagittal plane kinematics, and is often associated with spasticity of rectus femoris on clinical examination, i.e. a positive Duncan Ely test (Marks et al 2003). Rectus transfer can improve peak knee flexion and thus foot clearance problems. The muscle is transferred distally to sartorius or one of the hamstrings (Sutherland et al 1990). Its timing is unchanged but by changing the angle of pull it augments, rather than impedes, knee flexion in swing.

THE FUTURE

Single-stage multilevel orthopaedic surgery is now a procedure commonly performed in children with the spastic diplegic form of cerebral palsy. It aims to correct all deformities and improve ambulation while minimizing a child's exposure to repeated surgery and postoperative rehabilitation. Gait analysis has made this possible by providing a tool which allows objective evaluation of the patient's gait problems in a single assessment. Over the last 15–20 years various gait analysis studies have defined the indications for this type of surgery, established the efficacy of the multilevel single-stage approach and clarified the use of specific procedures. The 'birthday syndrome' (Rang 1990) has been eliminated: in this situation, children spent most of their childhood either having or recovering from surgery since the muscles were never balanced simultaneously.

Gait analysis studies have now progressed to evaluating the type of postoperative rehabilitation techniques that are most effective following multilevel surgery in cerebral palsy. In combination with other outcome measures, evidence is emerging of the importance of postoperative strengthening techniques to improve both gait and motor function (Thompson et al 2005).

Recent advances in the musculoskeletal models used in gait analysis are further improving treatment for children. The foot is a complex structure and until recently was modelled as a rigid segment which provided limited information on dorsi- and plantarflexion and foot progression angles only. Multisegment foot models are being developed for use in children and these models provide more detailed information on motion within the foot, so allowing for clinical assessment of foot deformities and their treatment (Theologis et al 2003, Stebbins et al 2005).

Computer simulations of the musculoskeletal system are important in explaining the biomechanical causes of movement abnormalities and the consequences of common treatments. Researchers are working towards creating biomechanical models that enable more accurate prediction of treatment outcomes. This is, however, a

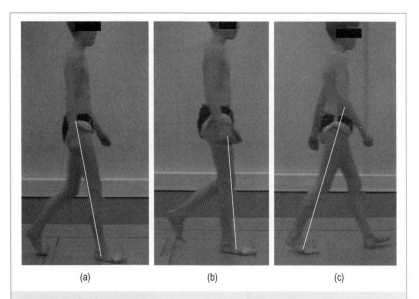

(a) (b) (c)

Figure 4.13 (a–c) In normal gait the ground reaction force acts close to hip, knee and ankle joint centres, so minimizing the moments about these joints in the interests of energy efficiency.

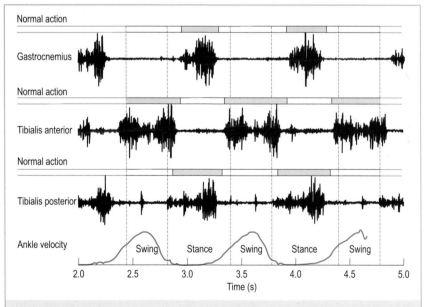

Figure 4.14 Normal electromyogram activity of the gastrocnemius, tibialis anterior and tibialis posterior reported in relation to the stance and swing phases of gait.

formidable challenge given the multifaceted cause of gait deviations in neurological conditions and some underlying limitations of the models. Progress has been made on modelling muscle lengths at the ankle and knee and their effect on gait (Delp et al 1995, Arnold et al 2006), as well as the potential causes of excessive hip internal rotation (Arnold & Delp 2001). The ultimate goal is to predict how an individual will ambulate following surgery.

CASE STUDY 4.1

The child in Figure 4.15a is a young girl with a lumbar-level spina bifida. She walked independently with a laboured gait and a right knee which frequently gave way. Clinical examination revealed antigravity knee extensor strength but significant proximal weakness at the pelvic girdle and flaccid feet bilaterally. During walking this distribution of weakness resulted in an increased range of pelvic rotation, and persistent knee flexion throughout stance, which together gave a valgus appearance to both knees during stance (Figure 4.15b). Although the knees had a similar valgus appearance visually, kinetic data revealed an abnormal internal varus knee moment or 'valgus thrust' on the right side, which explained the collapsing knee. Knee–ankle–foot orthoses were prescribed in which she walked well (Figure 4.15c), and the kinetic data show that by supporting the knee the abnormal knee moment is corrected (Figure 4.15d).

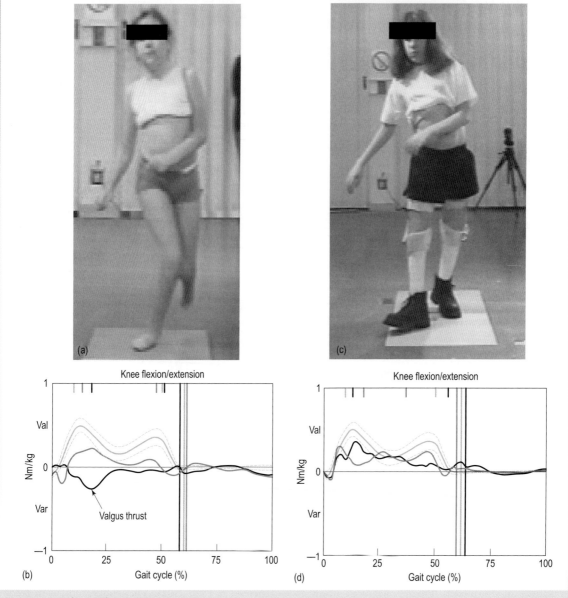

Figures 4.15 (a and b) An 11-year-old girl with lumbar-level spina bifida. Kinetics show an abnormal right internal varus knee moment or valgus thrust, resulting in frequent collapse of the knee. (c and d) Corrected knee moment when the knee is supported in knee–ankle–foot orthoses.

CASE STUDY 4.2

History

James is a 14-year-old boy with spastic diplegic cerebral palsy and has limited independent walking ability. He needs a wheelchair for long distances. He is complaining of a deteriorating crouch gait and walking distance is limited by bilateral anterior knee pain. He currently uses no orthoses and has previously had difficulty tolerating fixed ankle–foot orthoses and anterior ground reaction orthoses due to pressure problems at the feet.

James was born at full-term with a breech presentation with fetal distress on delivery. He had delayed milestones and walked from the age of 2 years on tiptoes. He attends a mainstream school. He has had no previous surgery. His physiotherapy management consists of a home programme of passive stretching for the lower limbs.

Observational Gait Analysis

Gait by observation shows an anterior pelvic tilt with crouch/stiff knee pattern and flat foot strike bilaterally. Foot progression angles are external to normal and there is the appearance of increased internal thigh rotation bilaterally (Figure 4.16).

Clinical Examination

Clinical examination reveals fixed flexion contractures at the hips and knees of 25° bilaterally and increased femoral anteversion of 30° bilaterally. There is severe hamstring tightness with popliteal angles of 80° bilaterally and bilateral patella alta. The Duncan Ely test is positive bilaterally. There are planovalgus foot deformities just correctable to neutral bilaterally. There is good muscle strength and selective control and moderate lower-limb spasticity.

3D Gait Analysis

Sagittal plane kinematics (Figure 4.16c) are consistent with multilevel spasticity/contracture. There is a double-bump pelvic pattern associated with overactivity/contracture of the hip flexors, incomplete hip extension in terminal stance bilaterally, and a crouch/stiff-knee pattern is confirmed. There is apparent dorsiflexion throughout the gait cycle consistent with planovalgus foot deformities.

There are no significant abnormalities in the coronal plane. Transverse plane kinematics reveal marginally increased internal thigh rotation on the right side only, and increased external foot progression angles, right more than left.

Sagittal plane kinetics show increased knee extensor moments bilaterally consistent with a crouch knee pattern. There are premature ankle plantarflexor moments consistent with overactivity of the gastrocnemius, but also reduced ankle power, indicating that the gastrocnemiei are additionally weak. Coronal plane kinetics reveal an abnormal valgus thrust bilaterally.

Temporal parameters show increased cadence due to reduced step and stride length, and mildly increased double support time.

Dynamic EMGs show prolonged activity of the hamstrings, indicating that in addition to being contracted they are also overactive. There is also some activity of rectus femoris in swing bilaterally. At the ankles there is premature activity of the gastrocnemiei.

Conclusions and Recommendations

In addition to knee pain there were multiple contractures as well as bone deformities at the feet. Furthermore motor control and muscle strength remained good, making him a good candidate for multilevel orthopaedic surgery. The internal rotation of the right hip was mild and not considered sufficient to warrant surgical correction. The valgus thrust at both knees was due to foot deformity rather than the mildly increased femoral anteversion. In summary (Table 4.3), the problems were: tightness of hip flexors, tight/overactive hamstrings, tight/overactive gastrocnemiei, rectus co-spasticity and valgus thrust at knees due to foot deformity. Based on this information the surgical plan included bilateral hamstring lengthenings, rectus femoris transfers, gastrocnemius lengthenings and calcaneal osteotomies.

Outcome of Treatment

At 1 year postoperatively James's gait is considerably improved. His knee pain has been eliminated and he no longer needs a wheelchair for long distances. Visual observation shows a generally more upright posture with improved hip and knee extension in stance and heel strike bilaterally. External foot progression angles are reduced (Figure 4.16d and e). Comparison kinematics (Figure 4.16c) confirms near-normal sagittal knee and ankle patterns in stance and swing, as well as foot progression angles within normal limits. Comparison kinetics show the valgus thrust has been eliminated due to improved foot position. The increased knee extensor moment and premature ankle moments are considerably improved and ankle power in terminal stance is within normal limits. Temporal parameters confirm cadence is within normal limits due to increased step and stride length.

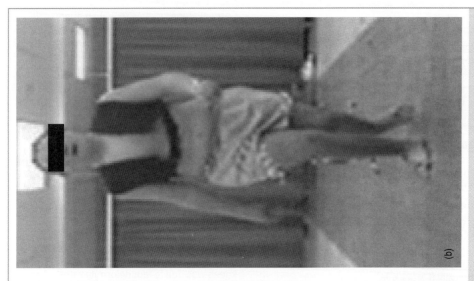

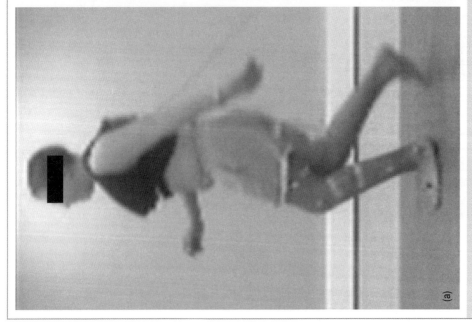

Figure 4.16 (a and b) Sagittal and coronal-plane video of James (case study 4.2) preoperatively.

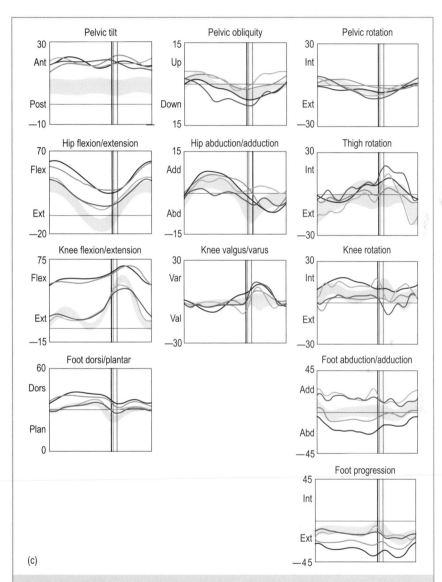

Figure 4.16c Kinematic graphs pre-operatively (black line = (R) leg, grey line = (L), and post-operatively (dark blue line = (L) leg, light blue line = (R) leg)

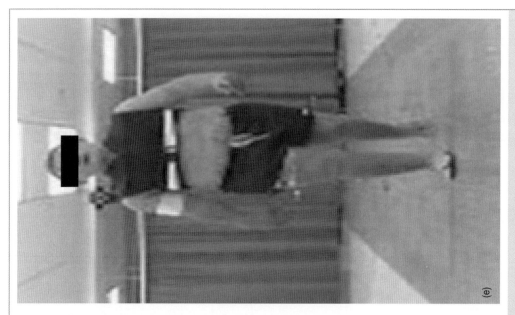

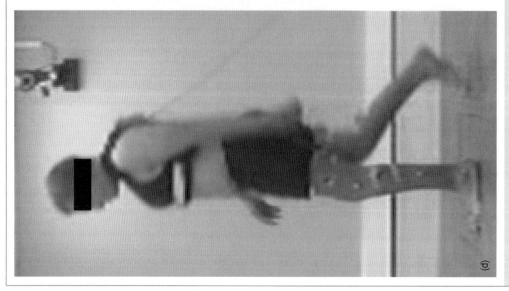

Figures 4.16 (d and e) Sagittal and coronal-plane video of James (case study 4.2) postoperatively.

Table 4.3				
	Sagittal	**Coronal**	**Transverse**	**Problems**
Trunk/pelvis	**Increased anterior pelvic tilt with mild double-bump pattern**			Poor pelvic femoral dissociation
Hip	**Increased hip flexion throughout and reduced range of motion (R) and (L)** **Incomplete hip extension in terminal stance (R) and (L)**		**Marginally increased internal-thigh rotation (R)**	Tight and overactive hip flexors (R) and (L) Slightly increased femoral anteversion (R)
Knee	**Crouch/stiff-knee pattern (R) and (L)** *Increased knee extensor moments (R) and (L) Electomyograms: prolonged hamstrings (R) and (L). Some rectus femoris activity in swing (R) and (L)*	*Valgus thrust (R) and (L)*		Tight and overactive hamstrings (R) and (L) Rectus femoris co-spasticity (R) and (L)
Ankle	**Flat-foot strike, apparent dorsiflexion throughout (R) and (L)** *Decreased ankle power (R) and (L)* *Premature ankle plantarflexor moments (R) and (L) Electromyograms: premature gastrocnemiei (R) and (L)*		**Increased external foot progression angles (R) > (L)**	Plano valgus foot deformities (R) and (L) Weak and overactive gastrocnemiei (R) and (L)

Bold type: 3D gait data and visual observations. *Italic* type: kinetic/EMG data.

REFERENCES

Arnold AS, Delp SI 2001 Rotational moment arms of the medial hamstrings and adductors vary with femoral geometry and limb position: implications for the treatment of internally rotated gait. *Journal of Biomechanics* 34: 437–447.

Arnold AS, Liu MQ, Schwartz MH, Oonpuu S, Delp SL 2006 The role of estimating muscle-tendon lengths and velocities of the hamstrings in the evaluation and treatment of crouch gait. *Gait and Posture* 23: 273–281.

Butler PB, Thompson N, Major RE 1992 Improvement in walking performance in children with cerebral palsy: preliminary results. *Developmental Medicine and Child Neurology* 34: 567–576.

Davies RB, Deluca PA 1996 *Clinical Gait Analysis*. New Jersey: IEEE Press.

Delp SL, Statler K, Carroll NC 1995 Preserving plantar flexion strength after surgical treatment for contracture of the triceps surae: a computer simulation study. *Journal of Orthopaedic Research* 13: 96–104.

Gage JR (ed.) 2004 *The Treatment of Gait Problems in Cerebral Palsy*. Mac Keith Press.

Krebs DE, Edelstein JE, Fishman S 1985 Reliability of observational kinematic gait analysis. *Physical Therapy* 65: 1027–1033.

Marks MC, Alexander J, Sutherland DH, Chambers HG 2003 Clinical utility of the Duncan-Ely test for rectus femoris dysfunction during the swing phase of gait. *Developmental Medicine and Child Neurology* 45: 763–768.

Perry J 1992 *Gait Analysis: Normal and Pathological Function*. Thorofare, NJ: Slack.

Read HS, Hazlewood ME, Hillman SJ, Prescott RJ, Robb JE 2003 Edinburgh visual gait score for use in cerebral palsy. *Journal of Pediatric Orthopedics* 23: 296–301.

Rose J, Gamble JG (eds) 2005 *Human Walking*. Maryland: Williams & Wilkins.

Stebbins JA, Harrington ME, Thompson N, Zavatsky A, Theologis TN 2006 Repeatability of a model for measuring multi-segment foot kinematics in children. *Gait and Posture* 23: 401–410.

Sutherland DH, Davids JR 1993 Common gait patterns of the knee in cerebral palsy. *Clinical Orthopedics* 288: 139–147.

Sutherland DH, Olshen RA, Biden EN, Wyatt MP 1988 *The Development of Mature Walking*. MacKeith Press.

Sutherland DH, Santi M, Abel MF 1990 Treatment of stiff knee gait in cerebral palsy: a comparison by gait analysis of distal rectus femoris transfer versus proximal rectus release. *Journal of Paediatric Orthopedics* 10: 433–441.

Theologis TN, Harrington ME, Thompson N, Benson MKD 2003 Dynamic foot motion in children treated for congenital talipes equinovarus. *Journal of Bone and Joint Surgery* 85: 572–577.

Thompson N, Seniorou M, Harrington M, Theologis TN 2005 The results of two strength training regimes on gait and function in cerebral palsy following multi-level surgery. *Gait and Posture* 22: S1.

Whittle MW 2001 *Gait Analysis: An Introduction*, 3rd edn. Butterworth-Heinemann.

Winters TF Jr, Gage JR, Hicks R 1987 Gait patterns in spastic hemiplegia in children and young adults. *Journal of Bone and Joint Surgery* 69: 437–441.

Neurology

5 Motor control in developmental neurology

Margaret Mayston

INTRODUCTION

The physical management of children with impairments of central nervous system (CNS) origin has evolved over the last century, from the predominantly orthopaedic approach of the early part of the twentieth century, through neurophysiological, educational, biomechanical and task-specific approach phases. In most parts of the world there is now a drive to achieve a client- or a child/family-centred approach, acknowledging the shift from a medical model of management to one which considers clients and their goals as the central focus. This is illustrated in Figure 5.1, which exemplifies the evolution of clinical practice over the last century. During this period, many names have become associated with particular approaches to therapy, such as Bobath (also known as Neurodevelopmental Therapy or

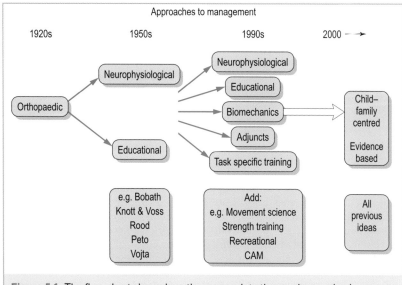

Figure 5.1 The flow chart shows how the approach to therapy has evolved over several stages during the last century according to current and emerging knowledge. CAM, complementary and alternative medicine; ICF, *International Classification for Functioning, Disability and Health*.

NDT), Pëto (Conductive Education), Jean Ayres (Sensory Integration), Roberta Shepherd and Janet Carr (motor learning/task-specific training). The possibilities for intervention now go far beyond those approaches already mentioned, and the internet provides a rich source of helpful, and in some cases not so helpful, advice for both families and therapists. Given this 'information-rich' climate it is essential that physiotherapists equip themselves with knowledge of the currently available options for physiotherapy and management. In addition they need to be acquainted with the advances in knowledge of motor control, the child's development of skills and advances in therapy and other interventions.

In this chapter we will explore the changing vista of motor control and views on infant development. The potentially useful *International Classification of Functioning Disability and Health* framework (ICF; World Health Organization 2001, 2002) as a basis for developing a rational evidence-based therapy approach will be discussed, in addition to some aspects of therapeutic options.

EVIDENCE-BASED PHYSIOTHERAPY

Until recently, physiotherapists have predominantly relied on named approaches on which to base their therapy intervention, often applied in an eclectic manner, and have primarily targeted the impairments of the child with cerebral palsy. It is becoming increasingly clear that no one approach applied in its 'pure' form can address all the needs of each child (Mayston 2004). As a result these approaches become altered and perhaps are no longer what they were originally intended to be. This is confusing to service providers, the therapy world and the wider management team community (Damiano 2004). Although aspects of these approaches are still useful, a lack of robust research evidence to support their use attracts criticism of their continued use.

The constant call to underpin therapy interventions with evidence of efficacy is essential to heed, and it has been suggested that only high-quality clinical research should be the requirement for evidence-based therapy (Herbert et al 2005). However, it needs to be recognized that as yet there is insufficient experimental evidence to do this. The evidence base for physiotherapy intervention in neurological movement disorders, in particular in paediatrics, is limited. Dromerick (2003) suggested that patients do not die from 'bad rehabilitation', and that because of this there have been fewer high-quality research studies in these areas. This may be true, but clinical research is difficult, particularly in paediatrics, given the ethical considerations, client preferences, financial restrictions and the lack of numbers to give adequate power to the statistical calculations for significance of results. Unless the study has been well planned and carried out and is repeatable, the question often arises as to whether it was the intervention that made a difference, or rather that significant changes were

due to the usual course of growth and development. This does not mean, however, that therapists should ignore the challenge: we all have a responsibility to our clients and service providers to use the available evidence and seek answers for what we do not yet know.

Sackett et al (1996) have suggested that evidence-based practice is not based solely on experimental evidence; rather, it is the integration of these findings with therapists' expertise and the client values which together provide the information needed. Therapists' expertise is valuable, the client is acquiring a greater voice, and experimental evidence is emerging, but even so, this evidence needs to be critically assessed. There is an interest in applying the findings from the emerging evidence base which supports the use of modalities such as muscle strengthening, sports/ fitness training, task-specific training (e.g. constraint-induced therapy, treadmill training), to name a few (Damiano 2004). But even these studies require critical evaluation as most of them are carried out on children who are more able, often category I–III of the Gross Motor Functional Classification System (GMFCS, Palisano et al 1997). Nevertheless, there is an encouraging movement towards a scientific-based approach to management of children with neurological movement disorders, the most common being cerebral palsy.

MOTOR CONTROL THEORIES AND THEIR RELEVANCE TO THERAPY INTERVENTION

One of the reasons for changes in the approach to therapy is that our understanding of motor control has vastly changed since the findings of Sherrington (1947), Hughlings Jackson (1958), Bernstein (1967) and others, although some of these early explorations of the neurological basis of motor control are still relevant. For example, the early work on reflex circuits in the spinal cord such as the stretch reflex is still of relevance. The actual circuitry of these reflexes as discovered by Sherrington and others remains as fact, but the role of these reflexes in motor control is differently understood. Rather than being a primary control for muscle activity and tone, it is now known that these reflexes are highly modifiable by supraspinal and other peripheral inputs, and thus of different functional relevance for the control of movement during sensorimotor tasks. There are a variety of models of motor control which have been described by various authors (Shumway-Cook & Woollacott 2001, Mayston 2002, Galea 2004). However it is this author's view that no one of these models can serve as a basis to understand the control of movement, for understanding the movement disorder, or as a basis for intervention.

The most commonly applied model currently is the dynamic systems model (Horak 1992, Galea 2004), based on the work of Bernstein (1967), and yet its reliance on the interactive nature of the various subsystems means that it is not always easy to identify the main locus of motor control. Dynamic systems gives less recognition to the significance of the contribution of the CNS to motor control, emphasizing more the environment and biomechanical factors, perhaps because these have been neglected in the past. Another useful model is the Information-Processing Model (Winstein 1999, personal communication) that in many ways encompasses all of the other models shown in Box 5.1. This model not only provides a means of understanding motor control, but also provides a framework for identifying deficits in the control of movement which can then be targeted for intervention.

The Information-Processing Model (Table 5.1) is based on the concepts of Bernstein (1967) and others (Brooks 1986, Rothwell 1994), and thus has its basis in the dynamic systems, neurophysiological and engineering models. This is a flexible model which can incorporate the useful aspects of models 1–7 shown in Box 5.1. For example, the plan for the performance of a particular

task is built up on the basis of a person's experience. The integration of innate and known actions with new experiences and subsequent adaptation of motor programmes resulting from novel sensory feedback forms the anticipatory or feedforward system. The concept of feedback and feedforward is based on the engineering model, and has been described by several authors, including Miall (in Arbib 1995). As an example, the task of drinking from a cup is used.

There are several stages in this process: firstly, there needs to be a stimulus generated, either internally or externally, for example, thirst or a social situation (Table 5.1, column 1). On the basis of past experience, the CNS organizes the required strategy to achieve the goal. Perceptual aspects such as the weight, shape and texture of the cup are essential in order for the correct grip and load forces to be computed by the CNS. Spatial concepts are important for the grading and timing of postural adjustments and the limb movements required to take the cup to the mouth. Oral and swallowing musculature need to be coordinated with breathing in order to have the drink without choking. All of these factors are included in the plan before it is executed (Table 5.1, column 2).

In order to perform a task effectively and efficiently, adequate strength and range of movement are needed, and the nervous system takes these into account when the plan is devised (Table 5.1, column 3). These biomechanical factors are seen to be highly significant for the movement science/motor learning and dynamic systems approaches, but are viewed as being complementary to the neurophysiological or CNS processes involved in motor control (Martenuik et al 1987). Once the execution of the task is underway, sensory feedback is generated.

Box 5.1 Models of motor control

1. Hierarchical
2. Reflex
3. Anatomical (wiring diagram)
4. Engineering model
5. Systems model/dynamic systems model
6. Ecological
7. Information-processing

Table 5.1 Simple plan giving an example of the different phases of motor control for drinking from a cup based on the Information-Processing Model

Idea	Plan	Execution	Appraisal
Desire Need Motivation	Motor programme Intrinsic factors Extrinsic factors	Muscle strength/length Skeletal system (e.g. alignment)	Sensory feedback during tasks to fine-tune/deal with unexpected events After task to update feedforward (plan)
e.g. have a drink Thirst Social: drink with friends	Reaching/oral motor programme Postural adjustment: before, during and after Haptic features: shape, size, texture, weight Environmental: self/object placement	Adequate muscle strength of grip/reach muscles, including postural/oral/motor muscles Effective posture: stand/sit	Effective sensory perception and processing to account for unexpected events, e.g. disturbed balance; unexpected contents of cup Also to monitor outcome

This sensory information has several vital roles. Firstly, it enables fine tuning during task performance; secondly, any errors in the transmitted programme can be corrected; thirdly, any unexpected events such as postural perturbation can be accounted for, and finally, if any adjustments are required for future performance of the task, the feedforward command can be updated (Table 5.1, column 4). The sensory system is vitally important for adaptation and learning: without the appropriate sensory experiences and processing, changes in motor control cannot be achieved. It has been said that we learn the sensation of a movement (Brooks 1986); thus appropriate sensory perception and processing are integral to the execution of finely tuned task performance, but more importantly for adapting already acquired movements and tasks to enable the learning of new skills. Thus, sensory function is a crucial factor to consider when the therapist is determining the possibilities for change in any particular child. Cognitive processing is also essential for successful task achievement. In the example given, a decision also needs to be made when sufficient liquid has been ingested and to determine whether the expected outcome has been achieved.

As in all tasks, the appropriate combination of motor, sensory, perceptual, cognitive and biomechanical components is necessary for optimal task performance. When any of these components is disordered or lacking, then other systems need to compensate for the deficient one(s), or, as may happen in extreme cases, the task cannot be carried out. For example, a child may have the necessary sensorimotor ability to perform a task such as walking independently, but a deficient spatial perceptual system will mean that independent gait is not possible due to fear of projecting the body into space. If spastic hypertonia is present, this may increase because of fear and could be erroneously identified as the main culprit preventing independence in gait. It is essential, therefore, to analyse task performance appropriately and correctly interpret the findings to enable specific intervention to target the primary areas of concern.

Changes in the understanding of motor control and of the complementary nature of neurophysiological and biomechanical contributions to skill performance have altered the way we view the impairments of the person with neurological movement disorder. Consideration of spasticity as part of the upper motor neurone syndrome shows that the significance of spasticity is less than previously thought, and that other aspects of the upper motor neurone syndrome cause more activity limitation. Rather than being 'overactive' and requiring inhibition, spastic muscles are weak (Damiano et al 2002, Rose & McGill 2005, Smits-Engelsman et al 2005) and often inappropriately activated due to other factors such as muscle stiffness and muscle imbalance. The emphasis on the task-specific nature of CNS function and activity-driven neuroplasticity necessitates that an active, meaningful, goal-directed intervention be provided.

CHANGES IN THEORIES OF DEVELOPMENT AND POSTURAL CONTROL

The other significant area of advancement of knowledge for the paediatric physiotherapist is that of typical development of the infant, and associated with this, changes in views on the development of postural control. In recent years different theories about development have emerged, and the reality of the milestone approach of Illingworth (1987) and others has been challenged. Hadders-Algra (2000a, b) has described the two main views of development and suggested that an additional model, the neuronal group selection theory (NGST), might offer a useful model for understanding the process of development and skill acquisition. She describes the traditional neural maturation theory (NMT) and the more recent dynamic systems theory (DST), and suggests that the main difference between these two models is the way in which they view the role of the developing nervous system's contribution to skill acquisition. The NMT places great emphasis on changes in the nervous system which enable development to proceed (i.e. nature), whereas in DST, the nervous system is only one of many subsystems. Thus the CNS is thought to have a necessary, although less significant, role in development, and it is a child's experience and interaction with the environment that emerge as the critical factor (nurture) (Hadders-Algra 2000a, Helders et al 2003). These two theories represent extreme views. the NGST has been suggested as a solution to the nature–nurture dilemma. This theory arises out of the work of Edelman, and has been described by Hadders-Algra and others (Thelen 1995, Forssberg 1999, Hadders-Algra 2000a, b, Helders et al 2003). This theory proposes that the infant has the capacity for self-generated activity due to the presence of innate, generally specified motor behaviour repertoires, which are subsequently refined by experience to enable the selection of the most effective motor patterns for successful achievement of a task (see Figure 1 in Forssberg, 1999).

In this model, development is seen to be the product of the infant's innate abilities/genetic make-up (nature), and the many experiences available to him/her (nurture). This theory can also be applied to postural control and speech development. For example, in postural control, rather than being organized by emerging reactions, as suggested by NMT, according to NGST the infant has an innate capacity for directionally specific responses (referred to as the first level: basic motor patterns). These responses are then adapted and modulated according to the infant's experience (the second level: Hadders-Algra et al 1996a; Hedberg et al, 2004, 2005). These responses can thus be modified by training (Hadders-Algra et al 1996b). Hadders-Algra (2000b) emphasizes the importance of sensory experience for motor development. This component is significant for children with neurological movement disorders for whom sensory dysfunction is often a significant impairment and correlates with the information-processing model of motor control (see previous section). Based on this view of development, in treatment the emphasis should be on practice of activities with trial-and-error performance for learning, with opportunity provided for variable sensorimotor experiences (Hadders-Algra 2000b). It is recognized, and has been shown, that a child with CNS dysfunction may need more practice than typically developing peers (Duff & Gordon 2003, Eliasson et al 2005). Exactly how much practice is needed remains unquantifiable (Bower & McLellan 1992, 1996), and is no doubt related to the potential for adaptation within the CNS, in addition to the motivational and cognitive processes of the child.

In addition to acceptance of these theories, it is also helpful to examine the great variety of ways that different infants develop their gross motor and fine motor skills, and the effects of personality on development in general. Bobath & Bobath (1975) challenged the milestone theory ('vertical development') and its phylogenetic emphasis as a result of experience in treating children with cerebral palsy. Clinical experience showed that children with spastic hypertonia who were not able to stand independently found it more difficult to learn to stand because of excessive flexion of hips and knees. By revisiting the developmental sequence, they observed that typically developing children do not kneel and half-kneel with extended hips, but rather with flexed hips and an anterior tilt of the pelvis. They observed that the ability to kneel and half-kneel with extended hips occurred after the child achieved independent walking, thus developing later than suggested by phylogenetic theory, at around 2–3 years of age. They also observed that when children start to crawl on all fours – if indeed they do crawl at all – they are also practising pull to stand and developing the skill of cruising around furniture. The presence of hip flexion makes it necessary for an infant to overuse the upper limbs and lateral flexion of the trunk in the task of pulling to stand (Figure 5.2).

Bobath & Bobath (1975) therefore assumed that the excessive flexion observed in a child with spastic cerebral palsy arose due to the practice of activities in crawling and kneeling, without the counterbalance of hip and knee extension usually practised in pull to stand and standing. Kneeling and half-kneeling are of course part of the important transition in getting up from the floor to standing. However, to practise kneeling and half-kneeling to gain hip extension for standing with a child who is not yet independently standing is inappropriate. This postural set requires the selectivity of hip extension combined with knee flexion, enabled by neutral pelvic tilt which is developed during the child's standing and independent walking practice. If the aim is to teach a transition from floor to stand for such a child, then it is an appropriate goal, but to practise kneeling with hip extension as a prerequisite for standing would be inappropriate.

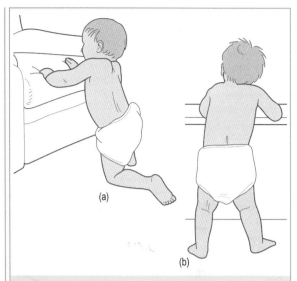

Figure 5.2 (a and b) This typically developing child overuses the trunk and shoulder girdle during pull to stand and cruising, to compensate for the lack of hip extension and pelvic/trunk control, which has not yet developed at the 9–10-month stage.

Rather, practice of the sequence should be encouraged in the best way that the child can manage to achieve that transition.

They regarded this horizontal view of development to be a more appropriate guide for intervention; that is, they suggested that it was important to determine the essential elements of development rather than trying to follow development per se (Bobath & Bobath 1975). These observations resulted in changed management of children with spastic cerebral palsy, in particular those with quadriplegia and diplegia. Children who could not yet stand and walk were not taught to practise crawling (quadruped) and high-kneeling as this would impede development of the ability to stand efficiently, already a challenge due to their variety of impairments. This does not mean, however, that children with cerebral palsy who can crawl should be stopped from doing so if this is their only form of independent mobility. Rather it gives the therapist a guide to work on that which counteracts the resultant flexion. This point is reinforced by Boyd & Ada (2001), who suggest that the motor patterns that can result in fixed contracture should be noted and counteracted by the therapist.

In addition to these observations, there have been attempts to describe the biomechanics of infant behaviour by Bly and others (Alexander et al 1993, Bly 1994, Thelen 1995), further recognizing the need to complement neural development with changes in biomechanical alignment and muscle activity and strength.

The previous discussion of changes in motor control theories and development suggest that skill-learning for children is multifaceted and has various requirements, including:

- Acceptance of the complementary nature of neuro-physiological processes and biomechanics in skill acquisition
- Interactive nature of all aspects of motor control: motor, sensory, cognitive, perceptual, behavioural, biomechanical
- Importance of environment
- Opportunity for experience
- Trial-and-error practice
- Varied practice: 'repetition without repetition'
- Meaningful goal: enjoyment of movement can be a goal in itself or it could be reaching a toy or communication
- Adequate sensory perception and processing to learn to adapt current behaviours to a new skill.

INTERNATIONAL CLASSIFICATION OF FUNCTIONING, DISABILITY AND HEALTH AND ITS RELEVANCE TO THERAPY INTERVENTION

With these essential components for skill acquisition in mind, we now turn to the question of how we can integrate these advances of knowledge into the management of the child with neurological movement disorders, to enable the application of a scientifically based, child-centred approach to intervention. The *International Classification of Functioning, Disability and Health* (ICF; World Health Organization 2001, 2002) may provide a means to do this. Although the ICF has been embraced in northern America and Australasia, it has perhaps been slower to become incorporated into clinical practice in Europe.

The ICF is intended to be a universal classification for health-related conditions, and is considered to be a multi-purpose tool for research, intervention, policy-planning and decision-making at all levels. The emphasis of this tool is on the positive aspects of function rather than the negativity of disability. The model has three basic areas of classification: body function and structure (e.g. sensory functions, structure of the nervous system respectively), activity (e.g. mobility) and participation (e.g. community/social life), all of which can be influenced by contextual factors. These can be personal (e.g. gender, character) and/or environmental (e.g. architecture, terrain). See the figure on p. 9, http://www3.who.int/icf/beginners/bg.pdf, which shows the interactive nature of these various categories. In the case of a health condition such as cerebral palsy, the three basic sections interact – body structure and function (impairments), activity (limitation) and participation (restriction) – and can be viewed in the context of personal and environmental factors. For example, reduced postural activity in sitting (impairment) may have an effect on the ability to use the hands for self-care and writing (activity limitation) and may result in difficulty in attending to activities in the classroom and playground (participation restriction). For many years physiotherapists have targeted intervention at the impairment level, but it is possible that intervention at an activity and participation level can also address impairments. This can result in an intervention which will be not only more meaningful, but of more value to a child and his/her family (Rosenbaum & Stewart, 2004), thus promoting the child-centred approach. For example, a study by Damiano et al (1995), which targeted the impairment level of muscle weakness, showed that a period of weight training for quadriceps and hamstrings increased muscle strength, and also resulted in an improvement in the Gross Motor Functional Measure (GMFM) scores in the activity domain of walking. The study by Schindl et al (2000) using treadmill training, an intervention aimed at the activity level, resulted in improvements in the activity of walking (shown by improvements in GMFM and Functional Ambulation Category scores) but also produced changes at the participation level (transfers for easier community access). One could also expect that there would be changes at the impairment level of muscle activation, although these were not measured in this study.

The ICF provides a useful summary of where the client 'is at', but it can be seen that the varied nature of the child's activity limitations and participation restrictions do not lie solely in the domain of the physiotherapist. The physiotherapist is one member of the multidisciplinary team which working cooperatively can provide optimal intervention for the child and family to enable the best possible outcome and progression to adult life. Given the need to strive for common language, goals and management aims, it is helpful if all members of the team adopt a similar framework for intervention. The ICF can be helpful in this respect; alternatively, or in addition to use of the ICF, regular team meetings, team assessments and invention seem to be essential.

SETTING THE GOALS FOR INTERVENTION FOR A CHILD WITH NEUROLOGICAL MOVEMENT DISORDER

What can the physiotherapist do given these diverse, complex conditions? The ICF, though extremely useful, can guide management but does not give sufficient detail of the 'hows and whys' of the child's activities to enable a specific therapeutic treatment plan to be devised. That is, it does not tell the therapist what to do.

A child with cerebral palsy has a variety of impairments which influence activity and participation (Mayston 2001) depending on the size, site and timing of the lesion (Wigglesworth 1990, Forssberg 1999). A child with cerebral palsy can be classified according to clinical signs (Paneth et al 2005), or assigned a functional level (e.g. using the GMFCS: Palisano et al 1997), but these classifications do not enable the therapist to decide which intervention might be beneficial. It should be possible to use the ICF with its stratification of impairments, activity and participation to guide management. This not only enables us to have an overview of the child and his or her possibilities but can also indicate what aspect of intervention might be required to improve quality of life and participation. For example, a child might have difficulty keeping up with games in the playground (participation) because he/she has insufficient balance (impairment). However, more detail of how the child performs various activities is usually required specifically to address the physical treatment goals of the individual (Figure 5.3).

The physiotherapist usually has excellent skills of observation, analysis and interpretation, to complement the various objective assessments available, for example, the GMFM, Functional Independence Measure for Children (WeeFim), Chailey Levels of Ability, Tardieu Scale for Spasticity, Movement Assessment Battery for Children, none of which is used routinely by all. Ideally, one could carry out a battery of objective tests of function, strength and range of movement, including motion analysis, e.g. gait analysis or upper-limb activity, postural control, sensory, perceptual and cognitive function, and assess CNS function and status using a range of neurophysiological tests. However, it is not practical to complete a full range of tests in a busy clinical or home/school environment where a child and family might be seen. Physiotherapists need to select appropriate practical assessment tools and in addition use their observational and analytical skills for their clinical reasoning. Figure 5.3 shows how these analytical skills may be incorporated into the ICF framework to assist the therapist in goal-setting and clinical reasoning for intervention. The focus of the assessment is on a child's abilities, activities and participation, but where these are absent then a consideration of the activity limitations and participation restrictions can be noted. The details of tone, patterns of activity, sensory/perceptual and cognitive function can then be added to the ICF, i.e. to look at the impairments in more detail to enable which aspect of impairment should be targeted if that is the level where intervention needs to start. Or there may be interdependence of the impairments which affect the activity level. For example, walking may be limited due to spatial–perceptual problems and increased spastic hypertonia associated with the fear of movement in space. In this case the primary problem to target is spatial perception, and the spastic hypertonia as a secondary problem needs to be managed in the context of the primary perceptual impairment. More detailed analysis at this level can assist the clinical reasoning process and enable specific intervention.

From this process, long-term goals for the therapy programme, in addition to short-term and sessional goals, can be determined (Damiano 2004). Box 5.2 exemplifies the stratification of goal-setting for an adolescent who has spastic diplegia and is a community walker, but in danger of increasing calf tightness, which will reduce walking capacity and require use of a walking aid.

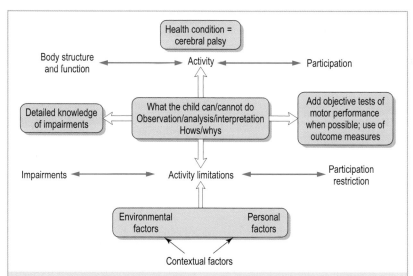

Figure 5.3 The *International Classification for Functioning Disability and Health* (ICF) provides a useful tool to analyse the participation, activity and impairments of the child with a neurological movement disorder and provides a framework for intervention. The upper half of the figure indicates the positive elements and the lower the negative, e.g. participation restriction.

Box 5.2 Goals can be set at all stages of the assessment/intervention process, including session goals which can enable the therapy session to be more focused

General management/long-term goals (based on Damiano, 2004)

- Reduce current musculoskeletal impairments to improve function and quality of life in short and long term: minimal calf shortness
- Enable children to function optimally given their existing impairments: able to participate in school sports and activities; manage classes in different locations
- Prevent or limit development of secondary impairments that may further limit function
- Alter the 'natural' course of disorder: maintain level of function so that walking aid is not needed
- Promote wellness and fitness over the lifespan: improve fitness, increase participation in school sports and activities

Short-term goals

- Improve distance walked in a given time
- Increase fitness, improve oxygen uptake during exercise
- Minimize calf contracture: improve or prevent loss of range of movement
- Improve strength in lower-limb muscles, especially quadriceps
- More symmetry of gait: improved single-leg stance and balance

Sessional goals

- Stretch calf and achieve plantar grade foot
- Improve dynamic standing balance on one leg for improved single-leg stance in gait
- Additional time on treadmill or in walking practice

THE 'THERAPY TOOLBOX' AND THE CHILD WITH CEREBRAL PALSY

Once the initial assessment has been carried out and the physiotherapy goals are determined, the physiotherapist has many tools to choose from in order to provide optimal intervention to the child and family, regardless of the child's level of activity and participation. Just as there is no one model for understanding motor control, neither is there one way to approach management of a child with a neurological movement disorder. To achieve child-centred

management, it is essential to put aside the philosophy approach, and from the determination of a child/family's goals and needs, to provide what is required. For example, an analysis of a child's skills based on Bobath/NDT training provides a framework for detailed task analysis, but then requires a look into the 'toolbox' to find the appropriate strategies to meet those needs. Some of these may be from a Bobath repertoire, but others, such as muscle strengthening, are taken from the emerging body of scientific evidence, which is beginning to underpin therapy intervention. Figure 5.4 is an attempt to show the variety of strategies/tools which the therapist has to use. By building on the process of analysis and organization of information outlined in the previous paragraph, the therapist can decide which strategies to use once the main area(s) for intervention are identified.

The level of ability will determine how much 'hands-on' therapy might be needed to enable optimal child-generated activity and participation. Figure 5.5 shows that, for the more able child, the most appropriate intervention would be active practice of agreed goal activities, whereas for a child who has significant activity limitation, hands-on for easier use of equipment and management is preferred. For the example given in Box 5.2, achievement of session goals could be by the following: use of physiotherapy handling techniques to reduce spastic hypertonia and stretch the calf muscle to achieve optimal alignment for activating stance muscles, training balance in single-leg stance, and a session on the treadmill walking at a velocity which enhances stride length, push-off and aerobic fitness. To achieve short-term goals, self-stretch calf in standing or with assistance of parent/carer, balance training and practice sessions on the treadmill at the local fitness centre, in addition to other aerobic activities like swimming. A programme of strengthening either using weights, or, if available, isokinetic dynamometry, could also be used to improve force generation for improved stance and swing. In the last 10 years a number of studies have provided evidence to show that a period of resisted muscle strength-training can improve muscle strength and function in independently ambulant children (Damiano et al 1995, MacPhail & Kramer 1995, Damiano and Abel 1998, Taylor et al 2004, Morton et al 2005) and less able adolescents (Dodd et al 2003, Allen et al 2004). Circuit training and treadmill training may also be a useful adjunct, although there is a lack of studies to support its use in children (Schindl et al 2000, Blundell et al 2003, Andersson et al 2004, Mayston et al, in press). Children and adolescents alike usually enjoy these types of training, which can also thus promote societal participation, and inclusion rather than exclusion (Allen et al 2004).

Balance training is an area of management for the more able child that has not been adequately researched. Limited evidence suggests that postural activity can be trained to improve consistency of postural responses in typically developing children and in some children with cerebral palsy (Hadders-Algra et al 1996b, Woollacott et al 2005).

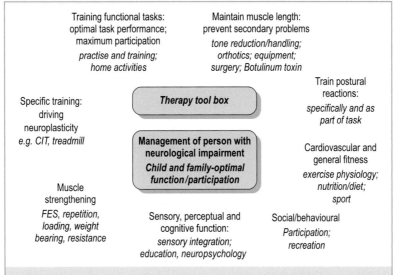

Figure 5.4 The therapy toolbox contains a range of possible interventions that can be applied to the child with a neurological movement disorder. Readers may like to add others. CIT, constraint-induced therapy; FES, functional electrical stimulation.

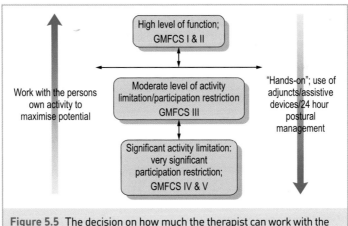

Figure 5.5 The decision on how much the therapist can work with the child's activity and participation depends on the child's level of ability. The Gross Motor Function Classification System (GMFCS) provides a guide to when it is appropriate for the therapist to use a more 'hands-on' therapy approach.

The achievement of long-term goals can be monitored by the use of the appropriate outcome measures, such as GMFM, 10-metre walk and goniometry to enable the adjustment of short-term and session goals as needed.

For a child with complex needs, the therapist would instruct those in the child's life in simple ways to optimize posture and movement for optimizing daily life activities. For example, to access a communication aid, to enable mealtimes to be less stressful, time-consuming and ultimately more enjoyable, or to optimize positioning for taking in information from the environment either visually or cognitively. In these cases, ease of assistance in daily life activities, 24-hour postural management and equipment needs are primary considerations for management. The principles of therapy handling to elongate stiff muscles for easier positioning, to gain either head control or upper-limb activity to access the communication device, can be applied to all activities of daily life. This type of therapy is more hands-on, but with the specific purpose of optimizing muscle length and activity for maximal participation and minimization of contracture and deformity via a consistent programme of postural management. Although there is little or no experimental evidence to support the idea that therapy handling makes positioning in equipment easier, it is the experience of most therapists, parents and carers that this is indeed the case. The evidence for management of the more complex child of GMFCS categories IV and V, particularly in the area of postural management, is another priority for research.

Whatever level the physiotherapy intervention is targeting, the priority should be to meet the task goals of the child/parent/carer. The intervention provided should also aim to access self-generated activity from the child, whether the goal is to improve walking or to use the head to access a switch to operate a computer, communication aid or other device.

It is now well known that the neuroplasticity of the CNS is driven by activity and experience, thus meaningful activities need to be practised. Another current example of task-specific training arises out of the work on constraint-induced therapy, or forced-use therapy for the upper limb. From the initial work using an animal model (Taub 1980, Nudo et al 1996), this work has extended to the management of adult stroke patients, and more recently to the paediatric hemiplegic population (Taub et al 1993, 2004, Gordon et al 2005, Naylor & Bower 2005). Like most aspects of therapy intervention, more robust evidence is needed to determine at what stage, for how long and at what frequency this type of training should be provided. However, initial reports show promise.

As research is expanded to investigate specific aspects of therapy intervention from functional, biomechanical and neurophysiological perspectives, the scientific basis of therapeutic intervention will enable a body of evidence to become available on which to structure rational and effective therapy programmes for the whole spectrum of the disorder known as cerebral palsy. It may take some time, but there is a growing confidence that sound evidence-based physical therapy can, and so will, become a reality.

REFERENCES

Alexander C, Boehme R, Cupps B 1993 *Development of Skill in the First 12 Months of Life*. Arizona: Therapy Skills Builders.

Allen J, Dodd KJ, Taylor NF, McBurney H, Larkin H 2004 Strength training can be enjoyable and beneficial for adults with cerebral palsy. *Disability and Rehabilitation* 26: 1121–1127.

Andersson C, Grooten W, Hellsten M, Kaping K, Mattsson E 2003 Adults with cerebral palsy: walking ability after progressive strength training. *Developmental Medicine and Child Neurology* 45: 220–228.

Arbib M 1995 *The Handbook of Brain Theory and Neural networks*. Cambridge, MA: MIT Press.

Bernstein N 1967 *The Co-ordination and Regulation of Movements*. Oxford: Pergamon.

Blundell SW, Shepherd RB, Dean CM, Adams RD, Cahill BM 2003 Functional strength training in cerebral palsy: a pilot study of a group circuit training class for children aged 4–8 years. *Clinical Rehabilitation* 17: 48–57.

Bly L 1994 *Motor Skills Acquisition in the First Year. An Illustrated Guide to Normal Development*. Tucson, AZ: Therapy Skill Builders.

Bobath B, Bobath K 1975 *Motor Development in the Different Types of Cerebral Palsy*. London: Heinemann Medical.

Bower E, McLellan DL 1992 Effect of increased exposure to physiotherapy on skills acquisition of children with cerebral palsy. *Developmental Medicine and Child Neurology* 34: 25–39.

Bower E, McLellan DL 1996 Assessing motor-skill acquisition in four centres for the treatment of children with cerebral palsy. *Developmental Medicine and Child Neurology* 36: 902–909.

Boyd R, Ada L 2001 Physiotherapy management of spasticity. In: Barnes MP, Johnson GR (eds) *Upper Motor Neurone Syndrome and Spasticity*. London: Cambridge Medicine, pp. 96–121.

Brooks V 1986 *Neural Basis of Motor Control*. New York: Oxford University Press, chapter 1.

Damiano DJ 2004 Physiotherapy management in cerebral palsy: moving beyond philosophies. In: Scrutton D, Damiano DJ, Mayston MJ (eds) *Management of the Motor Disorders of Cerebral Palsy*, 2nd edn. London: Mac Keith Press, pp. 161–169.

Damiano DL, Abel MF 1998 Functional outcomes of strength training in spastic cerebral palsy. *Archives of Physical Medicine and Rehabilitation* 79: 119–125.

Damiano DL, Vaughan CL, Abel MF 1995 Muscle response to heavy resistance exercise in children with spastic cerebral palsy. *Developmental Medicine and Child Neurology* 37: 731–739.

Damiano DL, Dodd K, Taylor NF 2002 Should we be testing and training muscle strength in cerebral palsy? *Developmental Medicine and Child Neurology* 44: 68–72.

Dodd KJ, Taylor NF, Graham HK 2003 A randomized clinical trial of strength training in young people with cerebral palsy. *Developmental Medicine and Child Neurology* 45: 652–657.

Dromerick AW 2003 Evidence-based rehabilitation: the case for and against constraint induced movement therapy. *Journal of Rehabilitation Research and Development* 40: vii–ix.

Duff SV, Gordon AM 2003 Learning grasp control in children with hemiplegic cerebral palsy. *Developmental Medicine and Child Neurology* 45: 746–757.

Eliasson AC, Krumlinde-Sundholm L, Shaw K, Wang C 2005 Effects of constraint-induced movement therapy in young children with hemiplegic cerebral palsy: an adapted model. *Developmental Medicine and Child Neurology* 47: 266–275.

Forssberg H 1999 Neural control of human motor development. *Current Opinions in Neurobiology* 9: 676–682.

Galea M 2004 Neural plasticity and learning. In: Scrutton D, Damiano DJ, Mayston MJ (eds) *Management of the Motor Disorders of Cerebral Palsy*, 2nd edn. London: Mac Keith Press, pp. 161–169.

Gordon AM, Charles J, Wolf SL 2005 Method of constraint-induced movement therapy for children with hemiplegic cerebral palsy: development of a child-friendly intervention for improving upper extremity function. *Archives of Physical Medicine and Rehabilitation* 86: 837–844.

Hadders-Algra M 2000a The neuronal group selection theory: a framework to explain variation in normal motor development. *Developmental Medicine and Child Neurology* 42: 566–572.

Hadders-Algra M 2000b The neuronal group selection theory: promising principles for understanding and treating developmental motor disorders. *Developmental Medicine and Child Neurology* 42: 707–715.

Hadders-Algra M, Brogren E, Forssberg H 1996a Ontogeny of postural adjustments during sitting in infancy: variation, selection and modulation. *Journal of Physiology* 493: 273–288.

Hadders-Algra M, Brogren E, Forssberg H 1996b Training affects the development of postural adjustments in sitting infants. *Journal of Physiology (London)* 493: 289–298.

Hedberg A, Forssberg H, Hadders-Algra M 2004 Postural adjustments due to external perturbations during sitting in 1-month old infants: evidence for the innate origin of direction specificity. *Experimental Brain Research* 157: 10–17.

Hedberg A, Carlsberg EB, Forssberg H, Hadders-Algra M 2005 Development of postural adjustments in sitting position during the first six months of life. *Developmental Medicine and Child Neurology* 47: 312–320.

Helders PJ, Engelbert RH, Custers JW, Gorter JW, Takken T, van der Net J 2003 Created and being created: the changing panorama of paediatric rehabilitation. *Pediatric Rehabilitation* 6: 5–12.

Herbert R, Jamtvedt G, Mead J, Hagen KB 2005 *Practical Evidence-based Physiotherapy*. Oxford: Butterworth Heinemann.

Horak F 1992 Motor control models underlying neurologic rehabilitation of posture in children. In: Forssberg H, Hirschfeld H (eds) *Movement Disorders in Children*. Medicine and Sport Science series, vol. 36. Basel: Karger.

Illingworth RS 1984 *The Development of the Infant and Young Child: Normal and Abnormal*, 8th edn. Edinburgh: Churchill Livingstone.

Jackson JH 1958 Evolution and dissolution of the nervous system: speech: various papers, addresses and lectures. In: Taylor J (ed.) *Selected writings of John Hughlings, Vol 2*. London: Staples Press.

MacPhail HEA, Kramer JF 1995 Effects of isokinetic strength training on functional ability and walking efficiency in adolescents with cerebral palsy. *Developmental Medicine and Child Neurology* 37: 763–775.

Martenuik RG, Mackenzie CL, Jeannerod M, Athenes S, Dugas C 1987 Constraints on human arm movement. *Canadian Journal of Psychology* 41: 365–378.

Mayston MJ 2001 Effects of and perspectives for therapy for people with cerebral palsy. *Neural Plasticity* 8: 51–69.

Mayston MJ 2002 Setting the scene. In: Edwards S (ed.) *Neurological Physiotherapy – A Problem Solving Approach*, 2nd edn. Edinburgh: Churchill Livingstone, pp. 3–19.

Mayston MJ 2004 Physiotherapy management in cerebral palsy: an update on treatment approaches. In: Scrutton D, Damiano D, Mayston M (eds) *Management of the Motor Disorders of Cerebral Palsy*, 2nd edn. London: MacKeith Press, pp. 147–160.

Mayston MJ, Beattie K, Gelkop N 2006 The effect of treadmill training on function and fitness in children with cerebral palsy: a preliminary study. *Developmental Medicine and Child Neurology* 48 (suppl. 105): 1B.1.

Morton JF, Brownlee M, McFadyen AK 2005 The effects of progressive resistance training for children with cerebral palsy. *Clinical Rehabilitation* 19: 283–289.

Naylor CE, Bower E 2005 Modified constraint induced movement therapy for young children with hemiplegic cerebral palsy: a pilot study. *Developmental Medicine and Child Neurology* 47: 365–369.

Nudo RJ, Wise BM, SiFuentes F, Milliken GW 1996 Neural substrates for the effects of rehabilitative training on motor recovery after ischaemic infarct. *Science* 272: 1791–1794.

Palisano R, Rosenbaum P, Walter S, Russel D, Wood E, Galuppi B 1997 Development and reliability of a system to classify gross motor function in children with cerebral palsy. *Developmental Medicine and Child Neurology* 39: 214–223.

Paneth N, Damiano D, Rosenbaum P, Leviton A, Goldstein M, Bax M 2005 Proposed definition and classification of cerebral palsy, April 2005. *Developmental Medicine and Child Neurology* 47: 571–576.

Rose J, McGill KC 2005 Neuromuscular activation and motor-unit firing characteristics in cerebral palsy. *Developmental Medicine and Child Neurology* 47: 329–336.

Rosenbaum P, Stewart D 2004 The World Health Organization International Classification of Functioning Disability and Health: a model to guide clinical thinking, practice and research in the field of cerebral palsy. *Seminars in Pediatric Neurology* 11: 5–10.

Rothwell J 1994 *Control of Human Voluntary Movement*, 2nd edn. London: Chapman Hall.

Sackett DL, Rosenberg WM, Gray AJM, Haynes RB, Richardson WSS 1996 Evidence based medicine: what it is and what it isn't. *British Medical Journal* 312: 71–72.

Schindl MR, Forstner C, Kern H, Hesse S 2000 Treadmill training with partial body weight support in nonambulatory patients with cerebral palsy. *Archives of Physical Medicine and Rehabilitation* 81: 301–306.

Sherrington CS 1947 *The Integrative Action of the Nervous System*. New Haven, CT: Yale University Press. First published 1906.

Shumway-Cook A, Woollacott M 2001 *Motor Control: Theory and Practical Applications*. Baltimore: Lippincott, Williams & Wilkins.

Smits-Englesman BCM, Rameckers EAA, Duysens J 2005 Muscle force generation and force control of finger movements in children with spastic hemiplegia during isometric tasks. *Developmental Medicine and Child Neurology* 47: 337–342.

Taub E 1980 Somatosensory deafferentation research with monkeys: implications for rehabilitation medicine. In: Ince LP (ed.) *Behavioural Psychology in Rehabilitation Medicine: Clinical Applications*. Baltimore, MD: Williams & Wilkins, pp. 371–401.

Taub E, Miller NE, Novack TA 1993 A technique for improving chronic motor deficit after stroke. *Archives of Physical Medicine and Rehabilitation* 74: 347–354.

Taub E, Ramey SL, DeLuca S, Echols K 2004 Efficacy of constraint induced movement therapy for children with cerebral palsy with asymmetric motor impairment. *Pediatrics* 113: 305–312.

Taylor NF, Dodd KJ, Larkin H 2004 Adults with cerebral palsy benefit from participating in a strength training programme at a community gymnasium. *Disability and Rehabilitation* 26: 1128–1134.

Thelen E 1995 Motor development. A new synthesis. *American Psychologist* 50: 79–95.

Wigglesworth JS 1990 Plasticity of the developing brain. In: Pape KE, Wigglesworth JS (eds) *Contemporary Issues in Fetal and Neonatal Medicine. No. 5: Perinatal Brain Lesions*. Boston: Blackwell Scientific.

Woollacott M, Shumway-Cook A, Hutchinson S, Ciol M, Price R, Kartin D 2005 Effect of balance training on muscle activity used in recovery of stability in children with cerebral palsy. *Developmental Medicine and Child Neurology* 47: 455–461.

World Health Organization 2001 International classification of functioning and disability and health. Available online at: http://www3.who.int/icf/icftemplate.

World Health Organization 2002 *International Classification of Functioning Disability and Health*. Available online at: http://www3.who.int/icf/beginners/bg.pdf.

6 Neonatal care

Anna Mayhew and Fiona Price

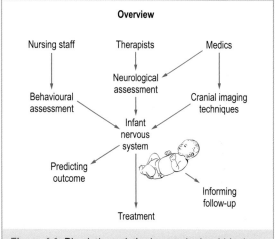

Figure 6.1 Physiotherapist's place and role within the wider team

INTRODUCTION

In the last 10–15 years, advances in modern medical care have resulted in the development of neonatology as a speciality. Where the neonatal unit was once the preserve of paediatricians and nursing staff, it has become multidisciplinary in nature, although the extent to which physiotherapists are involved varies considerably.

The physiotherapist is one member of a wider team and many of the roles may be shared with colleagues (Figure 6.1). That involvement can be purely based on a neonatal unit or may originate from within the community. It is therefore important to have effective liaison between the two settings, especially if several therapists are involved. Traditionally the physiotherapist's role has been in the management of respiratory conditions but more recently has extended to include neurological and behavioural assessment, therapeutic interventions and follow-up of high-risk infants.

BACKGROUND

Approximately 10% of babies will require admission to a neonatal unit following delivery (Macfarlane et al 1999). Reasons for admission may vary from observation of a term infant who has a mild degree of respiratory distress due to transient tachypnoea of the newborn, management of an infant with hypoxaemic–ischaemic encephalopathy to intensive care of an extremely premature infant (premature baby = baby born before 37 weeks).

Advances in medical care, particularly in terms of equipment, e.g. ventilators and incubators, and drug therapy, have made it possible to keep younger and smaller infants alive. Infants born below 1500 g are considered low birth weight (LBW), infants below 1000 g are termed very low birth weight (VLBW) and infants born below 750 g are extremely low birth weight (ELBW).

The younger the infants, the more vulnerable they are to complications of prematurity. These include respiratory distress syndrome (RDS), a condition primarily caused by a lack of surfactant resulting in non-compliant lungs, haemorrhagic or ischaemic brain damage (intraventricular haemorrhage (IVH) and periventricular leukomalacia (PVL) respectively) due to the immature structure of the brain and the infant's inability to self-regulate the autonomic nervous system. Other complications seen in the preterm infant are necrotizing enterocolitis (NEC), an inflammatory condition of the bowel often resulting in necrotic sections of bowel, jaundice and apnoeas and bradycardias of prematurity.

Table 6.1 Whom to assess in order of priority	
Whom to assess (in priority order)	**Details**
Babies born before 30 weeks' gestation	Some units assess all infants below 30 weeks. Others use either 32 or 28 weeks as a cut-off point. This variability is due to level of service provision
Babies less than 1500 g	This category can be used in conjunction with gestational age to determine assessment requirements
Severely growth-retarded infants	Below the second centile on growth charts and usually preterm
Hypoxic–ischaemic encephalopathy	Grades 2 and 3
Abnormal cranial ultrasound scans	Germinal matrix haemorrhage–intraventricular haemorrhage (GMH-IVH), parenchymal haemorrhagic infarct (PHI). Periventricular leukomalacia (PVL)
Syndromes	As appropriate and on discussion with the medical team
Chronic lung disease	Again, these infants usually fall within the first two categories
Severely hypotonic infants and/or poor feeders	These referrals are usually from the nursing staff and fall outside the above criteria

Despite the complications associated with premature birth, an increasing number now survive to discharge (Hack & Fanaroff 1999). However, the rate of cerebral palsy has remained relatively constant at around 10% (Pharoah et al 1998). There is growing evidence that premature infants are more at risk of behavioural and cognitive difficulties as well as neurological, medical and growth complications (Hack et al 1996).

This chapter aims to give an overview of the role of the physiotherapist in the assessment of the developing nervous system, respiratory care, and developmental and neurological interventions but will not include management of orthopaedic conditions.

ASSESSMENT OF THE NERVOUS SYSTEM

This section aims to cover:

- Whom to assess
- Neurological assessments (evidence for their effectiveness and training)
- When to assess
- Practical advice on assessment over time
- Specific conditions and their presentation.

An assessment must be practical to apply, reliable and valid and relevant to you as a clinician. Different professional groups may have designed assessments for different purposes. It may have been designed to determine follow-up requirements, predict neurological or behavioural outcome, target treatment or measure the effects of intervention. It is advisable to focus on one or two assessment

procedures which are most relevant to you as a clinician. Most importantly, build up practical skills by working with colleagues and visiting other units. It can be helpful to have a video to record assessments and then review these with colleagues. The most important tools are your eyes to observe babies whilst they are at rest or whilst they are being handled by staff or parents. Your own physical assessment is secondary to this ongoing observation.

Whom to assess

It can be difficult when you first enter a neonatal unit to know just whom to assess (Table 6.1). This will depend on the type of referral system you have. Some units will only allow you to assess infants referred specifically by the consultants. Ideally a blanket referral system should be in place with the opportunity to discuss specific referrals directly with staff. The criteria you set for assessment may change over time as you gain experience and depending on staffing levels. Table 6.1 is a suggested regime for whom to assess. This is based on the experience of several units over an extended period of time.

Neurological assessment

The assessments listed in Table 6.2 are not an exhaustive list but include the main assessment techniques. Many modified assessments exist, which suggests that neurological assessment is not straightforward. Table 6.2 summarizes

Table 6.2 Principal methods of assessing the nervous system in the neonate

	Principles	Equipment	Training	When
Imaging techniques				
Cranial ultrasound (US)	Portable, instant visualization, low cost. Performed in a series to monitor evolution of pathology. US is a useful tool, although not as predictive of outcome as once thought, as not all abnormal scans are associated with an abnormal outcome. PVL is most predictive, with many studies reporting 100% of cystic PVL, resulting in an abnormal outcome (Han et al 2002)	Portable US equipment can be used on ventilated infants in situ	Specific training required	From birth till the anterior fontanelle shuts at 3–15 months of age (average of 9 months)
Magnetic resonance imaging (MRI)	Requires dedicated MRI scanner. Infants must be taken to unit. Expensive and time-consuming analysis. More useful in term infants. Predictive ability similar to US	Required dedicated MRI local to NICU with experienced technician	Specific training required	Once infant is self-ventilating, as metal cannot be placed in the scanner
Neurological assessment Two similar approaches to neonatal neurological assessment (NNA) predominate, those of Dubowitz et al (1999) and of Prechtl (1977). Both have been standardized and validated and their diagnostic and prognostic value confirmed. Amiel–Tison (1995) has also developed an assessment for infants at term and, although the approaches are not identical, there are considerable similarities between them. All of these techniques are based on the assessment of passive and active tone and a series of elicited reflexes and reactions				
Dubowitz	Consists of a standardized proforma of 34 items assessing posture, tone, reflexes, orientation, behaviour and abnormal signs. Items are scored depending on the infant's response to the examination technique. An optimality score exists for its use in term infants but not in the preterm infant (Dubowitz et al 1998)	Rattle/black and white target/ red ball	None – textbook describes all the tests	From 28 weeks to 4 weeks postterm
Amiel–Tison	Amiel–Tison recommends serial assessment of infants. Significance is placed on physical signs as well as the usual assessment of posture, visual ability and tone in the limbs, head and trunk. The results of an examination are synthesized with the clinical pattern of the central nervous system injury such as seizures, global hypotonia, asymmetry of tone and the results of non-clinical investigations such as ultrasound or MRI. The assessment tends to relate to the term infant and above (Amiel–Tison 1995)	Rattle/black and white target/ red ball	None – some description in textbooks	From 28 weeks to 4 weeks postterm
Lacey	Based on Prechtl's NNA. Consists of a longitudinal assessment done over a period of weeks. Emphasis placed on observational skills. Documentation of antigravity movement and postures in addition to an analysis of the components and quality of spontaneous movements (Lacey & Henderson-Smart 1998)	Rattle/black and white target/ red ball	Training courses available	From 28 weeks/ once stabilized till term plus

continued

Table 6.2 *continued*

	Principles	Equipment	Training	When
Behavioural assessments				
Neurobehavioural Assessment Scale (NBAS) Brazelton	Assessment of a newborn infant's behavioural repertoire is based on 28 behavioural items, each scored on a nine-point scale. Neurological status is assessed on 18 reflex items, each scored on a four-point scale. The scale is designed to assess dynamic behavioural interaction between the infant and care-giver, which distinguishes it from other assessments (Brazelton & Nugent 1995)	Requires specific equipment	www.brazelton.co.uk Requires specific training as full course/introductory courses	From birth onwards
Assessment of Premature Infant Behaviour (APIB)	This assessment is a refinement of the NBAS			
Neonatal Individualized Developmental Care and Assessment Program (NIDCAP)	NIDCAP is based on the synactive model of development proposed by Dr Heidelise Als (Als et al 1994, 1996). It focuses on the continuous interaction of the infant's physiological motor state, self-regulatory and interactive state. NIDCAP is based on the careful observations of infant behaviours and responses to care-giving, and the formulation of individualized care plans appropriate for the infant's current developmental goals. Fundamental to NIDCAP is parental involvement in planning and executing care of their infant		Requires specific training	Mainly applied during the preterm period whilst the infant is on NICU
Neurobehavioural Assessment for Preterm Infants (NAPI)	A longitudinal assessment of neurobehaviour including motor development, orientation and alertness, irritability, asleep ratings and vigour of crying			From 32 weeks to term age
Quality of movement				
Observation of movements Prechtl	Prechtl suggests that the human foetus and young infant are characterized by a repertoire of distinct movement patterns, which occur spontaneously. One of these movement patterns he has defined as general movements (GMs). Assessment data are obtained by taking video recordings over time. Prechtl claims it is a quick, non-invasive method with high validity and high reliability. Analysis is done from the summary tape using your Gestalt perception to judge the quality of the GMs (Prechtl et al 1997, Einspieler et al 2004)	Video camera/ digital	www.general-movements-trust.info/	From 28 weeks till 10–12 weeks postterm age

PVL, periventricular leukomalacia; NICU, neonatal intensive care unit;

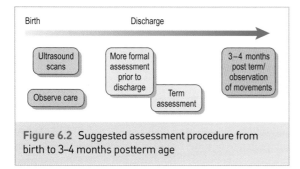

Figure 6.2 Suggested assessment procedure from birth to 3–4 months postterm age

each assessment method, the evidence for its effectiveness and any equipment needed and gives information on training.

Ideally a predictive test will identify both abnormal and normal measures accurately (see Ch. 3). Such a test will possess a high sensitivity and specificity, but will not detect too many false positives (positive predictive value: PPV) or false negatives (negative predictive value: NPV). PPV and NPV are both clinically useful measures but depend on prevalence, whereas sensitivity and specificity do not (see Ch. 3).

When to assess

It is important to spend your time wisely on what can be an all-consuming area. Once you have identified infants who need assessment you need to decide when to perform assessments. Figure 6.2 gives a suggested scheme. Keep records of when assessments are required. A simple table in front of your notes can guide you as to the quantity of work that needs doing from week to week.

It is important to combine the results from one examination with those of another. Ideally, a multidisciplinary meeting can deliver this most effectively.

Practical advice on assessment over time

Rather than describe each test, details of which can be gleaned from other textbooks (Amiel-Tison 1995, Dubowitz et al 1999), this section aims to direct you to the types of information you need to be gathering as an infant progresses through the neonatal intensive care unit (NICU), to the point of discharge and then the type of follow-up requirements once the baby is at home. Rarely do you gain a complete picture in one sitting. Change can occur rapidly in the maturing nervous system and assessment needs to be ongoing (Amiel-Tison 1995).

Early assessment

This early period may be a time fraught with difficulties, particularly for very preterm infants. It is therefore advisable

to discuss the baby with the nursing and medical team prior to approaching the family. This early information-gathering gives you an idea of the baby's neonatal history. Record in your notes maternal and antenatal details, birth history and ventilatory history during the ongoing weeks. Note number of days ventilated/continuous positive airway pressure (CPAP), and the need for low-flow oxygen.

Discuss with the doctors any scan results and seek clarification if necessary on their significance. Observe the baby during a care procedure and note the baby's posture in supine and prone, response to handling and the relationship of parents to their child. You may be asked for advice at this point on positioning and this is often your first opportunity to handle the baby, albeit briefly. Note colour changes on handling as well as cardiac and respiratory responses. Very preterm babies may become bradycardic on handling and desaturate significantly. Change a baby's position slowly and allow the child time to settle between each action. Have a nurse on hand if you need assistance or advice.

Ongoing assessment

Behavioural states

In order to carry out a neurological assessment the baby should ideally be in a quiet and alert state; the child should not have just been fed but should also not be very hungry. For some infants this will be a little after a feed, for others it is just before, and still others somewhere in between. Occasionally, no time is the right time for an unsettled or very 'sleepy' baby. Make a note of this.

Posture and muscle tone

Observe posture in the following positions: supine, prone, side-lying, and, for the older and more stable baby, ventral suspension and supported sitting (Figure 6.3). You may only complete one or two of these if the infant is still quite fragile. Make a note of the dominance of the asymmetrical tonic neck reflex (ATNR). See section on reflexes, below, for more detail. Assess the development of muscle tone. There are several different techniques for completing this part of the assessment. Dubowitz et al (1999) provide clear details of particular tests. These include arm recoil, traction, leg recoil and traction, popliteal angle, development of flexor and extensor neck tone and posture. Flexor tone, which is seen in term infants, develops from the feet upwards with flexor tone appearing in the legs first and then in the arms. The balance of tone is also important. Compare trunk flexor and extensor tone. A predominance of extensor tone is worth noting, although it is not uncommon in preterm infants.

Note head control in pull to sit. Take care to support the trunk and shoulders as you do this.

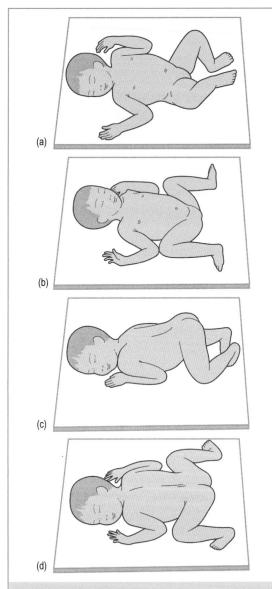

Figure 6.3 Supine lying. (a) Normal antigravity position; (b) flattened position. Prone lying. (c) Normal antigravity position; (d) flattened position

Reflexes

In the past, reflexes have played a considerable part in neurological assessment yet their value is uncertain. Their emergence and disappearance are related to gestational age. Palmar and plantar grasp may be tested and the suck and rooting reflex are important in prognosis. The Moro reflex should be performed with care but can be helpful in identifying lower motor neurone disorders. The stepping and placing reflexes do not contribute hugely to the overall assessment and their contribution to identifying abnormality is limited (Dubowitz et al 1999). The ATNR is a

normal pattern up until about 3 months of age but a dominant and fixed posture in a baby younger than this is an abnormal sign.

Abnormal signs

Note hand and foot postures, type and frequency of tremors and the presence of ankle clonus. It is not unusual to see tremors and a few beats of clonus in preterm infants. Indwelling thumbs are significant but only when seen in the presence of other abnormal signs. They do occur in the normal population (Dubowitz et al 1999).

Behavioural assessment

The tolerance of babies to handling is very significant. Take time to note their irritability, consolability, pitch of cry, response to visual targets and physiological response to handling. A detailed assessment of this can be made using Brazelton's assessment (Brazelton & Nugent 1995).

SPECIFIC CONDITIONS AND THEIR PRESENTATION

The following section summarizes key points and common problems associated with preterm infants and infants with chronic lung disease. The points below are based on clinical observations of a large number of infants. The list is not exhaustive and not every child will exhibit all the points.

Preterm infants

- Start out in a flattened antigravity posture as muscle tone is not sufficient to overcome gravity. As they approach term age, infants adopt a more flexed posture but a number never develop a typical term newborn posture and appear more extended (Mercuri et al 2003).
- Often present with tremors and some clonus in their ankles: this usually fades after term age
- Can develop shortening of gluteal muscles, which limits internal rotation at the hips, and/or shortening of trapezius muscles, which prevents protraction of the shoulder girdle
- Often have significant flattening of their heads – scaphocephaly
- Often more visually alert than their term counterparts and 'easily bored' as they mature
- Often like being up on their feet and are more likely to become children who walk on their toes.

Chronic lung disease

- Often have poor visual attention, which may be due to oxygen flow around their eyes from nasal prong oxygen
- Often adopt a hyperextended posture with excessive neck extension and arm retraction

- In the early stages weight gain is often not associated with growth so infants appear quite squat. Chest may be quite barrel-shaped
- Respiratory effort is often significant with visible recession
- Development generally slow, even with correction of age due to prematurity. Often make better progress once off nasal oxygen.

Early presentation of cerebral palsy

The early identification of cerebral palsy is not easy. That is why so many assessments exist. Isolated abnormal signs are not associated with a poor outcome. It is more usual for clusters of signs to indicate more significant problems. Prechtl's video assessment at fidgety movement age is a useful adjunct to identification of cerebral palsy. Video the infants at 8–10 weeks postterm, preferably on two separate occasions (Prechtl et al 1997).

DEVELOPMENTAL FOLLOW-UP OF THE HIGH-RISK INFANT

Follow-up is an integral part of the multidisciplinary service offered to children and families who are NICU graduates. It allows for monitoring of progress, timely advice and early referral to appropriate services. Physiotherapists may be involved in developmental follow-up or screening.

Physiotherapy follow-up is determined by the criteria for assessment, i.e. those most at risk of neurodevelopmental problems, by the findings of the assessment and the response to intervention. The frequency of follow-up should be based on the needs of a child and family and on clinical judgement and can range from frequent support immediately following discharge to screening the child at specific ages.

The physiotherapist uses knowledge of typical and atypical development in all domains to assess, monitor, advise, liaise and intervene. Screening and assessment can be aided by the use of standardized tests:

- Alberta Infant Motor Scales (AIMS) is an observational scale of infant motor performance incorporating theoretical concepts of motor development. It assesses the infant's sequential development of motor milestones from term to independent walking (18 months) in four postural positions: prone, supine, sitting and standing. It contains 58 items based on normative data. It is specifically designed to evaluate and treat at-risk infants, identifying atypical motor development (Piper & Darrah 1994)
- Bayley Scales of Infant Development, third edition (BSID-III) is designed to identify children with cognitive and motor delay aged between 1 and 42 months. The tests are administered on an individual basis and are divided into cognitive, language and motor scales. There is also the Bayley Infant Neurodevelopmental

Screener (BINS) for use with infants aged between 3 and 24 months at risk of developmental delay or neurological impairment containing age-specific items from the BSID-II (Bayley 2005)
- Peabody Developmental Motor Scales (PDMS-2) is designed to assess the motor skills of children from birth to 6 years in the following subsets: reflexes, stationary (posture control and equilibrium), locomotion, object manipulation, grasping, visual–motor integration (Folio & Fewell 2000).

Many professionals may be involved with a high-risk infant and their family following discharge from hospital. It is important to liaise closely with all the team members so as not to duplicate roles and put unnecessary demands on the family. Supporting the family means providing the relevant help from the relevant professional at the right time.

INTERVENTION

Early intervention covers the period that a baby is on the NICU through to the first months at home following discharge. You may not be involved in both these settings, or follow-up may be more clinic-based. The key to successful intervention is effective communication with the family and members of the multidisciplinary team.

Principles of intervention

The environment

The NICU is a stressful place as preterm infants are not yet mature enough to cope with the vast difference between the in utero and ex utero environment. A balance must be sought by all the staff on the NICU to provide the necessary life-saving interventions and care as well as creating a peaceful and calm environment in which babies can grow and develop to their full potential.

It is important to consider:

- Low-level lighting and individual lighting for cots
- The reduction of noise levels, especially bins, telephones, voices, ward rounds, alarms and the use of trolleys not incubator tops for care preparation
- Introducing cot covers for incubators to reduce sound and light
- The position of fragile infants away from busy positions in crowded rooms
- Appropriate pain management.

Positioning principles

Positioning is used to support respiration (Chang et al 2002a), minimize postural deformity (Downs et al 1991), promote physiological stability and facilitate self-regulatory strategies (Chang et al 2002b). There is increasing evidence of its effectiveness and importance in both the short and long term (Monterosso et al 2002, 2003).

Table 6.3 Treatment principles

For the unstable preterm infant	For the stabilizing preterm infant
• Minimal handling • Positioning to promote physiological stability • Positioning: respiratory versus developmental • Give boundaries and provide 'nesting' • For medical procedures, ensure adequate pain relief and provide containment. Encourage parental involvement and consider non-nutritive sucking to calm babies • Provide positive touch – not stimulation • Allow rest to grow – lots of it! • Provide families with appropriate booklets – see BLISS, under Contacts	• Infants start tolerating handling better – cues to inform all staff • May need to provide specific advice on head shape/moulding • Encourage kangaroo care: 'skin to skin' • Infants will start establishing feeding – assess ability to feed and non-nutritive sucking • Give specific positioning advice if infants have a strong head preference or there is any muscle tightness due to retraction of shoulders and externally rotated hips
Prior to discharge • It is important to prepare parents for home • Discuss the importance of the 'back to sleep' guidelines • Give advice on positions for play at home • Promote tummy time when the infant is awake • Seating – give advice and demonstrate supported sitting • Car seats – the advice from manufacturers is that no extra support should be placed in a car seat whilst driving. Some units monitor oxygen saturations of an infant in the car seat prior to discharge (American Academy of Pediatrics) • Feeding assessment by a trained speech and language therapist if necessary • Avoid baby walkers and limit the use of baby bouncers	Specific advice for: **Hypoxic–ischaemic encephalopathy (HIE) infants** • Positioning – they tend to push into hyperextension which may be so strong it cannot be contained by preterm positioning devices. Try 'bendy bumpers' which provide resistance or position them with their back against the cot side • Abnormal posturing – difficult to control. Bringing hips into flexion can be more effective in controlling hyperextension than trying to bring the head forward • Swaddling can be effective • Side-lying – soft toy in front, rolled-up towel against cot side behind **Irritable infants** These include some HIE babies, drug-dependent infants withdrawing, and some infants with chronic lung disease • Use a pram – rocking/patting • Swaddling can work • Hammock • Provide background music (not TV!) • Could be bored – try sitting up, visual stimulation • Offer extra parental support – help to arrange time out for parents if necessary

The following principles may be applied to all babies on a NICU. It is essential that these principles are applied to an individual in a way that is appropriate for the gestational age, medical condition and in response to a baby's behavioural cues (Table 6.3). These principles should be widely understood by all staff so on handling everyone returns an infant to a correct position or informs the nursing staff that the baby needs repositioning. Most importantly, once a baby is out of intensive care and is heading for home, the baby must be placed on its back to sleep. All staff must reinforce the importance of this position to parents according to the guidelines regarding sudden infant death syndrome (SIDS) as well as leading by example and placing the child on its back to sleep (Blair et al 2006).

Principles

- Flexion of the spine, legs and arms (but not overflexion of the cervical spine)
- Midline orientation: encourage hands together and prevent excessive hip abduction
- Symmetry: to prevent asymmetry which can become persistent if unchecked
- Containment: to promote physiological stability and emotional security
- Boundaries: this depends on an infant's preference but encourages flexion
- Variety of positions to promote good head shape
- Take into account respiratory versus developmental needs.

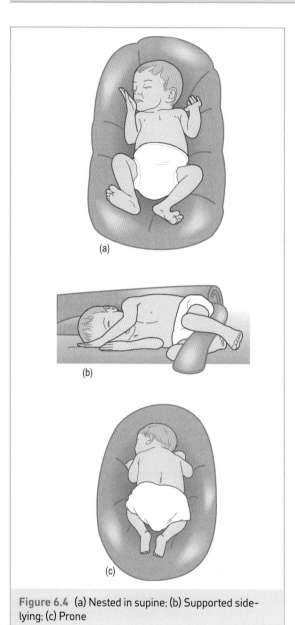

Figure 6.4 (a) Nested in supine; (b) Supported side-lying; (c) Prone

Practicalities

Several companies now produce aids to help position babies effectively but these can be costly. Rolled-up sheets and soft beanbag filled toys can often position babies well. Figure 6.4 gives some examples of good positioning for a baby in intensive care.

Sitting

As infants approach term age they may become more alert for longer periods and able to spend some time in a sitting position. It is not unusual for staff and parents to be anxious

to progress the infants in this way. To reassure all concerned, use a pulse oximeter to measure an infant's response to this change in position. The above positioning principles should be applied and preferably the chair used should have a firm back to prevent too much flexion in the trunk so as not to compromise respiratory effort. Rolled-up sheets make the best positioning aids in this instance.

Care times

These may be clustered to avoid excess handling and to give babies prolonged periods of uninterrupted sleep. Flexi cares make sense as they respond to the needs of the baby rather than set times for cares.

Handling

Handling refers to any process or procedure which involves touching the infant. Handling can be a stressful event, especially for the young, more vulnerable infant. The following principles can be applied in an effort to make handling as gentle and comfortable as possible an experience for the infant:

- Quantity: must be appropriate to the gestational age. Minimal for very fragile infants and increasing with age
- Quality: handling should be slow. Allow the baby periods of rest if the child is very upset with being handled. Offer containment holding to settle a baby during procedures
- Cues: reading a baby's stress signs can help staff understand a baby's behaviour. A more formal means of assessing a baby's behaviour and planning intervention can be learnt using Neonatal Individualized Developmental Care and Assessment Program (NIDCAP: sec Table 6.2)
- A good leaflet to refer parents to is the BLISS leaflet *Handle Me with Care* (see Contacts section, below)
- It is especially important to involve parents in the planning of care for their baby and relating positioning and handling principles to them. Take time to explain about appropriate levels of handling and how this will change, without making parents of a very fragile infant feel that they cannot touch their baby. Parents are often able to identify strategies to help their baby and these can be incorporated into care plans.

Early developmental advice

Your assessment may have identified certain shortfalls in a baby's motor skills or it may be age-appropriate to promote certain skills. You can show parents/carers how to facilitate:

- Pull to sit, to encourage early head control: make sure the head and shoulders are well supported
- Rolling, which can be linked with visual stimulation
- Stretching of shortened gluteal muscles restricting hip adduction and internal rotation

- Use of passive rotations with a baby who lacks trunk rotation can be done with the baby on your knee, or it can be introduced as part of rolling
- Vision and visual experience by promoting use of colour contrast toys and pictures. Before term age some professionals advise pastel colours only. Faces make the best visual aid so show parents how to promote attention with their baby on their lap: babies can fix and follow from as early as 36 weeks gestational age.
- Early communication/interaction
- Prone play.

Skill and competency in handling infants take time and practice. Practical training courses may be available but it is often useful to link up with other local staff to learn together and share experiences. Make use of booklets that are specifically published to help you, the parents and staff (see further reading section, below).

Conclusion

Intervention for the fragile preterm infant or the compromised term infant is a rewarding experience. The foundation work of developing a relationship with families can make a difference to the experience of a child and family, especially those transitioning to other professional services. Make sure their experience at this difficult time is a positive one. Provide good written information for parents and staff and keep records of child outcomes to inform your future practice. Create local networks of therapists interested in neonates and use the Association of Paediatric Chartered Physiotherapists Neonatal Group for peer support.

RESPIRATORY CARE

Introduction

The role of chest physiotherapy for the neonate is changing in response to advances in ventilation and surfactant therapy and in line with current evidence. Historically, chest physiotherapy was carried out routinely and early studies supported frequent treatment. Evidence that linked the incidence of brain lesions with chest physiotherapy led to a decline in the amount of physiotherapy performed. Although the work has since been questioned, it has led to significant changes that have benefited practice.

Preterm infants are extremely fragile and very different to the type of patients you would encounter in adult or even paediatric settings. It is therefore important to have knowledge of neonatal anatomy and lung development, common respiratory conditions and their pathology to treat these infants effectively (see Ch. 5). This section will cover the evidence base for chest physiotherapy, indications, precautions and contraindications for treatment, differences in assessment procedures and application of practical techniques relating to the neonate at different stages of recovery.

Evidence-based practice.

From the 1970s to 1990s chest physiotherapy was performed routinely and often frequently on premature infants with RDS. Observational studies published during this period show an improvement in arterial oxygenation, airway resistance and the number of hypoxaemic episodes after chest physiotherapy (Fox et al 1978, Tudehope 1980, Dall'Alba & Burns 1990). Other studies compared different manual techniques with suction and postural drainage alone and found an increased weight of secretions removed and improved oxygenation in treated infants, concluding that postural drainage combined with percussion were the most effective techniques in this population (Finer et al 1977, Etches & Scott 1978, Finer & Boyd 1978). Advances in practice and methodological issues with these studies mean that cautious generalizations and applications to practice should be made.

In 1998 an article was published by a group in New Zealand linking the incidence of encephaloclastic porencephaly, a bilateral full-thickness cortical necrosis of the brain, with frequent, routine chest physiotherapy in extremely premature and hypotensive infants (Harding et al 1998). This and subsequent investigations led to chest physiotherapy being banned in New Zealand. Similar incidences occurred in Birmingham, UK, but were significantly reduced once the practice of supporting the baby's head during treatment was adopted. A group in Australia found no correlation between chest physiotherapy and neurological damage (Beeby et al 1998), and the original authors have now questioned the link between encephaloclastic porencephaly and chest physiotherapy.

A systematic review of randomized trials suggests that chest physiotherapy may reduce extubation failure (Flenady & Gray 2002), although only if secretion retention is the reason for previous failures (Hudson & Box 2003).

Evidence for saline instillation is inconclusive but has been shown not to alter lung mechanics or cardiovascular parameters in newborns (Shorten et al 1991, Beeram & Dhanireddy 1992). There is no evidence supporting the use of chest physiotherapy to prevent endotracheal tube obstruction or to improve respiratory function, reducing the need for ventilatory support.

Current practice reflects the improvements in ventilatory strategies and medical management of these infants as well as taking into account research findings. Routine or prophylactic physiotherapy is not recommended and treatment is based on careful assessment and clear indications for intervention.

Indications, precautions and contraindications for chest physiotherapy

The following is an amalgamation of information from a variety of texts and articles (Parker 1985, Hough 1992, Prasad & Hussey 1995, Pryor & Prasad 2001, Greenough &

Milner 2003, Harden 2004). The literature is clear about the indications for chest physiotherapy but views on contraindications and precautions differ slightly.

Indications

- Thick, tenacious secretions not removed by suction alone
- Lobar collapse due to mucous plugging.

Precautions

The following should be considered when deciding how to treat an infant:

- In the presence of neonatal rickets, use positioning only
- Side-lying may not be well tolerated in infants with unilateral lung disease due to ventilation/perfusion mismatch
- Care should be taken during manual techniques in very preterm infants where the skin is fragile.

Contraindications

These are contraindications to postural drainage and manual techniques. In the presence of thick secretions but when active chest physiotherapy is contraindicated, consider nonspecific positioning, use of saline and check humidification.

- Very sick unstable infant
- Infants under 1500 g in the first week of life
- Cardiac instability/failure
- Recent IVH (within 24 hours)
- Low platelets ($>50 \times 10^9$/l) or blood-stained secretions obtained from the endotracheal tube
- Abdominal distension/NEC
- Pulmonary haemorrhage
- Early uncomplicated RDS/recent surfactant therapy

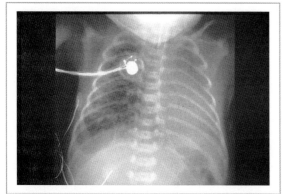

Figure 6.5 Neonatal chest X-ray depicting left-sided respiratory distress syndrome and right-sided pulmonary interstitial emphysema

- Undrained tension pneumothorax
- Pulmonary interstitial emphysema (Figure 6.5)
- Severe hypothermia
- Tracheo- and bronchomalacia
- Recent cranial or eye surgery
- Manual hyperinflation
- Head-down position.

Respiratory assessment and the neonate

Careful assessment is paramount. The physiotherapist must weigh up the benefits of chest physiotherapy against the risks to the infant of handling and intervention.

Principles of respiratory assessment are the same for neonates as for older children (see Ch. 17) but specific attention needs to be given to:

- Antenatal and birth history, including:
  - Administration of antenatal steroids
  - Birth history and resuscitation
  - Administration of artificial surfactant
  - Gestational age
  - Birth weight
  - Apgar score
  - Cord pH.

All of the above factors will give an indication of the condition of the baby, the state of the lungs and the likely pathology.

- Number of days since birth and medical history, including results of cranial ultrasound scans to rule out contraindications to treatment
- Chest X-ray:
  - Note anatomical differences between neonates and older children and adults
  - Check bone density by assessing opacity of ribs
  - Right upper lobe collapse/consolidation commonly seen
  - 'Ground-glass' appearance and air bronchograms are typical of RDS (see Figure 6.5)
  - Irregular honeycomb appearance with small cysts, patchy densities and hyperinflation is consistent with chronic lung disease
- Verbal handover from staff regarding:
  - Tolerance to handling during care times, especially response to suction
  - How long the infant takes to recover from handling
  - Need for preoxygenation.

Staff caring for the baby will know more about the baby's condition. The response to handling will help you weigh up the benefits of chest physiotherapy against the effect of handling on the infant.

- Cardiovascular stability
  - It is important to determine the infant's cardiovascular stability and the trend over time to assess respiratory status and the ability to tolerate treatment

- Neonates often exhibit apnoeas and bradycardias, either of central origin due to immaturity or in response to pathology
- Rule out the effect of a patent ductus arteriosus as this leads to swings in oxygen saturations
- Note that normal cardiovascular parameters for neonates differ from those of older children (see Ch. 17):
- Heart rate (normal = 100–180 beats/min)
- Respiratory rate (normal = 40–60 breaths/min)
- Blood pressure (normal = 60–85/40–50 mmHg)
- Appropriate oxygen saturation (90–96%)
- Blood gas and biochemistry levels
  - Normal values for preterm infants differ from those for term infants and older children
  - Check platelets and alkaline phosphate level to ensure safe levels for carrying out manual techniques
  - Babies with RDS/chronic lung disease can have a raised arterial carbon dioxide, which is normal for them; therefore assess trend over time

Auscultation

- Small babies are difficult to auscultate as sounds are easily transmitted
- If spontaneously breathing, breath sounds are very quiet
- Babies who have copious secretions often sound 'squeaky'
- Use palpation as another means of identifying the presence of secretions

Chest physiotherapy techniques

Techniques used in neonatal care are:

- Modified postural drainage positions
- Non-specific positioning
- Percussion
- Vibrations
- Saline instillation
- Suction.

The application of these techniques is discussed in relation to the unstable preterm infant, the stabilizing preterm infant and the ex-preterm infant later in this section.

Manual hyperinflation is not used as a therapeutic technique due to the risk of pneumothorax and barotrauma and is only used as a mode of resuscitation.

Coordinate treatment with care times or in between care times depending on the infant's tolerance to handling and recovery time. Most infants will be on continuous or bolus feeds. Treat prior to a feed, or, if on continuous feeds, stop the feed prior to treatment, and aspirate the nasogastric tube to minimize the risk of aspiration.

This section is divided into three summarizing practical techniques related to the neonate at different stages (Table 6.4).

The issue of competency

There is disparity between units on the level of service provided and on whether chest clearance techniques are performed by nursing staff or physiotherapists. This is partially related to the type of unit and level of care provided as well as the level of physiotherapy input. Where care is shared between nursing staff and physiotherapists it is important to have a robust education strategy and a competency framework, backed up by evidence-based protocols and guidelines. Where physiotherapists work as lone practitioners, regular peer review and clinical supervision are recommended to maintain clinical competence and provide portfolio evidence.

KEY POINTS

- The physiotherapist's role includes management of respiratory conditions, neurological and behavioural assessment, therapeutic interventions and follow-up of high-risk infants
- Neurological assessments are available to determine follow-up requirements, predict neurological or behavioural outcome, target treatment or measure effects of intervention
- Neurological assessment includes reflex development, posture, muscle tone, behavioural assessment and abnormal signs
- Criteria for assessment and follow-up are based on those most at risk of neurodevelopmental problems
- Early intervention includes environmental modification, advice on positioning, handling and early developmental advice
- The role of chest physiotherapy is changing in response to advances in ventilation and surfactant therapy and in line with current evidence
- Careful assessment is paramount; the benefits of chest physiotherapy must be weighed against the risks to the infant of handling and intervention
- Indications for treatment are secretion retention and lobar collapse to mucous plugging. There are several precautions and contraindications to treatment
- Techniques used are modified postural drainage positions, non-specific positioning, percussion, vibrations, saline instillation and suction

Table 6.4 Chest clearance treatment principles

	Key points
Unstable preterm infant	• Rarely need active treatment as the primary problem is lack of surfactant leading to non-compliant lungs and the need for respiratory support • Premature infants are not routinely paralysed and are on synchronized pressure or volume-controlled ventilation • Ventilators alarm when flow loop is interrupted, indicating when suction is required • Tend not to be productive for first 24–48 hours • Some units use closed-circuit suction to maintain pressures • Often too unstable to tolerate more than minimal handling • High risk of brain haemorrhage in the first week of life **Treatment strategies** • Postural drainage – may not tolerate specific positions due to compliant ribcage; consider head turns or quarter turns from prone or supine. Avoid the head-down position as it impedes venous return and increases the risk of brain haemorrhage • Use non-specific positioning – prone has been shown to stabilize the anterior ribcage and improve ventilation. Some units do not place babies prone if there is an umbilical artery catheter in situ due to the risk of bleeding and babies with distended abdomens/following surgery tend not to tolerate prone or side-lying • In the presence of thick secretions, check humidification, consider use of saline (0.2–0.4 ml dependent on gestation) and increase the frequency of position change and suction • When suctioning, stop the feed and aspirate the nasogastric tube to prevent aspiration of feeds. Ensure correct catheter size and suction pressures (6–8 kPa). Complete the suction in under 10–15 seconds
Stabilizing preterm infant	• More tolerant of handling and more able to maintain physiological stability • May be weaned on to trigger-assisted CPAP or flat CPAP **Treatment strategies** • May be able to tolerate modified postural drainage positions; as before, avoid the head-down position. Only use 1–2 positions at each treatment • Percussion – performed with middle three fingers in a 'tented' position, facemask or specially designed percussors (Figure 6.6). Stabilize the baby's head; often you can also contain the hand. Rest your forearm on the incubator porthole to ensure a relaxed wrist action. Treatment sessions should be short. For example, percuss for 15–30 seconds at a frequency of approximately 2 percussions per second, stopping if the infant becomes unstable. The older, more robust infant may tolerate a longer treatment session, for example percussing for 1–2 minutes • Vibrations – performed on expiration with the pads of 2 or 3 fingers every 2–3 breaths. Fast respiratory rate of the neonate makes this technique more difficult. May also de-recruit alveoli due to tendency of lungs to collapse • Preoxygenation – consider if saturations drop during handling at care times. Oxygen levels are carefully monitored due to the risk of retinopathy of prematurity • Suction, saline and non-specific positioning as before
Extubated ex-preterm infant at term/postterm age	• Most common problem is chronic lung disease leading to oxygen dependency • Not necessarily productive, therefore only treat if indicated • Should be demand feeding unless there is difficulty establishing feeding due to long-term ventilation • Time treatment sessions between feeds **Treatment strategies** • Can tolerate more vigorous treatments for longer • Consider treating on parent's knee • Be careful with the head-down position if the baby has gastro-oesophageal reflux • May need to swaddle if irritable and extending

continued

Table 6.4 *continued*	
	Key points
Role of respiratory care after discharge	• Ex-premature, especially LBW/VLBW infants and those with chronic lung disease, are more at risk of respiratory infections and have a high readmission rate • Rarely require prophylactic treatment at home • Importance of discharge planning, educating parents and preparing for home oxygen as a multidisciplinary team • Many units have designated teams and outreach nurses to monitor infants and support families at home

CPAP, continuous positive airway pressure; LBW, low birth weight; VLBW, very low birth weight.

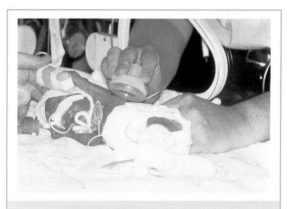

Figure 6.6 Chest physiotherapy. Percussion of a ventilated preterm infant's chest using a face mask

CASE STUDY 6.1

Developmental care case study

Katherine was born at 26 + 2 weeks' gestational age. She required resuscitation at birth and was intubated at 3 minutes of age and given curosurf (a porcine-derived surfactant). She was admitted to the neonatal intensive care unit (NICU) and has remained ventilated since birth. Following discussion with the nursing staff she was assessed with her parents present on day 5 of life.

Both the parents and nursing staff reported that she was still quite unstable and did not tolerate care-giving well, although the parents felt she settled when they offered her their finger to hold or if they contained her by cupping her head. On examination she was positioned in supine, was nested in a rolled-up sheet but was displaying frantic, diffuse movements. Her skin was a mottled colour and her saturation monitor was alarming. She was repositioned in side-lying, nested and contained using positioning aids and covered by a blanket.

Almost immediately her colour and oxygen saturations improved and movements became more coordinated as she was able to bring her hands together and towards her face.

Over the next days and weeks the physiotherapist continued to review and to advise on positioning and handling. She met with the parents occasionally and left advice for all the staff looking after Katherine on a chart attached to the hood of the incubator.

When she was 34 weeks corrected age (after 8 weeks on the NICU), she was assessed more formally using the Dubowitz assessment chart. (Dubowitz et al 1999). This showed that she was beginning to develop some good flexor tone in her arms and legs, bringing her knees up and able to bring her hands to her face. She was also developing a

continued

good suck, which the parents and nursing staff were encouraging by introducing both breast and bottle feeds. Her movements at times remained slightly frantic and she could appear quite upset, especially after feeds. She had a lot of wind,which her mum found difficult to get up. The physiotherapist showed parents some different positions in which to hold Katherine to help soothe her tummy and introduced some gentle massage techniques to aid digestion. She was reassessed at 36 weeks' gestational age and showed continuing development of flexor tone and greater visual awareness. Parents were shown how to position Katherine when she was alert and awake to encourage her ability to follow faces.

Parents were also given advice about early development and play and the importance of the 'back to sleep' campaign prior to discharge. She went home at 37 weeks corrected age, with delighted but anxious parents.

It was arranged for her to be seen in follow clinic at 3 months corrected age because, despite her good progress, ability to feed well and the fact that her head scan showed no abnormality, it is preferable to keep contact in case any problems evolve, which is possible over the first 12 months or so. However Katherine made good progress. Parents were taught some more massage techniques, which was something all the family benefited from. She was walking at 14 months corrected age and is into everything!

CASE STUDY 6.2

Respiratory case study

Jacob was born at 28 + 6 weeks' gestation. He weighed 1.44 kg and, although he required no resuscitation at delivery, he was on nasal continuous positive airway pressure for 4 days and placed in an incubator. During this time the nurses changed his position regularly, providing necessary support and containment. His parents spent long periods of the day helping the nurses care for him and bringing him out of the incubator for skin-to-skin cuddles. However, 23 days after he was born he deteriorated and was intubated with a nasal 3.5 mm endotracheal tube. The physiotherapist was asked to assess Jacob as his X-ray showed a right-sided consolidation over and above appearances consistent with a mild respiratory distress syndrome. There was mild uniform haziness with an air bronchogram.

The nursing staff reported that he tolerated handling well during care times, including suction, and did not require preoxygenation for suction or cares (he was only handled about every 3–4 hours for mouth and nappy care and for change of position and any medical intervention). However, they only removed a small quantity of secretions when performing suction.

On his first assessment the ventilator was on synchronized intermittent positive-pressure ventilation with airway pressures of 24/4 mmHg, a rate of 70 breaths/min and oxygen concentration of 35%. His heart rate was 150 beats/min, his respiratory rate was raised to 70 breaths/min and his oxygen saturations were 93%, an appropriate level. These readings had been stable over the last 24 hours. His temperature was 37.1°C. His last capillary gas was as follows: pH = 7.18, Po_2 = 4.2, Pco_2 = 10.7, HCo_3 = 23.6, base excess = 1.3. This suggested a sudden increase in Pco_2 and a drop in pH.

His most recent biochemistry was: platelets = 492, alkaline phosphate = 356, haemoglobin = 12.4, C-reactive protein <7, white cell count = 18.6. His fluid balance was not calculated.

The chest X-ray from that morning showed a right upper and lower zone shadowing with loss of diaphragmatic angles.

When the physiotherapist examined Jacob just before his 11 a.m. care, chest expansion was equal on the right and left but on auscultation there were decreased breath sounds on the right with no added sounds.

With the assistance of the nurse looking after him, Jacob was turned into left side-lying and percussion was performed to the right side twice for brief bursts of 30 seconds. He tolerated this well without desaturating. Suction was performed via the nasotracheal tube using 0.25 ml saline (0.9%), which removed moderate amounts of loose secretions with plugs of thick yellow secretions.

After treatment the physiotherapist reported increased breath sounds on right and the medical staff were able to wean ventilator pressures and oxygen over the next 2 days. Later that day the nursing staff repeated the treatment in conjunction with his care giving following the instructions of the physiotherapist. On day 26 he was extubated and made good progress, requiring no further respiratory care. He was discharged home with his parents when he was still 4 weeks early but he was feeding well and gaining weight.

REFERENCES

Als H, Lester BM, Brazelton TB et al. 1994 Individualized developmental care for the very low-birth-weight preterm infant. Medical and neurofunctional effects. *Journal of the American Medical Association* 272: 853–858.

Als H, Duffy FH, McAnulty GB 1996 Effectiveness of individualized neurodevelopmental care in the newborn intensive care unit. *Acta Paediatrica Supplement* 416: 21–30.

Amiel-Tison C 1995 Clinical assessment of the infant nervous system. In: Levene MI, Lilford RJ (eds) *Fetal and Neonatal Neurology and Neurosurgery*, 3rd edn. Edinburgh: Churchill Livingstone, pp. 83–104.

Bayley N 2005 *Bayley Scales of Infant and Toddler Development*, 3rd edn. San Antonio, TX: Harcourt Assessment.

Beeby PJ, Henderson-Smart DJ, Lacey JL, Rieger I 1998 Short- and long-term neurological outcomes following neonatal chest physiotherapy. *Journal of Paediatrics and Child Health* 34: 60–62.

Beeram MR, Dhanireddy R 1992 Effects of saline instillation during tracheal suction on lung mechanics in newborn infants. *Journal of Perinatology* 12: 120–123.

Blair PS, Platt MW, Smith IJ, Fleming PJ and the CESDI SUDI Research Group 2006 Sudden infant death syndrome and sleeping position in pre-term and low birth weight infants: an opportunity for targeted intervention. *Archives of Disease in Childhood* 91: 101–106.

Brazelton TB, Nugent JK 1995 *Neonatal Behavioral Assessment Scale*, 3rd edn. Cambridge: Mac Keith Press.

Chang YJ, Anderson GC, Dowling D, Lin CH 2002a Decreased activity and oxygen desaturation in prone ventilated preterm infants during the first postnatal week. *Heart and Lung* 31: 34–42.

Chang YJ, Anderson GC, Lin CH 2002b Effects of prone and supine positions on sleep state and stress responses in mechanically ventilated preterm infants during the first postnatal week. *Journal of Advanced Nursing* 40: 161–169.

Dall'Alba P, Burns Y 1990 The relationship between arterial blood gases and removal of airway secretions in neonates. *Physiotherapy Theory and Practice* 6: 107–116.

Downs JA, Edwards AD, McCormick DC, Roth SC, Stewart AL 1991 Effect of intervention on development of hip posture in very preterm babies *Archives of Disease in Childhood* 66: 797–801.

Dubowitz L, Mercuri E, Dubowitz V 1998 An optimality score for the neurologic examination of the term newborn. *Journal of Pediatrics* 133: 406–416.

Dubowitz LM, Dubowitz V, Mercuri E 1999 *The Neurological Assessment of the Preterm and Full-Term Newborn Infant*, 2nd edn. London: Mac Keith Press.

Einspieler C, Prechtl HF, Bos AF, Ferrari F, Cioni G 2004 *Prechtl's Method on the Qualitative Assessment of General Movements in Preterm, Term and Young Infants*. Cambridge: Mac Keith Press.

Etches P, Scott B 1978 Chest physiotherapy in the newborn: effect on secretions removed. *Pediatrics* 62: 713–715.

Finer N, Boyd J 1978 Chest physiotherapy in the neonate: a controlled study. *Pediatrics* 61: 282–285.

Finer N, Grace M, Boyd J 1977 Chest physiotherapy in the neonate with respiratory distress. *Pediatric Research* 11: 570.

Flenady VJ, Gray PH 2002 Chest physiotherapy for preventing morbidity in babies being extubated from mechanical ventilation. *Cochrane Database of Systematic Reviews*. Oxford: Update Software.

Folio MR, Fewell RR 2000 *Peabody Developmental Motor Scales (PDMS-2)*, 2nd edn. Oxford: Harcourt Assessment.

Fox W, Schwartz J, Shaffer T 1978 Pulmonary physiotherapy in neonates: physiological changes and respiratory management. *Journal of Pediatrics* 92: 977–981.

Greenough A, Milner R 2003 *Neonatal Respiratory Disorders*. London: Arnold.

Hack M, Fanaroff AA 1999 Outcomes of children of extremely low birthweight and gestational age in the 1990s. *Early Human Development* 53: 193–218.

Hack M, Klein N, Taylor HG 1996 School-age outcomes of children of extremely low birthweight and gestational age. *Seminars in Neonatology* 1: 277–288.

Han TR, Bang MS, Lim JY, Yoon BH, Kim IW 2002 Risk factors of cerebral palsy in preterm infants. *American Journal of Physical Medicine and Rehabilitation* 81: 297–303.

Harden B 2004 *Emergency Physiotherapy*. London: Churchill Livingstone.

Harding JE, Miles FK, Becroft DM, Allen BC, Knight DB 1998 Chest physiotherapy may be associated with brain damage in extremely premature infants. *Journal of Pediatrics* 132: 440–444.

Hough A 1992 *Physiotherapy in Respiratory Care*. London: Chapman & Hall.

Hudson RM, Box RC 2003 Neonatal respiratory therapy in the new millennium: does clinical practice reflect scientific evidence? *Australian Journal of Physiotherapy* 49: 269–272.

Lacey JL, Henderson-Smart DJ 1998 Assessment of preterm infants in the intensive-care unit to predict cerebral palsy and motor outcome at 6 years. *Developmental Medicine and Child Neurology* 40: 310–318.

Macfarlane A, Mugford M, Henderson J 1999 *Birth Counts. Statistics of Pregnancy and Childbirth*, 2nd edn. London: Stationery Office Books.

Mercuri E, Guzzetta A, Laroche S et al 2003 Neurological examination of preterm infants at term age: comparison with full term infants. *Journal of Pediatrics* 142: 647–655.

Monterosso L, Kristjanson L, Cole J 2002 Neuromotor development and the physiologic effects of positioning in very low birth weight infants. *Journal of Obstetric, Gynecologic, and Neonatal Nursing* 31: 138–146.

Monterosso L, Kristjanson LJ, Cole J, Evans SF 2003 Effect of postural supports on neuromotor function in very preterm infants to term equivalent age. *Journal of Paediatrics and Child Health* 39: 197–205.

Parker AE 1985 Chest physiotherapy in the neonatal intensive care unit. *Physiotherapy* 71: 63–65.

Pharoah PO, Cooke T, Johnson MA, King R, Mutch L 1998 Epidemiology of cerebral palsy in England and Scotland, 1984–9. *Archives of Disease in Childhood: Fetal and Neonatal Edition* 79: F21–F25.

Piper MC, Darrah J 1994 *Motor Assessment of the Developing Infant*. Philadelphia, PA: WB Saunders.

Prasad SA, Hussey J 1995 *Paediatric Respiratory Care*. London: Chapman and Hall.

Prechtl HF 1977 *The Neurological Examination of the Full-Term Newborn Infant*, 2nd edn. London: SIMPS/Heinemann Medical.

Prechtl HF, Einspieler C, Cioni G, Bos AF, Ferrari F, Sontheimer D 1997 An early marker for neurological deficits after perinatal brain lesions. *Lancet* 349: 1361–1363.

Pryor J, Prasad SA 2001 *Physiotherapy for Respiratory and Cardiac Problems*, 3rd edn. London: Churchill Livingstone.

Shorten DR, Byrne PJ, Jones RL 1991 Infant responses to saline instillations and endotracheal suctioning. *Journal of Obstetric, Gynaecologic and Neonatal Nursing* 20: 464–469.

Tudehope D 1980 Techniques of physiotherapy in intubated babies with respiratory distress syndrome. *Australian Pediatric Journal* 16: 226–228.

FURTHER READING

Intervention

Bly L 1994 *Motor Skills Acquisition in the First Year of Life*. Tucson, AZ, USA: Therapy Skill Builders (Psychological Corporation).

Cregar PJ 1989 *Developmental Interventions for Preterm and High-Risk Infants. Self-Study Modules for Professional*. Tucson, AZ, USA: Therapy Skill Builders (Psychological Corporation).

Finnie N 1997 *Handling the Young Child with Cerebral Palsy at Home*. Oxford: Butterworth-Heinemann.

Developmental

Sheridan M 1997 *From Birth to Five Years*. London: Routledge.

Parents

Bond C *Massage, A Silent Dialogue*. Arrohill.

Bradford N 2000 *Your Premature Baby 0–5 years*. London: Francis Lincoln.

Segal M 1999 *Your Child at Play*. London: Ebury Press.

Contacts

BLISS, 68 South Lambeth Road, London SW8 1RL. Telephone: 020 7820 9471. Fax: 020 7820 9567. e-mail: information@bliss.org.uk.

Neonatal SIG (subgroup of the APCP) can be contacted via APCP or www.interactivecsp.org.uk.

Parent Support Helpline freephone: 0500 618140 Monday to Friday 10 a.m.–5 p.m.

7 Cerebral palsy

Teresa Pountney

INTRODUCTION

In 1862, Little described spastic diplegia resulting from birth asphyxia and brain damage. However, Sigmund Freud suggested that infantile cerebral paralysis was caused by prenatal abnormalities, with birth asphyxia being a marker for, rather than a cause of, brain dysfunction (Pellegrino 1995). Little's views were widely accepted until the last 25 years, during which epidemiological studies have refuted the causation of cerebral palsy by birth trauma and asphyxia.

Greater understanding of genetic and other constitutional disorders has led to a change in the 'brain damage' model. This had been applied to a wide range of developmental disabilities ranging from cerebral palsy to mental retardation, learning disabilities and attention-deficit hyperactivity disorder. Although there was little proof of actual brain damage, there was an assumption that a milder degree of birth asphyxia or other brain-damaging event had resulted in a milder form of impairment. Cerebral palsy is now more commonly used as a description of the disability suffered due to an unspecified deficit rather than of the impairment itself.

A similar situation occurs with the less severe motor impairments seen as part of a generalized neurological dysfunction, such as in disorders of learning motor control and attention (see Ch. 9). These are now classified in the *Diagnostic and Statistical Manual of Mental Disorders* (American Psychiatric Association 2000) by descriptions of observable behaviour rather than by aetiology.

The lifestyle and opportunities available to people with cerebral palsy have improved remarkably and many adults live independent, though supported, lives and contribute to society through employment and further education. Legislation such as Special Education Needs Code of Practice and Disability Discrimination gives children with cerebral palsy a right to mainstream education, to be accepted by their peers, included in holidays and outings, and to take part in competitive games. Advances in technology have also made a significant contribution to increased independence, particularly in the areas of mobility and communication (see Ch. 10).

Since cerebral palsy and motor learning disorders have different aetiologies, manifestations and management, they will be addressed in separate chapters (see Ch. 9).

DEFINITION AND DIAGNOSIS

Cerebral palsy is 'an umbrella term covering a group of non-progressive, but often changing, motor impairment syndromes, secondary to lesions or anomalies of the brain arising in the early stages of its development' (Mutch et al 1992).

A diagnosis of cerebral palsy should not be made unless the motor disorder is obvious in comparison to other findings, such as developmental delay. This excludes most children with clumsiness and also children with a severe degree of learning difficulties and motor signs such as mild spasticity or mild hypotonia.

AETIOLOGY AND INCIDENCE

Until the early 1980s there were consistent reports of rises in the prevalence amongst live births of cerebral palsy and of its severity, particularly amongst preterm infants. These rises were accounted for largely by improvements in survival rate, since the incidence of low birth weight and the birth weight-specific prevalence rates of cerebral palsy amongst birth weights of 2500 g or more seem to be remaining largely stable. Recent data suggest that the rates of cerebral palsy are falling in very-low-birth-weight and very preterm infants (Hagberg et al 2001, Topp et al 2001). Data are documented from the UK, Western Australia and Sweden, which show a consistent trend from low to high cerebral palsy rates as birth weight falls. Within countries in the low-birth-weight populations, there is a trend to higher rates of cerebral palsy as mortality falls. The birth weight-specific prevalence of cerebral palsy in the highest-weight groups seems to remain stable within each population, despite falling mortality levels.

Some speculation still exists regarding the causes of cerebral palsy, largely because the expected drop in cases as obstetric care improved has not occurred. This has led to investigations that indicate there is a greater correlation between abnormalities during pregnancy and cerebral palsy than abnormalities during labour with cerebral palsy (Hagberg & Hagberg 1996). Birth asphyxia accounts for approximately 10% of all cases with cerebral palsy and only a small number of these are due to poor obstetric care (Rosenbloom 1995, Stanley et al 2000). Infrared and magnetic resonance imaging indicate that the normal infant withstands considerable hypoxia during a normal labour and delivery without ill-effect, suggesting that infants who suffer damage may have a pre-existing condition making them vulnerable to hypoxia (Stanley et al 2000).

Two 25-year studies of the changing epidemiology of cerebral palsy have shown a startling rise in the incidence of cerebral palsy amongst low- and very-low-birth-weight infants (Hagberg & Hagberg 1996, Pharoah & Cooke 1996). Such preterm infants now account for 50% of all cases of cerebral palsy compared to 32% at the start of the studies and are now considered to be the strongest predictor of cerebral palsy in newborn infants with a 30-fold increase in risk (see Ch. 6).

The developing brain of a foetus is a vulnerable organ; damage to it prior to birth is often dependent on the timing and type of insult, as well as the predilection of certain brain areas to certain types of insult (Stanley et al 2000). These include hypoxia, vascular accidents, infections and toxicity. Pre- and periconceptional causes include familial or genetic influences, teratogens, such as the viral infections of toxoplasmosis, rubella, cytomegalovirus and herpes simplex virus (TORCH), foetal malformation syndromes, iodine deficiency and consanguinity (Stanley et al 2000).

Multiple pregnancies are increasing within the developed countries and the higher rates of cerebral palsy reflect this increase (Pharoah et al 1996, Stanley et al 2000). Multiple pregnancy increases the risk of cerebral palsy to 4.5 times in a twin and to 18.2 times in a triplet pregnancy compared to singleton births (Stanley et al 2000). The reasons for this increase include placental malformations, foetal growth and birth weight, intrapartum factors and co-fetal death. A proportion of affected children have lost a twin perinatally or in utero (Pharoah et al 1996).

Cerebral palsy is also acquired postnatally in a significant number of cases, usually within the first year of life, the primary causes being cerebral infection, acquired brain injury and infantile spasms (Stanley et al 2000).

The changing aetiology of cerebral palsy has resulted in a changing pattern in the presentation of the condition, including increasing levels of visual impairment, eating and drinking difficulties, sleep disturbance and types of epilepsy.

CLASSIFICATION

It is traditional and clinically useful to classify cerebral palsy according to its type, distribution and severity. Type is categorized according to the impairment: spastic, dyskinetic, ataxic and hypotonic. Where a mixture of types is seen in one child, the classification will be made on the predominating form (McCarthy 1992). Approximately 70% of children with cerebral palsy have spasticity, 20–25% have dyskinesia and the remaining 5–10% have ataxia (McCarthy 1992).

The classical distribution of symptoms is:

1. Hemiplegia – one side of the body is primarily involved
2. Diplegia – the lower half of the body is primarily involved
3. Quadriplegia – the entire body is involved.

Common presentations include:

- **Spastic quadriplegia** – where a child has all four limbs involved with a mixture of spasticity and dyskinesia. Children in this group are usually at the severe end of motor disability and cannot sit or walk independently, and have little coordinated movement of their arms and hands.
- **Spastic diplegia** – where there is increased tone in the legs but little or no involvement in the arms. This group can usually walk with or without aids but tend to adopt a 'W' kneeling posture in preference to long sitting.
- **Spastic hemiplegia** is characterized by spasticity in the arm, leg and trunk on one side of the body. Most children walk independently but there is a wide variation in the function of the affected arm and hand.

Severity of cerebral palsy can be classified according to the Gross Motor Function Classification System (GMFCS). This is a five-level system, which ranks children according to the severity of motor involvement based on age, motor ability and use of assistive technology (Palisano et al 1997). The system is useful for both clinicians and families to determine a child's prognosis. It enables realistic expectations for future functional activity to be determined and the provision of appropriate treatment and assistive technology.

NATURAL HISTORY

The natural history of cerebral palsy has been documented by several authors, including Crothers & Paine (1988) and Freud (1968), who present a picture of a child generally below normal size, with poor motor and cognitive skills and beset by deformities of joints and bones. The initial neurological lesion a child sustains, which causes the cerebral palsy, in fact remains, by definition, unchanged throughout life (Griffiths & Clegg 1988). However, the effects of this lesion on other systems, including musculoskeletal and digestive systems, can be more debilitating than the original insult if left untreated.

There are associated complications of cerebral palsy, which include epilepsy, visual impairment, musculoskeletal deformities, growth delay, sleep disturbance and reduced life expectancy.

Epilepsy occurs frequently in children with cerebral palsy, with a higher incidence in children with quadriplegia than those with dyskinesia and spastic diplegia, especially preterm infants. Between 50 and 90% of children with quadriplegia experience seizures (Aicardi 1990). Epilepsy is linked with an increased risk of sensory impairment and cognitive impairment. Damage to the brain only occurs if seizures are prolonged or as a result of infantile spasms in the first year of life (Aicardi 1990). Seizures of this nature are often accompanied by developmental regression.

Most children with cerebral palsy experience some disorder of their sensory system, the most common of which is visual impairment (see below). Sensory deficits, which have a profound impact on movement coordination, are also found in the proprioceptive and tactile systems. Diminished anticipatory control and impaired tactile regulation in reaching and grasping objects have been demonstrated in children with cerebral palsy (Eliasson et al 1995). These studies suggest that children with cerebral palsy have a diminished ability to build internal models of objects and movement patterns, and may require additional environmental cues to execute movement successfully. This is reflected in the improved performance of children who are asked to undertake concrete rather than abstract tasks, e.g. raising the arm to shoulder height or reaching for a ball (van der Weel et al 1991).

Visual impairment in children with cerebral palsy is estimated at between 7 and 9%. Visual impairments can result from abnormalities of the eye but are more commonly a result of lesions in the retrochiasmatic visual pathway or the perceptual and processing areas of the brain responsible for visual stimuli (Guzzetta et al 2001). Visual impairment has an important role in motor development, particularly the acquisition of trunk and head control (Sonksen et al 1984).

It is commonly recognized that, as a group, children with severe cerebral palsy are considerably below the normal growth curves for height and weight. Nutritional problems in children with cerebral palsy are well recognized and can result in a failure to thrive and chronic ill health (Stallings et al 1993, Krick et al 1996). Nutritional factors and ability to walk have been shown to be significant factors in decreased bone mineral density in these children, making bones vulnerable to fracture (Henderson et al 1995).

The main causes of this growth delay are problems with the facial and bulbar muscles, making chewing and swallowing difficult, often requiring extended periods for eating amounting to several hours daily and constipation. Reflux may also occur, which can result in aspiration and consequent chest infection (Rogers et al 1994). Gastrostomy insertions to provide enteral feeding have improved the nutritional status of many children and relieved carers and children of the time-consuming task of eating (Bachlet et al 2002).

There is a high frequency of sleep disturbance in children with cerebral palsy and this has been attributed to a number of causes, including sleep hypoxaemia, upper-airway obstruction, decreased melatonin levels, nocturnal seizures, reflux and positional discomfort (Khan et al 1996). Hypoxaemia is probably due to brainstem dysfunction and upper-airway obstruction from hypertrophy of the tonsils and adenoids, and both are implicated in night wakening (Khan et al 1996). Children with visual impairment due to malformation of the eyes or abnormalities and malformations of the sleep centres in the brain may experience dysfunction of melatonin release, which regulates sleep onset and can in some cases be treated by exogenous melatonin (Hung et al 1998). Behavioural aspects may also cause sleep disturbance; anxious parents may find it difficult to set limits and boundaries in teaching good sleep hygiene (Dodge & Wilson 2001). Sleep is a learned neurological process and relates to the interpretation of environmental cues, e.g. sunlight, noise and social interactions, so where interpretation is difficult there will be a higher likelihood of sleep problems (Jan & Freeman 2004).

The life expectancy of children with cerebral palsy has been investigated in two well-researched studies by Crichton et al (1995) and Evans et al (1990), which both found high survival rates of around 90% into their teens and twenties. Immobility and severe learning difficulties were cited as the main factors influencing survival. Evans et al's study (1990) concluded that 'cerebral palsy is a condition with which one lives rather than a condition from which one dies' and that long-term planning is realistic to meet the needs of this group as adults.

As previously described, the GMFCS can be used as a guide to likely gross motor progress in children with cerebral palsy to help families and clinicians to prepare for the future (Rosenbaum et al 2002). The GMFCS is based on a population study of over 600 children whose gross motor function has been recorded over time. The GMFCS can be used to select appropriate interventions and identify the need for assistive technology and required environmental alterations. This scale measures only gross motor ability and was found not to reflect on a child's experience of pain or emotional state, as is sometimes assumed (Kennes et al 2002).

MUSCULOSKELETAL DEFORMITIES IN DIFFERENT TYPES OF CEREBRAL PALSY

The neurological lesion will slow the development of typical patterns of movement, often resulting in the adoption of asymmetrical postures and limited ranges of joint motion. Deformities can be classified either as postural, resulting from increased or decreased muscle tone, or positional, resulting from adopting habitual postures. Postural and positional deformities influence the muscle and bone to develop in different ways, resulting in imbalances in muscle groups, deformities of joints and bones, and often low bone mineral density in children unable to walk independently (Henderson et al 1995). The development of deformity is largely related to the child's motor activity, and consequently different distributions and type of cerebral palsy result in different patterns of deformities. The treatment and management of these deformities are through the use of hands-on therapy, postural management equipment, orthotics, botulinum toxin and surgery. These approaches and their use and efficacy will be described later in this chapter.

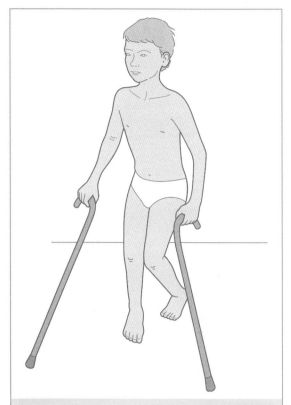

Figure 7.1 Diplegic gait with internal rotation, knee hyperextension and lack of heel strike.

Hemiplegia

Nearly all children with hemiplegia walk independently. However they often experience underdevelopment of the affected side, which results in smaller limbs and can result in leg shortening. Equinus of the foot and ankle, flexion of the elbow, wrist and fingers and adducted thumb are classical deformities of the child with hemiplegia.

Spastic diplegia

The deformities most commonly associated with spastic diplegia are contractures of the hip flexors and adductors and the hamstrings, and internal rotation of the hip and femoral anteversion. Most of this group of children walk independently and these deformities develop as a result of the crouch gait adopted by many children with spastic diplegia due to spasticity in the hip adductors and flexors, hamstrings and calf muscles. Children in this group may alternatively develop hyperextension of the knee to compensate for tight tendo-achilles (Figure 7.1). Kyphosis may develop as a sequela to tight hamstrings or hyperlordosis as a compensatory balance mechanism.

Quadriplegic cerebral palsy

The deformities seen in children and adults with quadriplegic cerebral palsy include the deformities described above but, in addition, many develop dislocation of their hip joints and spinal curvature (Scrutton & Baird 1997, Scrutton et al 2001). Hip subluxation or dislocation can cause significant morbidity in terms of pain and difficulty with postural control, creating limitations in sitting, standing and walking, and hygiene and personal care considerations. An association between hip dislocation and spinal curvature is well documented and children with a windswept deformity of the hip and pelvis, where the hip is subluxated or dislocated and the pelvis rests in obliquity and rotation, present as a precursor to spinal curvature (Letts et al 1984, Kalen et al 1992, Porter 2004).

In the group of children who do not walk independently, approximately 60% of this group will have one or both hips dislocated by age 5 years (Scrutton & Baird 1997, Scrutton et al 2001). It is recognized that dislocation continues to occur well into adolescence (Miller & Bagg 1992). Scrutton & Baird (1997) offered a protocol for the surveillance of hips in young children, which recommends

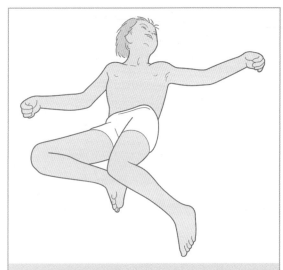

Figure 7.2 Posture showing pelvic asymmetry with subluxation of the left hip.

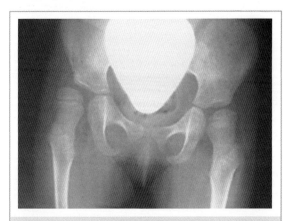

Figure 7.3 Hip and pelvic X-ray showing dislocation of the right hip.

a baseline X-ray at 30 months to determine risk (Figures 7.2 and 7.3).

Spinal curvature occurs in up to 70% of children with bilateral cerebral palsy, being most prevalent in those with quadriplegia. It is debilitating in terms of sitting stability, pain, pressure problems and respiration. Scoliosis is the most common curve seen but kyphosis and hyperlordosis are also common. Rotatory elements are present in many spinal curves and combinations of curve patterns, such as kyphosco-liosis, are frequently present. Spinal curvature can occur from a very young age and continue to progress well into adulthood, with individuals with the spastic form of cerebral palsy at greatest risk (Lonstein 1995, Saito et al 1998).

PAIN

Children and adults with cerebral palsy experience pain arising from, among others, musculoskeletal, gastrointestinal, muscle and respiratory sources. Its identification is essential to ensure that the pain is managed appropriately. Pain resulting from musculoskeletal deformities is common. Two large studies (93 and 234 participants) have investigated pain levels in adolescents and adults with cerebral palsy by interview and standardized pain questionnaires to identify sites and duration of pain. Hip pain was reported by 39% and 47% of interviewees respectively persisting over 20 years and consistent with sites of surgical interventions (Schwartz et al 1999, Hodgkinson et al 2001). Lower-limb and back pain were the most common areas where pain was experienced and in Schwartz et al's study 67% of their subjects had had pain in one or more areas for durations greater than 3 months.

A number of methods of measuring pain are now available and vary according to an individual's ability to communicate pain. Many children are able to self-report and scales such as the Brief Pain Inventory (Cleeland & Ryan 1994) and Faces scale (Wong & Baker 1988) can be used. Children who are unable to self-report are dependent on their care-giver's observational skills to recognize pain cues and determine a child's level of pain. The Paediatric Pain Profile is a valid and reliable tool for assessing pain in children with severe neurological and cognitive impairments (Hunt et al 2004).

MEDICATIONS

Medications are frequently used in children with bilateral cerebral palsy to control epilepsy, reflux and high muscle tone.

Anticonvulsants

Epilepsy is not necessarily a long-term condition and treatment with anticonvulsant therapy, such as carbamazepine or sodium valproate, is usually effective and many add-on medications are available to improve control. Surgical treatment is now an option for intractable seizures (Aicardi 1990). Damage only occurs if seizures are prolonged or as a result of infantile spasms. The use of anticonvulsants is a complex balance between controlling seizures and causing adverse side-effects.

Antiemetics

Antiemetics are used to control gastric reflux and are considered the first line of control for this problem.

MANAGEMENT OF SPASTICITY

Spasticity is one of the positive signs of upper motor neurone syndromes and persists as a focus for treatment, despite recent findings identifying the main problems in children with cerebral palsy related to the negative signs of weakness, fatigue and incoordination. Botulinum toxin and intrathecal baclofen (ITB) are two of the most frequently used medications for controlling spasticity.

Botulinum toxin

Botulinum toxins are protein products of the *Clostridium botulinum* bacterium, which are taken up by endocytosis at the cholinergic nerve terminals blocking release of synaptic vesicles. This effectively blocks the action of the synapse at the neuromuscular junction for several months until a new neuromuscular junction is established (Cosgrove et al 1994). Botulinum toxin in children with bilateral cerebral palsy is used to reduce increased tone for a period of time in selected muscles, to enable the establishment of new movement patterns and the reduction of contractures (Cosgrove et al 1994). Carr et al (1998) recommend criteria for patient selection, dosage, administration and likely long-term effects. This approach has gained popularity and has shown encouraging short-term results for improving gait in children with spastic hemiplegia and diplegia, improving upper-limb function and the management of hip pain (Koman et al 2000, Ubhi et al 2000, Baker et al 2002, Fairhurst 2004, Deleplanque et al 2002, Metaxiotis et al 2002, Speth et al 2005, Wasiak et al 2004). In terms of gait re-education there is some benefit in function in the short term but there is limited evidence of its long-term effect (Ubhi et al 2000, Ade-Hall et al 2002, Reddihough et al 2002, Gough et al 2005). Studies on upper-limb function are similarly inconclusive, showing very few significant changes (Wasiak et al 2004, Speth et al 2005). There have been few studies on the use of botulinum toxin for controlling hip migration and pain but three small studies found a reduction in pain and some increase in the Gross Motor Function Measure (GMFM) postinjection (Mall et al 2000, Deleplanque et al 2002, Fairhurst 2004).

The effect of botulinum toxin is to weaken the muscle and some researchers consider this to mask spasticity (Gough et al 2005). Recent studies on muscle fibres and exercise suggest that weakness may have a greater impact on a child's impairment than spasticity and some consider that interventions which further weaken muscles may be detrimental (Wiley & Damiano 1998, Shortland et al 2002, Fry et al 2004).

Baclofen

Baclofen, which can be taken orally or intrathecally, is one of the main pharmacological treatments for spasticity

and acts to inhibit the GABA-B receptors in the spinal cord by blocking the excitatory effect of sensory input (Ivanhoe et al 2001). Oral doses of baclofen can have side-effects, including drowsiness, which can outweigh its benefits.

Intrathecal baclofen (ITB) is increasing in popularity as it is thought to be more effective. The implantation of an ITB pump allows small doses to be used with greater effect and fewer side-effects. ITB aims to reduce levels of spasticity and improve range and ease of movement. Other effects include improved sleep, seating and nursing care. To date there is limited research evidence of the usefulness of ITB but several studies have reported improvement in GMFM scores, decrease in the Ashworth scale and perceived changes in motor control and positioning (Krach et al 2005).

SURGICAL AND ORTHOPAEDIC MANAGEMENT

The musculoskeletal deformities which can result from different types of cerebral palsy have been mentioned earlier. Every effort should be made to prevent the development of these deformities by conservative methods, but in many cases orthopaedic surgery is required at some point to alleviate deformities. Collaboration between paediatricians, therapists and surgeons is needed to ensure that there is an integrated approach to the management of deformities in children with cerebral palsy, which may involve the use of postural management equipment, botulinum toxin injections and surgery (Pountney & Green 2006). Low bone mineral density is common in children and young people with moderate and severe forms of cerebral palsy in whom walking is compromised, resulting in a high fracture rate (Henderson et al 1995). Up to 40% of non-ambulant children with spastic quadriplegia showed a history of documented previous fractures (King et al 2003). Other factors also contribute to low bone density, including poor nutritional intake, anticonvulsant medication, stiff joints and poor balance, leading to falls and violent seizures (Henderson and Madsen 1999, Henderson et al 2002).

If a fracture occurs, immobilization due to casting or postoperative treatment creates in turn the risk of further demineralization and substantially diminishes the quality of life for these children (Henderson 1997). New treatments for low bone mineral density in children with cerebral palsy include the use of bisphosphonates and active weight-bearing programmes (Chad et al 1999, Henderson et al 2002).

Orthopaedic surgery

Orthopaedic surgery needs to be undertaken in full consultation with a child, the family and/or carers so that they have an understanding of postoperative care and the long-term management required to prevent recurrence of the deformity. The surgery should form part of the individual's overall physical management programme.

Soft-tissue surgery involves the release of tendon, muscle or connective tissue and usually aims to equalize the muscle length balance across joints. By lengthening a muscle or tendon it is theorized that it effectively weakens its action and allows the opposing muscle group to become dominant. In the hip joint it will aim to help recentre the femoral head (Cottalorda et al 1998, Abel et al 1999). Bony surgery includes femoral osteotomy, pelvic osteotomy and open reduction which are designed to restructure the proximal femoral and acetabular anatomy to maintain the hip position. Outcomes from bony surgery are generally good when used to prevent progression of hip subluxation (Cornell 1995). A long-term review of 63 hips found that femoral osteotomy alone was not sufficient to maintain hip centration and acetabular reconstruction was also advised (Brunner & Baumann 1997). Cornell's (1995) review supports this and suggests that the development of the acetabulum is unaffected by femoral osteotomy. In many cases a combination of soft and bony surgery will be performed. Unilateral bony and soft-tissue surgery has been reported to cause an alteration in the direction of windsweeping and consequent increasing migration of the contralateral hip (Samilson & Carson 1967, Carr & Gage 1987).

Multilevel surgery involves bony and soft-tissue surgery at the hip, knee and ankle to correct deformities in a single stage. It is most commonly used in children with diplegia to improve their gait and requires an intensive postoperative exercise programme. This type of surgical intervention was introduced to overcome 'the birthday syndrome', where surgery at one level results in muscle contracture developing in the proximal muscles, which then require surgery the following year. Evans (2004) reviewed the available evidence on multilevel surgery and concluded that there was no consensus on the optimal age for surgery and, although there may be short-term improvement in gait patterns, the long-term prognosis is uncertain. Gait analysis is useful in determining accurately which muscles are affecting walking ability and which are most suitable sites for surgery (see Ch. 4).

There have been a number of studies undertaken to determine the outcome of different types of surgical interventions but many compounding variables, such as postoperative management, use of different surgical techniques, the measurement of outcome, the length of follow-up and heterogeneity of the sample in terms of age and physical ability, make analysis of the findings difficult (Reimers 1980, Moreau et al 1995, Cottalorda et al 1998, Song & Carroll 1998, Abel et al 1999, Turker & Lee 2000). Stott et al (2004) reviewed 27 studies and found little evidence for the efficacy of adductor releases due to the 'small sample sizes, heterogeneous interventions, poorly defined outcome measures and lack of statistical

analysis' and the need for further research to evaluate soft-tissue surgery was identified.

However, for hip surgery some criteria have been established, including indications that soft-tissue surgery is unlikely to be successful when the hip is migrated over 40% and that bony surgery is indicated at this level (Barrie & Galasko 1996, Association of Paediatric Chartered Physiotherapists 2001, Pountney & Green 2006).

Surgical correction of spinal curvature is considered when a curve is greater than 35–40° and there is an increasing difficulty in positioning, particularly for seating (Staheli 1992). Children whose pelvis forms part of the curve require correction of the pelvis and spine (Lonstein 1995). Spinal surgery is a large undertaking, with a number of possible complications, particularly in children with severe neurological impairment. Careful consideration needs to be given prior to surgery as to whether the risk is worth the improved outcome (Comstock et al 1998, Lipton et al 1999).

Selective dorsal rhizotomy

Selective dorsal rhizotomy is a neurosurgical technique to divide the posterior nerve rootlets in the lumbosacral region to reduce the level of spasticity, in particular in muscle groups of the lower limb. The roots are selected by stimulation to determine which are responsible for innervating each muscle. Results are dependent on the skill of the surgeon and pre and postoperative physiotherapy (Hare et al 1998). The technique is practised in only a few centres in the UK but is quite widespread in the USA (Heim et al 1995, Chicoine et al 1997). Several studies have reviewed the outcomes of selective dorsal rhizotomy, with little definitive evidence of its effectiveness and a possible risk of spinal deformity (Turi & Kalen 2000).

PHYSICAL MANAGEMENT

Motor assessment

Assessment of motor ability can be made by using the positive signs of the neurological lesion – tone, spasticity and reflex activity – or the negative signs of muscle weakness, fatigue and incoordination. Some physiotherapists will use a combination of these factors. Assessment needs to be objective and relevant and act as a guide to intervention. Many of the positive signs are subjective, due to the variability of the examiner's interpretation, and dependent on the position. Assessment of the biomechanical aspects of ability, e.g. position of head, shoulder and pelvis, and coordination are more likely to guide prescription of treatment. The normal model of motor activity provides our only consistent model and is therefore used as a basis for general motor assessments and gait analysis.

Commonly used tests

There exists a wealth of measures for assessing children with cerebral palsy. This is because assessments need to be selected according to the purpose of the assessment, e.g. prognosis, function, participation, pain, orthopaedic, the age of a child and his or her level of impairment. Some of the most commonly used tests include:

- Gross Motor Function Measure – GMFM 88 or 66 (Russell et al 2003)
- Chailey Levels of Ability – CLA (Pountney et al 2004)
- Bayley Scales of Infant Development – BSID (Bayley 1983)
- Pediatric Evaluation of Disability Index – PEDI (Haley et al 1992)
- Peabody Development Motor Scales – PDMS (Folio & Fewell 1983)
- Gait analysis.

Screening tools for the identification of children at risk of developing cerebral palsy are detailed in Chapter 6.

The GMFM is a structured test consisting of 66 or 88 items in five sections. It is scored according to how much of each specified skill the child achieves. The sensitivity of this test at the severe end of motor ability is limited.

The CLA offers a scale that is sensitive at low levels of ability up to independent standing (see section on postural management programmes, below). It does not include assessment of walking. This scale is a naturalistic assessment based on developmental biomechanics and assesses ability in lying, sitting and standing. Components of the levels clearly identify which aspect of postural development is hindering achievement of higher ability levels. The scale is widely used as a prescription for postural management equipment.

In adults with cerebral palsy there are fewer options, particularly for the more severely affected. The GMFM and CLA can continue to be used into adulthood, as well as functional measures such as the Barthel Index (Mahoney & Barthel 1965) and the Functional Independence Measure (FIM) (Granger et al 1986).

Assessment of walking is now increasingly undertaken in sophisticated gait laboratories (see Ch. 4). This method of assessment has led to a better analysis of the cause of gait abnormalities by distinguishing between the primary factors of motor control abnormalities and the secondary factors of inadequate muscle growth and bony deformity. Appropriate aspects of the abnormality can thus be corrected (Gage & Novacheck 2001). Simplified assessment using observation and video analysis can be useful for less complex gait problems.

The PEDI is a useful measure of a child's level of function with or without the use of assistive technology. It evaluates the areas of self-care, mobility and transfers, and social function (Haley et al 1992).

Treatment approaches

The treatment of children with cerebral palsy has seen the development of many treatment methods, such as Winthrop Phelps, Vojta, Conductive Education, Bobath and Doman Delacato (Scrutton 1984). In the mid-part of the twentieth century, treatment was largely orthopaedic in emphasis, concentrating on exercise, surgery and splinting. The late 1950s and early 1960s saw a swing towards a neurological emphasis (Bobath and Vojta), followed by a functional approach (Conductive Education) and finally a synthesis of all these methods, with the Chailey approach (Pountney et al 1990, 2004) and Hare approach (Hare et al 1998) considering biomechanical aspects. More recently, the role of exercise and muscle-strengthening has been shown to be effective and joined the repertoire of physiotherapy tools.

As yet, there is no evidence that any one method is superior to another. Hur (1995) reviewed 37 studies of therapeutic interventions for children with cerebral palsy and concluded that, although some studies showed some improvements, these were rarely sustained and for most the sample size or methodology was not rigorous enough to demand a change in practice. A more recent randomized controlled trial of intensities of treatment, goal-setting and current levels of physiotherapy found no significant differences between the groups (Bower et al 2001). Below are described some orthodox physiotherapy approaches and some alternative therapies now available.

Neurodevelopmental Therapy

The most widely used form of Neurodevelopmental Therapy (NDT) is the Bobath approach. Bobath, who originally devised this approach in the 1940s, suggested that moving and handling patients in a certain way could inhibit spastic patterns of movement, allowing the emergence of more normal patterns. The treatment techniques involve specialized handling, with control being given at key points to inhibit spasticity and guide movements. Such techniques are taught to the parents of a child in order that they may be continued at home. A rationale to support these practical findings was developed around the idea that brain lesions result in the release of abnormal movement patterns of coordination, abnormal postural tone and disordered reciprocal innervation (Bobath 1984).

The theoretical hierarchical rationale for this approach has been refuted by more recent studies on the nervous system (Thelen & Fisher 1982, Fetters et al 1989, Green et al 1995). Bobath methods of handling continue to provide a cornerstone for physiotherapeutic treatment but a review of the evidence on NDT by Butler & Darrah (2001) concluded that there was no consistent evidence that it facilitated more normal motor development or functional activity, or changed the amount of abnormal movement. Butler & Darrah (2001) suggested that not all therapists have 'kept pace with the evolution of the approach', which recognizes the importance of the interaction between biomechanical and neurological aspects of motor development (Neilson & McCaughey 1982, Carr et al 1995, Mayston 1995).

Conductive Education

Conductive Education, also known as the Peto method, is an approach to the treatment of children with cerebral palsy which was brought to the UK from Hungary. Users of this approach describe it as a system of education which encompasses motor development and aims to engage children in active learning (Hari & Tillemans 1984). Conductive Education programmes are provided in structured groups led by a conductor, who combines the roles of a teacher and therapist. In younger children, songs and rhythmic intention are used to encourage movement. Older children use task analysis. Studies in Australia and the UK have found little difference between the progress of children using traditional approaches and those involved in Conductive Education (Bairstow et al 1993, Reddihough et al 1998). There have been some criticisms of this approach because of its intensive nature, with little evidence of improved outcomes (Oliver 1990).

Hare approach

The Hare approach to assessment and treatment focuses on the underlying disorder of posture and movement rather than neurological signs. Assessment is made in all positions, with attention paid to the relationship between the trunk and body parts, and the supporting surface. Levels of ability are identified on fundamental postural skills. Treatment techniques aim to encourage a child's ability to control movement of the trunk by the use of arm and leg gaiters, below-knee plaster boots, aids and adapted furniture. The approach is applicable for all ages (Hare et al 1998).

Strength-training

There is a growing evidence of the benefits of strength-training programmes in improving functional ability in individuals with cerebral palsy. A number of studies have investigated different approaches and settings for strength-training programmes, mainly in children with diplegia from 4 years of age into adulthood (MacPhail & Kramer 1995, Blundell et al 2003). The results have been overwhelmingly positive, demonstrating gains in strength and speed of walking (Dodd et al 2003). A qualitative study identified that children perceived themselves to be stronger, more flexible, able to negotiate stairs more easily and had a greater sense of well-being (McBurney et al 2003). There has been limited research into the use of strength-training in children with severe cerebral palsy but static bicycle training was found to demonstrate significant improvements in GMFM scores following a 6-week programme (Williams & Pountney 2005). Concerns regarding the increase of spasticity following muscle-strengthening have been refuted. Damiano et al (2002) stressed the importance of differentiating between repetitive practice and specific training programmes designed to increase muscle strength. This approach has many advantages: exercise is a normal activity which can be undertaken in a variety of settings, it improves feelings of well-being and improves cardiovascular system. It is non-invasive and provides an activity which can be continued into adulthood.

Recent work on the gastrocnemius muscles supports the role of exercise and suggests that muscle strength may have an important role to play in the maintenance of muscle length (Shortland et al 2002). The study of children with spastic diplegia found that muscle fibre length was not reduced and it was suggested that decreased fibre diameter may shorten the aponeuroses to cause contracture.

Constraint-Induced Movement Therapy

Constraint-Induced Movement Therapy (CIMT) is based on the theory that a child's brain is plastic and can respond to intense training. It has been used since the mid-1990s for adults following a stroke and research studies are showing significant improvements in children with hemiplegia or a stroke (Taub et al 2004, Naylor & Bower 2005, Gordon et al 2006). The therapy involves constraining the use of a child's unaffected arm whilst encouraging increased activity of the affected limb. To date there are no definitive guidelines on the length of time the limb needs to be constrained on a daily basis, the period of training and its intensity. In the three studies quoted constraint was used from 1 to 6 hours during play activities and for 6 hours per day training. The period of intervention lasted from 4 to 7 weeks. The affected arm is restrained using either a mitt and a sling or a removable splint (Figure 7.4).

Eclectic approach

Limitations imposed by time restraints and service delivery options mean in reality that most physiotherapists select from the variety of treatments available which best meet a child's and family's situation. Elements of the Bobath approach are used in individual sessions, whereas Conductive Education ideas may be useful in group work. Children react in different ways to different approaches and play often provides the vehicle for delivering treatment to maintain interest and motivation.

Parental ability to continue treatment programmes outside sessions is variable and strict adherence to specific treatment methods can therefore be limited. Bower et al (2001) found little difference between the type and intensity of treatment in the change of GMFM score, suggesting that eclectic approaches, which fit into family lifestyles, are appropriate.

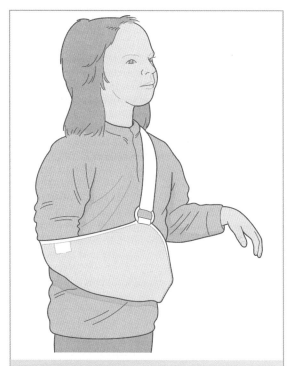

Figure 7.4 Child with sling on unaffected arm to encourage activity of affected aim

---

KEY POINTS

- There is no evidence that any one treatment method is superior to another
- Therapists select from the variety of treatments available those that best meet the child's and family's needs.

Alternative therapies

There is a burgeoning number of alternative therapies available to parents, often at great personal expense. The most widely used of these are hyperbaric oxygen therapy (HOT), acupuncture and cranial sacral therapy (CST). Very few studies have been undertaken to establish the effectiveness of these approaches. A randomized multi-centre trial of HOT in Canada found no differences in GMFM scores between children receiving minimal air pressures and those receiving HOT (Collet et al 2001).

With lack of firm evidence for the efficacy of any one current therapy approach, there is a need to look more closely at theories of motor development and motor learning, and compare outcomes of other rehabilitation approaches, such as muscle-strengthening and assistive technologies.

MANAGEMENT STRATEGIES

Management strategies differ from treatment approaches, as they reflect the need for ongoing interventions which support the individual beyond the confines of individual physiotherapy sessions. Examples of these strategies will be orthotics, postural management, positioning programmes, medications, botulinum toxin and orthopaedic management. These management strategies often require multi-professional collaboration, which includes the child and often the family along with a pooling of resources to achieve the desired outcomes. Many of these strategies will begin early in life and continue through childhood and adulthood to meet the individual's changing needs.

Postural management programmes

For children at GMFCS levels III–V, a postural management programme is often put in place to try and integrate the provision of equipment and treatment interventions. It has been defined as 'a planned approach encompassing all activities and interventions which impact on an individual's posture and function. Programmes are tailored specifically for each child and may include special seating, night-time support, standing supports, active exercise, orthotics, surgical interventions, individual therapy sessions' (Gericke 2006). A consensus statement on postural management has been published to guide clinicians on appropriate provision of postural management equipment and includes the following recommendations:

- Children in GMFCS groups IV–V should start 24-hour postural management programmes in lying as soon as appropriate after birth, in sitting from 6 months, and in standing from 12 months
- Children with a motor disorder at GMFCS level III require postural management programme that emphasizes postural activity from an early age
- Close surveillance should be maintained for the development of postural or positional deformity
- Postural care pathways and training are needed to enable the active understanding and involvement of all those directly involved with the child, professionals, parents, wheelchair services, education and respite carers.

The role of positioning and management of posture begins in the neonatal unit. Grenier (1988) described the early effects of muscle-shortening and bony malformation, which can be aggravated in the neonatal period by the 'frog-lying' position commonly adopted by premature infants. This posture results in shortening of the iliopsoas and adductor muscles, and exerts a rotational force leading to excessive anteversion. Protocols for positioning infants at this stage are available (Harrison, 1998) (see Ch. 6).

From the earliest possible age, parents should be taught and encouraged to carry, position and move their child in a way that promotes appropriate postures and development and discourages stereotypical patterns of movement. This type of approach should be incorporated into a child's normal activities and not occur as an isolated daily activity. This should also become a lifelong approach and be complemented by postural management equipment.

Postural management equipment forms an essential element of a physiotherapy programme for children and adults with cerebral palsy who are unable to maintain the lying, sitting or standing posture independently, cannot change position or require extra support to maintain their postural stability when active. Without appropriate support, these individuals are unable to participate in many activities or do so in postures which are likely to lead to deformity.

At Chailey Heritage Clinical Services, a 24-hour approach to postural management has been developed to prevent musculoskeletal deformities, whilst improving the ability of individuals with low motor abilities to participate more actively in life, with the use of powered mobility and communication aids (Pountney et al 2004). The approach combines postural control in the positions of lying, sitting and standing with hands-on therapy and active exercise programmes such as cycling, horse-riding and swimming and is supported by education programmes for users, parents and professionals.

The postures simulate a higher level of physical ability by changing the load-bearing surface and positioning the head, shoulder girdle, trunk, pelvis and legs. The postures adopted within the Chailey postural management equipment are based on a scheme of assessment – the CLA (Green et al 1995, Pountney et al 2004). The levels detail the position of the head, shoulder and pelvic girdles and limbs, and the load-bearing pattern of infants from birth through lying and sitting to achieving independent standing.

These biomechanical data have informed the design of this equipment. Lying, sitting and standing supports provide a starting position for movement and allow a range of movement within which a child can move and recover balance. With a stable base, a child's use of his/her head, arms and legs can be more controlled. Control of the hip, pelvis and spine is achieved by applying corrective forces via the supporting surface, lateral thoracic and pelvic control and kneeblocks. Figure 7.5 illustrates the effect of seating on balance and movement (Pountney et al 2004). The use of the Chailey 24-hour postural management approach prior to hip subluxation has been shown to reduce the level of hip subluxation significantly (Pountney et al 2002).

The neuronal group selection theory (NGST; see Ch. 5) suggests that the selection of motor patterns is dependent on behaviour and experience. The use of positioning through equipment and hands-on activities, which promote the experience of normal movement, should logically improve movement pattern selection in young children (Hadders-Algra 2000). These effects occur early in development and intervention should begin as soon as motor impairments are identified. A symmetrical lying position is achieved at approximately 3 months in the normal infant and persistence beyond this age should alert clinicians to possible

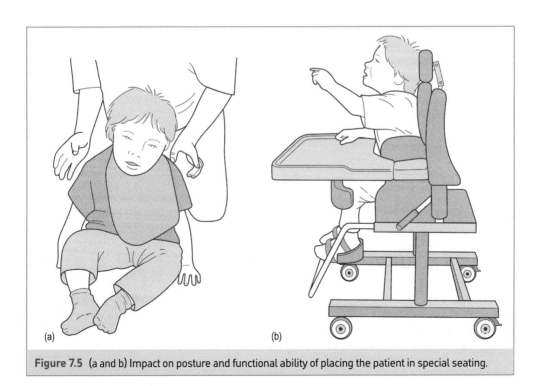

(a)   (b)

Figure 7.5 (a and b) Impact on posture and functional ability of placing the patient in special seating.

motor impairment. In the older population, neuroplastic adaptation can occur at a peripheral level. In both instances, more time needs to be spent in the postures which promote the desired movement than those that do not. The effect of postural management equipment in improving functional ability may be explained by the theory of reducing the degrees of freedom during skill acquisition. This has been a long-recognized method of achieving motor skills (Turvey et al 1982, Vereijken et al 1992). Higher levels of function are possible within postural management equipment, as the number of motor tasks requiring attention at any one time is reduced and concentration can be focused on specific motor or cognitive tasks.

Night positioning

Night positioning for sleep appears to be a crucial element of the programme, possibly because it offers a substantial time period of gentle muscle stretch while muscle activity is quiet. Several studies indicate that periods of between 5 and 7 hours are required to change muscle length (Tardieu et al 1988, Lespargot et al 1994). Postural support at night must promote good-quality sleep, which can be compromised by a number of factors, such as nocturnal seizures, reflux oesophagitis and nocturnal hypoxaemia. Supine positioning can aggravate some of these conditions, and investigation and observation of these conditions must be carried out prior to allowing a child to sleep unattended in a postural support (Cartwright 1984, Martin et al 1995). A sleep questionnaire which can be used by physiotherapists identifies risks and causes of sleep disturbance in children with cerebral palsy and can be used prior to the provision of a lying support or sleep system (Khan & Underhill 2006).

Seating

A variety of seating options are available, from corner seats, forward-lean seats and 90/90 systems, and evaluation of these products needs to be made to ensure that appropriate postures are achieved (Pope 2002). Older children and adults who have fixed deformities may require more complex systems, which are contoured to the body's shape to accommodate the deformities. Every effort should be made to prevent further deterioration of posture and this may include the use of sleep systems (see Ch. 10).

Standing

The opportunity to stand has long been cited as important in the development of bone joint development but there is limited evidence to support this. Stuberg (1992) recommended that children should weight-bear for an hour four to five times a week in order to enhance bone density and joint development (Figure 7.6). Other studies

have investigated the role of standing in increasing bone mineral density but these have not been conclusive (Wilmshurst et al 1996, Caulton et al 2004).

ASSISTIVE TECHNOLOGY

Assistive technology is an umbrella term for a wide range of equipment which ranges from simple devices such as walking sticks to complex electronic equipment, such as environmental control equipment or communication aids (Cook & Hussey 1995). Assistive technology offers individuals an opportunity to achieve a level of independence in a number of areas, including play, environmental controls, mobility and communication (see Ch. 10).

Orthotics

Orthotic management offers a conservative approach to prevent deformity, improve joint alignment and biomechanics and improve function. Orthoses provide intimate control of joints, which is not possible in positioning equipment. Evidence is available of the immediate impact of orthotics on gait but very little rigorous evidence exists on the long-term effect of orthotics (Morris 2002).

Lower-limb orthotics can be used to provide stability in standing transfers, clearance in swing and support for children with limited walking ability. Orthoses need to

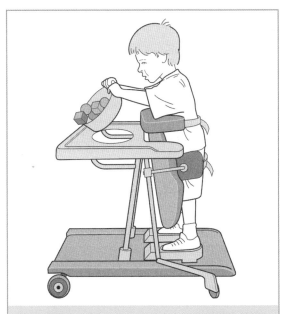

Figure 7.6 Use of standing support enabling functional activity.

be used with care, as excessive use can lead to immobility and consequent muscle weakness and atrophy (Shortland et al 2002). Prescriptions for orthoses need to made in the light of the theories of muscle and bone adaptation, and joint biomechanics to ensure that satisfactory outcomes are achieved.

Hip and spinal orthoses (HASO) are prescribed to control hip and spine position but there is no literature to support their effectiveness.

Thoracolumbosacral orthoses (TLSO) are used to control spinal curvature during growth. The construction of these jackets varies widely between orthotists and includes front or side opening, complete shells or shells with selected areas cut away. There is no evidence that spinal orthoses can reduce the rate of progression in scoliosis but studies have only introduced bracing when the degree of spinal curvature exceeded 25°. A clinical benefit of improved sitting balance has been cited (Miller et al 1996, Terjesen et al 2000) (see Ch. 10).

MULTIPROFESSIONAL AND MULTIAGENCY AGENCY WORKING

Cerebral palsy is a condition that requires multiprofessional and multiagency involvement to meet the needs of the individual and family. Children and adults with cerebral palsy are likely to be involved with a variety of health professionals, possibly from more than one centre, social services and education. Local health commissioners are responsible for ensuring that clear methods for collaboration exist between social services and the local education authority to fulfil their joint responsibilities of meeting children's needs.

This form of collaborative working requires liaison between agencies at both senior organizational levels and at operational levels to ensure frameworks and resources are in place, including pooling of budgets and integration of commissioning which can best support services for individuals with cerebral palsy. For children, the current Special Educational Needs Code of Practice (Department of Education and Skills 2001) aims to increase the number of children with disabilities in mainstream education and, as such, necessitates much closer working between agencies.

The transition to adult services often results in a reduction of medical and therapy input, and therefore preparation in terms of equipment provision and therapy needs to be put in place before leaving children's services.

CASE STUDY 7.1

Cerebral Palsy

SA was one of twins born at 28 weeks' gestation at his local maternity unit, where he was ventilated at 3 minutes for respiratory distress. After 3 days he was weaned off the ventilator but reintubated due to increasing apnoeas and desaturations. At 10 days he was transferred to a tertiary unit for neonatal care. He continued to be ventilated until day 14, when his condition became more stable. He had a stormy neonatal period during which he developed periventricular leukomalacia. At 7 weeks of age he returned home and came under the care of his local team.

Initial involvement included physiotherapy on a weekly basis at the local child development centre. Physiotherapy included parental advice on handling SA to promote normal motor development; positioning for play, sleep and feeding; and stretches to maintain muscle length. At 7 months of age he was able to achieve symmetry in supine and prone but unable to sit independently. When held in sitting he had a rounded spinal profile and a tendency to push back into extension. At this time concerns were raised regarding level of

useful vision. At home he had a simple contoured seat which was used for play, eating and drinking.

At 12 months of age there was little change in his physical ability and it was decided to prescribe a modular seating system, which maintained hip and pelvic position, and provided good position for hand control and a standing support.

From 2 years he used an adapted tricycle and began to attend a swimming group, using a head flotation aid. He tried a variety of walkers, none of which were found to be useful in terms of mobility or exploratory activities.

SA continued to have difficulty with eating and drinking, and mealtimes were prolonged. He gained weight slowly but steadily and had high-calorie supplements to help with weight gain.

At this age he still did not have an established sleep pattern. Investigation of sleeping habits revealed some behavioural issues but also the possibility of upper-airway obstruction. His adenoids were removed and consequently his sleep pattern improved.

At 2½ years he joined a multidisciplinary therapy group at the Child Development Centre with input from

continued

the occupation therapist, physiotherapist and speech and language therapist to work on physical, play and communication skills. A simple picture-based communication system was devised to enable him to make choices.

At 30 months he had a routine X-ray to screen for hip and spinal problems. His hips showed only limited migration and were deemed not to be at risk. Clinically he had a postural scoliosis with a curve to the left from the lumbar region. This was completely correctable and therefore no intervention was taken at this time but annual monitoring was implemented.

At $3^1/_2$ years he joined a nursery attached to a special school and his medical and therapy care were transferred there. He was beginning to show decreased range of movement at his ankles and stood on his tiptoes. Ankle–foot orthoses were prescribed to maintain the length of the tendo-achilles.

He continued to use his seating and standing supports, and was introduced at this stage to switches to facilitate his ability to play with toys, access a computer and begin independent mobility.

At school age he joined the mainstream primary school with a specialist unit for children with special educational needs which his twin was attending. He had a full-time learning support assistant (LSA) who enabled him to access most of the curriculum with the help of assistive technology. He received weekly physiotherapy sessions at school and a daily programme of stretches by the LSA.

At home, adaptations were made to his house to provide a downstairs bathroom and bedroom. Doors and corridors were made wide enough to manoeuvre a wheelchair.

Respite care with a local family was introduced for one weekend a month to relieve family stresses, and as a new baby was due.

At age 11 he transferred to a residential school for weekly boarding. His parents were struggling with his full-time care and his mother had a back problem and was unable to help with lifting. At 13 his spinal curve increased to about 25° and a thoracolumbosacral orthosis was prescribed. He was also exhibiting equinus deformity of the foot and some mild contractures of the upper limb. None of these had an impact on functional activity and therefore only the stretching programme was increased. He continued with use of his ankle–foot orthoses.

He used a powered chair and computer with specialized switches. At 15 years, the standing programme was stopped due to manual handling issues and a reluctance on the part of SA to stand.

At 19 years he left school and returned home with care assistance. He attended local tertiary college for a course in computing skills. Employment prospects were limited. He moved into a small unit for adults with disabilities with carer support. At this stage, physiotherapy input was on a needs-led basis with intervention on request. No regular treatment was available and his carers were encouraged to do passive movements. SA was encouraged to take part in some active exercise, such as swimming, if possible.

REFERENCES

Abel MF, Blanco JS, Pavlovich L et al 1999 Asymmetric hip deformity and subluxation in cerebral palsy: an analysis of surgical treatment. *Journal of Pediatrics and Orthopedics* 19: 479–485.

Ade-Hall RA, Moore AP 2002 Botulinum toxin type A in the treatment of lower limb spasticity in cerebral palsy [Cochrane review]. In: *Cochrane Database of Systematic Reviews*, issue 1.

Aicardi J 1990 Epilepsy in brain injured children. *Developmental Medicine and Child Neurology* 32: 191–202.

American Psychiatric Association 2000 *Diagnostic and Statistical manual of Mental Disorders: DSM IV.* Arlington, VA: American Psychiatric Publishing.

Association of Paediatric Chartered Physiotherapists (2001; updated 2005) *Hip Subluxation and Dislocation in Children*

with Cerebral Palsy – An Evidence Based Summary. York: Association of Paediatric Physiotherapists.

Bachlet A, Thomas AG, Eltumi M et al 2002 A 12 month prospective study of gastrostomy feeding in children with disabilities. *Developmental Medicine and Child Neurology* 44 (Suppl. 92): 12–13.

Bairstow P, Cochrane R, Hur JJ 1993 *Evaluation of Conductive Education for Children with Cerebral Palsy.* London: HMSO.

Baker R, Jasinski M, Maciag-Tymecka I et al 2002 Botulinum toxin treatment of spasticity in diplegic cerebral palsy: a randomized, double-blind, placebo-controlled, dose-ranging study. *Developmental Medicine and Child Neurology* 44: 666–675.

Barrie JL, Galasko CSB 1996 Surgery for unstable hips in cerebral palsy. *Journal of Pediatric Orthopaedics* 5: 225–231.

Bayley N 1983 *Bayley Scales of Infant Development*. San Antonio, TX: Therapy Skill Builders.

Blundell SW, Shepherd RB, Dean CM et al 2003 Functional strength training in cerebral palsy: a pilot study of a group circuit training class for children aged 4–8 years. *Clinical Rehabilitation* 17: 48–57.

Bobath KA 1984 *Neurological Basis for the Treatment of Cerebral Palsy. Clinics in Developmental Medicine*, no. 75, 2nd edn. London: MacKeith Press.

Bower E, Michell D, Burnett M et al 2001 Randomized controlled trial of physiotherapy in 56 children with cerebral palsy followed for 18 months. *Developmental Medicine and Child Neurology* 43: 4–15.

Brunner R, Baumann JU 1997 Long term effects for interthrochanteric varus-derotation osteotomy on femur and acetabulum in spastic cerebral palsy: an 11–18 year follow up study. *Journal of Pediatric Orthopaedics* 17: 585–591.

Butler C, Darrah J 2001 Effects of neurodevelopmental treatment (NDT) for cerebral palsy: an AACPDM evidence report. *Developmental Medicine and Child Neurology* 43: 778–790.

Carr C, Gage J 1987 The fate of the non operated hip in cerebral palsy. *Journal of Pediatric Orthopaedics* 7: 262–267.

Carr J, Shepherd R, Ada L 1995 Spasticity: research findings and implications for intervention. *Physiotherapy* 81: 421–429.

Carr LJ, Cosgrove AP, Gringras P et al 1998 Position paper on the use of botulinum toxin in cerebral palsy. *Archives of Disease in Childhood* 79: 271–273.

Cartwright RD 1984 Effect of sleep position on sleep apnea severity. *Sleep* 7: 110–114.

Caulton JM, Ward KA, Alsop CW et al 2004 A randomised controlled trial of standing programme on bone mineral density in non-ambulant children with cerebral palsy. *Archives of Disease in Childhood* 89: 131–135.

Chad KE, McKay HA, Zello GA et al 1999 The effect of a weight-bearing physical activity program on bone mineral content and estimated volumetric density in children with spastic cerebral palsy. *Journal of Pediatrics* 135: 115–117.

Chicoine MR, Park TS, Kaufmann BA 1997 Selective dorsal rhizotomy and rates of orthopaedic surgery in children with spastic cerebral palsy. *Journal of Neurosurgery* 86: 43–49.

Cleeland CS, Ryan KM 1994 Pain assessment:global use of brief pain inventory. *Annals of Academy of Medicine* 23: 129–138.

Collet J-P, Vanasse M, Marois P et al 2001 Hyperbaric oxygen for children with cerebral palsy: a randomised multicentre trial. *Lancet* 357: 582–586.

Comstock CP, Leach J, Wenger DR 1998 Scoliosis in total body involvement cerebral palsy: analysis of surgical treatment and patient and caregiver satisfaction. *Spine* 23: 1412–1424.

Cook A, Hussey S 1995 *Assistive Technologies Principles and Practice*. London: Mosby.

Cornell MS 1995 The hip in cerebral palsy. *Developmental Medicine and Child Neurology* 37: 3–18.

Cosgrove AP, Corry IS, Graham HK 1994 Botulinum toxin in the management of the lower limb in cerebral palsy. *Developmental Medicine and Child Neurology* 36: 386–396.

Cottalorda J, Gautheron V, Metton G et al 1998 Predicting the outcome of adductor tenotomy. *International Orthopaedics* 22: 374–379.

Crichton JU, Mackinnon M, White CP 1995 The life expectancy of persons with cerebral palsy. *Developmental Medicine and Child Neurology* 37: 567–576.

Crothers B, Paine R 1988 *The Natural History of Cerebral Palsy*. London: MacKeith Press.

Damiano DL, Dodd K, Taylor NF 2002 Should we be testing and training muscle strength in cerebral palsy? *Developmental Medicine and Child Neurology* 44: 68–72.

Deleplanque B, Lagueny A, Flurin V et al 2002 Toxine botulinique dans la spasticité des adducteurs de hanche chez les enfants IMC et IMOC non marchants. *Revue de Chirurgie Orthopédique* 88: 279–285.

Department of Education and Skills 2001 *Special Educational Needs Code of Practice*. Nottingham: DfES Publications.

Dodd JK, Taylor FN, Graham HK 2003 A randomized clinical trial of strength training in young people with cerebral palsy. *Developmental Medicine and Child Neurology* 45: 652–657.

Dodge NN, Wilson GA 2001 Melatonin for treatment of sleep disorders in children with developmental disabilities. *Journal of Child Neurology* 16: 581–584.

Eliasson A, Gordon AM, Forssberg H 1995 Tactile control of isometric fingertip forces during grasping in children with cerebral palsy. *Developmental Medicine and Child Neurology* 37: 72–84.

Evans P 2004 A review of the evidence in favour of and against multi-level surgery in the management of childhood disability. *Association of Paediatric Chartered Physiotherapy* 110: 7–14.

Evans P, Evans SJW, Alberman E 1990 Cerebral palsy: why we must plan for survival. *Archives of Disease in Childhood* 65: 1329–1333.

Fairhurst CBR 2004 *Analgesic Effect of Botulinum Toxin*. London: MacKeith Press, p. 22.

Fetters L, Fernandez B, Cermak S 1989 The relationship of proximal and distal components in the development of reaching. *Journal of Human Movement Studies* 17: 283–297.

Folio MR, Fewell RR 1983 *Peabody Developmental Motor Scales and Activity Cards*. Austin, TX: PRO-ED.

Freud S 1968 *Infantile Cerebral Palsies*. Coral Gables: University of Miami Press.

Fry NR, Gough M, Shortland AP et al 2004 Three-dimensional realisation of muscle morphology and architecture using ultrasound. *Gait Posture* 20: 177–182.

Gage J, Novacheck TF 2001 An update on the treatment of gait problems in cerebral palsy. *Journal of Orthopaedics* 10: 265–274.

Gericke T 2006 Postural management for children with cerebral palsy: consensus statement. *Developmental Medicine and Child Neurology* 48: 244.

Gordon AM, Charles J, Wolf SL et al 2006 Efficacy of constraint-induced movement therapy on involved upper-extremity use in children with hemiplegic cerebral palsy is not age-dependent. *Pediatrics* 117: 363–373.

Gough M, Fairhurst C, Shortland AP 2005 Botulinum toxin and cerebral palsy: time for reflection? *Developmental Medicine and Child Neurology* 47: 709–712.

Granger CV, Hamilton BB, Keith RA 1986 Advances in functional assessment for medical rehabilitation. *Topics in Geriatric Rehabilitation* 1: 59–74.

Green EM, Mulcahy CM, Pountney TE 1995 An investigation into the development of early postural control. *Developmental Medicine and Child Neurology* 37: 437–448.

Grenier A 1988 Prevention of early deformation of the hip in brain-damaged neonatals (in French). *Annales de Pédiatrie* 35: 423–427.

Griffiths M, Clegg M 1988 *Cerebral Palsy: Problems and Practice.* London: Souvenir Press.

Guzzetta A, Mercuri E, Cioni G 2001 Visual impairment associated with cerebral palsy. *European Journal of Paediatric Neurology* 5: 115–119.

Hadders-Algra M 2000 The neuronal group selection theory: promising principles for understanding and treating developmental motor disorders. *Developmental Medicine and Child Neurology* 42: 707–715.

Hagberg B, Hagberg G 1996 The changing panorama of cerebral palsy – bilateral spastic forms in particular. *Acta Paediatrica* (Suppl 416): 48–52.

Hagberg B, Hagberg G, Beckung E, Uvebrant P 2001 Changing panorama of cerebral palsy in Sweden. VIII. Prevalence and origin in the birth year period 1991–94. *Acta Paediatrica* 90: 271–277.

Haley SM, Coster WJ, Ludlow LH et al 1992 *Pediatric Evaluation of Disability Inventory.* Boston: New England Medical Center Hospital.

Hare NS, Durham S, Green EM 1998 The cerebral palsies and motor learning disorders. In: Stokes M (ed.) *Neurological Physiotherapy.* London: Mosby, p. 320.

Hari M, Tillemans T 1984 Conductive education. In: Scrutton D (ed.) *Management of the Motor Disorders of Children with Cerebral Palsy.* London: Spastics International Medical Publications.

Harrison M 1998 *Positioning the Neonate.* 10th Annual Meeting of the European Academy of Childhood Disability, Helsinki. Available from Physiotherapy Department, St James University Hospital, Leeds.

Heim RC, Park TS, Vogler GP et al 1995 Changes in hip migration after selective dorsal rhizotomy for spastic quadriplegia in cerebral palsy. *Journal of Neurosurgery* 82: 567–571.

Henderson RC 1997 Bone density and other possible predictors of fracture risk in children and adolescents with spastic quadriplegia. *Developmental Medicine and Child Neurology* 39: 224–227.

Henderson RC, Madsen CD 1999 Bone mineral content and body composition in children and young adults with cystic fibrosis. *Pediatric Pulmonology* 27: 8755–8863.

Henderson RC, Lin PP, Greene WB 1995 Bone-mineral density in children and adolescents who have spastic cerebral palsy. *Journal of Bone and Joint Surgery* 77: 1671–1681.

Henderson RC, Lark RK, Gurka MJ et al 2002 Bone density and metabolism in children and adolescents with moderate severe cerebral palsy. *Pediatrics* 110: e5.

Hodgkinson I, Jindrich ML, Duhaut P, Vadot JP, Metton G, Berard C 2001 Hip pain in 234 non-ambulatory adolescents and young adults with cerebral palsy: a cross-sectional multicentre study. *Developmental Medicine and Child Neurology* 43: 806–808.

Hung JCC, Appleton RE, Nunn AJ et al 1998 The use of melatonin in the treatment of sleep disturbances in children with neurological or behavioural disorders. *Journal of Pediatric Pharmacy Practice* 3: 250–256.

Hunt A, Goldman A, Seers K et al 2004 Clinical validation of the Paediatric Pain Profile. *Developmental Medicine and Child Neurology* 46: 9–18.

Hur JJ 1995 Review of research on therapeutic interventions for children with cerebral palsy. *Acta Neurologica Scandinavica* 91: 423–432.

Ivanhoe CB, Tilton AH, Francisco GE 2001 Intrathecal baclofen therapy for spastic hypertonia. *Physical Medicine and Rehabilitation Clinics of North America* 12: 923–937.

Jan JE, Freeman RD 2004 Melatonin treatment for circadian rhythm sleep disorders in children with multiple disabilities: what have we learned in the last decade? *Developmental Medicine and Child Neurology* 46: 776–782.

Kalen V, Conklin MM, Sherman FC et al 1992 Untreated scoliosis in severe cerebral palsy. *Journal of Pediatric Orthopaedics* 12: 337–340.

Kennes J, Rosenbaum P, Hanna SE et al 2002 Health status of school-aged children with cerebral palsy: information from a population-based sample. *Developmental Medicine and Child Neurology* 44: 240.

Khan Y, Underhill J 2006 *Identification of Sleep Problems by Questionnaire in Children with Severe Cerebral Palsy.* Barcelona, Spain: European Academy of Childhood Disability.

Khan Y, Kuenzle C, Green EM et al 1996 *Sleep Problems and Overnight Oxygen Saturation in Children with Cerebral Palsy.* Dublin: European Academy of Childhood Disability, p. 69.

King W, Levin R, Schmidt R et al 2003 Prevalence of reduced bone mass in children and adults with spastic quadriplegia. *Developmental Medicine and Child Neurology* 45: 12–16.

Koman LA, Mooney JF, Paterson-Smith BP et al 2000 Botulinum toxin type a neuromuscular blockade in the treatment of lower extremity spasticity in cerebral palsy: a randomised, double blind, placebo-controlled trial. *Journal of Pediatric Orthopaedics* 20: 108–115.

Krach LE, Kriel RL, Gilmartin DM et al 2005 GMFM 1 year after continuous intrathecal baclofen infusion. *Pediatric Rehabilitation* 8: 207–213.

Krick J, Murphy-Miller P, Zeger S et al 1996 Pattern of growth in children with cerebral palsy. *Journal of the American Dietetic Association* 96: 680–685.

Lespargot A, Renaudin E, Khouri M et al 1994 Extensibility of hip adductors in children with cerebral palsy. *Developmental Medicine and Child Neurology* 36: 980–988.

Letts M, Shapiro L, Mulder K et al 1984 The windblown hip syndrome in total body cerebral palsy. *Journal of Pediatric Orthopaedics* 4: 55–62.

Lipton GE, Miller F, Dabney KW et al 1999 Factors predicting postoperative complications following spinal fusions in children with cerebral palsy. *Journal of Spinal Disorders* 12: 197–205.

Lonstein JE 1995 The spine in cerebral palsy. *Current Orthopaedics* 9: 164–177.

MacPhail HE, Kramer JF 1995 Effect of isokinetic strength-training on functional ability and walking efficiency in adolescents with cerebral palsy. *Developmental Medicine and Child Neurology* 37: 763–775.

Mahoney F, Barthel D 1965 Functional evaluation: the Barthel Index. *Maryland State Medical Journal* 14: 61–65.

Mall V, Heinen F, Kirschner J et al 2000 Evaluation of botulinum toxin a therapy in children with adductor spasm by gross motor function measure. *Journal of Child Neurology* 15: 214–217.

Martin SE, Marshall I, Douglas NJ 1995 The effect of posture on airway caliber with the sleep apnea/hypopnea syndrome. *American Journal of Respiratory Care Medicine* 152: 721–724.

Mayston M 1995 Developments in neurology – some aspects of the physiological basis for intervention techniques. *Association of Paediatric Chartered Physiotherapists Journal* 15–21.

McBurney H, Taylor NF, Dodd KJ et al 2003 A qualitative analysis of the benefits of strength training for young people with cerebral palsy. *Developmental Medicine and Child Neurology* 45. 658–663.

McCarthy GT 1992 Cerebral palsy: definition, epidemiology, development and neurological aspects. In: McCarthy GT (ed.) *Physical Disability in Childhood – An Interdisciplinary Approach*. London: Churchill Livingstone.

Metaxiotis D, Siebel A, Doederlein L 2002 Repeated botulinum toxin A injections in the treatment of spastic equinus foot. *Clinical Orthopaedics and Related Research* 394: 175–185.

Miller F, Bagg MR 1992 Age and migration percentage as risk factors for progression in spastic hip disease. *Developmental Medicine and Child Neurology* 37: 449–455.

Miller A, Temple T, Miller F 1996 Impact of othoses on the rate of scoliosis progression in children with cerebral palsy. *Journal of Pediatric Orthopaedics* 16: 332–335.

Moreau M, Cook PC, Ashton B 1995 Adductor and psoas release for subluxation of the hip children with spastic cerebral palsy. *Journal of Pediatric Orthopaedics* 15: 672–676.

Morris C 2002 A review of the efficacy of lower-limb orthoses used for cerebral palsy. *Developmental Medicine and Child Neurology* 44: 205–211.

Mutch L, Alberman E, Hagedorn R et al 1992 Cerebral palsy epidemiology: where are we now and where are we going? *Developmental Medicine and Child Neurology* 34: 547–555.

Naylor CE, Bower E 2005 Modified constraint-induced movement therapy for young children with hemiplegic cerebral palsy: a pilot study. *Developmental Medicine and Child Neurology* 47: 365–369.

Neilson PD, McCaughey J 1982 Self regulation of spasm and spasticity in cerebral palsy *Journal of Neurology, Neurosurgery and Psychiatry* 45: 320–330.

Oliver M 1990 *The Politics of Disablement*. London: MacMillan.

Palisano R, Rosenbaum P, Walter S et al 1997 Gross Motor Function classification system for cerebral palsy. *Developmental Medicine and Child Neurology* 39: 214–223.

Pellegrino L 1995 Cerebral palsy: a paradigm for developmental disabilities. *Developmental Medicine and Child Neurology* 37: 834–839.

Pharoah POD, Cooke T 1996 Cerebral palsy and multiple births. *Archives of Disease in Childhood* 75F: 169–173.

Pharoah POD, Platt MJ, Cooke T 1996 The changing epidemiology of cerebral palsy. *Archives of Disease in Childhood* 75F: 169–173.

Pope PM 2002 Postural management and special seating. In: Edwards S (ed.) *Neurological Physiotherapy: A Problem Solving Approach*, 2nd edn. London: Churchill Livingstone, pp. 189–217.

Porter D 2004 *Study of Patterns of Postural Deformity in Non-Ambulant Subjects with Cerebral Palsy. Orthopaedic and Trauma Surgery*. University of Dundee. PhD thesis.

Pountney TE, Green EM 2006 Hip dislocation in cerebral palsy. *British Medical Journal* 332: 772–775.

Pountney TE, Mulcahy CM, Green EM 1990 Early development of postural control. *Physiotherapy* 76: 799–802.

Pountney TE, Mandy A, Green EM et al 2002 Management of hip dislocation with postural management. *Child: Care, Health and Development* 28: 179–185.

Pountney TE, Mulcahy CM, Clarke S et al 2004 *Chailey Approach to Postural Management*, 2nd edn. Birmingham: Active Design.

Reddihough DS, King J, Coleman G et al 1998 Efficacy of programmes based on Conductive Education for young children with cerebral palsy. *Developmental Medicine and Child Neurology* 40: 763–770.

Reddihough DS, King JA, Coleman G et al 2002 Functional outcome of botulinum toxin A injections to the lower limb in cerebral palsy. *Developmental Medicine and Child Neurology* 44: 820–827.

Reimers J 1980 The stability of the hip in children. *Acta Orthopaedica Scandinavica* (Suppl. 184).

Rogers B, Arvesdon J, Buck G et al 1994 Characteristics of dysphagia in children with cerebral palsy. *Dysphagia* 9: 69–73.

Rosenbaum PL, Walter SD, Hanna SE et al 2002 Prognosis for gross motor function in cerebral palsy: creation of motor development curves. *Journal of the American Medical Association* 288: 1357–1363.

Rosenbloom L 1995 Diagnosis and management of cerebral palsy. *Archives of Disease in Childhood* 1995; 72: 350–353.

Russell D, Rosenbaum R, Avery LM 2003 *Gross Motor Function Measure User's Manual*. London: Mac Keith Press.

Saito N, Ebara S, Ohotsuka K et al 1998 Natural history of scoliosis in spastic cerebral palsy. *Lancet* 351: 1687–1692.

Samilson RL, Carson JJ 1967 Results and complications of adductor tenotomy and obdurator neurectomy in cerebral palsy. *Clinical Orthopaedics* 54: 61–73.

Schwartz L, Engel JM, Jensen MP 1999 Pain in persons with cerebral palsy. *Archives of Medical Rehabilitation* 80: 1243–1246.

Scrutton D 1984 *Management of Motor Disorders of Children with Cerebral Palsy*. London: Spastics International Medical Publications.

Scrutton D, Baird G 1997 Surveillance measures of the hips of children with bilateral cerebral palsy. *Archives of Disease in Childhood* 56: 381–384.

Scrutton D, Baird G, Smeeton N 2001 Hip dysplasia in bilateral cerebral palsy: incidence and natural history in children aged 18 months to 5 years. *Developmental Medicine and Child Neurology* 43: 586–600.

Shortland AP, Harris CA, Gough M et al 2002 Architecture of the medial gastrocnemius in children with spastic diplegia. *Developmental Medicine and Child Neurology* 44: 158–163.

Song HR, Carroll NC 1998 Femoral varus derotation osteotomy with or without acetabuloplasty for unstable hips in cerebral palsy. *Journal of Pediatric Orthopaedics* 18: 62–68.

Sonksen PM, Levitt S, Kitsinger M 1984 Constraints acting on motor development in young visually disabled children and principles of remediation. *Child: Care, Health and Development* 10: 273–286.

Speth LAWM, Leffers P, Janssen-Potten YJM, Vles JSH 2005 Botulinum toxin A and upper limb functional skills in hemiparetic cerebral palsy: a randomized trial in children receiving intensive therapy. *Developmental Medicine and Child Neurology* 47: 68–473.

Staheli LT 1992 *Fundamentals of Pediatric Orthopaedics*. New York: Raven Press.

Stallings VA, Charney EB, Davies JC et al 1993 Nutrition-related growth failure of children with quadriplegic cerebral palsy. *Developmental Medicine and Child Neurology* 35: 126–138.

Stanley F, Blair E, Alberman E 2000 *Cerebral Palsies: Epidemiology and Causal Pathways*. London: Mac Keith Press.

Stott NS, Piedrahita L and AACPDM 2004 Effects of surgical adductor releases for hip subluxation in cerebral palsy: an AACPDM evidence report. *Developmental Medicine and Child Neurology* 46: 628–645.

Stuberg W 1992 Considerations to weight bearing programs in children with developmental disabilities. *Physical Therapy* 72: 35–40.

Tardieu CA, Lespargot A, Tabary C et al 1988 For how long must the soleus be stretched each day to prevent contracture? *Developmental Medicine and Child Neurology* 30: 3–10.

Taub E, Landesman R, De Luca S et al 2004 Efficacy of constraint-induced movement therapy for children with cerebral palsy with asymmetric motor impairment. *ProQuest Medical Library* 113: 305–312.

Terjesen T, Lange JE, Steen H 2000 Treatment of scoliosis with spinal bracing in quadriplegic cerebral palsy. *Developmental Medicine and Child Neurology* 42: 448–454.

Thelen E, Fisher DM 1982 Newborn stepping: an explanation for a 'disappearing' reflex. *Developmental Psychology* 18: 760–775.

Topp M, Uldall P, Greisen G 2001 Cerebral palsy births in eastern Denmark, 1987–90: implications for neonatal care. *Paediatric and Perinatal Epidemiology* 15: 271–276.

Turi M, Kalen V 2000 The risk of spinal deformity after selective dorsal rhizotomy. *Journal of Pediatric Orthopaedics* 20: 104–107.

Turker RJ, Lee R 2000 Adductor tenotomies in children with quadriplegic cerebral palsy: longer term follow-up. *Journal of Pediatric Orthopaedics* 20: 370–374.

Turvey MT, Fitch HL, Tuller B 1982 The Bernstein perspective: the problems of degrees of freedom and context conditioned variability. In: Kelso JAS (ed.) *Human Behaviour*. Hillsdale, NJ: Erlbaum, pp. 239–252.

Ubhi T, Bhakta BB, Ives HI et al 2000 Randomised double blind placebo controlled trial of the effect of botulinum toxin on walking in cerebral palsy. *Archives of Disease in Childhood* 83: 481–487.

van der Weel FR, van der Meer ALH, Lee DN 1991 Effect of task on movement control in cerebral palsy: implications for assessment and therapy. *Developmental Medicine and Child Neurology* 33: 419–426.

Vereijken B, Whiting HTA, Newell KM 1992 Free(z)ing degrees of freedom. *Journal of Motor Behaviour* 24: 133–142.

Wasiak J, Hoare B, Wallen M 2004 Botulinum toxin A as an adjunct to treatment in the management of the upper limb in children with spastic cerebral palsy. Cochrane Database of Systematic Reviews, Issue 4. Art No.: CD003469. DOI: 10. 1002/14651858.CD003469.pa63

Wiley ME, Damiano DL 1998 Lower extremity strength profiles in spastic cerebral palsy. *Developmental Medicine and Child Neurology* 40: 100–107.

Williams HA, Pountney TE 2005 Static bicycle training for non-ambulant adolescents with cerebral palsy: effect on muscle strength and functional ability. *Developmental Medicine and Child Neurology* 47 (suppl. 103): 61–62.

Wilmshurst SW, Adams K, Langton CM, Mughal MZ 1996 Mobility status and bone density in cerebral palsy. *Archives of Disease in Childhood* 75: 164–165.

Wong D, Baker C 1988 Pain in children: comparison of assessment scales. *Pediatric Nursing* 14: 9–17.

Neural tube defects

Teresa Pountney and Gillian McCarthy

INTRODUCTION

Neural tube defects (NTDs) are a group of developmental abnormalities in which the neural tube fails to fuse somewhere along its length from the spinal cord to the brain (McCarthy 1992). Spina bifida is the commonest NTD, where the lesion occurs in the spine. Hydrocephalus commonly occurs in association with spina bifida and is the condition where excess cerebrospinal fluid (CSF) circulates in and around the brain. This chapter describes the different NTDs and then focuses on the management of patients with spina bifida.

MECHANISM OF NEURAL TUBE DEFECTS

The neural tube develops from the neural plate early in embryonic development. Fusion normally occurs smoothly so that only the ends of the tube remain open. This means that the central canal remains in communication with the amniotic fluid. The upper (head) end of the tube develops into the brain and the lower end into the spinal cord. The lower end of the cord normally closes at 26 days of embryonic life (Levene 1988).

The tube can fail to fuse anywhere along its length but this occurs most commonly at the lower end. The vertebrae develop from ectodermal tissue and normally close over the cord at 11 weeks of embryonic life. In spina bifida there may be associated abnormality of the skin, bone, meninges and neural tissue. If only skin, bone and dura meninges are involved, a meningocele occurs (Figure 8.1a). This is relatively uncommon and may be associated with hair or a naevus. In spina bifida cystica the skin, dura and spinal cord are involved, and this is termed a myelomeningocele (Figure 8.1b); this occurs in 80% of spina bifida lesions. When the neural tissue of the spinal cord is displaced and exposed on the surface of the lesion, the term rachischisis is used (Figure 8.1c). In some cases the defect of the spinal cord and vertebrae may be covered by skin and hidden from sight, producing spina bifida occulta, which is a more minor abnormality.

At a higher level in the neural tube, the posterior part of the brain may fail to develop and fuse normally, producing an encephalocele. Of these lesions, 75–80% occur in the occipital region; however, lesions can be anterior, including over the bridge of the nose. If the whole of the anterior aspect of the neural tube fails to develop, anencephaly occurs, when there is complete absence of the cerebral hemispheres; this is incompatible with life after birth.

It is possible for both major and subtle abnormalities of the central nervous system (CNS) to accompany the spinal manifestations of spina bifida. The commonest problem is hydrocephalus, caused by obstruction of the outflow of CSF from the cerebral ventricles through the narrow canal or aqueduct, or the small exit foramina that allow the passage of CSF to the surface of the brain (Figure 8.2).

Another common problem is the Arnold–Chiari abnormality, in which the brainstem and cerebellar vermis are herniated through the foramen magnum. This can be associated with cysts, or dilation of the central canal of the spinal cord, syringomyelia, which may present with neurological abnormalities affecting swallowing, phonation, and power and sensation in the arms.

GENETIC ASPECTS

There is known to be a genetic element to the occurrence of NTDs, with a risk of recurrence of spina bifida of 1 in 20 following the birth of a first affected child. The risk of recurrence increases to around 1 in 10 if a second affected child is born. Thereafter, risk increases to 1 in 4. There is

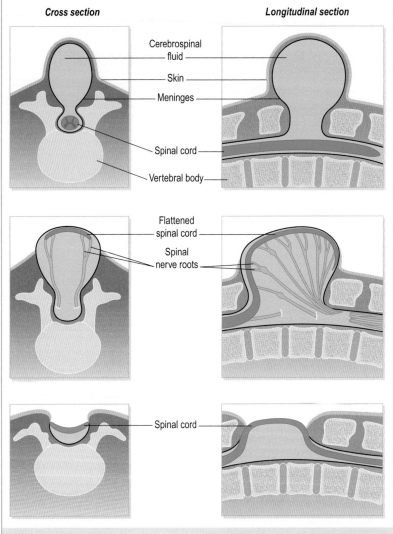

Cross section   **Longitudinal section**

Cerebrospinal fluid

Skin

Meninges

Spinal cord

Vertebral body

Flattened spinal cord

Spinal nerve roots

Spinal cord

Figure 8.1 Types of spinal lesion in spina bifida. (a) Meningocele: no neural tissue outside the vertebral canal. (b) Myelomeningocele: neural tissue and nerve roots may be outside the vertebral canal. (c) Rachischisis: there is no sac and the neural tissue lies open on the surface as a flattened plaque. CSF, cerebrospinal fluid. Reproduced from McCarthy (2002), with permission.

known to be a racial bias in the occurrence of NTDs. The Welsh and Irish have a higher incidence than the English, and Europeans have a higher incidence than Asians.

PREVALENCE

In the UK the prevalence of NTDs has been falling steadily over the past 30 years. Since it was unclear what part prenatal screening played in the reduced prevalence, a survey was carried out to clarify the position in relation to practice in 1985 (Cuckle et al 1989). The information available in

1985 showed that only 36% of the decline in prevalence of spina bifida could be accounted for by terminations of pregnancy. It was concluded that an NTD register should be set up to monitor the situation accurately. Figures from the National Congenital Abnormality Survey show a continuing decline in the UK (Table 8.1). The trend continued between 1995 and 1999 (Botting 2001).

In the mid-1970s, next to Ireland, the UK had the highest birth prevalence of NTDs in the world; now it has one of the lowest rates. Prenatal screening and diagnosis have been largely responsible for this but do not give the whole answer.

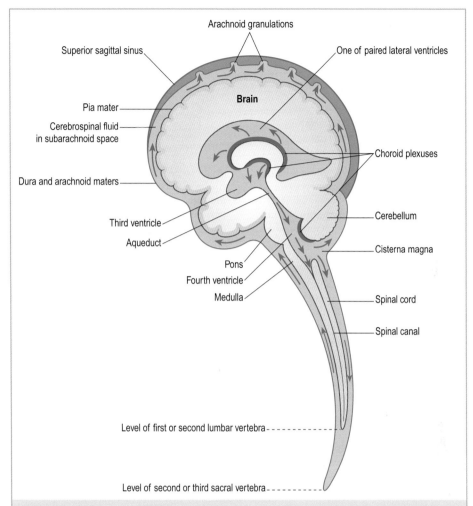

Figure 8.2 Cerebrospinal fluid (CSF) pathways. CSF is made by the choroid plexus in the lateral ventricles and flows through the third ventricle, aqueduct, fourth ventricle and, via the foramina of Magendie and Luschka and basal cisterns, over the surface of the brain, where it is absorbed by the arachnoid granulations. It also passes through the cisterna magna and spinal canal to circulate around the spinal cord. Reproduced from McCarthy (2002), with permission.

Folic acid has been shown to have a beneficial effect in preventing the occurrence of NTDs in a population of women at risk of producing further affected babies. An intake of folic acid of 4 mg/day before conception and for the first 3 months of pregnancy was sufficient to reduce the risk of recurrence of NTDs if there was a history of NTDs in the parents or first-degree relatives (Expert Advisory Group 1992). Since at least 30% of pregnancies are unplanned there is an argument for the fortification of flour with folic acid (Wald & Bower 1995). In the USA fortification of all enriched grain products such as flour has resulted in a population-wide increase in the concentration of serum folate (Lawrence et al 1999). It has been suggested that an increased intake of folic acid by the population in the UK of 0.4 mg/day could be sufficient to reduce the incidence of NTDs by approximately 1000 per year. However, there is still delay in implementing the proposal in the UK and continental Europe (Oakley 2002).

MANAGEMENT OF THE SPINAL LESION AFTER BIRTH

The neonate with open spina bifida needs to be carefully assessed after birth but it is not necessary to rush into rapid surgical intervention. Experience has shown that full assessment of the neurological, orthopaedic and medical problems should be carried out, together with social and emotional aspects of the family. The parents should be

Table 8.1 The incidence of anencephaly and spina bifida in the UK

	Rates per 10 000 births				
	1975–1979	1980–1984	1985–1989	1990–1994	1995–1999
Anencephaly	9.8	3.0	0.6	0.3	0.4
Spina bifida	15.1	8.5	3.3	1.3	1.0

fully involved with decision-making, including when not to treat babies with severe problems (Charney 1990).

The higher the neural lesion and hence the level of paralysis, the worse the prognosis for morbidity and mortality. The outlook is poor if severe hydrocephalus is present at birth, or there is marked spinal deformity or additional birth injury.

Active surgical treatment of myelomeningocele consists of closure of the lesion on the first or second day of life. The sac is opened, the neural placode mobilized and the dura then closed over the placode to form a watertight cover that is then covered by skin. Early closure reduces the risk of infection but the back can be covered by a sterile moist dressing and the sac will eventually epithelialize over. It is important to treat hydrocephalus at the same time as the closure of the back lesion, as pressure in the system rises and the back incision may leak CSF and fail to heal (see below).

HYDROCEPHALUS

The hydrocephalus associated with spina bifida is caused by obstruction to the normal pathways of flow of CSF in the brain, usually at the aqueduct, although it can occur at any point in the CSF circulation (Figure 8.2).

The CSF is produced by the choroid plexuses in the ventricles and normally circulates through the ventricular system and around the surface of the brain, where it is absorbed by the arachnoid granulations into the sagittal sinus. CSF also circulates around the spinal cord and down the central canal (Figure 8.2). If circulation of CSF is blocked, the fluid cannot be absorbed and pressure builds up.

Hydrocephalus develops in about 80% of children with spina bifida but is less likely to occur in those with lower spinal lesions (McCarthy & Land 1992). Hydrocephalus often develops after birth when the lesion on the back is closed (see above). This is caused by the rise in pressure caused by closure of the fluid-filled sac, which was previously able to absorb pressure rises. In addition, the Arnold–Chiari malformation may be displaced downwards by rising pressure in the cranium, obstructing the outflow of the foramen magnum and the posterior cisterns.

In the infant, pressure rises are more easily absorbed because the cranium is more flexible, the bones of the skull can be stretched and the head size increases rapidly. In the older child the skull becomes more rigid and the pressure is transmitted to the brain. The ventricular system dilates in three dimensions, stretching the brain and disrupting the architecture. The lateral ventricles themselves can increase the obstruction at the aqueduct by curling round and pressing directly on it.

There was no effective treatment for hydrocephalus until 1956 when John Holter, an engineer who had a son with hydrocephalus, working with Eugene Spitz, a neurosurgeon, perfected a valve and shunt system. This system was designed to provide a bypass for CSF from the cerebral ventricles to the right atrium of the heart, the ventriculoatrial shunt. Since that time many other types of shunt have been developed with the same principle of providing a bypass for the excess CSF. The most common route now used is from the cerebral ventricle to the peritoneum, a ventriculoperitoneal shunt, but shunts can also be drained into the lumbar theca, the pleura, or even into a gastric pouch.

In addition to bypasses for CSF, efforts have been made to place a tube into the aqueduct, using neuroendoscopy, or to reduce production of CSF by cauterizing the choroid plexus. The use of neuroendoscopy to make a window in the third ventricle to bypass the aqueduct, third ventriculostomy, has been successful in avoiding shunts in some children. This technique can also be used to make windows in cyst walls, or between the ventricles through the septum pellucidum, which is helpful if there is an uneven CSF flow between the two lateral ventricles. This is an exciting way to avoid long-term shunts but is only possible if the ventricular system is very dilated at the time of neuroendoscopy.

MECHANISMS OF ASSOCIATED NEUROLOGICAL PROBLEMS

If hydrocephalus is treated effectively from birth, neurological problems are likely to be reduced. However, some problems are undoubtedly caused by structural neurological abnormalities occurring during brain development and can be identified with magnetic resonance (MR) imaging. The effects of disruption of the immature brain can be inferred from the commonly encountered learning

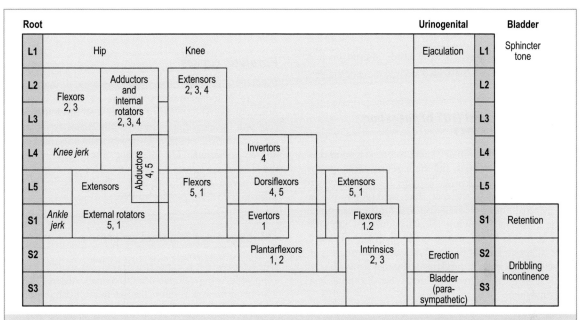

Figure 8.3 Segmental nerve supply of the lumbar (L1–L5) and sacral (S1–S3) nerve roots. Reading across from the nerve roots listed on the left of the diagram, the associated muscles of the lower limbs and bladder, bowels and sexual function can be seen. Reproduced from Pountney & Green (2004) with permission.

difficulties and problems of attention seen in children with hydrocephalus.

Vision

Pressure on the optic nerve can cause optic atrophy, which reduces visual acuity and can cause blindness. The optic pathways can be disrupted and the visual cortex may be damaged by huge dilatation of the ventricles, causing visual field defects or more subtle visual association difficulties. Eye movements can be affected by pressure on the oculomotor nerves, especially the sixth nerve, which has a long intracranial route, producing a convergent squint. Upward gaze can also be affected, causing the 'setting-sun' appearance. Cognitive visual problems are common in children with shunted hydrocephalus and should be sought by taking a structured history (Fixsen 1992).

Muscle power and sensation

The spinal lesion can affect innervation of the skin, muscles, bladder and bowel in many ways. Since MR scanning became widely available it has become clear that spinal cord abnormalities are very common. The cord may be divided by a bony spur or surrounded by fatty tissue. There may be a cystic swelling of the central canal, a syrinx, which occurs most commonly in the cervical or

lumbar regions. The cord may be adherent to the dural sac or stuck down by abnormally sited tissue. This tethering can cause gradual neurological damage and changes in neurological signs as the child grows, for example, loss of muscle power, altered skin sensation, or changes in bladder and bowel control.

SPINAL LEVEL OF THE LESION IN SPINA BIFIDA

The spinal level of neurological damage determines the functional abnormality, e.g. which muscles are affected and whether the bladder or bowel function is involved, although it is rare to get the precise cut-off level seen in spinal injury (Figure 8.3).

Neurological basis of orthopaedic problems

The spinal cord function may be impaired at a certain level or, more commonly, there may be interruption of the corticospinal tracts with isolated reflex activity present. A spastic paraplegia may occur, with some preservation of voluntary movements and sensation. Some children have a hemimyelomeningocele, with one leg affected and usually some bladder and bowel involvement.

Occult spinal dysraphism occurs when there is disordered closure of the neural tube or its coverings but the lesion is covered by skin. There may be external clues, such as a fatty swelling or hairy tuft or haemangioma, a dermoid or dermal sinus. There is usually no neurological abnormality at birth but the lesion should be fully investigated with MR imaging as neurological complications develop with growth.

Low lesions: sacral (10% of cases) or lumbosacral (20%)

With low lesions, there may appear to be very good neurological function at birth and the legs may look normal. It is important to examine the hips for instability and look at movement of the feet. The weakness of plantar flexion, small muscles of the feet and hip extension may not be immediately obvious. Sensory testing is also difficult but should be attempted in the neonatal period in order to get an idea of the level of lesion. Testing is performed using a firm pinprick from the toes upwards until a pain reaction is elicited. This indicates the spinal level of involvement.

Talipes equinovarus (TEV) deformities of the feet may be present at birth and it is important to initiate strapping or splinting to maintain a good position. The knees may be either flexed or hyperextended and there may be instability of the hips or frank dislocation, which requires immediate treatment (conservative management) in this group of children who have a good prognosis for walking independently.

Lumbar lesions (20%)

In higher lesions, muscle activity may be limited to hip flexion and adduction with some knee extension. The hips may be dislocated at birth but surgery in these circumstances is not indicated (Fixsen 1992).

High lesions: thoracolumbar (50%)

If the lesion is above L1 there is usually no useful muscle activity in the legs. Isolated reflex activity may be present, causing flexion contractures and flexor spasms that are difficult to manage and interfere with postural management and the use of orthoses.

Spinal deformity

Spinal curvature may be congenital or may occur as the child develops; the principles of management are similar for both.

Congenital curve

Spinal deformity may be present at birth, particularly in children with high lesions. There may be a kyphosis with a prominent forward curve. This is usually caused by the underlying vertebral, and sometimes rib, fusion abnormalities.

Paralytic curves

Paralytic curves are often associated with syringomyelia; they are related to muscle imbalance and appear later than other curves. About 75% of patients with myelomeningocele will develop a spinal curve; the majority of curves are paralytic or mixed, with fewer than one-third being entirely congenital. The incidence of scoliosis is related to the level of the lesion. All patients with a defect at T12 or above have a scoliosis, with the incidence reducing steadily to around 25% at L5 (Morley 1992).

Management of spinal deformity

During growth it is important to hold the spine as straight as possible, using a thoracolumbar spinal orthosis (TLSO). The anaesthetic skin can make bracing difficult, especially in the presence of kyphosis.

Conservative management of spinal deformity is, wherever possible, the best treatment. For this to be effective, the curve must be detected early and referred for specialist management. Bracing is the most commonly used treatment for curves which are flexible and less than 40°, and for children with remaining growth potential (Morley 1992).

Where surgery is indicated it is usual to carry out an MR scan of the spinal cord preoperatively to exclude any underlying abnormalities, including tethering of the cord. Assessment of respiratory function is important, especially in curves involving the chest, which may cause reduction of ventilatory capacity (see Ch. 18). Spinal fusion is carried out at the optimum time, usually between 10 and 13 years, carrying out anterior release, distracting the spine with a Harrington rod and fusing the spine posteriorly by excising the posterior joints and laying on bone grafts (Morley 1992).

Postoperative physiotherapy is vital to ensure that a child returns to full function as quickly as possible. Immediately postoperatively no form of spinal brace is worn, but when the child resumes sitting a removable polypropylene brace must be worn at all times for about 6 months to provide stability. When the child is sitting, care must be taken to prevent traction of the spine during lifting and transferring. Support must be given under the bottom during these procedures either by the lifter or by the use of transfer boards. There is a risk of pressure sores developing on anaesthetic skin and the child must be positioned and lifted to relieve pressure regularly (see below).

The child can usually begin sitting 4–7 days after surgery. While the child is in hospital a programme of exercises needs to be implemented to maintain muscle length and joint range in the lower limbs and to maintain the strength of arm and trunk muscles. Positioning of the ankles and knees to prevent muscle contractures is necessary, with passive movements to prevent decrease in joint ranges (see section on physical management, below). Significant postoperative complications of spinal surgery in children with spina bifida are higher than any other type of spinal deformity (Leatherman & Dickson 1988).

Neuropathic bladder

Bladder function may also be affected by the spinal lesion, depending on its anatomical site. If the sphincter is unable to relax during the normal sequence of micturition, there may be incomplete emptying of the bladder. This is often associated with high-pressure contractions of the bladder muscle, the detrusor, which can lead to back-pressure on the kidneys – detrusor sphincter dyssynergia. The combination of high pressure and infection can cause kidney damage, which may occur silently, eventually leading to renal failure.

Bladder activity can be monitored with urodynamic studies, which can be repeated at intervals. Renal function can also be monitored using different types of scan, e.g. dimercaptosuccinic acid nuclear scan, radionucleotide diethylenetriamine penta-acid (DTPA) scan or glomerular filtration rate scanning.

In general there are three types of bladder behaviour: contractile, intermediate and acontractile. The contractile problem of detrusor sphincter dyssynergia, which causes obstruction to outflow at the level of the distal sphincter, is recognized as the commonest cause of impaired renal function in children with congenital spinal cord problems. The most vulnerable times for renal function are in the first 5 years of life and the late teens (McCarthy et al 1992).

Management of the neuropathic bladder

The aims of management are to achieve continence and preserve renal function. Continence management depends on bladder function. Clean intermittent catheterization (CIC) is an effective method of management for some children, particularly with the use of medication to reduce bladder contractions and increase sphincter tone. Children can be taught to catheterize themselves from the age of about 6 years. If the bladder is small and contracts continuously, CIC is not helpful. If medication is not successful in reducing contractions, surgery may be necessary to increase bladder size or correct sphincter weakness.

Neuropathic bowel

Management of bowel incontinence can be a major problem, particularly for children with low spinal lesions who have poor anal sphincter tone and are active on their feet. The importance of early toileting to develop a pattern of

bowel emptying, even if it is through an incompetent sphincter, cannot be overemphasized. Other basic areas, such as appropriate diet, high fluid intake and the use of laxatives to aid the programme, need to be addressed.

The anocutaneous reflex, which has been used in planning bowel movement, is seen in 40% of children with spina bifida regardless of the level of the spinal lesion (Agnarsson et al 1993). Biofeedback has been used in the treatment of faecal incontinence in myelomeningocele (Whitehead et al 1986) and relies on the presence of some rectal sensation and a capacity to squeeze the external anal sphincter. Motivation and intelligence are also important for patient selection.

PHYSICAL MANAGEMENT

As with any disability, the physical management of a child with an NTD requires that the parents and therapists work in partnership to help the child achieve his or her full potential. Ultimately the parents' day-to-day care will have the greatest impact on the child's development and it is therefore vital that they are presented with a positive approach that puts value on their child's life and their ability to influence it. Professionals can give negative attitudes to disability that can be highly influential in shaping parental attitudes (French 1994). The physiotherapist needs to develop a lasting relationship with the child and family, and recognize the valuable role the parents play in this, by working with them to develop management programmes that can become part of their lifestyle.

The overall objective of physiotherapy in a child with a neural tube lesion is to promote normal development within the limits of the neurological constraints and achieve as much independence as possible.

The main aims of physiotherapy at all stages of an individual's life will include:

- Development of physical skills leading to independence
- The achievement of independent mobility, either walking or in a wheelchair
- Prevention of the development of deformity.

Management at different stages from birth to adulthood will now be considered.

Neonatal physiotherapy

An initial assessment should be made to determine the likely severity of the child's disability. Assessment of the baby's sensation and movement can be the responsibility of either the paediatrician or the physiotherapist. This assessment will give a fairly accurate picture of the child's future physical ability.

The assessment needs to be done quickly and efficiently, as the child will be in an incubator and unable to tolerate excessive handling. The physiotherapist should first record the baby's resting posture, any active movements and any abnormalities or deformities. Reflexes and muscle groups, rather than individual muscles, are then tested. A definite movement of the tendon or joint must be seen as an indication of the muscle's activity. The examiner should work from the toes upwards, as once normal activity is seen, the areas above this should be normal.

The test of sensation needs to be of protopathic (deep) feeling, as testing epicritic feeling (light touch) is not conclusive at this stage. Movements may be elicited due to uncontrolled reflex activity and a reaction to pain is a much more definite sign of sensation. This testing is best done using a firm pinprick.

Once the assessment is completed, a programme of passive movements and stretching exercises can be implemented to maintain and improve muscle length and joint range.

The most common deformities in the neonate with spina bifida are TEV and congenital dislocation of the hip. The management of TEV follows the same protocol as for idiopathic TEV and varies according to the severity of the deformity and between orthopaedic consultants (see Ch. 13). The most frequently adopted treatments are strapping with zinc oxide tape, the application of a corrective splint and serial plastering. Great care must be taken during these techniques as there may be impaired skin sensation and circulation that can lead to the development of pressure sores (see below).

The management of the baby with a congenital dislocation of the hips is conservative unless the lesion is low and the child will be an active independent walker (Fixsen 1992). The use of abduction splints is thought (from clinical observation) to lead to contractures of the abductors, causing later difficulties, and is not recommended.

During the neonatal period, early positive involvement by parents in their baby's care can aid acceptance of the disability. The main priorities will be the daily programme of stretching exercises and passive movements and care of the skin.

Preschool physiotherapy

The physiotherapist will often provide an ongoing link between home and hospital. Following the child's discharge from hospital, the parents will need regular support as the realities of the child's disability become evident. Visiting the family at home will reduce the unnecessary travelling and allow the child to be treated in a familiar environment. It also enables the physiotherapist to make a clearer assessment of the child's needs in the context of the family.

The physiotherapy programme started in hospital will need to continue and, as the child begins to develop, be updated. Between the ages of 6 and 12 months it is useful to update the muscle chart so that preparations can be made to provide the necessary orthotic equipment.

Passive movements to all lower-limb joints should be done at each nappy change to maintain joint range and stimulate the circulation. Once the child begins active arm and upper-body movements, these should be encouraged and strengthened. Children with spina bifida are often reliant on their arms for ambulation with sticks or crutches so they need to be strong. The child should be positioned as any normal infant in prone, supine and sitting positions to promote the normal developmental milestones of rolling and sitting (see Ch. 5) and maintain muscle length. The physiotherapist should educate parents in strategies to help their child develop and this is more successful through play and stimulation rather than rigid exercise programmes.

Children with high lesions may find developing sitting balance difficult and may require help with positioning so that they can free their hands for play. Trunk support or a wider sitting base may aid balance.

The normal child begins to explore the environment towards the end of the first year and it is important that the child with spina bifida is offered this opportunity, even if he or she cannot do it independently. Various items of equipment, such as prone trolleys and small carts, enable the child to propel himself or herself.

Children with spina bifida and hydrocephalus often experience difficulties with perception (Dunning 1994), including spatial difficulties, impaired hand function, and poor lateralization and figure-ground discrimination (the ability to identify details from a background and ignore irrelevant information). They may also have poor visual tracking skills so that they cannot track horizontally across the midline and converge and diverge rapidly. The combination of motor and perceptual deficits may result in the child having difficulty with walking as these skills are all needed to manoeuvre in relation to a stable and moving environment. An early opportunity to move about in the environment and experiment with movement may help to reduce these difficulties in later life.

A thorough occupational and physiotherapy assessment should be made to assess the level of the child's perceptual and motor skills, so that the necessary strategies can be implemented to overcome any deficits. Such tests are difficult to perform in detail in the preschool child but activities involving spatial awareness, e.g. moving over and under objects without touching them, judging speed of moving objects and general ability to move around in the environment, should be observed and any difficulties noted. Occupational therapists use a range of tests from the age of 4 years.

The child is usually ready to begin standing between the ages of 18 months and 2 years. An assessment of the degree of support needed can be made and the type of orthoses required discussed with parents. There are many benefits to standing, even if functional walking is not achieved. Mazur et al (1989) suggest that early mobility and the upright posture are valuable in promoting independence and mobility, decreasing the occurrence of pressure sores, reducing obesity and contractures, and are beneficial to the child's psychosocial well-being.

Children with a more severe disability who cannot walk will use a wheelchair and will be at high risk of developing postural deformities, so it is important that an assessment of their posture is made. The assessment should consider the child's needs in lying, sitting and standing. For a child who is sitting most of the day there is a risk of hip flexion deformities developing alongside windswept hips and scoliosis. The child should be controlled in a variety of symmetrical postures during the day and night to reduce the risk of developing deformity (see below), and sitting should be limited.

Before the child starts school an assessment of his or her physical and educational needs is made. The physical environment needs to be adapted to allow children with disabilities to move around freely and access all areas of the school. The addition of ramps, wider doorways and improved toilet facilities may be required. Consideration of the specific learning difficulties experienced by a child with hydrocephalus needs to take into account perceptual difficulties that involve figure-ground discrimination, spatial awareness, motor organizational skills, poor lateralization of skills, reasoning ability and number work. These factors may necessitate different learning strategies and the teacher needs to be made aware of these problems.

The 2001 Special Educational Needs (SEN) Code of Practice reinforces the 'stronger rights of children with SEN to be educated in mainstream school' (SEN Code of Practice 2001). Following assessment, parents and professionals will consider the available educational options based on the child's needs.

School-aged child

Once the child is in school, the physiotherapist will need to provide ongoing support to the parents and teaching staff. In many instances physiotherapists provide the link between the medical, home and school environments.

All staff working with children with hydrocephalus must be made aware of the signs that indicate shunt problems; these may include headache, vomiting, weakness or loss of dexterity, decreased levels of consciousness, irritability, slowing of performance, visual problems and worsening of any squint.

During the school years children develop their independence and begin to branch out from their families. This is a worrying time for parents and they need support in allowing their children opportunities to do this within safe boundaries. Teaching staff also need to recognize that a child with spina bifida experiences the same feelings and expectations as other children and should not allow the disability to interfere with the child's development. A child's attitude to his or her disability is likely to reflect the attitude of the adults encountered. If adults perceive the child as a difficulty to be endured, the child's

self-esteem will plummet. Imagination is often needed to enable the child to participate in all activities, but solutions can usually be found.

The school environment is much larger than home and the choice of walking or using a wheelchair for different activities may need to be made. Many children find that a wheelchair provides a speed and freedom they do not have when walking. For physical education and games, a wheelchair can be a real asset, as the child's hands are free. Physiotherapists or occupational therapists are responsible for teaching basic wheelchair skills.

During the school years, as a child is expected to take on more daily living and educational tasks, any difficulties with learning will become evident. Dressing and putting on orthoses, intermittent catheterization, learning the way to and around the school, as well as school work may prove arduous for children with perceptual, concentration or organizational difficulties. Tasks need to be broken down into manageable units and the use of visual cues introduced. Classroom assistants are invaluable in implementing such programmes. The physiotherapist needs to visit the school and/or home regularly to update these programmes.

A child's independence rests to a large extent on mobility, both moving around and transferring. Children need to develop strength and stamina in their arm muscles whether they wish to walk or use a wheelchair as their main form of mobility. To maintain this strength, children should be encouraged to do a regular programme of strengthening exercises, such as push-ups in prone or sitting positions, alongside an active sporting programme, which could include activities such as swimming, cycling with a hand-propelled or low-geared tricycle and wheelchair basketball. Not only do these activities strengthen muscles, they also increase the circulation and help with weight control, which are both contributory factors in the development of pressure sores.

Children should be taught to transfer safely to and from surfaces at different heights, e.g. from floor to chair, from wheelchair to toilet. It is important that the child is careful not to damage anaesthetic skin during transfers by clearing the surface over which they are moving and not dragging the skin. When a child is not wearing orthoses, he or she needs to make sure the legs are supported during the transfer.

Children who are walking with sticks or crutches need to practise how to fall safely and be able to regain the upright position. They must learn to release their crutches quickly and use their arms to protect themselves. Practice should begin on a soft crash mat and gradually move towards firmer surfaces. Reducing fear of falling is an important confidence booster for entering busy environments.

As the child grows, there is a risk of developing deformity and this must be monitored carefully. The most common deformities seen are hip dislocation and kyphoscoliosis. For children who have high lesions and spend most of their time in a wheelchair, it is essential that they are seated to maintain a symmetrical posture with an even distribution over the weight-bearing surfaces. Although seating cannot correct an existing deformity, it can contain postures and decrease the rate of progression (see below).

Muscle contractures of the hip flexors, hamstrings and calf muscles can develop due to spasticity if the child does not continue with a programme of stretching activities. The child needs to stand or lie prone for at least half an hour daily to stretch the hip flexors, to sit in the long-sitting position, preferably with orthoses to stretch the hamstrings and to position the feet in the plantigrade position when sitting or standing.

During the years at primary school, most children with hydrocephalus will undergo a revision of the shunt to lengthen the drainage tube. If a total revision is needed there may be some deterioration in physical skills. Intensive physiotherapy will be needed during these periods to restore the children to their previous levels of function.

Adolescence

The onset of puberty in children with spina bifida is often early and this can cause problems, as they tend to be socially and emotionally immature. Parents and teachers need to be aware of the conflict this creates within children and help them through this confusing period.

By the time children are in their teens, they should be able to take responsibility for much of their day-to-day care. They should also have an understanding of their disability and the implications of leading an independent lifestyle. Time should be spent on educating children in all self-management skills: physical management, catheterization, application of orthoses and skin care. They should also know where to seek help.

As children grow they need to take more responsibility for their health and fitness. They should learn to check their skin for signs of pressure, using inspection mirrors, when putting their orthoses on and off, and know the likely danger spots, i.e. toes, heels, behind the knees, buttocks and hips. If they are in wheelchairs for long periods they must do regular lifts, e.g. half-hourly, to relieve the pressure on the buttocks.

During the teenage years, many children will decide to increase the amount of time they use a wheelchair or opt to become a full-time wheelchair-user. A wheelchair can be liberating in terms of increasing speed and distance covered. This change can be a difficult decision to make and the child should ultimately make this decision.

The growth spurt experienced in adolescence will accelerate the progression of spinal deformities. Orthopaedic surgery of the spine and hips is often undertaken when the growth period is almost over. Preoperative physiotherapy is important to prepare a child physically for surgery. He or she must be prepared for a change in posture and the need to develop a different sense of balance. Some activities, such as moving the legs for transfers and putting on socks and shoes, may be limited after surgery.

With the decreasing incidence of NTDs and increasing inclusion in mainstream education, many children and teenagers lack the opportunity to socialize with others with similar disabilities. Such opportunities can be beneficial in terms of sharing experiences and learning more about the practical management of their condition. In the USA summer camps have proved a popular way of achieving this.

Adulthood

Transition to adulthood can prove difficult as the level of physiotherapy advice decreases and responsibility for care transfers to the young adult. Education can go some way towards enabling a young adult to be capable of caring for him-/herself, or of seeking care. Technological advances mean that adults can often achieve a high level of independence. However, where hydrocephalus has caused specific difficulties, such as short-term memory loss, the ability to cope may be severely compromised. In these cases appropriate care plans should be put in place for young adults who wish to live independent lives (Figure 8.4).

The young adult should be introduced to an adult physiotherapy team before leaving paediatric services so that there is a clear understanding of when and where to seek help. It may be useful for the physiotherapist to undertake an annual review to maintain contact (see Ch. 2).

Obesity and pressure sores are the main problems encountered in adults and it is important that opportunities to keep fit are offered via sports clubs for their active participation.

Orthoses

Orthoses that enable the child to achieve independent walking need to become an integral part of the child's life and should be introduced to the child and family in a positive, enthusiastic manner. The child should be encouraged, but not forced, to wear them and a gradual increase in their use advised. Edwards & Charlton (1996) reviewed orthotic devices used in adult neurological patients. Table 8.2 outlines the level of orthotic support required for different levels of lesion.

Children who require support above the pelvis frequently opt to use a wheelchair as an adult and it is important to be realistic in terms of walking for these children. The support required for a high lesion will include thoracic, lumbar, sacral and lower-limb orthoses. The child usually begins walking with a swivel movement, transferring weight from leg to leg, but progresses to a swing-through gait as strength and balance improve. Initially a rollator is used for support but the aim is to move to

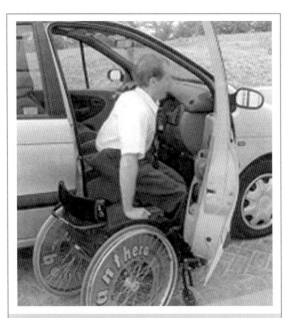

Figure 8.4 Independent young adult preparing to go to work in his adapted car. Reproduced from Pountney & Green (2004) with permission.

Table 8.2 Ambulatory support according to level of paralysis

Level of paralysis	Equipment required
Above L1	Thoracolumbar spinal orthosis (TLSO) with knee–ankle–foot orthoses (KAFOs) and hip guidance orthosis (HGO)
Below L2	TLSO with KAFOs and lumbar–sacral orthosis (LSO)
	LSO with KAFOs
Below L3–L4	LSO with KAFOs
	KAFOs alone
Below L5	KAFOs or ankle–foot orthoses (AFOs)
Below S1	AFOs

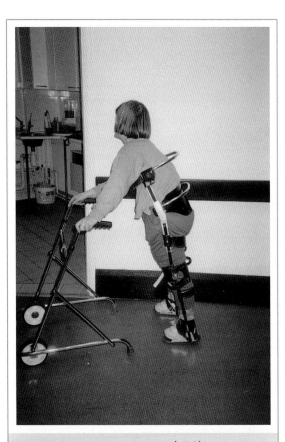

Figure 8.5 Hip guidance orthosis (HGO) in use with a rollator. The HGO is available under various brand names. Reproduced from Pountney & Green (2004) with permission.

quadruped sticks and eventually to crutches. The rate of progress will depend on the child's motivation to walk, parental input and physical limitations. The hip guidance orthosis (HGO) was developed for children with high lesions who experience difficulty with walking (Rose et al

1981). It enables the child to walk at a reasonable speed with a low energy output. The brace consists of a rigid body and leg brace with a fixed hip abduction of 5° that allows hip articulation during walking of between 5° and 10° on a shoe rocker (Figure 8.5).

Swivel walking plates may also aid the development of walking by enabling the child to move in an upright position before walking is possible.

The provision of orthoses to a child adds another very important dimension to the parental care that is already in place. It is important that parents understand how to apply the orthoses correctly and the need to make regular checks on the child's skin. Anaesthetic skin can easily develop pressure sores and care must be taken to prevent this.

The following guidelines should be implemented:

- A daily check of all anaesthetic skin areas
- Smooth clothing must be worn under orthoses and cover the whole area of skin contact; vest and socks should fit well and be worn with seams out

- Toes need to be uncurled when putting shoes on by running a finger underneath them
- Regular checks on the fit of orthoses and boots should be made.

A more definitive method is needed to assess the energy consumption of children with spina bifida who are walking, in order to assess their prognosis for long-term ambulation and as an indicator as to when ambulation should cease. Reliable predictive factors could reduce unnecessary surgery for children who will not be ambulant as adults. The Cosmed K2 system is a reliable method that can be used to measure energy cost in children with spina bifida (Duffy et al 1996).

Pressure care, posture and seating

The main factors in the development of tissue trauma are:

- Excessive force, causing tissue deformation and restriction of the blood supply
- Shear forces from friction of retaining a position or changing position
- Temperature: warm tissues have a better blood supply and therefore are at less risk of developing pressure sores
- Humidity: wet skin is more vulnerable to damage.

Children with spina bifida are at great risk of developing pressure sores, as most of the above factors are applicable, and where there is anaesthetic skin they are unaware of them. From birth the parents, and later the individual, must be vigilant in reducing these factors. Daily inspection is vital to spot areas that are developing redness. If reddened areas do not subside within 20 minutes of removing the pressure, then there is a real risk of sores developing and the pressure should not be reapplied.

Excessive force can arise from: uneven distribution of weight in sitting; failure to relieve pressure; poorly fitting orthoses; and creased clothing. Relieving pressure during long periods of sitting needs to become a habit alongside frequent orthotic checks.

Shear forces can be created when the person's sitting position does not maintain him or her in a stable posture and there is a tendency to slide down the chair or bed. Postural control systems that distribute pressure evenly and provide sufficient support are needed to prevent this (Pountney et al 2004). Seating systems for enhancing good posture in wheelchairs are discussed in Chapter 10 and have been reviewed by Pope (1996). Light-weight, high-performance wheelchairs are now available that are more functional and aesthetically pleasing than older models. Transfers by the child or carer can cause friction if the surface across which he or she is moving is not adequately cleared.

Temperature is difficult to assess where there is no sensation and is likely to fall in non-moving muscles and joints. The child should always be kept warm and learn to feel the skin regularly to check its temperature. Massage can be beneficial in warming the tissues and increasing blood flow. Sheepskin-lined boots can be worn in the winter.

Wet skin can be a danger area in children and adults who are incontinent. This, combined with excessive pressure or shearing forces, can be disastrous for anaesthetic skin. Skin hygiene in susceptible areas must be meticulous and, for later independence, wash-and-dry toilets are recommended.

Conservative management of pressure sores is achieved by relieving pressure on the affected area. For buttocks, contoured cushions and/or use of a self-propelled trolley is indicated. For legs, plaster of Paris or Baycast splinting, changed weekly, can be effective. Minor or plastic surgery is indicated for sores that do not respond to conservative management. Measures must be taken following healing to prevent pressure redeveloping in the same area.

CASE STUDY 8.1

JF was born in April 1989 with a myelomeningocele in the sacral region, L5/S1. The myelomeningocele was closed at 2 days and a shunt to control hydrocephalus inserted at 4 days.

An assessment of her muscle power at 10 days indicated that she would be an active walker with the help of orthoses. To maintain muscle length and joint range, a daily regimen of passive movements to the lower limbs was implemented.

Physiotherapy assessment at 2 months showed an infant with general low muscle tone and poor prone extension. There was no fixed calcaneus deformity; active dorsiflexion was present but there was no plantarflexion. Stretching of the ankles was recommended at each nappy change. Parents were advised to place JF in the prone position once a day to stretch hip flexors and to encourage active movement with stimulating play activities.

Equinus deformities were seen to be developing at 8 months and night splints to control ankle inversion were fitted. Parents were taught to check her skin regularly for marked areas.

continued

At 12 months JF could roll, sit unaided and take weight in standing. She was attending a specialist nursery once a week and developing into a happy and sociable little girl.

At 17 months she was beginning to pull to standing and at 21 months ankle–foot orthoses were prescribed, but she disliked them and preferred to walk without them, exhibiting an asymmetrical gait with hip-hitch and inverted feet. At 22 months knee–ankle–foot orthoses (KAFOs) were prescribed and gait education begun. Although able to walk without a rollator, she was encouraged to use it to develop a more symmetrical gait pattern.

At 2 years 8 months, JF suffered major shunt problems with infection and disconnection that lasted 4 months and included a bout of peritonitis. This was a very stressful period for her parents and left JF very weak. An intensive period of physiotherapy followed to regain lost muscle strength and mobility. Her left foot had developed an equinus deformity due to lack of splinting while she was ill, so splinting and frequent passive movements were encouraged.

At 4 years 3 months, JF was able to walk independently with KAFOs and a rollator but needed to hip-hitch to gain swing-through and later implications for her spine were noted. A physiological cost index (PCI) of 1.92 (normal 0.4) indicated that a great deal of effort was required to walk at this stage.

During this year preparations for JF to enter a mainstream school were made and she was awarded a statement of educational needs with ancillary help for 15 hours a week. This time was for educational support for specific learning difficulties related to hydrocephalus and physical support for moving around the school and toileting. At 5 years, JF began mainstream first school where staff were very concerned about accepting JF, and the specialist health visitor and physiotherapist spent a great deal of time liaising to support her entry into school.

Poor bladder function was successfully controlled with intermittent catheterization and JF was taught to perform the technique herself. This was a combined gradual approach, led by the specialist health visitor, with the parents and JF's non-teaching assistant.

JF had learnt to use quadruped sticks by the age of 6 years. She was managing well in school, walking independently and beginning to introduce crutches. She could walk independently but the asymmetry of her gait was reduced with sticks. She used a self-propelled wheelchair for long distances and games, rode a low-geared tricycle and swam weekly. These activities contributed to the promotion of specific muscle strength, general fitness and weight control.

At 6 years 6 months, problems with her shunt recurred. This was evident due to a loss of dexterity and general fatigue. She had a shunt revision, which was unsuccessful, followed by 2 weeks' exteriorization of the shunt due to infection. Another very stressful period with a long hospitalization occurred. Following this there was a considerable loss of balance and strength. JF returned to using a rollator for several weeks and increased her wheelchair use. Physiotherapeutic intervention was aimed at maintaining independent mobility whilst rebuilding muscle strength and fitness to previous levels.

REFERENCES

Agnarsson U, Warde C, McCarthy G et al 1993 Anorectal function of children with neurological problems. *Developmental Medicine and Child Neurology* 35: 893–902.

Botting B 2001 Trends in neural tube defects. *Health Statistics Quarterly* 10: 5–13.

Charney EB 1990 Parental attitudes toward management of newborns with myelomeningocele. *Developmental Medicine and Child Neurology* 35: 14–19.

Cuckle HS, Wald NJ, Cuckle PM 1989 Prenatal screening and diagnosis of neural tube defects in England and Wales in 1985. *Prenatal Diagnosis* 9: 393–400.

Duffy CM, Hill AE, Cosgrove AP, Corry IS, Graham HK 1996 Energy consumption in children with spina bifida and cerebral palsy: a comparative study. *Developmental Medicine and Child Neurology* 38: 238–243.

Dunning D 1994 *Children with Spina Bifida and/or Hydrocephalus at School*. Peterborough: Association for Spina Bifida and Hydrocephalus.

Edwards S, Charlton P 1996 Splinting and the use of orthoses in the management of patients with neurological disorders. In: Edwards S (ed.) *Neurological Physiotherapy: A Problem Solving Approach*. London: Churchill Livingstone, pp. 161–188.

Expert Advisory Group 1992 *Report on Folic Acid and the Prevention of Neural Tube Defects*. London: Department of Health.

Fixsen JA 1992 Orthopaedic management. In: McCarthy GT (ed.) *Physical Disability in Childhood*. Edinburgh: Churchill Livingstone, pp. 198–201.

French S 1994 Attitudes of health professionals towards disabled people. A discussion and review of the literature. *Physiotherapy* 80: 687–693.

Lawrence JM, Pettiti DB, Watkins M, Umekubo MA 1999 Trends in serum folate after food fortification. *Lancet* 354: 915–916.

Leatherman KD, Dickson RA 1988 *The Management of Spinal Deformities.* London: Wright, p. 191.

Levene MI 1988 The spectrum of neural tube defects. In: Levene MI, Bennett MJ, Punt J (eds) *Fetal and Neonatal Neurology and Neurosurgery.* Edinburgh: Churchill Livingstone, p. 267.

Mazur JM, Shurtleff D, Menelaus MB, Colliver JJ 1989 Orthopaedic management of high level spina bifida. *Journal of Bone and Joint Surgery* 71A: 5661.

McCarthy GT (ed.) 1992 *Physical Disability in Childhood.* Edinburgh: Churchill Livingstone, pp. 189–212.

McCarthy GT 2002 Cerebral palsy: the clinical problem. In: Squier W (ed.) *Acquiring Damage to the Developing Brain: Timing and Causation.* London: Arnold, p. 14.

McCarthy GT, Land R 1992 Hydrocephalus. In: McCarthy GT (ed.) *Physical Disability in Childhood.* Edinburgh: Churchill Livingstone, pp. 213–221.

McCarthy GT, Cartwright RD, Jones M 1992 Spina bifida. In: McCarthy GT (ed.) *Physical Disability in Childhood.* Edinburgh: Churchill Livingstone, pp. 189–212.

Morley TM 1992 Spinal deformity in the physically handicapped child. In: McCarthy GT (ed.) *Physical Disability in Childhood.* Edinburgh: Churchill Livingstone, pp. 356–365.

Oakley GP 2002 Delaying folic acid fortification of flour. *British Medical Journal* 324: 1348–1349.

Pope PM 1996 Postural management and special seating. In: Edwards S (ed.) *Neurological Physiotherapy: A Problem Solving Approach.* London: Churchill Livingstone, pp. 135–160.

Pountney T, Green E 2004 Neural tube defects: spina bifida and hydrocephalus. In: Stokes M (ed.) *Physical Management in Neurological Rehabilitation,* 2nd edn. Edinburgh: Elsevier.

Pountney TE, Mulcahy CM, Clarke S, Green EM 2004 *Chailey Approach to Postural Management.* East Sussex: Chailey Heritage Clinical Services, pp. 96–97.

Rose J, Gamble JG, Lee J et al 1981 Energy expenditure index: a method to quantitate and compare walking energy expenditure for children and adolescents. *Journal of Paediatric Orthopaedics* 11: 571–578.

SEN Code of Practice 2001 London: Department for Education and Skills, HMSO.

Wald NJ, Bower C 1995 Folic acid and the prevention of neural tube defects. *British Medical Journal* 310: 1019–1020.

Whitehead WE, Parker L, Basmajian L et al 1986 Treatment of faecal incontinence in children with spina bifida: comparison of biofeedback and behaviour modification. *Archives of Physical Medicine and Rehabilitation* 67: 218–224.

9

Developmental coordination disorder

Judith M. Peters and Ann Markee

CHAPTER CONTENTS

INTRODUCTION

The present chapter aims to provide paediatric physiotherapists with information about children with developmental coordination disorder (DCD) in terms of historical background, terminology and differential diagnosis and to offer a guide to service provision, including assessment and an outline of intervention approaches. Trends in current research are summarized and it is hoped that the chapter will reflect the present national and international picture of DCD and provide a useful resource of references.

DCD (American Psychiatric Association 1987, 1994, 2000) is a developmental condition in which there is marked impairment in the performance of motor skills. The impairment compromises success in everyday activities and school progress. The condition is idiopathic and the child has no identifiable medical, cognitive, psychological, social or other obvious condition or reason for the movement difficulty.

Health and educational professionals have long been aware of the existence of 'able' children who experience motor coordination difficulties that affect their ability to cope with the demands of everyday life. Longitudinal studies have demonstrated that such children do not simply 'grow out of' their difficulties (Hellgren et al 1993, 1994, Henderson & Hall 1982, Losse et al 1991). Without intervention the difficulties persist into adulthood and are frequently accompanied by other problems, both at home and at school (Cantell et al 1994). Of particular concern to physiotherapists is that this group of children tend to avoid normal physical activity (Bouffard et al 1996). This compromises fitness directly and in turn could make some children vulnerable to future disease, including osteoporosis, cardiovascular conditions, obesity, musculoskeletal disorders, accidents, type 2 diabetes mellitus and mental health problems (British Heart Foundation 2000, Department of Health 2004). The adverse effects of DCD are not always apparent to others, but may be doubly frustrating to a child whose potential in other learning domains may be normal. It is important that therapeutic intervention starts early and, as well as instigating thc foundations for an ongoing active lifestyle, should include guidance on the selection of appropriate physical and leisure activities. This can help alleviate motor problems during the school years and may also help improve quality of life and prevent later demands on physiotherapy and other services in adulthood.

HISTORICAL BACKGROUND AND A CONFUSION OF DIAGNOSTIC LABELS

Clumsiness that could be viewed as abnormal goes back at least to Galen (131–200 AD), who is reported to have spoken of some children as being 'ambilevous, that is, doubly left-handed' (Orton 1937, p. 120). In France, Dupré & Merklen (1909) reported clumsiness in children, which they viewed as a 'forme fruste' of, or at the very mild end of, a cerebral palsy continuum.

'Clumsy' is a descriptive word that derived from medieval Norse, meaning 'benumbed' or 'stiffened' with cold (*Compact Oxford English Dictionary* 1991). All of us are clumsy on occasion so it is not surprising that a colourful choice of synonyms has evolved in common English, e.g. 'awkward', 'clumsy' and 'uncoordinated', as well as expressions such as 'all fingers and thumbs'. However, it was not until 1962 that the term 'clumsy' became 'medicalized' as 'the clumsy child syndrome' following an editorial in the *British Medical Journal* (1962). For many years, this term appeared consistently in medical, paramedical, educational and psychological literature (Walton et al 1962, Dare & Gordon 1970, Gubbay 1975, Arnheim & Sinclair 1975, Gordon & McKinley 1980, Baker 1981) but due to its derogatory connotations it is now condemned in professional circles and by parents.

In contrast to 'clumsy', the term 'dyspraxia' (or developmental dyspraxia) has moved from its original medical usage to become a rather muddled lay term that lies uneasily alongside more specific use by professionals. Dyspraxia stemmed from 'apraxia' in adult neurology (Gonzalez Rothi & Heilman 1997), was adopted into paediatric vocabulary and entered everyday language officially in 1997 (Knowles & Elliott 1997). Speech and language therapists define the term in the context of specific language impairment (SLI). Similarly, within the sensory integration concept (Ayres 1972, Fisher et al 1991), dyspraxia is used quite specifically to denote difficulty in the ideation and planning of actions rather than a primary fault in the final execution of movement. Dyspraxia is used and defined much less precisely by parent support groups around the world (e.g. dyspraxia websites for Australia, Canada, Ireland, New Zealand and the UK).

The next term that deserves mention is 'minimal neurological dysfunction', which grew from the now firmly rejected diagnosis of minimal brain damage/dysfunction (Kalverboer et al 1978). Terms derived from these have retained popularity in parts of Australia (Williams & Unwin 1997). Another recent term, mainly confined to Scandinavia, is DAMP. The acronym stands for *d*isorder of *a*ttention, *m*otor control and *p*erception and denotes DCD plus attention-deficit disorder (ADD) (Gillberg 2003).

Non-specific terms such as 'movement difficulties' and 'poorly coordinated' are descriptive but 'motor learning difficulty' (Stephenson et al 1991) perhaps captures the crux of the problem by its emphasis on education rather than focusing only on the medical aspect of clumsiness.

Finally, the term 'sensory integration disorder/dysfunction', coined by Jean Ayres, an occupational therapist, is widely used following assessment on the Sensory Integration and Praxis Tests (SIPT) (Ayres 1989).

The above section reviewed a selection of terms applied to children with movement difficulties that are sometimes used synonymously with DCD. For further discussion on terminology, readers are referred to Henderson & Barnett (1998) and Peters et al (2001).

DSM-IV and official criteria for DCD

Two classifications systems attempt to provide definitions of childhood disorders as a standard yardstick for diagnosis.

The condition we are concerned with here, a motor learning difficulty (DCD), is now officially recognized by both the American Psychiatric Association (1987, 1994, 2000) and the World Health Organization (1992) in their formal classification manuals. The World Health Organization classifies childhood clumsiness as 'specific developmental disorder of motor function' (SDD-MF) in the *International Classification of Disease* (ICD-10) (World Health Organization 1992). However, this cumbersome term has never gained popularity. The *Diagnostic and Statistical Manual of Mental Disorders* (DSM-IV: American Psychiatric Association 1994, 2000) criteria for DCD are provided below. It should also be noted that entries for DCD and SDD-MF are not identical and the reader is referred to Henderson & Barnett (1998) for a critical review. Publication of an international consensus statement following a meeting in London, Ontario in 1994 moved toward clarification and standardization by proposing that the term 'developmental coordination disorder' be officially adopted and listed as a key term in published research on DCD (Polatajko et al 1995).

In the following section physiotherapists are reminded of the criteria for the use of the label DCD. DSM-IV-TR (American Psychiatric Association 2000, p. 58), documents the essential features of DCD under four criteria, *all* of which should be met for a diagnosis of DCD to be made.

Criterion A

Performance in daily activities that require motor coordination is substantially below that expected given the person's chronological age and measured intelligence. This may be manifested by marked delays in achieving motor milestones (e.g. walking, crawling, sitting), dropping things, 'clumsiness', poor performance in sports or poor hand-writing.

Criterion B

The disturbance in criterion A significantly interferes with academic achievement or activities of daily living.

Criterion C

The disturbance is not due to a general medical condition (e.g. cerebral palsy, hemiplegia or muscular dystrophy) and does not meet the criteria for a pervasive developmental disorder.

Criterion D

If mental retardation is present, the motor difficulties are in excess of those usually associated with it.

DSM further states that symptoms may vary with age. Younger children may show clumsiness, delayed motor milestones or difficulty buttoning clothes, tying shoelaces or using a knife and fork. Older children may present with difficulties with the motor aspects of assembling puzzles, building models, playing ball or hand-writing. Speech and language problems are commonly associated with the condition.

For physiotherapists, the following comments that appear in either or both of the official manuals are relevant: the coordination difficulty should have been present since early development (i.e. not an acquired deficit); it should be significant and measurement on a standardized motor test is recommended; although there is no diagnosable neurological disorder, in many cases 'soft' neurological signs and symmetrically altered reflexes may be elicited; and there may be a history of perinatal complications, e.g. prematurity or very low birth weight.

Researchers and clinicians are urged to follow the official international criteria as a basis for standardizing communication of what constitutes DCD. As will become clear, however, there are many problems in applying the criteria, especially when it comes to criterion C and the exclusion of other conditions.

Heated argument continues worldwide about disparate use of labels and how one interprets the official criteria for DCD. Physiotherapists should be careful to use objective methods to compare a child's motor performance with age peers, and interpret information provided by a child, parents/carers and professional colleagues to determine whether the movement difficulty actually amounts to a problem (criteria A and B). Criterion C is the most difficult to interpret. There is often argument about what amounts to a medical condition and especially around the ill-defined boundary area between very mild cerebral palsy and DCD.

Does a child with co-occurring Asperger's syndrome (a pervasive developmental disorder) automatically become excluded from having a diagnosis of DCD? Yes, according to current DSM criteria. A recent series of seminars attended by a panel of experts working in the field of DCD resulted in the Leeds Consensus Statement (Sugden 2006). The delegates acknowledged DCD as a unique and separate neurodevelopmental disorder that often co-occurs with other disorders such as attention-deficit disorders, autistic spectrum disorders and dyslexia. They considered it inappropriate to exclude a dual diagnosis of DCD and pervasive developmental disorder and that both diagnoses should be given if appropriate. Generally, a child with an IQ below 70 would not be diagnosed as DCD (criterion D) in current practice, although DSM does not provide an exact guide. There are ongoing attempts to bring some consistency across research internationally, but clinically there is still a lack of diagnostic standardization.

Physiotherapy intervention should be based on reliable evidence and as a starting point a child's condition must be clearly and consistently identified according to agreed criteria. Physiotherapists must examine published research studies critically to determine the characteristics of the participants and whether the movement difficulty was the primary core problem or whether a child had additional diagnoses, which might influence the results. A valid and reliable outcome measure may suggest whether intervention has brought about change but this is only relevant to a child's initial condition as clearly defined. A child with 'pure' DCD meeting DSM criteria may be very different from a child with 'clumsiness' associated with an autistic spectrum disorder (pervasive developmental disorder). All too often articles are published on ill-defined groups of children with so-called DCD, within which are a variety of children with mixtures of cerebral palsy, attention deficits or perhaps mild mental handicap and the conclusions are therefore not necessarily applicable for DCD as officially defined. However it is encouraging that there are now many studies with better-defined groups.

PREVALENCE

Prevalence figures vary from under 3% to over 15% depending on criteria used, but a figure of 5–6% of children in mainstream primary education is quoted in DSM-IV (American Psychiatric Association 1994). DCD occurs worldwide and boys are identified around two to three times as often as girls. However it is important not to overlook symptoms in girls. They may be underrepresented, often blending into the classroom without displaying externalizing behaviour that draws attention to their difficulties.

AETIOLOGY

The precise causes of DCD are not yet known but appear to be multifactorial. DCD co-occurs or is associated with other developmental conditions including SLI, ADD and/or hyperactivity (ADD/HD), reading difficulty (dyslexia) and Asperger's syndrome (Ghaziuddin et al 1994, Kaplan et al 1998). When one considers that some of these conditions further overlap with other disorders, e.g. tic disorders/Tourette syndrome, joint hypermobility syndrome, obsessive-compulsive disorder and conduct disorder, to name just a few, the scene becomes quite complex! Researchers are looking at genetic causes and in some children with DCD premature birth, low birth weight and other prenatal factors are implicated (Hadders-Algra & Gramsbergen 2003). Children are affected to varying degrees and do not all present with the same features. Sometimes the problem mainly affects gross motor actions; in others manipulative skill is affected. In many cases a child has motor dysfunction with associated language, attention and/or behaviour problems. The physiotherapist is likely to be primarily involved with the core motor difficulty but the associated problems must always be borne in mind and should determine and influence the approach to intervention.

PROGNOSIS

Although movement skills tend to improve with maturity, research has shown that DCD may persist and associated educational, social and emotional problems often continue into adult life (Losse et al 1991, Cousins & Smyth 2003). There is no magic cure, but children can be helped to understand and improve their movement skills and develop self-confidence and coping strategies.

PRESENTATION

The formal entry in DSM, already mentioned, outlines the main presenting features. Children with DCD have much greater difficulty than other children in acquiring the fluent movement needed to function in everyday life. Motor milestones may have been delayed, but not always. At home, dressing, especially tying shoelaces or fastening buttons, and using a knife and fork are frequent problems. Often, younger siblings overtake the child with DCD, with consequences for family dynamics. At school, they struggle with activities such as hand-writing, drawing diagrams and using scissors. They often hate physical exercise and balancing, hopping, skipping, catching a ball or pedalling a bicycle are all difficult skills to learn. They may become loners in the playground, not enjoying the rough and tumble and physical activities and games enjoyed by their peers. Lack of movement skill often interferes with school progress and many children do less well than would be expected of them, given their cognitive and language abilities (Cantell et al 1994). This gives rise to frustration for a child, teachers and parents alike. Even more puzzling and frustrating is that children with DCD are generally healthy and bright with no other obvious medical, psychological or cognitive reason for their difficulties.

DIFFERENTIAL DIAGNOSIS: THE 'RED FLAGS'

The first and most important step in the management of any child presenting with possible DCD is to rule out a differential diagnosis such as muscle/neurological diseases or cerebral palsy by a thorough medical examination, ideally by a specialist paediatrician. Physiotherapists play a major role in the identification process. This includes differentiating between typical and atypical motor development. Physiotherapists who treat a wide variety of movement conditions will be well aware that 'clumsiness' is not an uncommon observation; however, in order to recognize abnormality, the physiotherapist must be thoroughly familiar with *typical patterns* of development in the context of different socioeconomic backgrounds, experiences and cultures. The average 2-year-old often tumbles, is not expected to tie shoelaces or fasten buttons and will not be able to hop, skip or write letters. Many physiotherapists, however, have vast knowledge about *atypical function* but insufficient understanding of exactly how and when typically developing children learn and achieve different motor skills. Children mature at different rates and follow a variety of developmental trajectories. Some walk early at 7 months and talk late after 2 years, some never crawl, others speak early but may be slower than their peers to walk. There is a wide range of normal variability and it is unwise to label a child formally as having DCD in the preschool period. Physiotherapists are key professionals trained with specific skills which enable them to recognize subtle deviations and concerns about motor progress during this early developmental period; a period when intervention may be most effective.

Clumsiness may be associated with deficits in vision or hearing, musculoskeletal problems such as tibial torsion or hypermobility syndrome. However, poor motor function may also indicate a deteriorating condition such as muscular dystrophy or a neurological condition. The physiotherapist may be the first professional who meets with a child and should look out for 'red flags' (Box 9.1) that might point to serious pathology that requires further investigation.

Referral depends upon presenting problems, local facilities and protocols. Best practice is based on a transdisciplinary model with good interprofessional communication, liaison and skill mix. There is considerable overlap between services offered by physiotherapy, occupational therapy and speech and language therapy. Occupational therapy waiting lists have been reported to be up to 4 years in some areas of the UK (Dunford & Richards 2003). The use of screening protocols, including one-stop clinics, has been explored recently (Stephenson et al 2002, Green et al 2005). Increasing links are developing between health, psychology and education in addressing the complex needs of the

---

Box 9.1 Red flags to alert physiotherapists

- Sudden appearance of clumsiness in an otherwise typically developing child
- Muscle weakness, especially if localized, asymmetrical or becoming more marked
- General fatigue and listlessness, which may indicate systemic illness or depression
- Abnormal reflexes that might point to a neurological condition
- Café-au-lait marks and freckling, which may indicate neurofibromatosis
- Joint pain, which may indicate juvenile idiopathic arthritis or haemophilia
- Spine, hip or foot deformities that may underlie the movement problem Unusual bruise patterns that could be associated with abuse

whole child and new approaches to the management of DCD are less focused on the clinic and extend into education and community settings.

FEATURES OF DCD

Developmental variability means that the physiotherapist must decide whether the 'clumsiness' identified is significantly out of line with age peers and family and cultural trajectories. The following are some features to look out for at different ages.

Preschool: 0–4 years

Concern should be raised when there is motor delay in an otherwise medically healthy infant with normal neurological and cognitive development, especially when combined with mild language delay and/or unusual locomotion. Frequent falls, poor rolling, bottom shuffling and/or low tone may be observed. At this stage the main features that the parents note are that a child's motor function is slower than and/or different from that of siblings and a child may be described as 'accident-prone'. The infant may be fussy and respond unusually to sensation and may be either excessively hyperactive or noticeably hypoactive and unwilling to explore. It is important to determine whether the child has had an opportunity to move and been encouraged to play freely. Following recommendation that babies should be placed in a supine sleeping position, some infants lack experience of play in the prone position, which may affect early development (Majnemer & Barr 2005). Sometimes a child has been carried, fed, dressed and generally overprotected, and his or her lack of motor independence and organization reflects immaturity and inexperience rather than DCD. Although many children with learning difficulties have poor movement skills, the label DCD is not usually appropriate. This does not mean, however, that their 'clumsiness' should not or cannot be helped by intervention.

Primary school: 5–11/12 years

Physiotherapists are likely to receive referrals of children with gross motor delay in the preschool period. However, it is at primary school, at around 6 or 7 years, when parents and/or teachers raise concerns, that children showing signs of DCD are most often referred to physiotherapy by the general practitioner, school doctor, paediatrician or therapy colleague. Referral to a physiotherapist is usually on account of gross/fine motor incoordination. A child drops things, is described as 'clumsy' and difficulty is noticed in learning to hop, skip, ride a bicycle or catch a ball. Teachers notice that a child avoids or is poor at physical education and may lack strength and/or stamina

and be unfit (or even overweight) due to lack of appropriate regular physical activity.

'Soft' neurological signs such as mild muscle hypotonia or hypertonia (but not asymmetrical in distribution) may be noted. There is often language delay and a child may have been referred for speech and language therapy (Stephenson et al 1991, Peters & Wright 1999). Some children with DCD may also display features of autistic spectrum disorder and require further investigation (Ghaziuddin et al 1994, Green et al 2002).

Subtle signs, such as fear of movement or dislike or avoidance of certain textures (e.g. clothing, food or 'messy' play), may indicate that a child is uncomfortably stressed by sensations from the environment. These factors must be taken into consideration for the classroom, home and therapy setting.

Hand-writing is one of the most frequent concerns for children with DCD and at least 60% of children with DCD are reported as having hand-writing difficulty (Peters et al 2004). Unless the problem is addressed early, such children will struggle in school as increasing demands are made for writing production. The nature of hand-writing difficulties includes difficulty in control of the pen, an uncomfortable grip with complaint of aching, poor posture and problems with the concept of letter formation. There are also children whose difficulties are more subtle and hard to define whose problems with the motor aspects of hand-writing may be linked with other problems, e.g. with language, attention, social communication and reading. A child may be slow to adopt a preferred hand and may remain ambidextrous. Often such children have problems in direction (distinguishing right from left). A child may also have problems in handling other tools such as scissors, rulers and cutlery.

Self-care activities of daily living, e.g. eating tidily, putting on socks, tying shoelaces, doing up buttons or zips, may be problematic. The tasks may need breaking down into achievable components to ensure success.

The child with DCD may have primary or secondary behavioural and emotional difficulties which compromise friendships. At playtime a child may be ostracized and become isolated from the peer group. Yet again the opportunity for physical activity is reduced. Reports of underachievement in school combined with increasing lack of self-esteem are frequent, especially as transfer to secondary education approaches (Schoemaker & Kalverboer 1994, Smyth & Anderson 2000).

Secondary school

Problems continue but in addition there are demands for greater self-organization, the need to cope with using more intricate tools (in craft, science, maths), the demands of a competitive physical education curriculum and the need for legible fast writing sustained over long periods of time. The student must also be able to carry schoolbooks around and swim competently and peer acceptance usually expects reasonable proficiency in leisure activities such as dancing or cycling. Approach to adolescence raises the importance of looking good and fundamental to this is grooming, e.g. nails and hair, postural control and stance. As a student enters the adult world the impact of under-achievement and lack of enjoyment and participation in physical activity may lead to feelings of anxiety, helpless-ness and depression (Hellgren et al 1994).

WHOLE-CHILD APPROACH TO ASSESSMENT

DCD is a complex condition in which paediatric medi-cine, psychology and education overlap and is of major concern to physiotherapists, occupational therapists and speech and language therapists. It is important that pro-fessionals from health, educational and/or psychological backgrounds involved in the assessment process form a team, which shares knowledge/experience and informa-tion yet avoids unnecessary duplication of skills. A whole-child approach is essential with the child and the family/carer as vital members of that team (see Ch. 2).

Evaluation of perceptual motor function is most often carried out by paediatric-trained occupational and/or phys-iotherapists. Concerns in the domain of communication and oral function should be assessed by a speech and lan-guage therapist. It is important that a child undergoes psy-chometric tests of cognitive function and that possible associated specific learning difficulty be identified early on. Vision and hearing should be tested to exclude dysfunction.

Physiotherapy assessment

It is appropriate to consider assessment as an ongoing cyclical process involving the identification, classification and description of the motor difficulties, leading to plan-ning of intervention and reassessment and evaluation of outcome (Figure 9.1).

Several factors determine the format of the physiother-apy assessment, one of the most important being whether the assessment is uni- or multidisciplinary. Ideally profes-sionals from different disciplines will each contribute toward assessment in their own area of expertise either jointly or individually. There is sometimes overlap of knowledge but more often there is a dearth of suitably experienced professionals. In the following section assess-ment is addressed from the physiotherapy perspective but appreciating the value of a multidisciplinary approach.

Background information and medical history

Information about particular areas of difficulty and school progress may be gathered via the child, parents and teachers using a variety of informal or published checklists, e.g.

Developmental Coordination Disorder Questionnaire (DCDQ) (Wilson et al 2000); Movement Assessment Battery for Children (M-ABC) checklist (Henderson & Sugden 1992) and Strengths and Difficulties Questionnaire (SDQ) (Goodman 1999).

It is important to record relevant details concerning the child's birth history (gestation, pre- peri- or postnatal problems), developmental milestones and significant medical details. Always ask whether a child is currently taking medication and note especially whether this has been administered prior to physiotherapy assessment. A child's behaviour and performance on perceptual motor tests may be affected by medication.

Neurodevelopmental clinical observation

The assessment should include examination of muscle tone and power. Manual muscle testing based on the Medical Research Council scale (Medical Research Council 1943) provides a useful guide. Recent technological advances in myometry provide reliable objective measures, e.g. fist grip measurement using an instrument such as the Cytec dynamometer has been used in the management of patients with muscular dystrophy (Bushby et al 2004). It is important to assess flexibility of the musculoskeletal framework as it affects core stability and may account for a child losing balance, tiring easily and having difficulty stabilizing a pencil for writing. Flexibility depends on sev-eral factors, including age, ethnicity and gender. Beighton criteria (not yet standardized for children) give a simple guide to flexibility/laxity and joint range (Maillard & Murray 2003, p. 36). However, recent research questions the cut-off scores that are most used and recommends that stricter criteria should be adopted when assessing children (Jansson et al 2004). Figure 9.2 shows an athletic boy aged almost 8 years with asymptomatic joint flexibility and normal motor function. This contrasts with other cases where connective tissue elasticity severely affects muscle function and stability throughout the body.

It is important to observe movement patterns, postural control and girdle stability, comparisons between perfor-mance of unilateral versus bilateral actions and a child's abil-ity to sequence a series of individual actions during the physiotherapy assessment. Box 9.2 provides examples and a guide to the types of observations that are useful.

A standardized norm-referenced test of general motor competence (e.g. M-ABC) is recommended as a measure of general motor competence and as a basis from which to derive evidence of the effectiveness of subsequent intervention. The child completes a series of fine and gross motor tasks in the domains of manual dexterity, aiming and catching and balance. The M-ABC not only gathers quantitative data (normed scores) but also pro-vides the opportunity to record qualitative observations in a structured framework of how the child performs the motor actions. Many informal and subjective measure-ments are used in clinical practice and supply useful

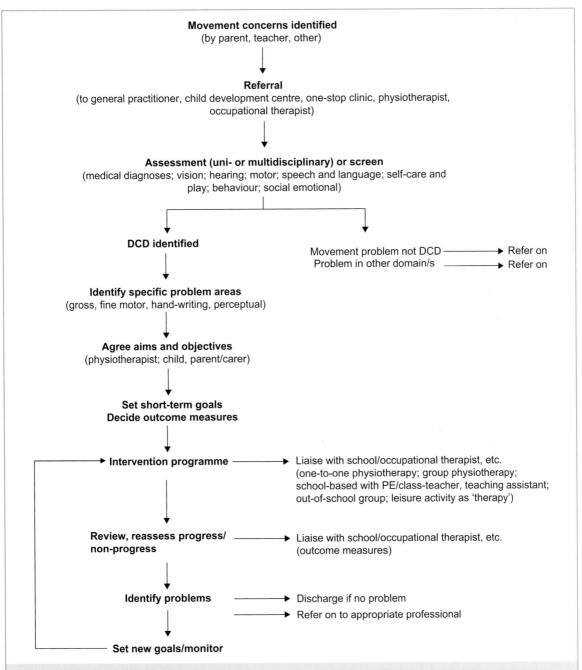

Figure 9.1 Flow chart to demonstrate cyclical process of identification, classification, intervention planning and evaluation of outcome. DCD, developmental coordination disorder.

qualitative information. These do not provide sufficiently reliable objective data for the justification or effect of intervention.

An attempt should be made to evaluate what may be termed 'praxis' or the more cognitive aspects of motor skill, including ideation and planning of movement. Tests such as Sensory Integration and Praxis Test (SIPT) (Ayres 1989) and Miller Assessment for Pre-schoolers (MAP) (Miller 1988) have been designed to examine perceptual motor function within a broader context. These include execution of novel movement sequences, gesture, imitation of postures and tests of tactile, proprioception, visual and auditory perception. The physiotherapist may find that it is helpful to include a test of visual motor function to assist in teasing out a child's difficulties. The developmental test of Visual Motor Integration (VMI) (Beery 1997) now includes a main test and subtests of visual perception and motor coordination

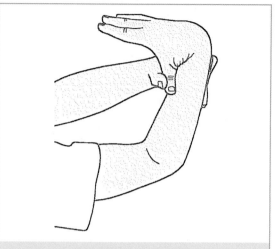

Figure 9.2   Joint hypermobility identified at physiotherapy assessment.

(see Ch. 3). This and observations of a child's drawings may highlight underlying visual spatial difficulties. Figures 9.3 and 9.4 illustrate confusion in body perception and planning that children with DCD often show in their drawings.

Functional activities and goal-setting

DCD may be associated with lack of fitness and/or obesity. Physiotherapists have access to a range of gym equipment to evaluate fitness and anthropomorphic measures such as body mass index. Assessment in a clinic is far removed from real life and it is important to evaluate the impact of a child's lack of coordination in terms of everyday pursuits. Tools are available that focus on function (e.g. Pediatric Evaluation of Disability Inventory (PEDI): Haley et al (1992); Peabody Developmental Motor Scales, 2nd edn: Folio & Fewell (1983); the Perceived Efficacy and Goal-setting System (PEGS): Missiuna et al (2004). These may be used to help determine a child's attitude and interest in physical activity and leisure pursuits and can help the child and therapist to set relevant goals. Functional tools reflect the move away from classification of handicap and impairment toward health and well-being (World Health Organization 2001).

Box 9.2   Observations that are part of a physiotherapy assessment of a child with developmental coordination disorder

Movement patterns

- Are these symmetrical and fluent or are there marked overflow movements and associated reactions that might suggest neurological damage?
- Does child appear weak at the 'core' but with excess twitching or associated movements distally in face and fingers?
- Does child walk with normal heel–toe action and symmetrical arm-swing?
- Can child run, jump, hop (on either leg) with adequate explosive muscle action?

Postural control and girdle stability

- Can child rise to stand from supine lie without reliance on hands?
- Can child move from half-kneel to stand via either leg?
- Can child maintain four-point kneel with stability while moving one or two limbs?
- Can child achieve and sustain supine flexion or prone extension?
- Can child balance on either or both legs on various surfaces with or without vision occluded?
- Are head, shoulders, pelvis and spine in alignment?

Unilateral versus bilateral action

- How does child perform action – unilaterally or bilaterally? Many children struggle with bimanual tasks such as holding paper while cutting with scissors, using a knife and fork, buttoning clothes or coordinating reciprocal actions such as skipping
- Is there hesitation when crossing midline of the body? Does the child change hands?
- Can child move tongue rapidly side to side without coupled jaw action?

Action sequences (depending on age)

- Can child carry out a series of actions such as threading a lace; copying a clapping/jumping sequence; constructing a brick model; folding paper and placing it in an envelope; unwrapping a sweet or taking apart and putting together a biro or simple toy?
- Can child copy a sequence of hand postures/gestures?
- Can child write the letters of the alphabet in sequence?
- Can child repeat 'pat-a-cake' clearly?

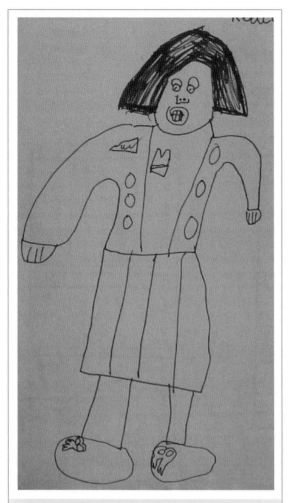

Figure 9.3 Drawing by a girl with developmental coordination disorder: note asymmetry of arms reflecting her visual perceptual difficulty.

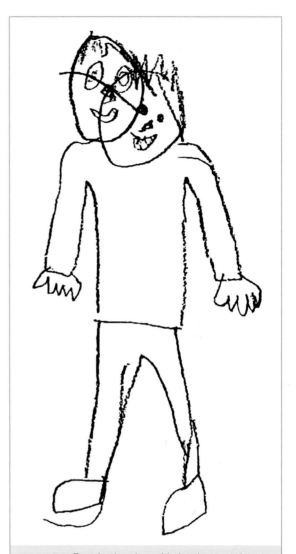

Figure 9.4 Drawing by a boy with developmental coordination disorder: note his perceptual and planning difficulty.

Behaviour, attention, arousal, communication

It is important also to be aware of function outside the motor domain (Chesson 1998). The physiotherapist should observe behaviour, including activity level, cooperation, ability to modulate arousal response (reactivity) (e.g. using the Short Sensory Profile: Dunn 1999) and attention. Observe non-verbal and verbal communication, listening skills, appropriate eye contact and social interaction. The SDQ is a screening tool which provides useful information across a breadth of domains. There are also specific tools to screen children for the likelihood of an associated autistic spectrum disorder (e.g. the high-functioning Autism Spectrum Screening Questionnaire (ASSQ) (Ehlers et al 1999).

Hand-writing

Hand-writing is described as 'language by hand' (Berninger 2004). It is a complex cognitive, perceptual motor skill which, unlike other motor skills, is not acquired automatically but needs to be well taught. It is also different from other graphic skills and involves many non-motor components (Barnett & Henderson 2004). Hand-writing as a motor skill is pertinent to physiotherapists due to their expert knowledge of the anatomy of the hand and understanding of the development of manipulation. They have specific awareness of musculoskeletal function, the development of balance and postural control, which provides the essential proximal stability for writing.

Hand-writing evaluation, often in conjunction with an occupational therapist, is an inherent part of the assessment for any child with DCD. Prerequisite hand-writing skills may be observed during graphomotor items in the VMI, M-ABC or by watching a child scribble, draw a person/picture or write letters of the alphabet in sequence. Pencil grip should be observed and, although the dynamic tripod grasp (support by thumb, first and second fingers) is the most common and natural grasp, many different grasps are acceptable provided they are functional and do not result in muscle strain (Benbow 2002). Variation in pen hold is normal and does not seem to predict legibility or speed of writing (Berninger 2004). Sequential finger movements are needed for producing letters in isolation and in written communication. As the child faces increased demands to produce longer scripts it may be useful to utilize speed writing

tests for the older child in order to evaluate constraints on writing production (Wallen et al 1996). The physiotherapist should observe posture, especially tension around the wrist, shoulder and neck that may signal potential problems later in life. Figures 9.5 and 9.6 show the tense, left-handed grip and hand-writing sample of a boy in secondary school who types proficiently and who rarely reverts to hand-writing.

Evaluation of hand-writing is a complex and specialist area that includes observing posture, pen control, pressure exerted, letter formation, legibility and spacing as well as speed, effort and efficiency. At a different level, research studies may use sophisticated technology to examine fine motor deficiencies, including detection of tremor and influency (Smits-Engelsman et al 2001).

PUBLISHED ASSESSMENT TOOLS

A selection of published tools that are commonly used in physiotherapy assessment are included in Table 9.1. For more detailed test reviews, see Burton & Miller (1998) and Barnett & Peters (2004).

MOTOR LEARNING

There have been many recent advances in theories of motor control and motor learning. Fifty years ago traditional theories were based on hierarchical models of information-processing and neuromaturation, where predetermined skills unfolded and emerged in a cephalocaudal sequence in stages as the neuromuscular system matured. More recent theories emphasize the self-organizational characteristics of the biological system and its dynamic interaction with the environment. One of the fundamental assumptions of dynamic systems theory is that individuals are composed of many complex, cooperative systems (Thelen 1995, Thelen & Spencer 1998) that together are responsible for motor control. These include both motor and non-motor factors, any one of which can facilitate or limit performance on a particular task. Dynamic systems theory suggests that movement variability is an

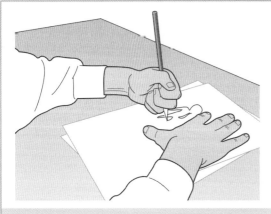

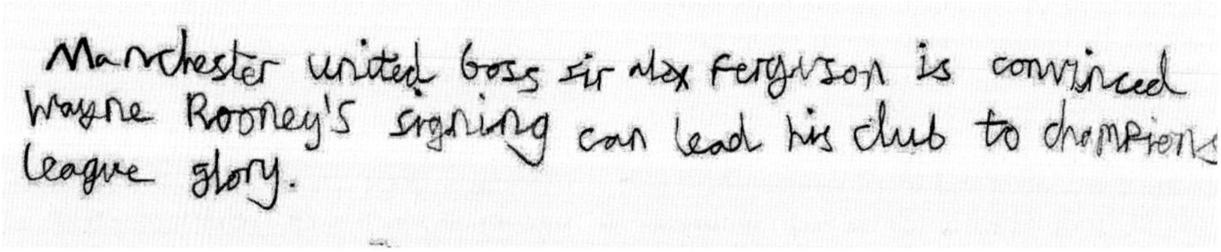

Figure 9.5 Awkward grip, wrist tension (boy, aged 11:11 years).

Figure 9.6 Hand-writing sample (same boy, aged 11:11 years).

Table 9.1 Published assessment tools commonly used by physiotherapists

Assessment tool	Reference
The high-functioning Autism Spectrum Screening Questionnaire (ASSQ)	Ehlers et al (1999)
Bayley Scales of Infant Development (BSID) (motor scale)	Bayley (2001)
Bruininks Oseretsky Test of Motor Proficiency (BOTMP2)	Bruininks & Bruininks (2005)
Clinical Observation of Motor and Postural Skills (COMPS)	Wilson et al (1994)
Developmental Coordination Disorder Questionnaire (DCDQ)	Wilson et al (2000)
Developmental test of Visual Motor Integration (VMI)	Beery (1997)
Miller Assessment for Preschoolers (MAP)	Miller (1988)
Movement Assessment Battery for Children (M-ABC) plus (M-ABC Checklist)	Henderson & Sugden (1992)
Peabody Developmental Motor Scales (2nd edn)	Folio & Fewell (1983)
Pediatric Evaluation of Disability Inventory (PEDI)	Haley et al (1992)
Perceived Efficacy and Goal-setting System (PEGS)	Missiuna et al (2004)
Short Sensory Profile	Dunn (1999)
Sensory Integration and Praxis Tests (SIPT)	Ayres (1989)
Strengths and Difficulties Questionnaire (SDQ)	Goodman (1999)
Test of Gross Motor Development (TGMD2)	Ulrich (2000)
Hand-writing Speed Test	Wallen et al (1996)

intrinsic feature of skilled motor performance, as the variability provides the flexibility required to adapt to complex dynamic environments. Motor skills develop as a continuous dynamic interaction between the child, the tasks and challenges he/she meets and solves and the impact or constraints of the environment. Knowledge of motor control and motor-learning theories is vital in planning physiotherapy intervention and in harnessing the processes involved in learning to ensure that a child may be facilitated toward full movement competence.

The learning process in all areas is founded on understanding the rules of the task and acquiring and practising the skill until this becomes automatic and may be generalized and applied in different contexts (Henderson & Sugden 1992). Figure 9.7 presents a flow diagram of the four phases of learning. The physiotherapist as teacher helps the child to identify and understand the rules by demonstration and instruction (e.g. in order to catch a ball attention, stance and hands are appropriately prepared). The child may then be encouraged to practise the skill and explore his/her success or failure and correct errors and refine performance toward success. Initially

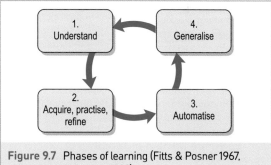

Figure 9.7 Phases of learning (Fitts & Posner 1967, Henderson & Sugden 1992).

the child has to think hard about the rules but gradually the skill requires less cognitive processing and becomes automatic. Finally the child is able to generalize the skill with fewer constraints. For example, the child becomes competent to catch a large or small ball, with either or both hands, from any height or direction while stationary or moving and thus can adapt according to the demands of the task. Another example applies to hand-writing: a child needs to know what is required and understand the rules such as how letters are formed, the direction, shape, orientation and spacing until fluent, cursive writing is automatic, effortless and attention may be given to content and literary expression.

INTERVENTION

Research suggests that intervention, including specialist intervention from occupational and physiotherapists and programmes provided in collaboration with schools and parents, improves function in this group of children. However, no one intervention method has yet been shown to be superior (Schoemaker et al 1994, Sugden & Chambers 1998, Peters & Wright 1999, Pless & Carlsson 2000, Ayyash & Preece 2003). A whole-child approach grounded in sound neurophysiological/developmental psychological theory is important.

THERAPEUTIC APPROACHES

Therapists often use an eclectic approach drawn from a mixture of theoretical concepts and are sometimes even rather unsure of the principles upon which their treatment method is based. One way of categorizing intervention approaches is into process-oriented (bottom-up) or task-oriented (top-down) methods. The former are aimed at processes deemed to underlie the difficulties, e.g. sensory motor processes, and methods include Sensory Integration (SI) therapy (Ayres 1972, Fisher et al 1991); Neurodevelopmental Therapy (NDT) (Bobath 1969) and Perceptual Motor Training (Laszlo & Bairstow 1985). In contrast, task-oriented approaches are primarily aimed at improving skills, usually through problem-solving and breaking down tasks into smaller component steps in order to work toward achieving the task goal. Examples include the Cognitive Motor Approach (Henderson & Sugden 1992), Cognitive Orientation to daily Occupational Performance (COOP) (Mandich & Polatajko 2005; Missiuna et al 2001) and Neuromotor Task Training (NTT) (Schoemaker & Smits-Engelsman 2005). A meta-analysis of 13 intervention studies gave support to a task-oriented approach but was not able to find significant support for SI for children with DCD (Pless & Carlsson 2000). Currently a Cochrane review of occupational therapy and physiotherapy for DCD is nearing completion (Lipson et al 2003). Unfortunately, many studies published in both physiotherapy journals and elsewhere lack rigorous experimental design. There is a great need for well-designed, controlled studies on children with DCD who meet accurate diagnostic criteria, and undergo clearly defined therapeutic intervention.

The overall objective of therapists is to help children acquire the skills they need to function successfully in everyday life. Paediatric physiotherapists focus on the development or rehabilitation of movement and posture. The authors of this chapter do not propose to provide a 'cookbook' of prescriptive therapy but rather to outline key points for the management of children with DCD. Children develop and learn in different ways and, similarly, physiotherapists have their own individual preferred styles of interaction with the child, his/her family and teachers. We consider that an important part of physiotherapy is the highlighting, based on assessment findings, of daily functional home activities that are specifically designed and recommended by the physiotherapist as *therapeutically* valid for that child. For example, if the physiotherapist assesses a child and finds that core postural muscles lack strength, an explanation of the importance of head/neck/shoulder girdle stability for looking, listening and for aiming/catching a ball and hand-writing may be a revelation to the family. They become motivated by a purpose. The therapist and family may then develop a plan of suitable activities that the child is keen to try and will therefore practise. These might include games involving rolling, wheelbarrow walks, tug-of-war, visits to the playground with encouragement to climb, travel along a bar using arms, underarm pull-ups and swimming.

Physiotherapy may be provided individually or in a group and may be clinic-based, school-based or cascaded through out-of-school activity via the parent/carer, family or teacher. Sometimes regular daily or weekly intervention is indicated, sometimes periods or blocks of more intense therapy are warranted and at other times management may be contained within ongoing advice and monitoring discussion of progress. However, a family-centred approach is recommended and therapy must be fun and motivate the child to practise appropriate activities.

Self-confidence helps a child's motivation so it is really important to encourage and provide understanding, positive support and opportunities for success mediated through physical activity. Physiotherapy management for children with DCD includes enabling educators and parents to integrate therapeutic advice into the curriculum and home activities. In-service training might outline the types of difficulties commonly met and suggest useful activities.

Children with DCD are often denied access to therapy due to their comparatively high level of function. They develop strategies for avoiding doing things that they find hard and their problems frequently go unrecognized and children are labelled as being lazy or not trying. Research shows that without intervention they do not improve and their difficulties compromise school achievement, behaviour and self-esteem (Losse et al 1991, Cantell et al 1994). They are often bright, frustrated youngsters who have much to lose by failing to reach their potential. It is essential that waiting lists are reduced by multidisciplinary best practice and that continued effort

---

KEY POINTS

- Assess and identify problems, then set aims/objectives/goals with a child and family
- Provide a report with minimum jargon which is accessible and circulate it, with the parents' consent, to the wider team involved
- DCD is a motor learning disorder rather than a medical problem: avoid encouraging learnt helplessness or identifying the child as 'sick'
- Provide positive feedback and encouragement rather than criticizing a child or making comparisons, especially with siblings and peers
- Note: ribcage stability and good breathing control are the foundation for respiration and oxygen transfer
- Analyse tasks and break them down into achievable components
- Build these up toward goals that are important for the child
- Avoid pointing out what the child cannot do
- Emphasize positive problem-solving and strategies for success
- Encourage and adapt tasks such as catching/throwing/hitting/kicking a ball by use of a larger bat or ball
- Prepare ahead: a child with DCD can be helped by parents and therapists preparing a child ahead for skills such as skipping, cycling and swimming
- Motivate by making therapy fun and extend physiotherapy through everyday home-based activities that interest the child
- Be creative – juggling, circus skills, archery, horse-riding, playing a musical instrument all demand coordination, strength, organization and offer a greater variety of motor actions which will motivate a child to practise far more than visits to a clinic
- Encourage daily activities: walking, dressing, helping around the house
- Encourage organization through forward-planning strategies – pack school bag, lay clothes ready
- Structure is important and frequent short sessions of practice (little and often) have been shown to be more valuable than longer, widely interspersed sessions
- Maintain close liaison with the child's school. Teachers and assistants will often incorporate physiotherapy advice and deliver motor programmes within the classroom or playground with individual children or small groups
- Be familiar with a school's hand-writing policy
- Encourage pre-writing skills: mark-making, messy play with water, finger paints, cutting, pasting, threading, pencil and paper games, construction toys and puzzles
- Formal hand-writing is best started when a child is ready to write and has sufficient neuromuscular control
- Keyboarding is now an essential life skill. It will be essential for some children with DCD
- Voice-activated software may be used where manipulative skills are exceptionally poor
- Praise effort and successes. It's easy for a child with DCD to lose self-esteem

---

is made to evaluate the effect of physiotherapy and that service delivery is evidence-based.

SUMMARY

This chapter has outlined issues related to the identification, assessment, intervention and evaluation of DCD for physiotherapists in the context of the current national and international situation. The field of DCD is constantly growing and physiotherapists are urged to maintain a vigil over new information and keep abreast of the changing picture. National and international meetings are held regularly and further information may be obtained from papers published in special issues of journals (Henderson 1994, Barnett et al 1998, Geuze et al 2001, Hadders-Algra & Gramsbergen 2003) and websites related to DCD (www.dcd-uk.org).

REFERENCES

American Psychiatric Association 1987 *Diagnostic and Statistical Manual of Mental Disorders: DSM III*, 3rd edn. Washington, DC: American Psychiatric Association.

American Psychiatric Association 1994 *Diagnostic and Statistical Manual of Mental Disorders: DSM IV*, 4th edn. Washington, DC: American Psychiatric Association.

American Psychiatric Association 2000 *Diagnostic and Statistical Manual of Mental Disorders: DSM IV*, 4th edn. Text revision (DSM-IV-TR). Arlington, VA: American Psychiatric Association.

Arnheim DD, Sinclair WA 1975 *The Clumsy Child: A Program of Motor Therapy*. St Louis: CV Mosby.

Ayres AJ 1972 *Sensory Integration and Learning Disorders*. Los Angeles, CA: Western Psychological Services.

Ayres AJ 1989 *Sensory Integration and Praxis Tests*. Los Angeles, CA: Western Psychological Services.

Ayyash FA, Preece PM 2003 Evidence-based treatment of motor coordination disorder. *Current Paediatrics* 13: 360–364.

Baker J 1981 A psycho-motor approach to the assessment and treatment of clumsy children. *Physiotherapy* 67: 355–362.

Barnett A, Henderson SE 2004 Assessment of hand-writing in children with developmental coordination disorder. In: Sugden D, Chambers M (eds) *Children with Developmental Coordination Disorder*. London: Whurr, pp. 168–188.

Barnett A, Peters JM 2004 Motor proficiency assessment batteries. In: Dewey D, Tupper E (eds) *Developmental Motor Disorders: A Neuropsychological Perspective*. New York: Guilford Press, pp. 66–109.

Barnett AL, Kooista L, Henderson SE (eds) 1998 'Clumsiness' as syndrome and symptom. Special issue. *Human Movement Science* 17: 679–737.

Bayley N 2001 *Bayley Scale of Infant Development*, 2nd edn. Motor scale kit. New York: Psychological Corporation.

Beery KE 1997 *The Beery-Buktenica Test of Visual-Motor Integration with Supplemental Developmental Tests of Visual Perception and Motor Coordination*. Parippany, NJ: Modern Curriculum Press.

Benbow M 2002 Hand skills and hand-writing. In: Cermak SA, Larkin D (eds) *Developmental Coordination Disorder*. Albany, NY: Delmar, pp. 248–279.

Berninger VW 2004 Understanding the 'graphia' in developmental dysgraphia. In: Dewey D, Tupper E (eds) *Developmental Motor Disorders: A Neuropsychological Perspective*. New York: Guilford Press, pp. 328–350.

Bobath B 1969 The treatment of neuromuscular disorders by improving patterns of coordination. *Physiotherapy* 55: 18–22.

Bouffard M, Watkinson EJ, Thompson LP 1996 A test of the activity deficit hypothesis with children with movement difficulties. *Adapted Physical Activity Quarterly* 13: 61–73.

British Heart Foundation 2000 *Coronary Heart Disease Statistics*. London: British Heart Foundation.

British Medical Journal 1962 Clumsy children. *British Medical Journal* Dec 22: 1665–1666.

Bruininks RH, Bruininks BD 2005 *Bruininks–Oseretsky Test of Motor Proficiency*, 2nd edn. NfER-Nelson.

Burton AW, Miller DE 1998 *Movement Skill Assessment*. Champaign, IL: Human Kinetics.

Bushby K, Muntoni F, Urtizberea A, Hughes R, Griggs R 2004 Report on the 124th ENMC International Workshop. Treatment of Duchenne muscular dystrophy; defining the gold standards of management in the use of corticosteroids 2–4 April 2004, Naarden, The Netherlands. *Neuromuscular Disorders* 14: 526–534.

Cantell MH, Smyth MM, Ahonen TP 1994 Clumsiness in adolescence: educational, motor and social outcomes of motor delay detected at five years. *Adapted Physical Activity Quarterly* 11. 115–129.

Chesson R 1998 Psychosocial aspects of measurement. *Physiotherapy* 84: 435–438.

Compact Oxford English Dictionary, 2nd edn 1991 Oxford: Clarendon Press.

Cousins M, Smyth MM 2003 Developmental coordination impairments in adulthood. *Human Movement Science* 22: 433–459.

Dare MT, Gordon N 1970 Clumsy children: a disorder of perception and motor organisation. *Developmental Medicine and Child Neurology* 12: 178–185.

Department of Health 2004 *At Least Five a Week: Evidence on the Impact of Physical Activity and its Relationship to Health*. London: Department of Health.

Dunford C, Richards S 2003 'Doubly Disadvantaged': Report of a Survey on Waiting Lists and Waiting Times for Occupational Therapy Services for Children with Developmental Coordination Disorder. London: College of Occupational Therapists and National Association of Paediatric Occupational Therapists.

Dunn W 1999 *Sensory Profile*. San Antonio, TX: Harcourt Assessment.

Dupré E, Merklen P 1909. L'insuffisance pyramidale physiologique de la première enfance et le syndrome de débilité motrice. *Revue Neurologique* 17: 1073–1074.

Ehlers S, Gillberg C, Wing L 1999 A screening questionnaire for Asperger syndrome and other high-functioning autism spectrum disorders in school age children. *Journal of Autism and Developmental Disorders* 29: 129–141.

Fisher A, Murray EA, Bundy AC (eds) 1991 *Sensory Integration, Theory and Practice*. Philadelphia, PA: FA Davis.

Fitts PM, Posner MI 1967 *Human Performance*. Belmont, CA: Brooks/Cole.

Folio M, Fewell R 1983 *Peabody Developmental Motor Scales*, 2nd edn. Austin, TX: Pro-Ed.

Geuze RJ, Jongmans MJ, Schoemaker MM, Smits-Engelsman BCM 2001 (eds) Special issue: developmental coordination disorder: diagnosis, description, processes and treatment. *Human Movement Science* 20: 1–210.

Ghaziuddin M, Butler E, Tsai L, Ghaziuddin N 1994 Is clumsiness a marker for Asperger syndrome? *Journal of Intellectual Disability Research* 38: 519–527.

Gillberg C 2003 Deficits in attention motor control and perception: a brief review. *Archives of Disease of Childhood* 88: 904–910.

Gonzalez Rothi LJ, Heilman KM (eds) 1997 *Apraxia: The Neuropsychology of Action*. Hove: Psychology Press.

Goodman R 1999 The extended version of the Strengths and Difficulties Questionnaire as a guide to child psychiatric caseness and consequent burden. *Journal of Child Psychology, Psychiatry and Allied Disciplines* 40: 791–799.

Gordon N, McKinley I 1980 *Helping Clumsy Children*. London: Churchill Livingstone.

Green D, Baird G, Barnett AL, Henderson L, Huber J, Henderson SE 2002 The severity and nature of motor impairment in Asperger's syndrome: a comparison with Specific Developmental Disorder of Motor Function. *Journal of Child Psychology and Psychiatry* 43: 655–668.

Green D, Bishop T, Wilson B et al 2005 Is questionnaire-based screening part of the solution to waiting lists for children with DCD? *British Journal of Occupational Therapy* 68: 2–10.

Gubbay SS 1975 *The Clumsy Child. A Study of Developmental Apraxic and Agnosic Ataxia*. London: Saunders.

Hadders-Algra M, Gramsbergen A 2003 (eds) The clumsy child. *Neural Plasticity* Special Issue 10: 1—178.

Haley SM, Coster WJ, Ludlow LH, Haltiwanger J, Andrellos PJ 1992 *Pediatric Evaluation of Disability Inventory*. Boston: New England Medical Center Hospitals.

Hellgren L, Gillberg C, Gillberg IC, Enerskog I 1993 Children with deficits in attention motor control and perception (DAMP) almost grown up: general health at sixteen years. *Developmental Medicine and Child Neurology* 35: 881–893.

Hellgren L, Gillberg IC, Bagenholm A, Gillberg C 1994 Children with deficits in attention, motor control and perception (DAMP) almost grown up: psychiatric and personality disorders at age 16 years. *Journal of Child Psychology and Psychiatry* 35: 1255–1271.

Henderson S (ed.) 1994 Special issue: developmental coordination disorder. *Adapted Physical Activity Quarterly* 11: 111–244.

Henderson SE, Barnett AL 1998 The classification of specific motor coordination disorders: some problems to be solved. *Human Movement Science* 17: 449–469.

Henderson SE, Hall D 1982 Concomitants of clumsiness in young school age children. *Developmental Medicine and Child Neurology* 24: 448–460.

Henderson SE, Sugden DA 1992 *Movement Assessment Battery for Children*. London: Psychological Corporation.

Jansson A, Saartok T, Werner S, Renström P 2004 General joint laxity in 1845 Swedish school children of different ages: age- and gender-specific distributions. *Acta Paediatrica* 93: 1202–1206.

Kalverboer AF, van Praag HM, Mendlewica J 1978 *Minimal Brain Dysfunction: Fact or Fiction?* Basel, Switzerland: S Karger.

Kaplan BJ, Wilson BN, Dewey D, Crawford SG 1998 DCD may not be a discrete disorder. *Human Movement Science* 17: 471–490.

Knowles E, Elliott J (eds) 1997 *Oxford English Dictionary of New Words*. Oxford: Oxford University Press.

Laszlo J, Bairstow P 1985 *Perceptual-Motor Behaviour: Developmental Assessment and Therapy*. London: Holt, Rhinehart and Winston.

Leeds Consensus Statement 2006 *Economic Science Research Council Seminar Series: Developmental Coordination Disorder as a Specific Learning Difficulty; 2004–2006.*

Lipson A, Edwards P, Logan GS 2003 Occupational therapy and physiotherapy for developmental coordination disorder (protocol). *Cochrane Database of Systematic Reviews* issue I. Article no. CD004256. DOI:10.1002/14651858. CD004256.

Losse A, Henderson SE, Elliman D, Hall D, Knight E, Jongmans M 1991 Clumsiness in children – do they grow out of it? A 10-year follow-up study. *Developmental Medicine and Child Neurology* 33: 55–68.

Maillard S, Murray KJ 2003 Hypermobility syndrome in children. In: Keer R, Grahame R (eds) *Hypermobility Syndrome*. Edinburgh: Butterworth Heinemann, pp. 33–50.

Majnemer A, Barr RG 2005 Influence of supine sleep positioning on early motor milestone acquisition. *Developmental Medicine and Child Neurology* 6: 370–376.

Mandich AJ, Polatajko HJ 2005 A cognitive perspective on intervention for children with developmental coordination disorder: the Co-Op experience. In: Sugden D, Chambers M (eds) *Children with Developmental Coordination Disorder*. London: Whurr, pp. 228–241.

Medical Research Council 1943 *Aids to the Investigation of Peripheral Nerve Injuries*. War memorandum no. 7, 2nd edn. London: HMSO.

Miller L 1988 *Miller Assessment for Preschoolers*. San Antonio, TX: Therapy Skill Builders.

Missiuna C, Mandich AD, Polatajko HJ, Malloy-Miller T 2001 Cognitive Orientation to Daily Occupational Performance (COOP): part I – theoretical foundations. *Physical and Occupational Therapy in Pediatrics* 20: 69–81.

Missiuna C, Pollock N, Law M 2004 *Perceived Efficacy and Goal Setting System (PEGS)*. San Antonio, TX: Psychological Corporation.

Orton ST 1937 *Reading, Writing and Speech Problems in Children*. New York: Norton.

Peters JM, Wright AM 1999 Development and evaluation of a group physical activity programme for children with developmental coordination disorder: an interdisciplinary approach. *Physiotherapy Theory and Practice* 15: 203–216.

Peters JM, Barnett AL, Henderson SE 2001 Clumsiness, dyspraxia and developmental coordination disorder: how do health and educational professionals in the UK define the terms? *Child: Care Health and Development* 27: 399–412.

Peters JM, Henderson SE, Dookun D 2004 Provision for children with developmental coordination disorder (DCD): audit of the service provider. *Child: Care Health and Development* 30: 463–479.

Pless M, Carlsson M 2000 Effects of motor skills intervention on DCD: a meta-analysis. *Adapted Physical Activity Quarterly* 17: 381–401.

Polatajko HJ, Fox M, Missiuna C 1995 An international consensus on children with developmental coordination disorder. *Canadian Journal of Occupational Therapy* 62: 3–6.

Schoemaker MM, Kalverboer AF 1994 Social and affective problems of children who are clumsy: how early do they begin? *Adapted Physical Activity Quarterly* 11: 130–140.

Schoemaker MM, Smits-Engelsman BCM 2005 Neuromotor task training: a new approach to treat children with DCD. In: Sugden D, Chambers M (eds) *Children with Developmental Coordination Disorder*. London: Whurr, pp. 212–227.

Schoemaker MM, Hijlkema MGJ, Kalverboer AF 1994 Physiotherapy for clumsy children: an evaluation study. *Developmental Medicine and Child Neurology* 36: 143–155.

Smits-Engelsman BCM, Niemeijer AS, van Galen GP 2001 Fine motor deficiencies in children diagnosed as DCD based on poor grapho-motor ability. *Human Movement Science* 20: 161–182.

Smyth MM, Anderson H 2000 Coping with clumsiness in the school playground: social and physical play in children with coordination impairments. *British Journal of Developmental Psychology* 18: 389–413.

Stephenson E, McKay C, Chesson R 1991 The identification and treatment of motor/learning difficulties: parents' perceptions and the role of the therapist. *Child: Care, Health and Development* 17: 91–113.

Stephenson E, Chisholm D, Chesson R 2002 Children with developmental coordination disorder (DCD): is screening assessment effective? Glasgow: College of Occupational Therapists Annual Conference.

Sugden DA (ed.) 2006 *Leeds Consensus Statement*. ESRC Research Seminar Series. Cardiff: Discovery Trust.

Sugden DA, Chambers ME 1998 Intervention approaches and children with developmental coordination disorder. *Paediatric Rehabilitation* 2: 139–147.

Thelen E 1995 Motor development: a new synthesis. *American Psychologist* 50: 79–95.

Thelen E, Spencer JP 1998 Postural control during reaching in young infants: a dynamic systems approach. *Neuroscience Behavioral Review* 22: 507–514.

Ulrich DA 2000 *Test of Gross Motor Development*, 2nd edn. Examiner's manual. Austin, TX: Pro-ed.

Wallen M, Bonney MA, Lennox I 1996 *The Hand-Writing Speed Test*. Adelaide: Helios.

Walton JN, Ellis E, Court SDM 1962 Clumsy children: a study of developmental apraxia and agnosia. *Brain* 85: 603–612.

Williams J, Unwin J 1997 Physiotherapy management of minimal cerebral dysfunction in Australia: current practice and future challenges. *Australian Physiotherapy* 43: 135–143.

Wilson B, Pollock N, Kaplan BJ, Law M 1994 *Clinical Observation of Motor and Postural Skills*. San Antonio, TX: Psychological Corporation.

Wilson B, Kaplan B, Crawford S, Campbell A, Dewey D 2000 Reliability and validity of a parent questionnaire on childhood motor skills. *American Journal of Occupational Therapy* 54: 484–493.

World Health Organization 1992 *The ICD-10 Classification of Mental and Behavioural Disorders: Clinical Descriptions and Diagnostic Guidelines*. Geneva: World Health Organization.

World Health Organization 2001 *International Classification of Functioning, Disability and Health (ICF)*. Geneva: World Health Organization.

10 Assistive technology

Donna Cowan and Alice Wintergold

WHAT IS ASSISTIVE TECHNOLOGY?

Assistive technology (AT) is an umbrella term for a wide range of products. A commonly accepted definition is 'any item, piece of equipment or product system whether acquired commercially off the shelf, modified or customized that is used to increase, maintain or improve functional capabilities of individuals with disabilities' (US Statute 1988). Therefore in terms of devices or equipment it includes from walking sticks to environmental control systems (ECS), or simple dressing aids to communication aids.

One chapter cannot outline the functionality and purpose of such a wide range of equipment and therefore we will cover the range of products which a physiotherapist is most likely to come across when involved with families and children. There will be additional details with the equipment that a physiotherapist is likely to be involved with assessing.

The AT described will be divided into two sections;

1. Mechanical (i.e. seating, lying, standing equipment and personal care/activities of daily living (ADL)
2. Electronic (i.e. computer access, communication aids, powered mobility and environmental control).

WHY PROVIDE ASSISTIVE TECHNOLOGY?

The benefits and purpose of AT are in many respects self-evident. When appropriate equipment is provided in a timely manner it allows children to move around their environment, communicate with others and take part in developmentally appropriate activities that they would be unable to do without this technology. It also enables the family and carers to look after a child in activities which the child cannot undertake independently, such as personal care, e.g. hoisting, bathing and toileting (Audit Commission 2000, Beresford 2003, Mountain 2004).

Physiotherapists are routinely involved in the prescription of some AT devices such as standing supports or orthoses. However it is important to have an understanding of a wider range of AT so that one can recognize the role that AT plays in family life and when it might be a solution to a problem. It is not necessary to hold information about the details of each device but it is important to have an overview of such equipment as an ECS and how to refer the family to the appropriate service for further information (Beresford 1995, Mitchell & Sloper 2000, Cowan & Khan 2005).

> **KEY POINT**
>
> - It is important to have knowledge of local equipment services so that information can be passed on to families

It is also important to have an awareness of the wide range of technology a child and family use in everyday life in order to understand the impact that your work can have on all the other areas in a child's life. An example may be when the use of botulinum toxin is recommended to improve a child's ability to extend his/her arm. Such an intervention may decrease pain and facilitate easier care routines for the child. It may also affect the way in which a child accesses powered mobility, communication aids and their computer for schoolwork. Therefore there is a need to inform other members of the team to review these systems so that the child can continue to function optimally in all environments.

ASSESSMENT

AT and its prescription and provision have historically been the domain of the therapist. However with the increasing numbers of children with complex disability and the increasing range, complexity and options within AT that are possible it is becoming more necessary to include other disciplines to participate in the prescription and provision.

Members of the team can include:

- Paediatrician
- Therapists (occupational, physiotherapist and speech and language therapist)
- Engineer (rehabilitation, clinical)
- Prosthetist/orthotist.

The child and family must be central to this team. It is vital for them to be and feel part of the decision-making process. Apart from ensuring the child's and family's needs are met, it also allows them to gain the most understanding on the importance and potential effect of equipment. For example, a family may simply be looking for an appropriate seat so that a child can be placed safely at home. If engaged in the assessment and choice of equipment they will also understand that it can reduce the risk of deformity, offer the child the opportunity to develop fine motor skills as he or she can use the hands and arms more effectively, and that the child can eat safely and engage in activities with greater independence. In this way the seat provided is more likely to be used appropriately and the family can see the positive effects in many other areas of the child's life.

The team approach is required to ensure that all the needs of the client, in this case the child and family/carers, are considered in a coordinated way and that the provision of equipment and care for the child is appropriate and useful. This reduces the likelihood of abandonment of equipment and increases the compliance of families using equipment as recommended (Korpela et al 1993).

In order for a child to achieve his or her potential, whatever that may be, the team must be aware of each other's role and have knowledge of who else should be involved with respect to the assessment and provision of AT. Each member of the team needs to have an understanding of what AT can offer and be able to access or offer basic information/advice.

A key factor in the transition from recommendation to realization is the existence of a local team to work with the family. This local multidisciplinary team needs to understand the service delivery systems involved as well as the therapeutic, medical and engineering aspects of AT relevant to this child. They need to continue to review the child's needs and make the changes to the equipment provided as needs change.

OUTCOME MEASURES

Having provided equipment, it is then important that as clinicians we have an objective method of determining whether the equipment is meeting the need expressed by the child and family and whether the goals identified are being aided by the provision of the equipment. Outcome measures are discussed in depth in Chapter 3; however the literature over the past 5–10 years has reported the development of some outcome measures in the evaluation of AT. These can be used to determine outcomes such as whether the equipment meets the needs of the client, whether the service provided is satisfactory and also the impact of the equipment on the client's life.

Quebec User Evaluation of Satisfaction with assistive Technology (QUEST) (Demers et al 1996) was developed to allow the user to determine the important attributes of the device and score against those accordingly. This prevents the clinician being the person deciding what is important about the device and relies on users being able to make that judgement themselves. This tool looks at the device itself and how appropriate it is for the user. It also enables the team to investigate the success of the delivery process, i.e. it can give feedback on service delivery. QUEST 2 (Demers et al 2002) is a revised version of this tool to demonstrate its use routinely gaining user evaluation of equipment and services.

Psychosocial Impact of Assistive Devices (PIAD) (Jutai & Day 2002) is a self-report questionnaire designed to assess the effects of an assistive device on functional independence, well-being and quality of life. PIAD has also been used by care-givers to give proxy ratings of device impact.

The development of outcome measures is a growing field and of increasing importance, with the resource implications AT provision brings with it.

MECHANICAL ASSISTIVE TECHNOLOGY

This section provides an overview of the range of mechanical AT available and is considered in the following areas:

- Postural management equipment
- Equipment for active exercise
- Wheeled mobility
- Equipment for ADL
- Protective devices
- Prosthetics and orthotics.

Introduction

In this section mechanical AT is used to describe the equipment that may be used by a child with a disability that is not controlled electronically. It includes equipment such as manual wheelchairs, postural management equipment, orthoses and aids for daily living. Some technology has both mechanical and electronic aspects and this will be discussed where it is most appropriate. Mechanical AT may be of a simple design or may be very complex.

Assessment is required for the provision of all mechanical AT but some equipment requires a more thorough assessment than others. This is not necessarily due to the complexity of the equipment but has more to do with how it will be used. For example, a simple dressing hook may be used by a child to assist with pulling up trousers but a complex assessment could be required if hand function was compromised by the child's disability and he or she could not hold and grip a dressing stick in the hand.

The complexity of the assessment also depends on how a piece of equipment will be used. The assessment for the same type of attendant-controlled manual wheelchair used for occasional use by a child who is able to walk short distances outside and the assessment of a child who is not able to stand independently and sits in the same wheelchair all day will be very different.

Once new equipment has been issued it is important that the most appropriate person takes on the responsibility for monitoring it. Depending on the equipment this person may be the child, family or carers or a therapist. The equipment should be comfortable to use, although it may feel different. As some equipment is designed to support

and correct the body structure there may be a risk of pressure sore development. Pressure sore development is also a consideration for those with reduced or absent sensation such as a child with a spinal cord injury or spina bifida. The skin should be regularly checked in the early stages of provision for red marks and possible areas where pressure sores may form. It is also important to monitor the function of a child and the equipment to ensure they are working together as intended.

Provision of mechanical AT for children has its own unique challenges. Children are constantly changing as they grow and their abilities change and develop. Equipment therefore needs to be chosen with these aspects in mind. Adjustable equipment enables changes to be made according to a child's needs. Adjustability within a device does tend to make equipment heavier, more complex and expensive but it will last longer and may be adjusted to fit the constantly changing needs of a child.

Postural management equipment

As previously discussed in Chapter 7, postural management programmes encompass all activities and interventions that impact on an individual's posture and function. These activities and interventions may require the support of postural management equipment such as special seating, nighttime support and standing supports. Other types of mechanical AT, such as adapted tricycles, orthoses and walking aids, may be used as part of a postural management programme. For the purposes of this chapter they have been described in their own separate sections.

One of the most important aspects of postural management equipment is the quality of posture achieved. A good posture can only be achieved by assessment and use of equipment that has been specifically designed to fulfil the purpose. A large range of equipment has been developed to cover the 24-hour period.

KEY POINT

- The quality of the posture achieved is one of the most important aspects of postural management equipment

---

With the provision of equipment, biomechanics should be considered. It is important to think about how a piece of equipment will alter joint position and forces. The equipment selected for an individual should provide a symmetrical position, even load-bearing under the area of support, a neutral or anteriorly tilted pelvis with neutral joint positions and a stable base that provides a starting point for movement.

Assessment

When providing postural management equipment for children with disabilities a multiprofessional assessment is essential. The assessment should include a thorough physical examination looking at range of motion, level of physical ability, biomechanics and the postures adopted and achievable. Postures should be assessed both in a static position and dynamically as some children require a different level of support depending on the activity they are performing. For example, a boy may be able to sit in a symmetrical posture with the pelvis anteriorly tilted, the shoulder girdle protracted and the chin tucked with the arms resting at their sides. As soon as he tries to lift an arm to reach a toy then his posture may become asymmetrical with his pelvis posteriorly tilted and his arm that is not reaching may be used to balance or prop.

A tool such as the Chailey Levels of Ability (Pountney et al 2004) should be used during the assessment to provide a baseline measure, give guidelines for the type of equipment required and measure the effectiveness of the equipment on the child's posture (see Ch. 3). The assessment should include discussions with a child and family in order to choose equipment that will fit in with a child's priorities and lifestyle. Outcomes of what the equipment should achieve should be decided and then used to measure the effectiveness of equipment.

Once the choice of equipment has been decided then measurements will be taken from a child so that equipment of the correct size can be provided. The measurements must be accurate. This may seem an obvious statement but

often measurements are dependent on posture. For example, a child with a posteriorly tilted pelvis in sitting (with a correctable slumped posture) will have an apparent longer seat depth requirement. If the seat is supplied with the longer seat depth then the child's pelvis is likely to roll back into posterior tilt in order to use the back rest.

Seating

Seating equipment is often the most important piece of postural management equipment that a child has as he or she is likely to spend a considerable amount of time in this position (for mobility and function). Good seating can have a dramatic effect on aspects of function such as propulsion of the wheelchair and access to switches.

A variety of seating options are available, including corner seats, forward-lean seats and 90/90 systems, and evaluation of these products needs to be made to ensure appropriate postures are achieved (Pope 2002). Seats may be simple, such as a wheelchair canvas or simple wooden school chair, or complex, such as a modular adjustable seating system.

Children may require a different level of support in seating depending on the activity they are doing. Some children are able to achieve a position but are unable to participate in an activity while in this posture, as all their attention is focused on maintaining their posture. When they begin the activity their posture deteriorates.

Functional seat

A functional seat may provide postural support and offers a child a starting position for activities. The ideal position depends on factors including disability, level of ability, comfort and body shape but there are certain elements that are relevant for all. The child should be seated with the pelvis upright, the femurs horizontal with the hips, knees and ankles at 90°, the spine straight in the lateral plane and natural curves in the anterior posterior plane (slight lumbar lordosis and thoracic kyphosis). The hips should be neutral or slightly abducted (Ham et al 1998).

Children who are typically developing will be able to achieve the above posture but will constantly be able to move. They may choose to adopt this posture when concentrating on tasks such as writing at school (Sents & Marks

1989). A child with a physical disability but with a high level of ability may require minimal assistance to achieve this posture. An example of this would be a chair at the correct height to ensure the feet are placed firmly on the floor and a conforming top surface. They may require a back rest and some pelvic lateral support to encourage a symmetrical position. A child with a low level of ability would require a much more comprehensive piece of equipment.

When supplying seating for a child with a low level of ability, certain aspects of posture require particular attention. These include control of the pelvis for tilt, rotation and obliquity, control of the trunk anteriorly, posteriorly and laterally, and foot and head support. Control of the pelvis may be achieved using a variety of different methods such as using an anteriorly tilted seat to encourage an upright pelvis and reduce the pull on the hamstrings (Ham et al 1998). Another option is to use a seat with a cushion with a pre-ischial bar, a ledge that is designed to retain the ischial tuberosities and prevent them from sliding forwards, in conjunction with a sub-anterior superior iliac spines (ASIS) bar, a solid support located in front of the ASIS to prevent the pelvis rotating or moving forwards.

The solution that has been developed and successfully used at Chailey Heritage Clinical Services is a seating system that provides adjustable control for the whole sitting posture (Pountney et al 2004). This is achieved by having a seating system that has a horizontal area under the pelvis to ensure that the pelvis is horizontal without obliquity and the spine is straight laterally, a ramp to ensure the femurs are horizontal, a curved sacral pad to block the pelvis stepped back to a curved back rest to allow for the difference in pelvic and thoracic dimensions, lateral pelvic and thoracic supports (Figure 10.1). A firm lap strap keeps the pelvis back in the seat and knee blocks work in conjunction with the sacral pad and pelvic pads to prevent the pelvis rotating or tilting posteriorly. In order to achieve this control the seat has an adjustable seat depth to ensure the correct seat length, adjustable footplate height to ensure the 90° angle at the hips and knees and adjustable width to ensure the pelvis is supported symmetrically and laterally.

Floor sitting seat

As part of their early development children learn to sit and play on the floor. Children with a physical disability, developmental delay or learning difficulties may not be able to adopt this position or if they can it is unlikely that they do so with a stable base and can release their hands for play. Some floor sitting seats are a simple planar shape and may provide support for children who have a good floor sitting posture but require boundaries to work within. For a child with a lower level of ability an appropriately prescribed floor sitting seat will provide a stable base with a good pelvic position (Figure 10.2). This will enable a child to move the trunk and limbs and safely play on the floor in this typical developing position. In order to achieve this posture the seat requires a firm, snug, curved sacral support;

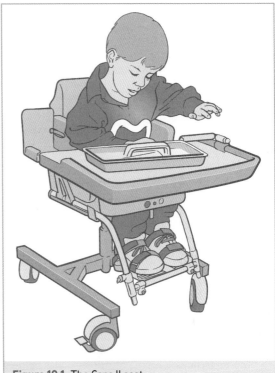

Figure 10.1 The Caps II seat.

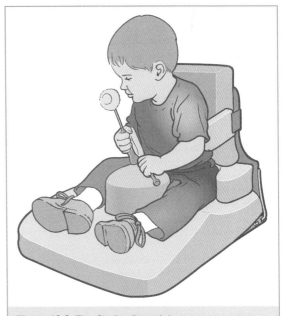

Figure 10.2 The Chailey floor sitting seat.

a flat area under the pelvis; a ramp up to the knees and back down from the knee to the ankle; a pommel to encourage abduction and external rotation; a curved back rest; thoracic lateral support and a tray to prop or play on.

Relaxing seat

For older children a comfy chair may be beneficial to provide a supported but relaxed position for leisure time. The seat should be adjustable in the seat depth and width as a minimum and provide some postural support. This type of seat is unlikely to be useful for children who require a high level of postural control as they are not supportive enough to achieve this.

Lying

Children sleep for up to 12 hours a day. Providing a good posture whilst sleeping provides a substantial period of gentle muscle stretch while muscle activity is quiet. Several studies indicate that periods of between 5 and 7 hours are required to change muscle length (Tardieu et al 1988, Lespargot et al 1994). Postural support at night must promote good-quality sleep, which can be compromised by a number of factors, such as nocturnal seizures, reflux oesophagitis and nocturnal hypoxaemia (Cartwright 1984, Martin et al 1995). Supine positioning can aggravate some of these conditions, and investigation and observation of these conditions must be carried out prior to allowing a child to sleep unattended in a postural support. A sleep questionnaire (Newman et al 2006) may assist in identifying sleep problems and overnight oximetry may be used to compare oxygen levels in different sleep positions.

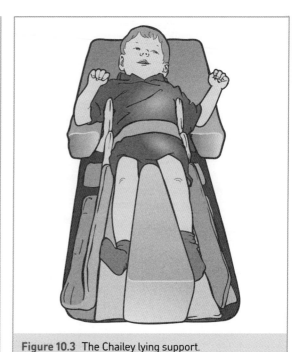

Figure 10.3 The Chailey lying support.

> ### KEY POINTS
> - Nighttime postural support should provide good-quality sleep but medical considerations must be addressed first
> - Lying can be a good position for play, particularly for younger children and those with a lower level of ability

A lying support should provide a symmetrical position with the load-bearing areas shifted downwards towards the pelvis, anterior pelvic tilt, the knees in slight flexion and a protracted shoulder girdle. One method of achieving this posture is with the use of the Chailey lying support (Figure 10.3). The contoured firm base alters the load-bearing surface, with the lumbar support encouraging anterior pelvic tilt and the knee supports providing slight flexion at the knee. The abducted, symmetrical hip position is achieved by an abduction block in conjunction with lateral supports and the pelvic strap. The head and shoulder girdle support promotes a protracted shoulder girdle, with the hands together and chin tucked.

Custom-made and commercial side-lying equipment is available for children who are not able to tolerate lying in prone or supine due to medical or postural reasons. In side-lying it is not possible to achieve complete symmetrical correction and some pelvic obliquity and rotation are inevitable. Supine and prone-lying have the benefit of complete correction being possible and gravity assisting the symmetrical posture.

Standing

Standing supports are routinely prescribed for children with physical disabilities and many reasons are cited for their use, including musculoskeletal, biomechanical, physiological, sensory, psychological, emotional and social factors.

In practice the benefits of standing have been appreciated but the evidence is limited, with the studies often being small and providing conflicting information on effectiveness. An example of the conflicting results is the effect of standing on increasing bone mineral density (Wilmshurst et al 1996, Caulton et al 2004). Stuberg (1992) recommended that children should weight-bear for an hour four to five times a week in order to enhance bone and joint development but there is limited evidence for these recommendations.

The posture that is achieved in a standing support depends not only on the ability of the child but also on the postural control offered by the support. There is currently no evidence that provides guidance on the most effective posture that should be achieved within supported standing. Nor is there consideration of opportunities for movement within the support and how this may impact on function and development.

Many different types of standing supports are available and used by therapists. A questionnaire found physiotherapists most commonly used standing supports that

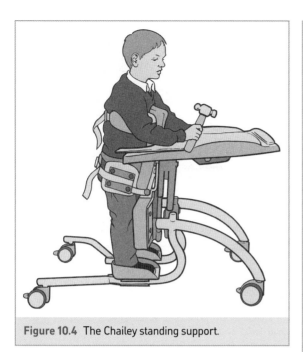

Figure 10.4 The Chailey standing support.

provide a position in prone and upright. Supine, tilt table and developmental positions are also used but less frequently (Wintergold 2006). Standing equipment has been developed at Chailey Heritage Clinical Services that supports the typical development model (Figure 10.4). The child stands with the feet on a horizontal base with adjustable foot position; the femurs are supported vertically and the trunk support is angled forwards from vertical at the hips to enable the weight to be forwards over the base. The chest support is narrow and soft to enable shoulder protraction and movement and a tray for forearm propping or activities is placed at elbow height. A pelvic strap stabilizes the pelvis in a neutral/anterior tilt (Green et al 1993).

Custom-made equipment

Not all children are able to use commercially available equipment. This may be due to health issues or fixed deformity. For these children custom-made equipment is required. If a child has a fixed deformity then they may require a complex system contoured to the body's shape to support and accommodate the deformities.

Assessment should be carried out by a multiprofessional team and medical input in these instances has additional importance. Following the assessment the design must be specified. The design should aim to prevent further deterioration where possible. The equipment is manufactured and then fitted and supplied with appropriate information and instructions. It is important that once custom-made equipment has been provided, there is

initial checking by the child's family and local team and regular review.

Equipment for active exercise

Children with a complex disability such as quadriplegic cerebral palsy often do not have the opportunity to participate in active exercise. This in turn may lead to muscle weakness. Equipment to support children in these activities should provide a balance between function and good posture. The exercise should be designed to strengthen muscles as children with a disability, particularly those with a neurological impairment, often have weak muscles.

> **KEY POINT**
> • Active exercise provides an opportunity for participation and muscle-strengthening

Tricycles

A tricycle can be used in place of a bicycle for children with disabilities. A tricycle has the benefit of being stable so that a child does not have to balance as with a bicycle. For children with complex physical disabilities tricycles with support have been developed to enable children to be appropriately positioned and supported so that they can cycle. At Chailey Heritage Clinical Services adaptations have been developed that can be fitted to standard children's tricycles and provide postural support (Mulcahy et al 1991). The adaptations consist of a saddle seat to support the pelvis and provide a slightly abducted hip position and an anterior support so the child's weight can be brought forwards over the base and bring the hands forward to the straight handle bars (Figure 10.5). Wrist supports, footplates and foot straps can be used if additional support is required. Similar adaptations are available from other commercial companies with various elements of support. Some of the supports for these trikes provide trunk support from behind the child.

Walkers

Walking is an important experience for children with a disability. Children with a disability may not be able to walk unassisted at the typical developmental age or they may never be able to achieve independent walking. Available AT includes simple items such as walking sticks and rollators that may be used on their own or in conjunction with orthotics, such as the hip guidance orthosis or reciprocating gait orthosis. More comprehensive walking aids include the David Hart walker made from an adjustable modular brace and a wheeled frame that supports part of the body weight,

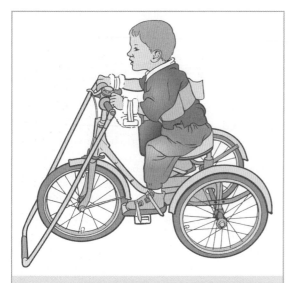

Figure 10.5 Tricycle with Chailey trike adaptations.

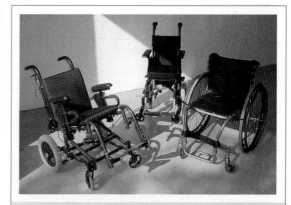

Figure 10.6 Selection of wheelchairs. (Courtesy of Sussex Care Centres)

providing a handsfree walking aid, and is suitable for children with cerebral palsy (Wright et al 1999). The swivel walker has a frame that provides stabilization to the body and swivelling footplates that allow progression as the child leans from side to side and is suitable for young children with spina bifida for facilitating walking on flat surfaces (Stallard 2005).

Swimming aids

Children with a physical disability may enjoy the freedom from gravity that swimming allows. For some children with complex disabilities additional support is required in the water for safety. Arm bands and swim rings are commonly used pieces of equipment by babies and toddlers who are not yet able to swim but these are often not suitable for older children with a disability or for children with poor head control. Equipment that they may require could be a flotation aid for their head so that as they lie on their back the head is safely supported above the surface of the water. Waistcoats are also available that add buoyancy to the trunk.

Wheeled mobility

There is a large range of wheelchairs and buggies available. Those with a long-term need that meet a clinical requirement can be supplied through the National Health Service via the local wheelchair service. Wheelchairs may also be loaned on a temporary basis from organizations such as the British Red Cross or they may be purchased privately; this may be with the assistance of charity funding.

Wheelchairs may be: (1) of a standard design and provide a basic seat and a method for mobility; or (2) designed for a specific purpose such as a high-performance wheelchair for a child who has a spinal cord injury and is very active; or (3) a specialist sports wheelchair for basketball or wheelchair racing. Wheelchairs may have additional facilities such as a tilt-in-space or recline mechanism. To enable the occupant to reach items at different levels, some wheelchairs have elevating seats and others have a stand-up function (Kelsall et al 1993, Ham et al 1998).

A wheelchair may be self-propelled, attendant-propelled or powered (Figure 10.6). Powered wheelchairs may be occupant- or attendant-controlled and are described in the electronic AT (EAT) section of this chapter.

When choosing a wheelchair there are several factors that should be considered, including the method of propulsion, stability, fit of seating components/system, manoeuvrability, aesthetics and cost. The importance of the correct choice of wheelchair cannot be underestimated.

> **KEY POINT**
>
> - The correct choice of wheelchair is very important. Consideration must be given to propulsion, stability, fit, manoeuvrability, aesthetics, features and cost

Aspects of a wheelchair can be altered depending on how the wheelchair is used or set up. For example, moving the rear wheels forward makes a wheelchair more unstable in the backwards direction. This would be an advantage for a user with a high level of ability wishing to climb kerbs but a disadvantage for those with a lower level of ability who cannot alter the position of their body weight and therefore require a more stable wheelchair for safety (Brubaker 1986, Engstrom 2002).

Wheelchair seating

The wheelchair seating may be simple, such as a canvas sling seat and back rest. This is fitted as standard to most wheelchairs. More supportive wheelchairs may have additional features such as a tension-adjustable back rest canvas and others come complete with contoured seat and back rest cushions providing the majority of support required. Some wheelchairs provide the wheelchair base only and require a seating system to be inserted into it.

There is an enormous range of cushions and back rests that can be added to wheelchairs to provide comfort, support and pressure reduction.

Wheelchair accessories

Wheelchairs have a range of accessories that may be fitted to them. These items include pelvic straps, arm supports, harnesses, elevating leg rests and trays (Kelsall et al 1993).

The choice of wheelchairs, seating and cushioning and accessories is constantly changing as new products are brought on to the market. Information about the equipment that is currently available can be gathered from the local wheelchair service, shops supplying wheelchairs or by carrying out a search on the internet.

Transfers

Assistance with transfers covers a large range of equipment and is an important consideration with the provision of AT. Transfer boards can be used for seated transfers, transfer turntables to facilitate rotation during transfers, transfer belts, slide sheets and hoists. This is a large field in itself and is beyond the scope of this book.

Transportation

Many children who use a seating system within a wheelchair full-time travel in a vehicle in their wheelchair. General guidelines recommend that, wherever possible, users should transfer to a vehicle seat but for those with a complex posture or where there are manual handling considerations this may not be possible. When wheelchairs are used in this way it is important that they are suitable for this purpose. Manufacturers of wheelchairs and seating systems state whether their equipment is transportable and ascertain this by 'crash testing' the equipment. A transport kit may be recommended and if required this should be purchased and attached to the equipment prior to travel so that the wheelchair may be safely restrained.

Wheelchair tie downs and occupant restraint systems should be used in order to secure the equipment and occupant safely in an adapted vehicle. The guidelines published by the Medicines and Healthcare Products Regulatory Agency (formally the Medical Devices Agency) stipulate that a person with a disability travelling in a wheelchair should have the same level of safety as other passengers travelling in the vehicle (Medical Devices Agency 2001).

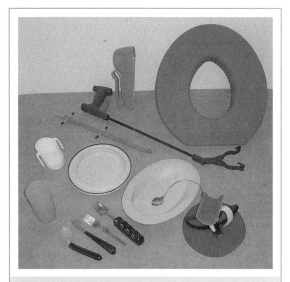

Figure 10.7 A selection of equipment for activities of daily living.

Equipment for activities of daily living

Equipment for ADL can be described as equipment that provides assistance with routine everyday activities. Some of the technology is simple but can make a difference between a child being able to complete an activity independently or being completely dependent for it. Use of AT may be as simple as using a non-slip material under a plate to prevent it from moving around. ADL equipment is often assessed for and supplied by occupational therapy services. There is a huge range of commercially available equipment (Figure 10.7). The Disabled Living Foundation has a database of equipment and many companies produce catalogues of products. Disabled living centres (DLCs) provide venues across the UK where a range of products can be seen before purchase, often with expert therapist assessment and advice available on site. Some DLCs are changing their name to reflect the independence that is enabled by their products and services.

Some children's needs cannot be met by commercially produced equipment and therefore require custom-made equipment. All equipment requires assessment but in order to provide custom-made equipment effectively the assessment should be carried out by a specialist multiprofessional team. In practice there are very few services where this is possible.

It is essential to involve a child and family in every step of the assessment process. For children in particular it is important to introduce equipment for ADL at the appropriate time for them to fit in with their social, educational and psychological stages of development. The motivation that the child has will go a long way in helping to ensure success.

KEY POINT

- Equipment for ADL promotes independence but must be introduced at the appropriate time for the child

---

Personal care

Dressing

To assist those with a disability a range of AT for dressing is available. The type of equipment that is available includes items such as shoe horns, sock aids and dressing sticks. For those with limited finger strength, reduced dexterity, muscle weakness, reduced range of mobility or absence of part of limbs, dressing frames can be used to place items of clothing on so that they can be positioned on the body more easily. Items of clothing may also be modified to assist with dressing, for instance, by replacing fastenings with Velcro in the place of buttons or elastic laces in shoes.

Individualized strategies should be used in conjunction with equipment where required to break down the dressing tasks into more manageable and meaningful steps.

Bathing

Depending on the age, interests and abilities of a child, AT for bathing may take many different forms. Some may use a long-handled sponge to reach parts of their body that they cannot reach with their hands. Children with a more complex disability may require a bath seat to support them in the bath. Some children require the complete support from a shower chair so that they are comfortable and secure while being washed by a parent or carer. Some children have specialist baths that have facilities such as drop-down sides for easy access or padding.

Children may also use devices such as toothbrush holders to hold the toothbrush securely so that children can bring their mouth to it rather than having to be able to grip the toothbrush and hold it close to their mouth.

A long-handled hairbrush can be used by a child who has reduced upper-limb mobility. It can be used for hairbrushing or if shampoo is placed on the brush the brush can then be used to apply shampoo to the hair. This would require an appropriate environment in order for the whole task to be completed independently.

Toileting

As children grow up privacy or independence in toileting often becomes a priority. For some children independence may be achieved with the use of a cleansing aid so that they can reach to wipe their bottom. The aids are often a simple paper-holder with a means of releasing the paper hygienically once used. Independence in toileting often requires consideration in conjunction with aspects of independent dressing.

Children may require toilet seats at a particular height or angle to give them a stable base to enable them to sit on the toilet or potty. In addition they may require assistance with getting on and off the toilet with a step.

Some children with a complex disability require a complete toilet seat that provides full postural support to give a safe, comfortable, effective environment. This can be used either over the toilet or with a potty. The seat may be mounted so that it is permanently attached to the toilet or mounted into a frame.

Eating and drinking

There is a wide range of AT that may be used to assist with eating and drinking. Again, it may be very simple, such as the use of a drinking straw for a child who cannot hold a cup. Other AT for drinking includes different shapes of cups with lids, handles and cut-outs to facilitate drinking without spilling fluids. There are different types of adapted plates and bowls available with lips or specially shaped. There are guards that can be clipped on to the edge of a standard plate. Various ranges of cutlery are available that have handles that are easier to grip and utensils that have modified shapes and can be used by children to enable them to feed themselves. More complex eating equipment such as a rocker spoon or an aid with a system of levers to enable a child with limited mobility and arm strength, such as arthrogryposis, is available commercially and can also be custom-made.

Writing and drawing

Children with a disability may not be able to hold a standard pen for writing or drawing but there are many writing aids available to assist with this. They may be in the form of devices that slip over the pen to make gripping easier. If children are not able to use their hands then a head pointer or mouth stick with a pen attachment may be used. The head pointer and mouth stick may also be used to press switches or a keyboard. Custom-made equipment can be made for a child who is not able to use commercially available equipment.

Play

Some children with a disability require AT in order to facilitate play. Much of the equipment uses switches and is therefore discussed in the EAT section. Toys with specific tactile or sensory features are available commercially from a variety of companies. Large items such as specialist playground equipment are available such as roundabouts and are designed for use with wheelchairs. Smaller items such as an indoor swing to provide sensory feedback are also available. The play environment may also require equipment such as padding to enable safe play.

Protective devices

Some children require equipment to help protect them. This may take the form of equipment such as helmets, mittens or devices to limit movement.

Helmets may be commercially available or custom-made. They may be made from a variety of materials. They can be used for children who may fall due to their disability and damage themselves, for example a child who has seizures. They can also be used for children who have a disability that causes them to have self-injurious behaviour, such as Lesch–Nyhan disease or some children with learning disabilities. Helmets may be used by children who have had a craniotomy as a result of a head injury. For these children small protective devices have been designed that can be woven into the hair to reduce the visual impact of having a protective device.

Children with some types of disability choose to wear mittens for protection. This will reduce the incidence of self-injury from biting fingers or scratching. The mittens will often need to be custom-made as the requirements of each child's protective requirements is often unique and not met by commercially available mittens that do not tend to be specifically designed for these purposes.

Equipment that is used to limit movement may take the form of wrist and ankle straps that allow freedom within a safe envelope of space. Children with athetosis or unwanted movements may prefer this option to using splints.

Prosthetics and orthotics

This is a specialist topic in itself and cannot be fully covered within this chapter and it is recommended that a specific text is used for more indepth information on this subject (Lusardi & Neilson 2000).

A prosthesis replaces an absent limb such as a leg, foot, arm or hand. The limb may be absent due to an amputation or as a result of a congenital deficiency. The prosthesis may be designed to replace a joint such as the knee, ankle, elbow or wrist. The prosthesis may be functional, such as providing a jointed leg to walk with or a hand to pick up objects, or it may be purely cosmetic. The limb should have the appearance and function as close as possible to a standard limb as technology allows.

Prosthetic limbs are made up of a number of different segments, joints and parts. The socket connects the limb to the body. It is custom-made to fit the shape of the residual limb and should be designed dependent on the forces that are to be applied to it in use. The socket is retained on the residual limb via a suspension system. This may be achieved using a vacuum system or a strapping system. The joints of a functional limb may be powered or non-powered. The prosthesis is finished with a cosmetic layer.

An orthosis supports an existing limb across a joint. It may be functional or resting. Orthotic management offers a conservative approach to prevent deformity, improve joint alignment and biomechanics and improve function. Orthoses provide intimate control of joints, which is not possible in positioning equipment. Evidence is available of the immediate impact of orthotics on gait but very little rigorous evidence exists on the long-term effect of orthotics (Morris 2002).

Lower-limb orthotics can be used to provide stability in standing transfers, clearance in swing and support for children with limited walking ability. Orthoses need to be used with care, as excessive use can lead to immobility and consequent muscle weakness and atrophy (Shortland et al 2002). Prescriptions for orthoses need to made in the light of the theories of muscle and bone adaptation, and joint biomechanics to ensure that satisfactory outcomes are achieved.

Hip and spinal orthoses (HASO) are prescribed to control hip and spine position but there is no literature to support their effectiveness. Thoracolumbosacral orthoses (TLSO) are used to control spinal curvature during growth. The construction of these jackets varies widely between orthotists and includes front or side opening, complete shells or shells with selected areas cut away. There is no evidence that spinal orthoses can reduce the rate of progression in scoliosis but studies have only introduced bracing when the degree of spinal curvature exceeded 25°. A clinical benefit of improved sitting balance has been cited (Miller et al 1996).

ELECTRONIC ASSISTIVE TECHNOLOGY

The following section covers equipment commonly known as EAT. Like mechanical AT, all EAT requires detailed assessment before provision.

Assessment

The assessment process and the time it takes vary depending on the activity and the needs of the child. In some circumstances children can be assessed for a device within a short time period provided there is background information from a team that knows that child; however, when the disability is more complex, in general a longer timeframe is required. Assessment will also vary depending on the purpose of the equipment, e.g. whether to build an understanding of cause and effect or to offer a child independence in an ADL.

Assessment for different types of EAT varies according to the activity. However there are a number of commonalities.

In order to use EAT children must first be motivated to undertake the activity. They must have a basic understanding of cause and effect and they need a reliable voluntary movement to be able to access the equipment. For equipment that is seeking to extend a child's independence rather than develop an understanding of cause and effect there is a need to have the ability to make choices.

The requirements of the child and family with regard to the activity need to be known and the child's abilities – physical, sensory and cognitive – need to be assessed. In order to identify potential solutions, knowledge of the range of products available is required to match those needs accurately to the equipment. Then a plan on how to introduce the equipment to the home and school in a way that ensures it fully meets those identified needs is also important.

Consideration of the child's changing needs cognitively, socially and physically has to be taken into account as well as the environments in which the child is placed. The support network around the child (are the family and school interested in having this technology in their home?) is also an important factor when considering EAT, as are the learning needs of the child in undertaking the activity.

KEY POINTS

Assessment requires knowledge of:

- Requirements of child and family
- Physical abilities
- Sensory abilities
- Cognitive abilities
- Support network around the child
- Range of equipment which map to child's abilities and child's/family's needs
- Learning needs of child in activity

Expectations

For some there is an assumption that technology is a cure-all – for example, the assumption that providing a communication aid to a child means that he or she will be able to talk. What the device can do is enhance communication by giving audible expression of what is already in the child's mind, providing the child has the appropriate skills both physically and cognitively in place to access the device. The issue of managing the expectation that comes with the assessment and provision of EAT is important, or else both child and family will quickly become disheartened. This is best addressed by keeping the child and family central to the decision-making process and encouraging realistic goals for the child.

KEY POINTS

Providing equipment to a child requires realistic expectations of that child's capabilities. This is aided by:

- Multidisciplinary assessment
- Critical eye to technology
- Matching the child's needs to equipment features
- Identifying the next steps

For all types of EAT, regular review is required to ensure that the equipment continues to meet those needs. For example, a child may start to operate a powered chair using a set of switches; however, over time an improvement in fine motor skills and awareness of directional control may make the introduction of a joystick appropriate. If this does not happen the children are left with their original access method. They are then not using the most efficient and fastest method for accessing a piece of equipment. The children's ability to participate in this activity is therefore limited by their equipment rather than enabling them to achieve their full potential.

Once the equipment has been provided it needs to be regularly maintained and training given to ensure that all those involved with the child are aware of how to operate it, charge it, basic fault-find and also whom to contact if it needs to be repaired.

After the equipment has been delivered there is often a need for a therapist to work with the child to develop understanding of the activity, control of the device and thus increase confidence in its use.

It should be recognized that the introduction of EAT can be both a bonus and a challenge for those around the child. For example, in order to integrate a communication aid into daily life changes may be required in the way others communicate with the child. At first additional time may be needed to wait for a response; questions must be phrased differently to encourage more than yes/no responses.

Another common assessment requirement for all types of EAT is determining the access method or how the child operates the equipment. For example, a typically developing child may access a computer using a standard keyboard and mouse, whereas a child with a physical disability can operate the same equipment and programs using adapted keyboards, a touch screen, a joystick or even just a single switch. For the child with complex physical disabilities this part of the assessment is particularly important.

Unless the interface between the user and the equipment is effective the use of the equipment is likely to be severely compromised. For children with complex physical disability the energy and effort required to operate a switch can be great. Therefore the method offered to access the device should be the fastest, most energy-efficient and reliable. This can sometimes mean a compromise in terms of positioning when undertaking a specific activity. This also means that therapeutic targets may not be paramount when thinking about access options for a child. For example, placing a switch centrally on a tray to encourage the child to move hands towards midline is not a fast or energy-efficient way of accessing equipment in comparison with placing the switch to one side where the child can easily reach.

> **KEY POINTS**
>
> Access methods used should be:
>
> - Fastest
> - Most energy-efficient for the child
> - Reliable

Alternative access options

There are many forms of switches commercially available, each being suitable for a particular client group. When undertaking the assessment there is a need to have knowledge of the different types of switches and controllers that exist, what inputs different equipment accept, how the options can be displayed on different devices and the user needs in order to match their abilities (Cook & Hussey 1995). The simplest types are mechanical switches (Figure 10.8). They have a number of characteristics which vary on different models to meet the physical needs of the child. These characteristics include size (larger switches for poor targeting skills), force required to activate the switch, feedback and amount of movement required to operate the switch.

> **KEY POINTS**
>
> Basic characteristics to consider in the choice of mechanical switch:
>
> - Force
> - Shape/size
> - Travel (movement to activate)
> - Feedback

As well as the array of mechanical switches available there is also a range of devices which can pick up body movements that activate a switch, e.g. eyeblink switches, movement (twitch) switches, sip and puff, sound and, more recently, eye gaze movements (Figure 10.9). These options tend to require a power supply in order to operate, e.g. a battery, and in some cases require more detailed set-up by a carer prior to each use.

It should be noted that not all methods are appropriate for all activities; however the availability of this spectrum of solutions offers potential independence in an activity for even the most physically challenged child.

Posture

A fundamental part of any assessment for EAT is consideration of the child's posture. Research shows that appropriate posture aids a child's ability to concentrate on a task (Sents & Marks 1989). This is particularly important with children with complex disability as posture affects the child's ability to control the movements of the trunk, arms, hands and head (Cowan 2005). The first part of this chapter elaborates on the ideal posture for a child,

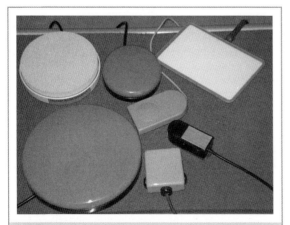

Figure 10.8 Selection of commercially available simple mechanical switches.

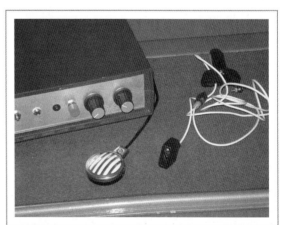

Figure 10.9 Sound-operated switch and infrared beam switch.

and in general this is true for establishing a good starting base for activities involving switches and EAT. However each child needs to be seen as an individual to determine appropriate posture for a given activity.

For some children consideration of accessing toys while lying down in a support may be appropriate or perhaps in a standing support wherever most effective use of their hands/arms or head is possible.

Young children learn through play and therefore introducing this technology in a play setting, e.g. switch-adapted toys, playing chase in a powered chair, has huge benefits. Sullivan & Lewis (2000) reported on the positive impact switch-activated AT has in developing a child's understanding that the environment is responsive and controllable. Smith (1994) reported on the important role communication aids play in a child's total communication system. Besio (2003) reported on the benefits of AT used in play to enhance social and cognitive development.

> **KEY POINT**
>
> ● Consideration of posture is an important part of the assessment of a child for any type of EAT

Powered mobility

Powered mobility offers children the opportunity to explore their environment independently. There is now a wide range of powered chairs available with differing capabilities. As well as controlling the movement of the chair, positioning of the seat can be altered such as recline and tilt and also raising and lowering the height of the seat, which allows interaction with peer group when standing or sitting on the floor (see Figure 10.10). For older children and young adults, when moving and handling become more challenging, chairs that allow the user to transfer to a standing position are also available.

Specialist features are available commercially and include options such as collision avoidance systems or SMART wheelchairs which offer track-following facilities or avoidance of obstacles (Figure 10.11). These can be used to offer additional support when some children are learning to operate a powered chair (Nisbet 2002).

As stated in the mechanical AT section, within the UK National Health Service wheelchair services are the main providers of mobility equipment and this includes powered mobility, although due to limited resources options are sometimes limited. Eligibility criteria can mean that in some services very young children are not provided with powered mobility (Durkin 2002, Staincliffe 2003). If a more elaborate chair is required, discussion with the child's local service can bring different funding and maintenance options.

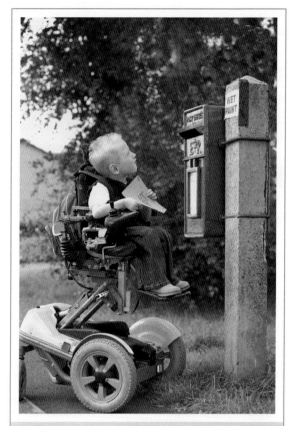

Figure 10.10   Child using powered wheelchair with seat riser. (Courtesy of Whizz Kidz Charity.)

Access options for powered mobility are also now very flexible. As well as the traditional joystick, a wide array (and number) of switches can be used to operate a chair.

In order to be able to operate a powered chair there is a need for the child to develop an array of skills which then have to be integrated to achieve what we call 'driving' a powered chair. A child with no experience of independent movement therefore has an enormous learning curve to climb when faced with operating a powered chair. There is a need for the team to introduce this activity just as one would other learning experiences. The activity needs to be graded appropriately for the child's skills, both physical and cognitive. For some children introducing powered mobility is straightforward and on being presented with a joystick they quickly gain an understanding of space, route-finding and problem-solving in order to drive from A to B. For others this can take several years and it is only by observing and presenting the child with opportunities to practise and gain experience and skills that powered mobility can be achieved.

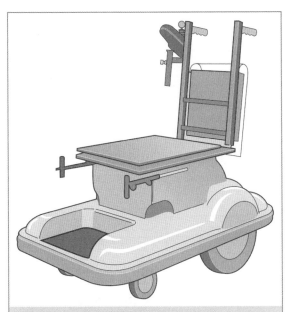

Figure 10.11 Smart wheelchair with bumper to detect when impact has been made and also track-following capability. (Courtesy of Call Centre, Edinburgh.)

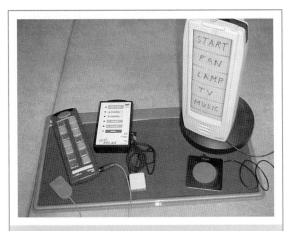

Figure 10.12 Environmental control systems.

ENVIRONMENTAL CONTROL SYSTEMS

ECS allow children to control aspects of their home/ school environment that they would normally be unable to control (Figure 10.12).

For example, children who have only one reliable voluntary movement, such as voluntary eyeblink or movement of one finger, can access a switch controlling a scanning array of options which allow them to operate

TV controls, audio equipment, toys, an alarm to call for help and for young adults control access through the front door and answer the telephone.

KEY POINTS

Environmental control can enable control of function in the following areas

Communication

- Simple voice output capabilities
- Access to a telephone
- Intercom systems
- Calling or paging for assistance

Comfort

- User can control operation of heating and cooling devices such as fans and heaters
- Operation of main overhead lighting and lamps
- Curtains
- Control of profiling beds and seats

Leisure

- Access to a computer
- Page-turners
- Television and music systems

The devices can be similar in size to standard TV remote controls and they operate equipment using infrared or radiofrequency signals. The child controls which device to operate by scanning through a menu of options.

To access a system offering all the above functions requires a range of physical and cognitive skills. For example, a single-switch user would need to have timing skills in order to access more than one option. The options are arranged in menu structures and therefore there needs to be an understanding of this structure. There needs to be an ability to anticipate and recall the location of options on different pages of the menu. For example, the volume-up option is on the TV page of commands.

Environmental control can be introduced at an early age by using simple items of equipment, for example, to turn on and off the mixer in the kitchen, or operate a set of Christmas tree lights (Figure 10.13). This more basic equipment is often funded in the early years by education for school purposes or sometimes provided by child development centres on a loan basis, or alternatively private/charity funding is sought. Again, early introduction of environmental control is important as children learn that they can affect their own environment. From an

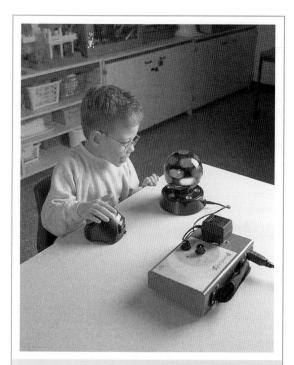

Figure 10.13 Child using simple environmental control to operate mains-operated light globe. (Courtesy of Inclusive Technology.)

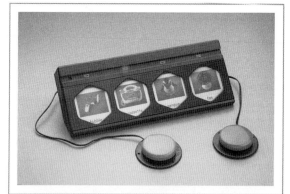

Figure 10.14 Simple voice output communication aid (Courtesy of Inclusive Technology)

early age typically developing children learn how to control their environment (e.g. television, opening and closing doors, switching on lights) and this equipment offers this opportunity to children with physical disability. Use of this equipment, like all AT, should be incorporated into all areas of the child's life. Some children are more motivated to access this type of technology than others as it offers an immediate and functional output.

National Health Service environmental control services are in place around the country. Some operate at a regional and others at a local level. Referral is generally through an occupational therapist.

The more complex systems which are more generally available through services can cover a variety of options and can be extended as the child's needs expand. Thus children could begin with a basic system which allows them control of the television. Then as their scanning and access skills increase, control of other remote controlled equipment could be added. Room set-ups can then be developed. With the system mounted on the child's wheelchair, for example, they can scan through menus offering them the control options for different rooms.

Consideration of all aspects mentioned in the earlier assessment section is required. The devices have differing sizes and offer different access options. For example, a child with visual impairment may require auditory scanning of the options or a screen where large symbols can

be displayed. The device chosen will therefore depend on a number of factors, including sensory needs and likely expansion of the system over time.

Consideration of where the main controller should be mounted is important as often operation of equipment while in bed is required as well as when in a wheelchair. This may require additional consideration of different switch access in different rooms as the child's physical skills in and out of postural control equipment may vary greatly. Again, the activity needs to be graded to meet the child's learning needs Therefore the size and the number of options in any menu have to be considered as well as position within the menu, i.e. all frequently used options near the top.

Once installed, training is required for both child and carers, with regular review to ensure the equipment continues to meet the child's needs.

COMMUNICATION AIDS

Around the UK, communication aid assessment centres offer assessment for different types of voice output communication aids (VOCAs: Figure 10.14). Some offer additional assessment expertise, advising on access to the curriculum (e.g. ACE centres) Often a 'library loan' system is in place which allows the child to trial a device before the local team and family seek funding.

VOCAs operate in a variety of ways and can offer simple recorded message output through to complex text to speech output.

The simplest system (e.g. BigMack) outputs a single short recorded phrase. This is often used as an introduction to VOCAS and enables the child to take part in simple story-telling activities and games during the school day. Others can offer a larger number of prerecorded digitized speech phrases which the child can access using one or more switches. The phrases can be recorded over depending on the child's needs.

Like ECS, more sophisticated devices have dynamic screens, i.e. using switches children can navigate their way through pages of menus filled with words or symbols to build up sentences as required. These systems tend to use synthesized speech as output rather than the digitized prerecorded option.

Support for both family and the child in the use of these systems has been identified as crucial to ensure success and extended use.

The devices are available in a range of sizes and have different display and access options to meet a wide range of needs. For ambulant users small devices can be purchased; these are accessed using a keyboard on a Personal digital assistant (PDA) type device or for non-ambulant users they can be mounted on a wheelchair. In this case care needs to be taken to ensure that the stability of the chair is not compromised and that users have a clear view of where they are going when driving their powered chair.

Assessment is usually undertaken by a specialist speech and language therapist and requires assessment of the child's basic communication skills. Device choice is based on a complex consideration of the child's current abilities and requirements, environments in which the system is to be used, access skills and sensory ability.

Computer access

For clients who cannot access a keyboard or mouse there is now a range of commercially available products which can enable access to all computer activities. For children of school age this aspect of access is generally addressed by the education provider. Keyboards of different shapes and layouts are available to assist those for whom the standard layout is not effective (Figure 10.15). Also key guards can be employed to provide access for those who have difficulty lifting their hand or fingers off the keys between strokes, thus preventing errors when using the keyboard. Standard operating systems such as Microsoft Windows also have accessibility options which can be set to accommodate some basic needs. For example, for those who accidentally hit the keys twice due to tremor, timeframes can be set up so that a given time has to elapse between keystrokes. Also for those who cannot manipulate a mouse, keys can be set to produce cursor movement around the screen.

For those who cannot access a keyboard at all, i.e. a one- or two-switch user, keyboard emulators are available (Figure 10.16). This is software which produces a keyboard (whose layout, size shape and colour can be adapted to meet the individual needs of the child) on the screen. Using a switch or switches, the child then scans through the keyboard to the letter required and continues generating a sentence in this way. Altering scanning patterns can dramatically speed up the access time for this method. For

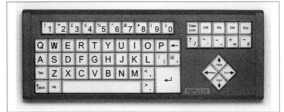

Figure 10.15 Example of alternative keyboard. (Courtesy of Inclusive Technology.)

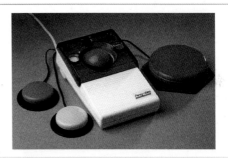

Figure 10.16 Examples of a trackball and switch alternative to a mouse. (Courtesy of Inclusive Technology.)

young children there are simple cause-and-effect type programs which are readily operated using one or two switches.

Having full access to the mouse can be a more challenging proposition. This entails being able to move around the screen, dragging, single- and double-click and scrolling. Different types of mouse are available with different shapes and sizes to accommodate some difficulties; also trackball-type devices can be used. These require the user to move a ball on top of the device instead of gliding the mouse over a surface. A joystick can also be used in place of a standard mouse. Other devices replace switches with each directional movement of the mouse, e.g. four switches allow movement in four directions (Figure 10.16).

For children with visual impairments, screen readers and magnifiers are available which allow access to standard software packages and the internet.

Again assessment is crucial and individual for each child.

Multifunctional devices

Increasingly, devices are being produced which are multifunctional (Figure 10.17). For example, communication aids have ECS capabilities; ECS have communication aid capability and also computer access options. This use of

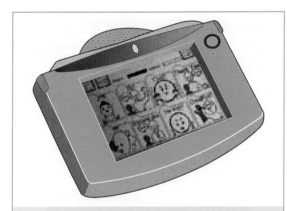

Figure 10.17 Multifunctional device incorporating communication and environmental control.

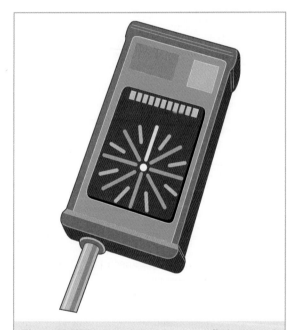

Figure 10.18 Integrated access scanner offering control of wheelchair and other devices using single-access method. (Courtesy of Novomed.)

multifunctional equipment has led to an increased need for teams and services to work more closely to ensure that resources are effectively used. For example, ECS services need to be informed if the child has a communication aid which has an ECS integrated within it as this could then be used as a main controller within the home and school.

As well as integrated devices, integrated control systems exist (Figure 10.18). These allow children who may only have one reliable voluntary movement to have real independence when operating a number of pieces of EAT, for example, a powered chair, communication aid and an ECS. With each piece of equipment comes a switch or access method. Therefore children using three types of equipment are left with three switches on their tray. With limited movement they then need someone to position each switch as it is required. The integrated control system allows the child independently to change the device the switch is operating. Guerette & Sumi (1994) and Nisbet (1996) have discussed these systems and developed criteria to determine when integrated control systems should be considered.

KEY POINT

- Children who have only one reliable access method or single voluntary movement which can be used to access a switch may benefit from using an integrated control system to enable full independent use of EAT

CASE STUDY 10.1

F is 6 years old. He has a diagnosis of quadriplegic cerebral palsy and he takes medication to control his seizures. He has used assistive technology since the age of 1.

Age 1

Following an assessment at a posture clinic (Table 10.1), F was issued with postural management equipment, including a lying support, supportive seating system and standing support.

Although F was able to lie in a symmetrical posture, a supine lying support was prescribed. This was because he lay with hips widely abducted and externally rotated. There was also concern for his breathing as he extended his head and neck. In the lying support F's hips were neutral for abduction/adduction and internal/external rotation. His head was supported with his chin tucked by the use of the head and shoulder girdle support.

F was prescribed with a Minicaps seat on a mobile base. He was able to sit on the floor with wide abduction and external rotation of his hips but he was not able to move and tended to fall backwards. The supportive seat enabled F to use his arms and practise control of his trunk within his base.

F was prescribed with a standing support that emulates the posture of a typically developing child. When assessed, F required full support under his axilla in order to stand. Within the standing support F was able to begin to take weight through his feet and to experience a typically developing standing posture.

Age 2

F was able to roll from supine to prone and move about from a lying position. The lying support was limiting his activity, therefore it was withdrawn.

F was issued with a tricycle with adaptations to provide postural support. This enabled him to explore his environment.

F continued to use the Minicaps on the mobile base and the standing support.

Age 3

F's ability was constantly improving and he continued to use his supportive seating system at school .The anterior and lateral supports on the standing support were removed as F had developed good trunk control in this position.

F was beginning to be able to stand unaided, although he stood with a poor posture with a very wide gait and with his pelvis posteriorly tilted. He was supplied with dynamic ankle–foot orthoses (DAFOs).

F was beginning to communicate more formally using Signalong and Makaton signs. He was issued with a Chailey Communication System (CCS) book.

Table 10.1 Chailey level of ability for F at age 1 (case study 10.1)

Supine	3
Prone	3
Floor sitting	3
Standing	2

Table 10.2 Chailey level of ability for F at age 6 (case study 10.1)

Prone	6
Supine	6
Floor sitting	7
Box sitting	7
Standing	8

Age 4

F continued to use the standing support as he could not free his hands to use them in standing.

F was able to walk short distances inside without assistance. He continued to use DAFOs to correct his foot position.

F was issued with a Blade self-propelling wheelchair with a cushion that he was able to propel outside over level ground.

F was provided with a potty chair to assist him with toilet training.

F used his Minicaps supportive seating system on occasions at home.

F was introduced to switches in order to operate switch toys. He used a one- or two-switch system.

Age 5

F was able to walk short distances outside and used a soft hat for outside play.

F continued to use his potty chair for toileting and was now able to get on and off independently.

The supportive seating system was no longer required and was withdrawn.

Age 6

F walks using DAFOs and, although much more confident, he continues to have difficulties with steps, slopes and uneven ground (Table 10.2).

continued

He continues to use his wheelchair for longer distances outside.

F is assessed for a school chair to enable him to stabilize his pelvis while working at school. He requires a seat at the correct height, with the correct seat depth, a conforming top surface and a lap strap.

F is using the computer at school. He is able to access it using two switches, a joystick or using the touchscreen facility.

The standing support is no longer required and is withdrawn.

CASE STUDY 10.2

Electronic Assistive Technology

S has cerebral palsy affecting all four limbs and seizures controlled by medication. She has no verbal communication. She is gastrostomy-fed and relies on others for all aspects of daily living.

Currently used mechanical assistive technology:

- Manual wheelchair with seating system
- Lying support
- Standing support
- Adapted trike
- Hoists at home and school
- Supportive armchair at home
- Adjustable-height bed
- Adapted toilet/shower seat.

She lives in an adapted house with her parents.

Age 1–3

S used wedge-shaped hand switches to activate toys and later on a tape player to listen to stories and songs. Although successful to some extent, with only gross movements of her arms S found it difficult to control movement and maintain pressure on switches regardless of positioning.

Communication progressed with development of reliable yes/no responses and use of communication book. S used a single switch in a power chair during play.

Age 3–8

S persisted with hand switches for a short period, as family and S indicated they were not ready to give up. She moved on to trail chin and head switches as an option. These offered more choices to meet her cognitive ability but she found it difficult to access these as extension and flexion of neck were difficult to initiate without great effort. A single head switch could be accessed but produced large movement and S could not grade the force with which she accessed the head switch. S used switches at home and school for different activities.

Access to computer was introduced using switches. S still found it difficult to target and slow to make choices but given time she was able to.

Powered chair progressed to using two directions (i.e. left and right) to keep the task simple and achievable but still enabling her to take part in chase games and games such as knocking over boxes. S also used the powered chair on a track system to manoeuvre around the school environment.

Age 8–11

S continued with all activities. S stopped using her hands to operate switches but still found accessing chin switches difficult. The head switch was used more reliably, although movements were still ungraded, but timing skills were emerging. S used a head switch mounted on a headrest to access the computer using a single switch and so could begin to access a menu of options using autoscanning (software scans through options rather than the user having to move through options using switch presses). S used switches to control racing cars and games on a computer. Voice output communication aids (VOCA) were introduced: access was slow in comparison with other communication methods but speed improved with increased timing skills. VOCA had environmental control integrated within the device so that it could be used for both communication and control of other devices. S used this at home to operate a simple TV control menu and a couple of mains sockets for devices such as a fan, a lamp and kitchen equipment.

During this period S's control of her rotational head movement from midline to right improved and she could control the extent of movement and force. S could also achieve midline to left rotation but without any timing skills or grading of force within movement. S quickly progressed to using this method on her communication aid. S used this in class and at home along with yes/no responses and a communication book. S accessed powered mobility using a scanner mounted on her chair and a single switch. S no longer needed the track system.

Extending the environmental control system to allow her to use equipment when in lying support and armchair was considered. However it was problematic to use the system when not in the seating system as S has less control of head movement.

continued

Age 12

S required help when she wanted to change from operating her chair to operating her communication aid. She was provided with an integrated control system. She used her reliable centre-to-right head movement as the main control and would change mode (or device to be operated by the main switch) by accessing a second switch placed on the left-hand side of the headrest.

Her environmental control system was extended so that she could control more aspects of her home, including the curtains in her room, doors around the house, TV (including Sky options), music system and mains sockets when seated in her wheelchair. Her integrated control system also had infrared input/output and so family could add codes to the device each time a new remote-control toy was bought or additional devices such as TVs were added around the home. S operated these as part of her integrated control system. S accessed the computer at home via the integrated control system and could contact her friends via the internet.

Age 13

S continues to use her system. She has requested an alternative communication aid as the current one obscures her vision when driving.

S chooses when she wants to use her technology. Sometimes she chooses to have someone operate her chair and communicate using her communication book and at others times she uses the equipment herself exclusively. She is aware of what the system can do and directs what she wants to control next.

S's parents feel she has the opportunity to express her personality, be naughty and be left alone to play.

The addition of the integrated system has improved interaction with her peer group and socially generally.

REFERENCES

Audit Commission 2000 *Fully Equipped*. London: Audit Commission.

Beresford B 1995 *Expert Opinions: A National Survey of Parent Caring for a Severely Disabled Child*. The Policy Press: Bristol

Beresford B 2003 *The Community Equipment Needs of Disabled Children and their Families*. Research works 2003-01. York: Social Policy Research Unit, University of York.

Besio S 2003 They play and learn to play. First results of the Italian research project on play and children with motor impairment. Proceedings of AAATE 2003 AT. Shaping the future, pp. 221–226. 105 Amsterdam Eds Buhler C, Krops H

Brubaker CE 1986 Wheelchair prescription: an analysis of factors that affect mobility and performance. *Journal of Rehabilitation, Research and Development* 23: 19–26.

Cartwright RD 1984 Effect of sleep position on sleep apnea severity. *Sleep* 7: 110–114.

Caulton JM, Ward KA, Aisop CW et al 2004 A randomised controlled trial of standing programme on bone mineral density in non-ambulant children with cerebral palsy. *Archives of Disease in Childhood* 89: 131–135.

Cook A, Hussey S 1995 Control interfaces for assistive technologies. In: *Assistive Technologies: Principles and Practice*. Mosby: Philadelphia pp. 311–373.

Cowan D, Khan Y 2005 Assistive technology for children with complex disabilities. *Current Paediatrics* 15: 207–212.

Demers L, Weiss-Lambrou R, Ska B 1996 Development of the Quebec User Evaluation of Satisfaction with assistive Technology (QUEST). *Assistive Technology* 8: 3–13.

Demers L, Weiss-Lambrou R, Ska B 2002 The Quebec User Evaluation of Satisfaction with assistive Technology (QUEST 2.0): an overview and recent progress. *Technology and Disability* 14: 101–105.

Durkin J 2002 The need for the development of a child led assessment tool for powered mobility users. *Technology and Disability* 14: 163–171.

Engstrom B 2002 *Ergonomic Seating. A True Challenge. Wheelchair Seating and Mobility Principles*. Germany: Posturalis Books.

Goodacre L, Turner G 2005 An investigation of the effectiveness of the Quebec User Evaluation of Satisfaction with assistive technology via a postal survey. *British Journal of Occupational Therapy* 68: 93–96.

Green EM, Mulcahy CM, Pountney TE et al 1993 The Chailey standing support for children and young adults with motor impairment: a developmental approach. *British Journal of Occupational Therapy* 56: 13–18.

Guerette P, Sumi EI 1994 Integrating control of multiple assistive devices: a retrospective review. *Assistive Technology* 6: 67–76.

Ham R, Aldersea P, Porter D et al 1998 *Wheelchair Users and Postural Seating. A Clinical Approach*. Singapore: Churchill Livingstone.

Jutai J, Day H 2002 Psychosocial Impact of Assistive Devices Scale (PIADS). *Technology and Disability* 14: 107–111.

Kelsall AD, Houghton RH, Cochrane GM et al 1993 *Wheelchairs*. Oxford: The Disability Information Trust.

Korpela R, Seppanen R-L, Koivikko M 1993 Rehabilitation service evaluation: a follow-up of the extent of use of technical aids for disabled children. *Disability and Rehabilitation* 15: 143–150.

Lespargot A, Renaudin E, Khouri M et al 1994 Extensibilitiy of hip adductors in children with cerebral palsy. *Developmental Medicine and Child Neurology* 36: 980–988.

Lusardi MM, Neilsen C (eds) 2000 *Orthotics and Prosthetics in Rehabilitation*. Boston: Butterworth-Heinemann.

Martin SE, Marshall I, Douglas NJ et al 1995 The effect of posture on airway caliber with the sleep apnea/hypopnea syndrome. *American Journal of Respiratory Care Medicine* 152: 721–724.

Medical Devices Agency 2001 *Guidance on the Safe Transportation of Wheelchairs*. Device bulletin MDA DB2001(3). Medical Devices Agency.

Miller A, Temple T, Miller F et al 1996 Impact of orthoses on the rate of scoliosis progression in children with cerebral palsy. *Journal of Pediatric Orthopaedics* 16: 332–335.

Mitchell W, Sloper P 2000 *User Friendly Information to Families with Disabled Children. A Guide to Good Practice*. York: YPS.

Morris C 2002 A review of the efficacy of lower-limb orthoses used for cerebral palsy. *Development Medicine and Child Neurology* 44: 205–211.

Mountain G 2004 Using the evidence to develop quality assistive technology services. *Journal of Integrated Care* 12: 19–27.

Mulcahy CM, Pountney TE, Billington GD et al 1991 Adapted tricycle. *Physiotherapy* 77: 660.

Newman CJ, O'Regan M, Hensey O et al 2006 Sleep disorders in children with cerebral palsy. *Developmental Medicine and Child Neurology* 48: 564–568.

Nisbet P 1996 Integrating technologies: current practices and future possibilities. *Medical Engineering and Physics* 18: 193–202.

Nisbet PD 2002Assessment and training of children for powered mobility in the UK. *Technology and Disability* 14: 173–182.

Pope PM 2002 Postural management and special seating. In: Edwards S (ed.) *Neurological Physiotherapy: A Problem Solving Approach*. London: Churchill Livingstone, pp. 189–217.

Pountney TE, Mulcahy CM, Clarke S et al 2004 *The Chailey Approach to Postural Management*. East Sussex: Chailey Heritage Clinical Services.

Sents BE, Marks HE 1989 Changes in preschool children's IQ as a function of positioning. *American Journal of Occupational Therapy* 43: 685–687.

Shortland AP, Harris CA, Gough M et al 2002 Architecture of the medial gastrocnemius in children with spastic diplegia. *Developmental Medicine and Child Neurology* 44: 158–163.

Smith MM 1994 Speech by any other name: the role of communication aids in interaction. *European Journal of Disorders of Communication* 29: 225–240.

Staincliffe S 2003 Wheelchair services and providers discriminating against disabled children? *International Journal of Therapy and Rehabilitation* 10: 151–159.

Stallard J 2005 Walking for the severely disabled. Research and development, experience and clinical outcomes. *Journal of Bone and Joint Surgery* 87: 604–607.

Stuberg W 1992 Considerations related to weight bearing programs in children with developmental disabilities. *Physical Therapy* 72: 35–40.

Sullivan M, Lewis M 2000 Assistive technology for the very young. Creating responsive environments. *Infant Young Child* 12: 34–52.

Tardieu CA, Lespargot A, Tabary C et al 1988 For how long must the soleus be stretched each day to prevent contracture? *Developmental Medicine and Child Neurology* 30: 3–10.

US Statute 1988 *Technology Related Assistance for Individuals with Disabilities Act* PL 100–407 title 29 USC 2201 et seq

Wilmshurst S, Ward K, Adams JE et al 1996 Mobility status and bone density in cerebral palsy. *Archives of Disease in Childhood* 75: 164–165.

Wintergold A 2006 The use of standing supports for children with disabilities. (in press). APCP Journal

Wright E, Belbin G, Slack M et al 1999 An evaluation of the David Hart Walker orthosis: a new assistive device for children with cerebral palsy. *Physiotherapy Canada* Autumn: 280–291.

Acquired brain injury

11 Acquired brain injury: acute management

Lesley Nutton

CHAPTER CONTENTS

INTRODUCTION

In children head injuries are very common: some are of a serious nature with consequences which will remain with them for the rest of their lives. In 2002 acquired brain injury (ABI) caused 2% of all deaths in those aged 0–14 years in England and Wales (Parslow et al 2005).

Although children have better survival rates compared with adults with ABI, the long-term sequelae and consequences are often more devastating in children due to their age and developmental potential. The costs involved in the care of a child with severe ABI, extended over a lifetime, are significant (Mazzola & Adelson 2002).

Although advances in emergency resuscitative treatment, improved neurosurgical facilities and diagnostic procedures (computed tomography (CT) scans, magnetic resonance imaging) have resulted in a reduction in mortality, there has been an increase in the number of children

who are surviving severe ABI who have major residual problems.

The aim of this chapter is to emphasize the importance of early physiotherapy intervention in respiratory, musculoskeletal and neurological care, highlighting the background knowledge, especially with emphasis on paediatric/developmental considerations, required to enable the physiotherapist to help optimize outcome for each child.

WHAT IS ACQUIRED BRAIN INJURY?

ABI is a non-degenerative injury to the brain that has occurred since birth, and can be classified into two groups:

1. Non-traumatic – strokes, other vascular accidents, tumours, infectious disease, hypoxia, metabolic disorders and toxic product inhalation/ingestion (www.headway.org.uk)
2. Traumatic brain injury (to be referred to as ABI throughout this chapter) is the commonest cause of acquired disability in childhood (Crouchman et al 2001) and will be the main topic of this chapter, but acute rehabilitation pathways are similar.

INCIDENCE

A recent study (Parslow et al 2005) found that:

- The prevalence rate for children (0–14 years) admitted to intensive care with ABI was 5.6 per 100 000 per year
- ABI was commonest in low socioeconomic class (overcrowding, decreased supervision, less secure play areas)
- In 65% of admissions ABI was an isolated injury
- There was a significant summer peak in admissions in children under 10 years
- Time of injury peaked late afternoon and early evening, a pattern that remained constant across the days of the week
- Prevalence of ABI is higher in males than females in all age groups, with a 2.5:1 male-to-female ratio (Felice 2005)

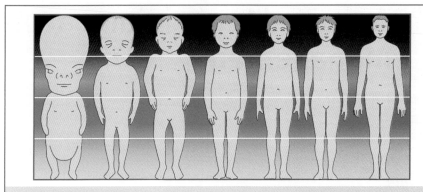

Figure 11.1 Change in body proportions from before birth to adulthood.

- Children with premorbid problems displayed a higher risk of ABI – behavioural (11%), learning (18%), both of these (42%) and neither (29%) (Rutter 1981)
- Children with existing behavioural problems are three times as likely to sustain ABI as compared to those without behavioural problems (Michaud et al 1993).

CAUSES

Causes of ABI vary considerably with the age of the child. Parslow et al (2005) also found that:

- The commonest mechanism of injury was a pedestrian accident (36%), most often occurring in children over 10
- Injuries involving motor vehicles have the highest mortality rates (23% of vehicle occupants, 12% of pedestrians) compared with cyclists (8%) and falls (3%)
- Infants fall from windows, furniture and down stairs, whereas older children fall from trees, roofs and playground equipment
- Cycling injuries account for 20% of all ABI in children (Powell 2005)
- Non-accidental injury is most common in infants (Billmire & Myers 1985).

The above causes and statistics give clear targets for injury prevention. Primarily accidents can be prevented by traffic calming. Airbags, soft playground surfaces, use of infant restraint harnesses and removal of pull bars have reduced ABI incidence and cycle-related ABI has been reduced by 85% since the promotion of cycle helmet use (Powell 2005).

DEVELOPMENTAL CONSIDERATIONS

A fundamental knowledge of age-related differences in cerebrovascular physiology and anatomy is essential in the application of adult-based head trauma protocols in paediatric patients. Anatomical differences in the skull, cervical spine, brain and chemistry render the child's brain more susceptible to injury than the adult. The outcome for children suffering ABI is far worse than the outcome for an equally injured adult (Anderson & Moore 1995).

Head-to-torso proportions

The brain has achieved 25% of its adult size at birth, 50% by the end of 1 year, 90% by the end of the fifth year and 98% by age 15 (Wong 1995) (Figure 11.1).

Height of child

The toddler's head is at the level of the motor vehicle front, and isolated severe head injury is subsequently common.

Skull

Children's skulls are only one-eighth as strong as adults and therefore more vulnerable to injury through deformation and fracture of the skull, leading to brain injury. Infants and young children tolerate increased intracranial pressure (ICP) better because open fontanelles and cranial sutures lead to a compliant intracranial space. The mass effect of, for example, a haemorrhage, is often masked by a compensatory increase in intracranial volume through fontanelles and sutures. Therefore increased ICP signs and symptoms present when the pathology is advanced. Mature suture closure occurs by 12 years but completion of fusion continues until the third decade (Ommaya et al 2002).

Brain growth and development rates

There are vast differences in the organization of the brain in different ages of childhood/adolescence. During the normal maturation of the brain plasticity and potential are most diverse and extensive remodelling will occur in developing children, thereby increasing their ability to learn. This has led many to expect a greater degree of recovery in younger children. However, babies and young children have very few matured functional pathways to tap into and this may well put the child at a disadvantage when compared to an older child who will have existing pathways for functional movement. Skills that are emerging or developing may be affected differently by brain injury than skills that are already established (Wedel-Sellars & Hill-Vegter 1997).

Some neurological deficits may not manifest for years after a head injury, e.g. frontal lobes develop relatively late in a child's growth, so that injury to frontal lobes may not become apparent until the child reaches adolescence as higher-level reasoning develops and social interaction and interpersonal skills are required (Tranel & Eslinger 2000).

Brain water content

The child's brain has a higher water content (88%) than the adult brain (77%), meaning that the brain is softer and more prone to acceleration–deceleration injury.

Blood supply

Cerebral blood flow (CBF) is the amount of blood in transit through the brain at a given point in time. A child has a larger percentage of cardiac output directed to the brain, as the head accounts for a larger percentage of body surface area and blood volume (Table 11.1). This can make maintenance of cerebrovascular stability difficult.

Pituitary gland

The pituitary gland can be damaged in moderate to severe ABI. If production of growth hormone is affected, hormone therapy may be needed to prevent the long-term ill effects of low pituitary output, which may affect the heart, the psychiatric state of the child and produce sexual dysfunction (Bondanelli et al 2005).

Table 11.1 Cerebral blood flow in normal unanaesthetized children (Zwienenburg & Muizelaar 1999)

Age	Cerebral blood flow (ml/100 g per min) (approximate)
0–6 months	40
3–4 years	108
9 years onwards	71

CLASSIFICATION OF HEAD INJURY

Injuries can be divided into primary and secondary injuries.

- Primary injury is due to direct mechanical damage inflicted at the time of injury. Except for preventive measures, little can be done to alter primary brain damage which is irreversible (Palmer 2000). If primary damage is not extensive, outcome becomes dependent upon the management of the secondary damage
- Secondary injury is represented by systemic and intracranial events that occur in response to primary injury and further contribute to neuronal damage and cell death.

Recovery from any type of brain injury depends on the extent of the initial injury and the secondary damage (Arbour 1998).

Injuries are also classified by mechanism (closed versus open), morphology (fractures, focal intracranial injury and diffuse axonal injury) and severity (mild, moderate or severe).

Mechanisms of injury

- Open – also referred to as penetrating injuries; these occur when both the skin and the dura are penetrated by a foreign object (e.g. bullet) or a bone fragment of a fractured skull. The most common (and most severe) type of injury to the brain is the diffuse injury
- Closed – are the most common type; the skin remains intact and there is no penetration of the dura. Closed ABI falls into two categories: focal and diffuse.

The severity of these injuries varies according to the velocity of impact and the vector (linear versus rotational) of forces applied. History of the accident is utilized to determine the velocity of the injury.

Low-velocity injuries include a child falling a short distance, an accidental blow to the head, e.g. with a bat, or an aggressive tackle in a football game. Injuries are usually mild and only require observation.

High-velocity injuries include a fall from an upper-storey window and a pedestrian being struck by a moving car. Even in the absence of neurological dysfunction children are usually observed in hospital.

Crushing injuries may also occur where the head might be caught between two hard objects (e.g. the wheel of a car and the road). This is the least common type of injury, and often damages the base of the skull and nerves of the brainstem rather than the brain itself (Duhaime et al 1995).

Morphology of injury

Skull fractures may be in the cranial vault or skull base and may be linear or stellate, depressed or non-depressed. The main significance of finding a fracture is that it is an indication of the force of the injury. Depressed skull fractures are invariably associated with high-velocity injury and may result in brain injury. A CT scan is mandatory. Basal skull fractures may involve the floor of the skull's brain cavity and are occasionally associated with cerebrospinal fluid (CSF) rhinorrhoea or otorrhoea (leakage of spinal fluid into the nose and ears). Bruising around the eyes, ears and back of neck may also be present.

Brain injuries arise from three characteristics of the brain/skull anatomy:

1. Rigidity and internal contours of the skull
2. Incompressibility of the brain tissue
3. Susceptibility of the brain to shearing forces.

The first and second points give rise to contusions or haematomas on the surface of the brain.

There are often two contusion sites. One occurs at the impact site – coup injury (frontal and temporal lobes are commonly involved). The other arises where the brain bounces off the skull when it has been moved away from the site of the original blow – contrecoup injury (Figure 11.2b). Some bleeding may also arise at the suture points where the dura mater, which serves to suspend the brain within the skull, is torn away from the inside of the skull. Contusions are usually multiple and may occur bilaterally. Multiple contusions do not in themselves contribute to depression of conscious level, but this may arise when bleeding into the contusions produces a space–occupying haematoma.

The third point, susceptibility of the brain to shearing forces, plays a role primarily in injuries that involve rapid and forceful movements of the head, e.g. motor vehicle accidents, shaken-baby syndrome. Rotational forces, associated with rapid acceleration–deceleration of the head, are smallest at the point of the rotation of the brain near the lower end of the brainstem and successively increase at increasing distances from this point The resultant shearing forces cause different levels in the brain to move relative to one another. This movement produces stretching and tearing of the axons (diffuse axonal injury; Figure 11.2a) and the insulating myelin sheath, injuries which are the major cause of loss of consciousness in a head trauma. Small blood vessels are also damaged, causing bleeding deep in the brain.

Collectively these injuries can result in swelling of the brain. If swelling continues the brain will gradually be pushed down through the foramen magnum (coning). Brainstem nuclei controlling breathing and cardiac function will eventually be compressed, resulting in death (Lindsay et al 1986, Wong 1995, Waugh & Grant 2005).

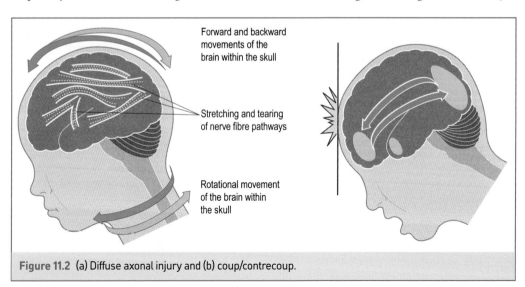

Forward and backward movements of the brain within the skull

Stretching and tearing of nerve fibre pathways

Rotational movement of the brain within the skull

Figure 11.2 (a) Diffuse axonal injury and (b) coup/contrecoup.

To summarize, the brain may be injured in a specific location or the injury may be diffused to many different parts of the brain. The indefinite nature of brain injury makes treatment unique for each child. It is important to understand that the brain functions as a whole by interrelating its component parts and its implications for rehabilitation. The injury may only disrupt a particular step of an activity that occurs in a specific part of the brain. The interruption of that activity at any particular step, or out of sequence, can reveal the problems associated with the injury (Table 11.2).

Severity of head injury

The Glasgow Coma Scale (GCS) is the most widely accepted tool to determine severity of head injury. It is a simple scale developed in 1974 to assess conscious levels and has a relatively high degree of interobserver reliability (Rowley & Fielding 1991, Gill et al 2004). It serves as an immediate prognostic guide and provides a useful baseline with which future examinations can be compared. The scale has been adapted for infants and young children – the Paediatric Coma Scale (Reilly et al 1988).

Table 11.2 Specific functions of different brain areas and problems associated with injury

Area of brain	Functions	Problems if damaged
Frontal	<ul><li>Motor cortex</li><li>Contralateral movement of face, arm, leg, trunk</li><li>Contralateral head- and eye-turning</li><li>Expressive centre for speech</li><li>Personality and initiative, and emotional response</li><li>Cortical inhibition of bladder and bowel voiding</li></ul>	<ul><li>Monoplegia/hemiplegia is dependent on extent of damage</li><li>Paralysis of head and eye movements to the opposite side</li><li>Inability to sequence a complex task, difficulty with problem-solving</li><li>Persistence of a single thought (perseveration)</li><li>Changes in personality with antisocial behaviour and loss of inhibitions</li><li>Loss of initiative and becomes uninterested and unconcerned</li><li>Emotionally labile</li><li>Expressive language problems</li><li>Incontinence of urine and faeces</li></ul>
Parietal	<ul><li>Appreciation of posture, touch and passive movements</li><li>Receptive speech area where language is understood</li><li>Visual attention</li><li>Manipulation of objects</li><li>Concept of body image and awareness of external environment</li><li>Mathematical skills</li></ul>	<ul><li>Postural and passive movement sensation disturbed</li><li>Receptive dysphasia</li><li>Lack of awareness of certain body parts or surrounding space</li><li>Difficulty distinguishing left from right</li><li>Difficulty with mathematics</li><li>Hand-eye incoordination</li><li>Difficulty reading, naming and drawing objects, locating words for writing</li><li>Can only attend to one object at a time</li></ul>
Occipital	<ul><li>Perception of vision</li></ul>	<ul><li>Cortical blindness</li><li>Visual field cuts</li><li>Difficulty identifying colours</li><li>Hallucinations</li><li>Visual illusions</li><li>Difficulty recognizing words and drawn objects</li><li>Reading and writing problems</li><li>Cannot put name to familiar face</li></ul>

continued

Table 11.2 *continued*		
Area of brain	**Functions**	**Problems if damaged**
Temporal	• Hearing of language, sounds, rhythm, music • Learning and memory • Some visual perceptions • Emotional/affective behaviour	• Cortical deafness • Difficulty in hearing spoken words, appreciation of rhythm/music • Short- and long-term memory • Inability to establish new memory • Aggressive and antisocial behaviour • Persistent talking (right lobe) • Difficulty recognizing faces and objects
Brainstem	• Breathing • Heart rate • Swallowing • Reflexes to seeing and hearing (startle response) • Controls seating, blood pressure, digestion, temperature (autonomic nervous system) • Affects level of alertness • Ability to sleep • Sense of balance (vestibular function)	• Decreased vital capacity for breathing, important for speech • Swallowing • Difficulty with organization/ perception of the environment • Problems with balance and movement • Dizziness and nausea • Sleep difficulties
Cerebellum	• Maintenance of gait • Maintenance of postural tone and coordination of voluntary movement • Maintenance of balance and equilibrium	• Unsteady gait • Tremor • Unable to perform rapid movements • Impaired fine–movement coordination • Dizziness • Slurred speech

Modified from Lindsay et al (1986), Wong (1995) and Waugh & Grant (2005).

The GCS is scored between 3 and 15, 3 being the worst and 15 the best (Table 11.3). It is composed of three parameters: best eye response, best verbal response and best motor response:

Best eye response (E)

1. No eye-opening
2. Eyes opening to pain
3. Eye-opening to verbal command
4. Eyes open spontaneously.

Best verbal response (V)

1. No vocal response
2. Incomprehensible sounds
3. Inappropriate words
4. Confused
5. Oriented.

Table 11.3 Grading of acquired brain injury (ABI) using the Glasgow Coma Scale (GCS) score

Grade of ABI	GCS score
Mild	13–15
Moderate	9–12
Severe	3–8

Motor response (M)

1. No motor response
2. Extension to pain (decerebrate posturing)
3. Flexion to pain (decorticate posturing)
4. Withdrawal from pain
5. Localizing to pain
6. Obeys commands.

To be useful the 'GCS of 12' needs to be broken down into its components, e.g. E4V3M5 = GCS 12 (Teasdale & Jennett 1974).

The GCS has limitations in the assessment of some children, including those who are intubated, dysphasic, have periorbital haematomas and facial swelling and immobilized broken limbs.

INTRACRANIAL DYNAMICS AND AUTOREGULATION

In order to plan appropriate intervention, it is essential for the physiotherapist to understand the importance of monitoring the patient's intracranial status. At present ICP and cerebral perfusion pressure (CPP) monitoring remain the most commonly used clinical parameters for assessing intracranial dynamics. By continuous observation and regulation of the ICP and mean arterial pressure (MAP), CPP can be maintained.

What is intracranial pressure?

It is the pressure exerted by the volume of the three intracranial components inside the skull:

1. Brain tissue: 80%
2. Blood: 10%
3. CSF: 10% (Andrus 1991).

Under normal conditions ICP ranges between 0 and 10 mmHg, although it will rise transiently with coughing or straining (Chudley 1994), with no significant pressure gradient between the two cerebral hemispheres or between supratentorial and infratentorial compartments (Dixon & Vyas 1999). Following trauma, this situation may change.

When the volume of any of the intracranial components increases, the volume of one or both of the others must decrease or the ICP will rise (Arbour 1998). Normally the brain has the ability to autoregulate its blood flow by dilation and constriction of blood vessels. This ensures a constant blood flow to all areas of the brain. Autoregulation is apparently preserved in the majority of head-injured children (Sharples et al 1995a).

Compensatory mechanisms for increased intracranial pressure

The brain may try to compensate for the increase in one of the intracranial components by shunting CSF to the spinal subarachnoid space, increasing CSF absorption or decreasing CSF production or shunting venous blood out of the skull. However, cerebral trauma may disrupt autoregulatory mechanisms and cause a sustained increase of ICP to

Table 11.4 Clinical signs of increased intracranial pressure in infants and children (Wong 1995)

Infants	Children
• Tense, bulging fontanelle • Separated cranial sutures • 'Cracked-pot' sound on skull percussion • Irritability • High-pitched cry • Increased occipitofrontal circumference • Distended scalp veins • Changes in feeding • Cries when held or rocked • 'Setting-sun' sign (impaired upward gaze)	• Headache • Nausea • Vomiting • Diplopia, blurred vision • Seizures • Changes in behaviour and personality **Late signs (all ages)** • Decreased consciousness • Decreased motor and sensory responses • Alteration in pupil size and reactivity (pupillary response changes*) • Decerebrate and cortical posturing • Change in respiration pattern • Papilloedema[†]

*Pupillary response changes: the light reflex tests oculomotor (III) nerve function and is a crucial indicator of an expanding intracranial lesion. The pupil dilates on the side of the expanding lesion and is an important localizing sign (Lindsay et al 1986).
†Papilloedema: swelling of the optic disc when intracranial pressure is raised.

15 mmHg or higher (Johnson 1999). Treatment is normally required >20 mmHg and can be measured by various monitoring devices.

Monitoring of ICP is important and this is closely linked to the maintenance of an adequate CPP and the importance of normovolaemia.

Clinical effects of increased intracranial pressure

A raised ICP will produce signs and symptoms but does not cause neuronal damage provided CBF is maintained (Table 11.4). Damage results from brain shift.

What is cerebral perfusion pressure?

CPP is the pressure at which the brain tissue is perfused with blood and is a measure of the adequacy of the cerebral circulation. It is maintained by supporting MAP and/or reducing ICP.

When autoregulation is impaired, the CBF fluctuates with changes in systemic blood pressure e.g. during suctioning, coughing, causing a rise in blood pressure and resultant increased ICP. An acutely injured brain has a higher metabolic rate and therefore requires a higher CPP (Sharples et al 1995b).

Normal CPP in paediatric patients is variable and dependent upon the age-related MAP. Monitoring of ICP as a means of calculating CPP is widely used, aiming for a CPP of >50 mmHg in infants under 1 year and 60 mmHg in children above that age (Table 11.5: Dixon & Vyas 1999, Hackbarth et al 2002).

SECONDARY BRAIN DAMAGE

Critical care management is focused on minimizing secondary brain injury caused by a cascade of cellular events that occur after the primary insult. Initial vascular and parenchymal disruption leads to ongoing neuronal degeneration, resulting in neuronal ischaemia and cell death (Bayir et al 2003).

Secondary brain damage is caused by several factors, including increased ICP and decreased CPP, which may follow:

- Haematoma
- Brain swelling
- Brain shift
- Ischaemia
- Infection

Haematoma

Intracranial bleeding may occur outside (extradural) or within the dura (intradural) (Figure 11.3):

- Extradural – a skull fracture may cause tearing of the middle meningeal vessels, causing a bleed into the extradural space. There may be a lucid interval after the injury, then increasing headache (the dura is pain-sensitive) and a subsequent clinical deterioration as the mass lesion increases in size.
- Intradural – which may evolve into a life-threatening mass as bleeding from the torn veins continues, consisting of a mixture of both subdural and intracerebral haematomas. Bridging veins may be ruptured following impact, producing a subdural haematoma. It is usually associated with high-velocity injury with immediate severe neurological dysfunction.

Brain swelling

This results from either vascular engorgement or an increase in extra- or intracellular fluid. A haematoma may or may not be present.

Brain shift

A progressive rise in ICP due to a supratentorial haematoma at first produces midline shift followed by a series of herniations, causing progressive midbrain and lower brainstem compression (Figure 11.4).

Table 11.5 Minimum cerebral perfusion pressure (CPP) to strive for (Chambers et al 2005)	
Age band (years)	**CPP (mmHg)**
2–6	53
7–10	63
11–16	66

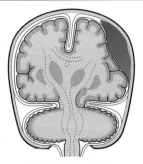 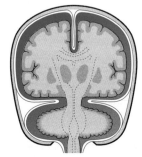 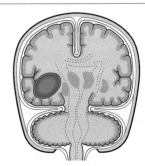

(a) Subdural haematoma   (b) Subarachnoid haemorrhage   (c) Intracerebral haemorrhage

Figure 11.3 Effects of different types of expanding lesion. (a) Subdural haematoma; (b) subarachnoid haemorrhage; (c) intracerebral haemorrhage.

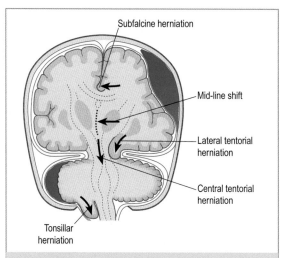

Figure 11.4 Supratentorial haematoma producing midline shift and herniation.

Ischaemia

This is caused by either hypoxia or impaired cerebral perfusion and may result in a drop in cerebral perfusion since autoregulation results in cerebral vasodilation.

Infection

Skull fractures may result in dural tearing which leaves the brain susceptible to a potential route for infection. Basal skull fractures may cause leakage of CSF from the nose (rhinorrhoea) or ear (otorrhoea) which requires immediate antibiotic therapy to prevent infection, leading to meningitis or cerebral abscesses.

PRIMARY MANAGEMENT AND INTERVENTIONS FOR ACQUIRED BRAIN INJURY

The first 24–72 hours is the vital period in management of ABI (Johnson 1999). Adequate oxygen delivery and haemodynamic stability in the child at the earliest moment remain the most important aspects of the management plan (Lam & MacKersie 1999).

Most patients who survive the first few hours after severe ABI require several days of intensive care, and ICP is usually measured during this time (Segal et al 2001).

The recognition that the combination of hypoxia (oxygen saturation < 90%) and hypotension (systolic blood pressure < 90 mmHg) is universally associated with unfavourable outcome underlies the importance of immediate action with airway protection, adequate ventilation and intravenous access and fluid replacement.

Hypotension has been shown to increase mortality rates significantly in children with ABI but isolated ABI rarely leads to hypotension. Blunt abdominal trauma and long-bone fractures frequently occur in association with ABI and may be a major source of blood loss. A child's blood volume should be restored with crystalloid solutions and/or blood products. These children should undergo aggressive fluid therapy resuscitation with isotonic fluids until appropriate fluid balance is achieved (Felice 2005).

Children who suffer multisystem trauma typically present with head injury, followed in decreasing frequency by limb fracture and trauma to the torso (Moulton 2000). Fracture management follows once medical stability is optimized.

Children suspected of head injury require an assessment of:

- GCS
- A neurological examination, including pupillary responses
- An examination of the head and neck for signs of bruising, lacerations and open fractures – bruising associated with basal skull fractures often takes several hours to develop.

Following initial assessment, repeated neurological observations are required to detect deterioration. Children in a coma (GCS < 8) require urgent intubation. Endotracheal intubation allows for airway protection and better control of oxygenation and ventilation. Oral (for base-of-skull fractures) or nasal intubation tubes should be taped and not tied in place to avoid jugular compression. Confused or agitated patients may also require controlled sedation, intubation and ventilation before CT scanning.

The detection of a skull fracture in combination with an impaired level of consciousness greatly increases the risk of intracranial haematoma formation. A fracture demonstrated on a skull X-ray is now a definite indication for a CT scan.

Hypoxia and hypercapnia are both potent vasodilators, resulting in increased CBF and increased ICP. Therefore mechanical ventilation should ideally keep the following levels:

SaO$_2$ 92–100%
PaO$_2$ 10–14 kPa
PaCO$_2$ 4–4.5 kPa

After issues involving oxygenation, ventilation and hypotension are addressed, focus is shifted towards other strategies that minimize intracranial oedema, limit intracranial hypertension, maintain adequate CPP and prevent secondary damage (Table 11.6). Most of the management will occur simultaneously, but it is important to assess each child's response to each intervention (Palmer 2000).

Table 11.6 Interventions to reduce intracranial pressure (ICP) and increase cerebral perfusion pressure (CPP)

Intervention	Details
Head midline	Prevents kinking of the jugular veins (Johnson 1999) Cervical collars and endotracheal tube ties not too tight as may impair cerebral venous drainage (Arbour 1998)
Nurse head elevated	15–30° of head elevation is optimal >30° elevation reduces CPP (Dixon & Vyas 1999)
Inotropes	May be indicated to maintain the MAP and CPP
Induced hypothermia	Fever (>38°C) can arise due to hypothalamic dysfunction or infection and decreases seizure threshold (Chambers 1999) Using cooling devices (32–34°C) decreases inflammatory responses, excitoticity, metabolic demands and oxidative stress (Marion et al 1993, Chambers 1999, Johnson 1999) Increases risk of bleeding and infection, arrhythmias and exacerbation of chest infection (Schubert 1995)
Sedation	Barbiturates (heavy sedation) cause a 'barbiturate coma' Decrease cerebral metabolic rate and ICP (Arbour 1998)
Anticonvulsants	Seizures impose major metabolic burden on the brain and increase ICP Used if seizure activity is identified clinically or on EEG (Dixon & Vyas 1999)
Hyperosmolar therapy	Reduces elevated ICP by creating an osmotic gradient that draws cerebral oedema fluid from brain tissue into the circulation Mannitol widely used Hypertonic saline solutions may also be used (Knapp 2005)
Hyperventilation	Decreases P_{CO_2} to between 4 and 4.5 kPa, producing a reflex cerebral vasoconstriction, therefore decreasing CBF and ICP (Arbour 1998) Effects noted less than 30 seconds from onset, and the peak effect is noted at approximately 8 minutes (Oh 1997)
Positive end-expiratory pressure (PEEP)	Used to maintain airway patency, but PEEP above 10 cmH$_2$0 mmHg may cause pressure decreased intracranial compliance (Dixon & Vyas 1999)
Paralysing agents	Can be given continuously or in intermittent boluses as required Disadvantages of use include masking of seizure activity (Dixon & Vyas 1999), prevention of coughing and decrease in effective secretion clearance (Felice 2005) and development of muscle weakness which may prolong ventilation (Dixon & Vyas 1999)
Analgesia	Reduction of painful stimuli (e.g. tracheal suction, intravenous cannulation)
Craniotomy	Removal of a section of the skull (bone flap) to access the traumatized brain underneath and then it is replaced (Lindsay et al 1986)
Burrhole	A small opening is made and minimally invasive procedures used, e.g. to drain a blood clot (Lindsay et al 1986)

MAP, mean arterial pressure; EEG, electroencephalogram; CBF, cerebral blood flow; PEEP, positive end-expiratory pressure.

DIFFERENT STAGES OF RECOVERY

As children progress out of their coma and wean from sedation/paralysing medication, most follow a general pattern of recovery after severe ABI The brain may be injured within a specific location or diffused to many parts of the brain. The indefinite nature of brain injury is unique for each child and follows the stages of recovery in a different way; the amount of time spent in each stage varies and recovery may stop at any stage.

The Wessex Head Injury Matrix (WHIM) is a useful behavioural scale to assess and monitor recovery in children after severe ABI. It can be used from the earliest stages of coma recovery onwards and can demonstrate subtle signs of recovery that enable realistic goal-setting (Shiel et al 2000).

A general understanding of the brain and its functions paves the way for the knowledge required to facilitate the physiotherapist to adapt assessment, treatment and goal-planning around these different phases (Appendix 11.1).

Recovery from ABI can be grouped into the following main stages:

1. Unresponsive/coma stage
2. Early responses stage
3. Agitated/confused stage
4. Higher-level responses stage.

Unresponsive/coma stage

Coma is a state of unawareness of self or environment, and the inability to sense or respond to bodily or environmental needs, caused by injury to the arousal centre in the brainstem. Coma is caused by brainstem damage and severe injury to both sides of the cortex. The brainstem is highly interconnected with other parts of the brain; therefore, when it is injured other parts of the brain are affected as well. The child's eyes remain closed, he or she is unable to communicate, fails to move in a purposeful manner or respond in a consistent or appropriate manner and a normal sleeping pattern is not re-established (Bateman 2001).

The auditory sense is often present in a state of coma, therefore discussion about the child's condition and thoughtless or derogatory remarks should be discouraged (Wong 1995).

Random movements of the arms and legs may occur for no specific reason. Families can become very fixated on any and very varied movements that the child starts to exhibit. The following stereotyped postures may also occur:

- Decerebrate posture – bilateral upper- and lower-limb extensor posture, usually the consequence of bilateral midbrain or pontine lesions. Opisthotonos, a severe muscle spasm of the neck and back, may accompany decerebrate posture in severe cases
- Decorticate posture – bilateral flexion of the upper limbs and extension of the lower limbs, usually the consequence of an upper-brainstem lesion. Although a serious sign, it is usually more favourable than decerebrate posture and may progress to a decerebrate posture, or the two may alternate
- Unilateral decerebrate or decorticate postures can be seen and are an indication of a unilateral lesion. This asymmetry has some localizing value (Bateman 2001).

Observation of spontaneous activity, resting posture and response to painful stimuli provides clues to the location and extent of the neurological damage, for example:

- Damage above the brainstem results in flaccidity of muscle tone, is asymmetrical and may be valuable in the localization of structural damage (Bateman 2001). Flaccidity can occur before spasticity appears but may persist indefinitely
- Limb weakness with decreased level of consciousness can be determined by comparing the response in each limb to painful stimuli
- Hemiparesis usually occurs in the limbs contralateral to the side of the injury but may also occur in the ipsilateral limbs. This is due to indentation of the contralateral cerebral peduncle by the edge of the tentorium cerebelli
- If eyes and head are deviated to the side opposite hemiparesis, this implies a hemisphere lesion, whereas deviation to the side of hemiparesis is indicative of a pontine lesion
- Using the GCS, if pain produces an asymmetrical motor response, the limb weakness is present on the side with the lower score, e.g. right-side weakness if right side extends, left side flexes or right side flexes, left side localizes (Lindsay et al 1986).

A child may start to appear to be 'more wakeful', with cycles of eye-opening and closing, but reveals no sign of awareness or wakefulness. This stage is sometimes referred to as the 'vegetative state', when the child is breathing spontaneously and has a stable circulation. The shorter the period of coma/vegetative state, the better the prognosis for recovery (Jennett 2002).

The use of coma arousal therapy, also known as sensory stimulation, is the subject of much debate. It is intended to promote awakening and enhance rehabilitative potential by using an intensive programme of visual, auditory, olfactory, gustatory, cutaneous and kinaesthetic sensory input. Sensory stimulation can start as soon as the child's medical condition is stable but there are conflicting views on its efficacy. There is limited reliable evidence to support its use (Lombardi et al 2002) and constant stimulation may even be detrimental (Wood 1991).

Early responses stage

Children will now be keeping their eyes open for longer and need less vigorous stimulation to wake them up, e.g. initially arouse only to painful stimuli, then touch, then sound. Children start to respond to the environment and responses will be more appropriate but may be inconsistent or slow. Localized responses, e.g. turn towards a sound, pull away from something uncomfortable, follow with eyes.

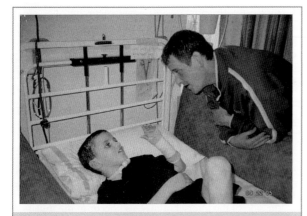

Figure 11.5 Encouraging eye contact in a child with severe acquired brain injury.

At this stage communication should be encouraged but children often experience fatigue and a short attention span. Tips for improving communication include:

- Speaking slowly and clearly
- Encouraging eye contact if possible (Figure 11.5)
- Clarifying names of body parts to help movement requests
- Using age appropriate language
- Blinking – once for yes, twice for no. Blinking is an involuntary action so must be done very definitely
- Simple commands, e.g. open and shut eyes
- Thumbs up and grip and release of hand
- Awareness of slow processing and be patient for a response
- Hand gestures or physical guidance with hands or with verbal cues.

At this stage the goal is to increase the consistency of responses. Recording achievements of recovery, however small, in a diary is a way for all carers to follow the child's progress. Rest periods are essential throughout the day with decreased stimulation of the surroundings if possible. However, within a busy ward setting this can prove difficult.

Methylphenidate appears to be an effective treatment to improve arousal in the minimally responsive child (Hornyak et al 1997).

Agitated/confused stage

Children will be responding more consistently at this stage. However, they will probably be confused and disoriented in time and place, with memory and behaviour difficulty. Many children display disinhibited behaviour and may yell, bite and swear and will often pull their nasogastric tubes and intravenous lines out. All carers need to be aware that at this stage the child's behaviour is (on the whole!) not intentional. A consistent approach to inappropriate behaviour is vital from all carers and family, e.g. not laughing at the patient's behaviour or language.

As the child becomes more aroused, it is important for all carers and visitors to speak to the child in an age-appropriate manner. Inappropriate language and actions can lead to inappropriate responses from the patient and may lead to future behavioural problems.

The goal at this stage is to help the child become more oriented and continue to treat the physical needs. The child may be moving about randomly in bed and trying to climb out of bed; padded cot sides can be helpful to prevent injury and/or tissue damage. Elbow and knee pads can also be useful. Children are very vulnerable at this stage, as once out of bed, they can be disoriented, lack safety awareness and have decreased balance reactions. At this stage they require constant supervision. A child may become very frustrated if not allowed to move about and mats on the floor can be useful where the patient can roll about or crawl. Sometimes the presence of a family member can be enough to calm the patient.

At this stage a child benefits greatly from low noise levels and short periods of activity with hopefully increased attention span times. Orientate the child to their surroundings using visual and verbal information. Clocks, calendars and diaries can be useful to write a child's daily schedule of timetable, mealtimes, therapy input, visitors and special appointments.

Sitting a child who is constantly moving may prove challenging and cause agitation to the child if repeatedly attempted. It is potentially unsafe unless the child is constantly supervised.

Higher-level responses stage

Routine tasks become easier but help is needed with problem-solving and making judgements and decisions. Children will have become aware of any residual physical problems and conscious of their body image. The goal at this stage is to decrease the amount of supervision needed and increase their independence (see Ch. 12).

THE PHYSIOTHERAPIST'S ROLE FOR CHILDREN WITH ACQUIRED BRAIN INJURY

Following ABI, the management of each individual child will vary enormously, depending on the extent of the head injury and any other injuries sustained. The clinical experience and problem-solving ability of the physiotherapist in the context of a knowledge and understanding of current research literature remain the main way to determine realistic goals for each child's management. Owing to the wide age range, developmental and premorbid neurodevelopmental backgrounds, there is little evidence to guide on the best assessment approaches.

The physiotherapist's roles include:

- Prevention of secondary respiratory problems, primarily in intensive care but also after transfer to the rehabilitation ward
- Prevention of secondary soft-tissue shortening and joint contractures.

In order to assess accurately, plan appropriately and carry out physiotherapy intervention effectively, it is vital for the physiotherapist to understand the effects of ABI on intracranial dynamics and how to interpret the interrelationships of vital signs, including ICP, MAP and CPP.

Physiotherapy needs to be combined with nursing interventions to ensure minimal disturbance. Sedation management, feeding regimes and effective pain relief all need to be discussed so that respiratory assessment/treatment times can be incorporated (Edwards 2002).

Irrespective of their conscious state, patients should be involved in any activity. Talking to a child and explanation of what cares are being carried out can help minimize any rise in ICP (Snyder 1983).

During the acute management of ABI, physiotherapy intervention is known to raise ICP, therefore:

- Short, more frequent and efficient treatments are essential
- Allow time for acute increased ICP to recover to acceptable values (15–20 mmHg) both between general procedures, e.g. position change, and in individual treatments (Johnson 1999)
- Monitor the child's reactions to different procedures and modify or avoid them accordingly.

An ICP of more than 20 mmHg for longer than 3 minutes requires immediate medical intervention. Elevations that return to baseline within 30 seconds are usually well tolerated (Prasad & Tasker 1990).

Prevention of secondary respiratory problems

Children with ABI who present with a GCS <8 are likely to have impaired respiratory function at the time of the injury or later on. There may be direct damage to the chest wall or fractured ribs, or lung damage in the form of contusions. The child may have vomited and aspirated at the time of the injury. Any damage to any part of the respiratory system may potentially lead to hypoxia and hypercapnia which ultimately leads to cerebral oxygenation problems.

Once ventilated a number of factors predispose to secondary respiratory complications:

- Introduction of the endotracheal tube promotes colonization of lower-respiratory tract with upper-respiratory organisms and increased mucus production (Coplin et al 2000)

- Paralysing the child inhibits the cough reflex and reduces the effective mucociliary function
- Sputum can often become thick and sticky if fluid restriction is required for ABI management; small airways may plug off easily
- Pooling of secretions also occurs in dependent lung areas (in supine posterior upper and lower lobes).

If a chest infection develops, management of the child becomes much more challenging. Infection causes fever and increases already overstretched metabolic demands. It is harder to achieve good ventilation, especially if positioning of the patient is limited due to ICP problems or multitrauma. Extubation and intensive care stay are prolonged. Weaning may proceed provided that the child is able to maintain and protect the airway and clear secretions (Coplin et al 2000), but can be more difficult because the ICP may increase as the child's cough returns.

Children needing prolonged ventilation for the management of intracranial hypertension or for respiratory complications (e.g. excess secretions) require a tracheostomy (Koh et al 1997, Gurkin et al 2002).

It is vital that the physiotherapist has a sound knowledge and understanding of intracranial dynamics to be able to assess accurately and treat effectively (Table 11.7).

Prevention of secondary soft-tissue shortening and joint contractures

In the acute stages following ABI, the child will be changing rapidly. Objective assessments must be done and outcome measures selected in order to monitor change. Physiotherapists have a leading role in this task, having the knowledge that there are likely to be changes in muscle tone following head injury.

Objective assessments may include:

- Muscle tone (Modified Ashworth Scale)
- Orthopaedic assessment (joint range and muscle length)
- Changes in functional status (Pediatric Evaluation of Disability Inventory: PEDI) (Dumas et al 2002).

Any measure of muscle tone may be affected by the child's medical status (e.g. pyrexia, coughing, pain), which may make repeatability of some measures unreliable. Spasticity, defined as 'excessive and inappropriate involuntary muscular activity in association with upper neurone damage' is probably the most common physical disorder following acute ABI and soft-tissue contractures commonly follow in its presence (Watkins 1999).

ABI can produce a number of key deformities, especially when prolonged abnormal posturing is encountered (Table 11.8). Equinovarus is the most common deformity associated with ABI because it appears in both decerebrate and decorticate posturing (Conine et al 1990). Sometimes, even with the optimal medication management and physiotherapy interventions, there may be some unavoidable loss of joint ranges. These may occur during the early

Table 11.7 Physiotherapy interventions and effect on intracranial pressure (ICP)

Physiotherapy intervention	Details
Positioning	Although patients with raised ICP are nursed with head elevation of 30°, postural drainage can be performed if needed when strict guidelines are followed (Imle et al 1997)
Changing position	Changes in head and body positioning can increase ICP (Chudley 1994) Log-rolling maintains head in relation to the body Side–lying may increase ICP with only small changes in CPP (Rising 1993) Hip flexion of >90° limits venous drainage and increases ICP (Arbour 1998)
Manual techniques	Percussion performed slowly does not increase ICP and may even lower it Shakes may increase ICP over time, whereas vibrations done in isolation have no effect on ICP (Imle et al 1997)
Manual hyperinflation	Known to increase ICP (Imle et al 1997) Should be interspersed with short-duration hyperventilation to decrease P_{CO_2} and ICP, prior to or following suction (Kerr et al 1997)
Suctioning	Causes a progressive rise in ICP with each insertion of the catheter. Elevations in ICP are transient and return to baseline levels within minutes (Kerr et al 1998) Stimulation of the cough due to the direct tracheal stimulation causes a rise in ITP, decreased cerebral venous return, increased CBV and ICP (Kerr et al 1998) Hypoxia can be minimized by use of closed–suction circuits and hyperoxygenation (Johnson 1999)

CPP, cerebral perfusion pressure; CBV, cerebral blood volume; ITP, intrathoracic pressure.

Table 11.8 Key deformities in acquired brain injury

Joint	Most common deformity
Shoulder	Adducted/internally rotated
Elbow	Flexed (decorticate) Extended (decerebrate)
Forearm	Pronated
Wrist	Flexed/ulnar-deviated
Fingers	Flexed
Thumb	Adducted/flexed into palm
Hip	Adducted/medially rotated Extended if mass extensor tone very high, or held flexed
Knee	Extended if decorticate/decerebrate posturing present Sometimes flexed
Ankles/subtalar	Plantarflexed/inverted (equinovarus)
Great toe	Flexed/extended

stages of recovery but can often be regained further down the rehabilitation pathway.

Physiotherapy treatment options include:

- Passive stretches/movement
- Positioning and postural management
- Serial casting.

Passive stretches/movement

Passive movements for unconscious/paralysed children and those presenting with hypertonus are required to maintain muscle and joint range of movement (ROM).

Changes in hamstring and quadriceps length will hamper forward pelvic tilt and impact on a child's ability to sit. Trunk and neck muscles can also become shortened if passive elongation is not performed.

Maintenance of nervous system mobility is also essential. Children who are unable to move or those dominated by hypertonic stereotyped postures are as likely to develop shortened neural structures as they are of loss of ROM of the musculoskeletal system (Shacklock 1995). Nerve pain may occur later into the rehabilitation process, and can be treated effectively with gabapentin. Often musculoskeletal pain relief fails to have any effect on this type of pain.

Passive movements are ideally done one to two times per day, especially in the intensive care setting. However, due to time constraints, other strategies must be developed for the rest of the day, especially for the child dominated by stereotyped patterns which maintain muscles in a shortened position, to produce more lasting effect in the control of body posture and movement.

Positioning and postural management

Postural management should extend to all aspects of care and be consistent throughout the 24-hour day (see Chapters 7 and 10).

The needs of the child will need reassessing and prioritizing on a daily basis. The physiotherapist should use skills and experience to anticipate the changes and carry out effective interventions to minimize the risk of secondary complications.

Choice of position, for both support and movement performance, must be considered in respect of tonal changes, influence of gravity, potential structural deformity and preservation of tissue viability.

A child will require varying degrees of external support to stabilize body posture and position relative to the supporting surface in lying, sitting and standing.

Serial casting

Once paralysis and sedation are reversed, ROM should be closely monitored and active intervention commenced as soon as ROM is at risk. Elbows and ankles are the most problematic areas due to stereotyped posturing in the early stages following ABI.

- Casts can be used prophylactically to maintain ROM, prevent development of muscle and tendon shortening, to correct alignment of joints and regain lost muscle length
- Removable splints such as ankle resting splints or wraparound arm gaiters can be beneficial. Carers needs to be shown the correct application and routine use of splints and the risk of pressure sores explained in children with poor sensation. Splints should not interfere with other team members' input, e.g. intravenous access.

Guidelines for use of serial casting:

- Children with increased muscle tone can be at risk of pressure areas. Medical management of tone should therefore be discussed before considering casting extremes of tone
- Casts may need padding on the outside when children are agitated or prone to hitting or kicking. Agitation may be too severe to be able to apply any form of cast or orthosis
- Arm casts need to be light-weight to prevent pulling on the shoulder
- Ideally casts should be left on for 5–7 days (Conine et al 1990) and be reapplied once reassessment of joint ranges and stretches to muscles have been done

- Use of casts over the weekend ensures maintenance of joint positions in the absence of the physiotherapist
- Advice on cast removal is essential if the cast causes increased agitation, or the child deteriorates, e.g. intravenous access is required.

Serial casting may enhance the treatment of children with ABI by reducing the abnormal sensory input. Children can weight-bear while casts are in place and thereby achieve a better postural alignment. Casting has been shown to be as effective as botulinum toxin A in the short-term treatment of spasticity (Corry et al 1998).

USEFUL ADJUNCTS TO PHYSIOTHERAPY

Useful adjuncts include medication and orthotic management.

Medication

The physiotherapist can work in conjunction with the paediatric neurologist to assess the efficacy of medication to reduce spasticity. The different medication options include:

- Muscle relaxants, which include baclofen delivered orally or intrathecally when oral medication has not been effective (Armstrong et al 1997) (see Ch. 12)
- Botulinum toxin A can be used to control increased tone by causing temporary paralysis and weakness (Graham et al 2000, Munchau & Bhatia 2000). It provides the physiotherapist with a window of opportunity to make changes in the pattern of movement and can be used in conjunction with serial casting/orthotics (Bottos et al 2003, Mackey et al 2003).

Orthotics

In order to facilitate prolonged stretching of muscles, the physiotherapist can work in conjunction with the orthotist using splints (e.g. ankle–foot orthosis) to maintain optimum positions, especially of distal joints (see Ch. 10).

THE MULTIDISCIPLINARY TEAM APPROACH FOR THE CHILD WITH ACQUIRED BRAIN INJURY

As in all paediatric settings, the service to a child is best delivered by a multidisciplinary team (MDT). Each child with ABI displays a unique and often rapidly changing recovery pathway; monitoring progress by the MDT is often described as 'chasing a moving target' (see Ch. 2).

Assessment, treatment and goal-planning

Assessment, treatment and goal-planning need to be adapted through all phases of recovery in conjunction with the child and family. It is essential to gather information to develop a care plan consistent with the problems and needs of the child.

It is impossible to gather all information in a single assessment. Use of standardized and objective assessments can prove difficult in the acute paediatric setting as the child can change on a daily basis. As a consequence, assessment can remain somewhat unstructured in format and subjective in content, relying on the skill and experience of the therapist to reassess continually, analysing changes in quality of movement, posture and function. Key issues should be clearly documented.

Support and involvement of the family

The unconscious phase and early recovery stages can be a time of great stress and uncertainty for parents, siblings, other family members and friends. There will be many different emotions that the family will naturally go through throughout the child's recovery, including panic, fear, shock, denial, anger, guilt, isolation and hope. The parents are faced with the uncertain outcome of the ABI. Intervention with parents depends upon the personality of the parents, and the parent–child relationship before the injury (Mercer 1994).

Involvement and training of family members early in the recovery process are critical for successful long-term outcome. Family members are best equipped to ensure treatment compliance and follow-through with treatment recommendations, in maintaining treatment gains, and in generalizing treatment effects beyond the medical setting (Beaulieu 2002).

Useful tips to guide the family:

- General information leaflets are useful, including the roles of different team members
- Help the family to put together a file of information about their child's injury and progress reports and to keep a diary. This will help the child make more sense of events as he/she recovers
- Encourage the family to become actively involved, so reducing any feeling of helplessness
- Families can attend the weekly team meeting and should be encouraged to express and discuss any concerns and anxieties
- Providing photographs or favourite toys or belongings and daytime clothes can make the bed space homely
- Encourage the family's role in controlling the environment and the number of visitors to avoid overstimulation (Appleton 1994)
- Family members also need 'time out' to spend time with the rest of the family rather than keeping a vigil at the bedside.

The family play a vital part in providing an accurate picture of a child's ability before an ABI (Williams 1992) to determine if there were predisposing problems or concerns which need to be considered in the management of a child, e.g. visual impairment. Unfortunately, brain injury is known to exaggerate pre-accident personality traits and disability (Vannier et al 2000).

Identification of the child's problems gives the rehabilitation team areas to focus treatment plans. Each problem area affects other areas and in many cases resolving one problem has a major impact on other problems.

Transfer from intensive care to the ward

Once weaned off life support and no longer needing intensive care, a child is transferred to the paediatric ward for ongoing neurorehabilitation. A range of clinical assessments is done by the MDT to provide an overall picture of the child's functional ability. Relevant information is communicated to health, social and education colleagues in the child's home area.

A rehabilitation programme is developed and tailored flexible to the child's individual needs, including a range of identified functional goals. It also starts to address discharge planning by looking forward to the child's anticipated needs at home and school.

The child will be seen by the hospital teacher daily for short periods. Therapists can advise on adaptation of some activities, e.g. positioning, which will help reinforce rehabilitation.

A daily programme of activities is useful to give children structure to their daily routine, which needs to incorporate periods of activity and rest. Following ABI many healing processes take place, especially if they have suffered other trauma. Fatigue sets in quickly and attention spans are short-lived.

Use of a central communication file (from day 1) is essential to:

- Keep the MDT and family all working towards the same goals
- Maintain consistency of care throughout the 24-hour period
- Encourage a vital team approach to all aspects of care to which everyone involved with a child can refer.

PREPARATION FOR DISCHARGE FROM HOSPITAL

Once the rapidly changing stage of recovery has started to stabilize and short-term goals have been achieved, plans for discharge home or to a local hospital should commence. Preparation for discharge is essential early on in the recovery phase, although it is impossible to predict the level of support a child and family will require once out of hospital. It is far better to oversubscribe services, e.g. equipment loans, and reduce the needs as required than to have prepared insufficient support, which will ultimately delay discharge plans. General ABI awareness training/training specific to the needs of the child may be required for all carers subsequently involved.

There are a variety of options for placements following discharge, including specialist rehabilitation units, a child's local hospital or a specialist hospital. There are advantages and disadvantages to these options, such as distance from home and the type of rehabilitation packages available in the different settings.

Arrangements can be made to enable the child to go home for short stays, which can then graduate to longer periods, allowing for slow reintegration at home, aiding the whole family in preparing for the child's long-term difficulties.

During the inpatient phase the team needs to liaise closely with a child's local community, social and health services to ensure a smooth transition of care into a suitably prepared environment.

OUTCOME FOLLOWING ACQUIRED BRAIN INJURY

Generally, within 6 months to 1 year after the injury, 90% of the long-term neurological outcome has been achieved. Some consequences are likely to remain as long-term impairments. Many children have problems that appear months – sometimes years – later as educational, behavioural or emotional disturbances (Reynolds 1992).

Although neuronal plasticity provides the potential for neuronal reorganization in a child's brain, it is the behavioural demands of the environment that allow the child to take advantage of this potential and to maximize recovery (Beaulieu 2002).

The ultimate long-term impact of ABI sustained in childhood depends on the child's ability to achieve developmental milestones following injury. Although injury-related and treatment-related factors are critical during the early stages of recovery, child-related factors such as

age and developmental achievement at time of injury, maturation and family involvement and resources impact the later stages of recovery.

Severe ABI has been found to be a source of considerable care-giver morbidity when compared with other traumatic injuries (Wade et al 1998) and psychosocial family functioning deteriorates in a substantial number of families (Tomlin et al 2002).

Therefore raising awareness of the consequences of ABI and providing a dedicated and integrated approach to assessment and provision of care across the domains of hospital, education and community are vital to facilitate family adaptation and for successful reintegration of these children back into the community.

KEY POINTS

- Children are not 'mini-adults'
- ABI displays an extremely varied spectrum of possible lesions and resulting potential disabilities. It is the indefinite nature of the brain injury that makes treatment unique for each individual child
- Fundamental knowledge of age-related differences in cerebrovascular physiology and anatomy, the child's premorbid ability and psychosocial situation is required
- An understanding of intracranial dynamics, medical and surgical interventions is essential to make accurate assessment and carry out appropriate effective treatment
- Physiotherapy intervention is vital from day 1 to optimize respiratory, musculoskeletal and ultimately neurological outcomes
- Family members are an integral part of the MDT
- Early communication pathways concerning referrals to community care are paramount
- An awareness of the consequences of ABI needs to inform the integrated approach to assessment and provision of care across health, education and community

CASE STUDY 11.1

Jamie, an 8-year-old boy, sustained a severe acquired brain injury (ABI) when he was hit by a car travelling at 30 mph whilst he was riding a pedal bike with no helmet. His Glasgow Coma Scale (GCS) at the scene was 7/15.

The injuries he sustained were:
- Fracture to right frontal bone of skull. Computed tomography scan showed a right frontal intracranial haemorrhage
- Fracture to mid-shaft right tibia

- Fracture to left elbow
- Laceration to right elbow
His management included:
- Intubated and ventilated (due to GCS < 8)
- Right frontal craniotomy and evacuation of traumatic haematoma
- External fixator applied to right tibia (non-weight-bearing)
- Above-elbow plaster cast left arm (set at 90°)

continued

- Repair to right-elbow laceration
- There was no medical history of note.

Jamie lives in a two-storey house with Mum, Dad and three siblings. The house has a downstairs toilet. His hobbies include Playstation and football.

He remained on the paediatric intensive care unit (PICU) for nearly 2 weeks. Intracranial pressure (ICP) remained <25 mmHg postoperatively. A failed extubation at day 10 resulted in a tracheostomy.

Physiotherapy input commenced immediately after his neurological status was stabilized on PICU. The main aims were to prevent secondary respiratory complications, maintain joint ranges and prevent joint contractures through passive stretches, positioning and splints.

On transfer to the rehabilitation ward the following problems were noted:

1. Decreased conscious state
2. Inability to communicate
3. Dysphagia
4. Impairment of respiratory function, tracheostomy, excess secretions
5. Decorticate posturing
6. Dense right hemiplegia (right-handed child)
7. No head or trunk balance
8. Non-weight-bearing right leg with external fixation in situ
9. Immobilized left arm in above-elbow plaster cast.

During the early stages of rehabilitation, Jamie was totally dependent upon others for all his functional needs. Following individual and joint assessments by members of the multidisciplinary team (MDT), the above problems were addressed:

1. Wessex Head Injury Matrix assessment was started to monitor change in conscious state. Position was regularly changed (lying and sitting) to encourage increased arousal and sensory awareness. A structured timetable to encourage a balance of activity and rest was commenced. The busy ward made it difficult to maintain a controlled environment to avoid overstimulation.
2. A personalized therapy file was issued to provide consistent communication input, which initially started as blinking, progressing on to yes/no and picture cards as eye-tracking/fixing and following returned.

3 and 4. The physiotherapist and speech and language therapist worked together to facilitate swallowing and maintain and restore respiratory function. Excess secretions required regular suctioning and repeated coughing impacted on overall muscle tone and posturing. Joint assessments for suitable seating and moving and handling procedures were also done with the occupational therapist, with subsequent carry-over into other treatment input. Tracheostomy removal was delayed due to the presence of granuloma formation in airways (causing stridor).

5. Repeated coughing caused increased muscle tone/decorticate posturing with subsequent tightness in elbow flexors and resultant equinovarus bilaterally. Passive stretches and provision of ankle splints maintained plantargrade but more intensive input was required for the upper limbs. The left arm was already immobilized in a plaster cast with the elbow at 90°; the right arm required serial casting to maintain optimal extension. Supine lying was avoided where possible.

6. As decorticate posturing became less dominant, a dense right hemiplegia became more apparent. His left side began to display random purposeless movements in all directions which maintained a reasonable overall left upper-limb joint range, but his right-sided muscle tone began to increase arm (flexor) greater than leg (extensor) with no active movement. Right shoulder girdle mobilizations, botulinum toxin injections and stretches were used to reduce tone and a hand splint was provided to maintain functional hand position. An ankle-foot orthosis was used on the left leg to prevent clonus and help with weight-bearing.

7. Side-lying and high sitting were encouraged with appropriate support for head and trunk in midline. A tilt-in-space chair with full head, trunk and pelvic support was chosen so that support and chair angles could be gradually reduced as head and trunk control improved.

Trunk mobilizations were performed in sitting over the edge of the bed to maintain trunk and pelvic mobility, and encourage midline orientation, head and trunk activity.

Movements from lying to sitting and vice versa were actively assisted via both sides and transfers into a chair were done via the left side with maximal assistance to support head, trunk and non-weight-bearing right leg. This support was gradually reduced as activity returned. The hoist was used by carers to transfer from bed to chair, due to the specialized handling techniques required at this stage.

A supportive wheelchair was provided to allow some mobility away from the ward.

8. The right lower leg required elevation to prevent swelling which created asymmetry in the sitting position. In discussion with the orthopaedic team it was agreed that for short periods it would not be detrimental to allow the lower leg to rest down.

9. The immobilized left elbow maintained range of movement of the elbow at 90° but on removal of

continued

the cast the elbow had a moderate degree of fixed flexion due to underlying tone and prolonged immobilization limiting active elbow extension.

Treatment progression

Over the next few weeks, intensive rehabilitation continued, consisting of:

- Establishment of more advanced communication (tracheostomy in situ/speaking tube. Tracheostomy in situ for 2 months overall)
- Re-established gag and swallow, allowing sitting for meals
- Appropriate family involvement
- A balanced timetable with activity and rest periods encouraged
- Joint treatment sessions with physiotherapist, occupational therapist, speech and language therapist and teacher
- Increased time spent out of bed to promote activities of daily living
- Active movements encouraged to optimize functional movement
- Moving and handling reviewed as return of activity evolved
- Facilitation of active sitting, transfer and standing work, gradually increasing weight-bearing on the right leg
- Mirror used to provide visual feedback on posture and movements and to maintain attention
- Weekly MDT meeting including family.

As active movement returned, Jamie became very agitated, especially by the tracheostomy/coughing. When awake he constantly moved randomly about the bed, requiring padded cot sides to prevent injury (especially to external fixator). He required supervision when sat out as he chose to sit in an asymmetrical manner (premorbid favourite sitting posture) and became agitated if attempts were made to reposition him. He resisted passive stretches to encourage elbow extension and splints and casts were not tolerated due to his agitation.

Once the external fixator was removed from his right leg and full weight-bearing was re-established, activities were encouraged to promote weight transference to his right side.

Jamie displayed a good physical recovery and was eventually independently mobile, but still had the following residual problems:

- Impulsiveness
- Poor safety awareness of his surroundings, especially on the stairs
- Reduced proprioception in his right leg, resulting in poor awareness of lower-limb/foot placement
- He continued to favour using his left side for many activities
- Communication – problems with word-finding and occasional slurring of speech
- Reduced attention span and easily distracted
- Poor motor planning skills, especially with hand-writing (letter formation).

Outcome

Jamie has made a good physical recovery over a 4-month period, but still requires some ongoing assessment and therapy input.

No major home adaptations were required and phased discharge was beneficial, including visits to school and weekend leave, allowing his family and community carers to prepare for his physical, psychosocial and educational needs appropriately as follows:

- Continued supervision from carer, especially on stairs
- A working environment to reduce distractions and maintain attention
- Encouragement to use right side in a variety of activities
- Gait re-education
- Balance and coordination activities
- General muscle strengthening and return of physical fitness
- Ongoing assessments of perceptual needs and sensory processing
- Motor planning skills, especially hand-writing.

REFERENCES

Anderson V, Moore C 1995 Age at injury as a predictor of outcome following paediatric head injury. A longitudinal perspective. *Child Neuropsychology* 1: 187–202.

Andrus C 1991 Intracranial pressure: dynamics and nursing management. *Journal of Neuroscience Nursing* 23: 85–92.

Appleton R 1994 Head injury rehabilitation for children. *Nursing Times* 90: 29–32.

Arbour R 1998 Aggressive management of intracranial dynamics. *Critical Care Nurse* 18: 30–40.

Armstrong RW, Steinhok P, Cochrane DD et al 1997 Intrathecally administered baclofen for treatment of children with spasticity of cerebral origin. *Journal of Neurosurgery* 87: 409–414.

Bateman DE 2001 Neurological assessment of coma. *Journal of Neurology, Neurosurgery and Psychiatry* 71: 13–17.

Bayir H, Kochanek PM, Clark R 2003 Traumatic brain injury in infants and children: mechanisms of secondary damage and treatment in the intensive care unit. *Critical Care Clinics* 19: 529–549.

Beaulieu CL 2002 Rehabilitation and outcome following paediatric traumatic brain injury. *Surgical Clinics of North America* 82: 393–408.

Billmire M, Myers PA 1985 Serious head injury in infants: accident or abuse. *Paediatrics* 75: 340–342.

Bondanelli M, Ambrosio MR, Zatelli MC et al 2005 Hypopituitarism after traumatic brain injury. *European Journal of Endocrinology* 152: 679–691.

Bottos M, Benedetti MG, Salucci A et al 2003 Botulinum toxin with and without casting in ambulant children with spastic diplegia: a clinical and functional assessment. *Developmental Medicine and Child Neurology* 45: 758–762.

Chambers IR, Stobbart L, Jones PA et al 2005 Age related differences in intracranial pressure and cerebral perfusion pressure in the first six hours of monitoring after children's head injury: association with outcome. *Child's Nervous Systems* 21: 195–199.

Chambers S 1999 Induced hypothermia for head injury. *Nursing in Critical Care* 4: 112–116.

Chudley S 1994 The effect of nursing activities on intracranial pressure. *British Journal of Nursing* 3: 454–459.

Conine, TA, Sullivan T, Mackie T et al 1990 Effect of serial casting for the prevention of equines in patients with acute head injury. *Archives of Physical Medicine and Rehabilitation* 71: 310–312.

Coplin WM, Pierson DJ, Cooley KD et al 2000 Implications of extubation delay in brain injured patients meeting standard weaning criteria. *American Journal of Respiratory and Critical Care Medicine* 161: 1530–1536.

Corry IS, Cosgrove AP, Duffy CM et al 1998. Botulinum toxin A compared with stretching casts in the treatment of spastic equines: a randomised prospective trial. *Journal of Paediatric Orthopaedics* 18: 304–311.

Crouchman M, Rossiter L, Colaco T, Forsyth R 2001 A practical outcome scale for paediatric head injury. *Archives of Disease of Childhood* 84: 120–124.

Dixon H, Vyas H 1999 Management of intracranial hypertension and cerebral oedema. *Current Anaesthesia and Critical Care* 10: 236–240.

Duhaime AC, Eppley M, Margulies S et al 1995 Crush injuries to the head in children. *Neurosurgery* 37: 401–406.

Dumas HM, Haley SM, Ludlow LH et al 2002 Functional recovery in paediatric traumatic brain injury during inpatient rehabilitation. *American Journal of Physical Medicine and Rehabilitation* 81: 661–669.

Edwards S 2002 *Neurological Physiotherapy: A Problem Solving Approach*, 2nd edn. Edinburgh: Churchill Livingstone, p. 125.

Felice S 2005 Neurointensive care for traumatic brain injury in children. Available online at: www.eMedicine.com.

Gill MR, Reiley DG, Green SM 2004 Interrater reliability of Glasgow Coma Scale scores in the emergency department. *American Emergency Medicine* 43: 215–223.

Graham HK, Aoki R, Autti-Ramo I et al 2000 Recommendations for the use of botulinum toxin A in the management of cerebral palsy. *Gait and Posture* 11: 67–79.

Gurkin SA, Parikshak M, Kralovich KA et al 2002 Indicators for tracheostomy in patients with traumatic brain injury. *American Surgery* 68: 324–328.

Hackbarth RM, Rzeszutko KM, Sturm G et al 2002 Survival and functional outcome in paediatric traumatic brain injury: a retrospective review and analysis of predictive factors. *Critical Care Medicine* 130: 1630–1635.

Hornyak JE, Nelson VS, Hurvitz EA 1997 The use of methylphenidate in paediatric brain injury. *Paediatric Rehabilitation* 1: 15–17.

Imle PC, Mars MP, Eppinghaus CE et al 1997 The effect of chest physical therapy on intracranial pressure and cerebral perfusion pressure. *Physiotherapy Canada* 49: 48–55.

Jennett B 2002 The vegetative state. *Journal of Neurology, Neurosurgery and Psychiatry* 73: 355–357.

Johnson L 1999 Factors known to raise intracranial pressure and its associated implications for nursing management. *Nursing in Critical Care* 4: 117–120.

Kerr ME, Rudy EB, Weber BB et al 1997 Effect of short duration hyperventilation during endotracheal suctioning on intracranial pressure in severe head injured adults. *Nursing Research* 46: 195–201.

Kerr ME, Sereika SM, Orndorff P et al 1998 Effect of neuromuscular blockers and opiates on the cerebrovascular response to endotracheal suctioning in adults with severe head injuries. *American Journal of Critical Care* 7: 205–217.

Knapp JM 2005 Hyperosmolar therapy in the treatment of severe head injury in children: mannitol and hypertonic saline. *AACN Clinical Issues* 16: 199–211.

Koh WY, Lew TWK, Chin NM et al 1997 Tracheostomy in neuro-intensive care setting: indications and timing. *Anaesthesia and Intensive Care* 25: 365–368.

Lam WH, MacKersie A 1999 Paediatric head injury: incidence, aetiology and management. *Paediatric Anaesthesia* 9: 377–385.

Lindsay K, Bone I, Callander R 1986 *Neurology and Neurosurgery Illustrated*. Edinburgh: Churchill Livingstone, p. 31.

Lombardi F, Tarrico M, De Tanyti A et al 2002 Sensory stimulation of brain injured individuals in coma or vegetative state: results of a Cochrane systematic review. *Clinics in Rehabilitation* 16: 464–472.

Mackey A, Walt S, Stott SN 2003 Botulinum toxin type A in ambulant children with cerebral palsy. *Physiotherapy* 89: 219–232.

Marion DW, Obrist WD, Carlier PM et al 1993 The use of moderate therapeutic hypothermia for patients with severe head injury: a preliminary report. *Journal of Neurosurgery* 79: 354–362.

Mazzola CA, Adelson PD 2002 Critical care management of head trauma children. *Critical Care Medicine* 30: 393–401.

Mercer A 1994 Psychological approaches to children with life threatening conditions and their families. *ACCP Review and Newsletter* 16: 56.

Michaud LJ, Rivara FP, Jaffa KM et al 1993 Traumatic brain injury as a risk factor for behavioural disorders in children. *Archives of Physical Medicine and Rehabilitation* 74: 368–375.

Moulton SL 2000 Early management of the child with multiple injuries. *Clinical Orthopaedics and Related Research* 376: 6–14.

Munchau A, Bhatia KP 2000 Uses of botulinum toxin injection in medicine today. *British Medical Journal* 320: 161–165.

Oh TE 1997 *Intensive Care Manual*, 4th edn. Oxford: Butterworth Heinemann, p. 923.

Ommaya AK, Goldsmith W, Thibault L 2002 Biomechanics and neuropathology of adult and paediatric head injury. *British Journal of Neurosurgery* 16: 220–242.

Palmer J 2000 Managemant of raised intracranial pressure in children. *Intensive and Critical Care Nursing* 16: 319–327.

Parslow RC, Morris KP, Tasker RC et al 2005 Epidemiology of traumatic brain injury in children receiving intensive care in the UK. *Archives of Disease in Childhood* 90: 1182–1187.

Powell T 2005 *Head Injury: A Practical Guide*. UK: Speechmark, p. 8.

Prasad A, Tasker R 1990 Guidelines for the physiotherapy management of critically ill children with acutely raised intracranial pressure. *Physiotherapy* 76: 248–250.

Reilly PL, Simpson DA, Sprod R et al 1988 Assessing the conscious level in infants and young children: a paediatric version of the Glasgow Coma Scale. *Child's Nervous System* 4: 30–33.

Reynolds E 1992 Controversies in caring for the child with a head injury. *American Journal of Maternal Child Nursing* 17: 246–251.

Rising C 1993 The relationship of selected nursing activities to ICP. *Journal of Neuroscience Nursing* 25: 302–307.

Rowley G, Fielding K 1991. Reliability and accuracy of the Glasgow Coma Scale with experienced and inexperienced users. *Lancet* 337: 535–538.

Rutter M 1981 Psychological sequelae of brain damage in children. *American Journal of Psychiatry* 138: 1533–1544.

Schubert A 1995 Side effects of mild hypothermia. *Journal of Neurosurgical Anaesthesiology* 7: 139–147.

Segal S, Gallager AC, Shefler AG et al 2001 Survey of the use of ICP monitoring in children in the United Kingdom. *Intensive Care Medicine* 27: 236–239.

Shacklock M 1995 Neurodynamics. *Physiotherapy* 81: 9–16.

Sharples PM, Stuart AG, Matthews DS et al 1995a Cerebral blood flow and metabolism in children with severe head injuries. Part 1: relationship to age, GCS, outcome, ICP, and time after injury. *Journal of Neurology, Neurosurgery and Psychiatry* 58: 145–152.

Sharples PM, Matthews DS, Eyre JA 1995b Cerebral blood flow and metabolism in children with severe head injuries. Part 2: cerebrovascular resistence and its determinants. *Journal of Neurology, Neurosurgery and Psychiatry* 58: 153–159.

Shiel A, Horn SA, Wilson BA et al 2000 The Wessex Head Injury Matrix (WHIM) main scale: a preliminary report on a scale to assess and monitor patient recovery after severe head injury. *Clinics in Rehabilitation* 14: 408–416.

Snyder M, 1983 Relationship of nursing activities to increased ICP. *Journal of Advanced Nursing* 8: 273–279.

Teasdale G, Jennett B 1974 Glasgow Coma Score. *Lancet* ii: 81–83.

Tomlin P, Clarke M, Robinson G et al 2002 Rehabilitation in severe head injury in children: outcome and provision of care. *Developmental Medicine and Child Neurology* 44: 828–837.

Tranel D, Eslinger PJ 2000 Effects of early onset brain injury on development of cognition and behaviour. *Developmental Psychology* 18: 273–280.

Vannier A, Brugel DG, De Agostini M 2000 Rehabilitation of brain injured children. *Childs Nervous System* 16: 760–764.

Wade SL, Taylor HG, Drotar D et al 1998 Family burden and adaptation during the initial year after traumatic brain injury in children. *Paediatrics* 102: 110–116.

Watkins C 1999 Mechanical and neurophysiological change in spastic muscles. *Physiotherapy* 85: 603–609.

Waugh A, Grant A 2005 *Anatomy and Physiology in Health and Illness*, 9th edn. Edinburgh: Churchill Livingstone, Chapter 7.

Wedel-Sellars C, Hill-Vegter C 1997 *Pediatric Brain Injury*. Houston, TX: HDI.

Williams J 1992 Assessment of head injured children. *British Journal of Nursing* 1: 82–84.

Wong DL 1995 The child with cerebral dysfunction. In: Campbell S, Glasper EA (eds) *Children's Nursing*. Edinburgh: Mosby, pp. 660–681.

Wood RL 1991 Critical analysis of the concept of sensory stimulation for patients in vegetative states. *Brain Injury* 5: 401–409.

Zwienenburg M, Muizelaar JP 1999 Severe paediatric head injury: the role of hyperaemia revisited. *Journal of Neurotrauma* 16: 937–943.

WEBSITES

www.headway.org.uk

www.includemein.org

APPENDIX 11.1: CRANIAL NERVE DAMAGE

Basal skull fracture or extracranial injury can result in damage to the cranial nerves (CN). Evidence of damage (except for CN III lesion) does not usually help immediate management but must be recorded. Damaged CN may have an impact on functional recovery. It is important for the physiotherapist to be aware of some of them:

- Damage to CN II may cause visual acuity and field problems
- Damage to CN III, or IV and VI may cause problems with coordinated movements of the eyes. Loss of one parameter of eye movements may lead to double vision and cause visual disturbance to the patient with true and false images. This may be problematic when doing many functional tasks. The patient may have to tip the head in a certain way to minimize the diplopia, e.g. in CN IV palsy the patient complains of double vision when looking downwards when descending stairs or reading. Use of eye patches may be beneficial
- Damage to CN III may cause ptosis (droopy eyelid) which hinders full vision.

Damage to CN IX and X is considered jointly since their actions are seldom individually impaired. Impaired swallowing and gag reflexes need to be closely observed due to the risk of aspiration. Head positioning is therefore very important (Lindsay et al 1986).

12 Acquired brain injury rehabilitation

Patricia Wilcox

INTRODUCTION

Following discharge from hospital a rehabilitation placement can be appropriate for a child once he or she is medically stable. Therefore, a child can enter a rehabilitation unit whilst having high health and nursing needs: the child may have a tracheostomy, a gastrostomy or a nasogastric tube in situ. Alternatively the patient may be independently mobile with, for example, some mild balance problems, muscle weakness or altered muscle tone. However the majority of children entering a rehabilitation unit are likely to be in a wheelchair, to have some muscle tone and joint range problems and to have emerging movement in their limbs and emerging sitting balance.

Although a child who has suffered an acquired brain injury may present with similar problems to a child who has cerebral palsy, there are some important differences. Children with an acquired brain injury usually have a history of normal development and have experienced normal movement. They are therefore retrieving skills rather than learning them for the first time. They are in a changing situation so they have greater potential for improvement, especially in the first years following their injury.

Rehabilitation is a much more active process than a child may have experienced in the acute stage. Children need to be able to share the therapist's goals to enable them to work with commitment. As the children's ability and awareness improve, depending on their age, they may take the lead in goal-setting.

The family may have spent the time since their child's injury at the bedside, totally involved in their child's care. The transition to a rehabilitation setting may necessitate a change in the family's role, as parents return to work and spend more time with siblings. It is important, however, that the family maintains an active role in their child's care and rehabilitation. They can be involved in goal-setting, carrying out exercise programmes and the appropriate use of postural equipment (Demellweek & O'Leary 1998).

AIMS OF REHABILITATION

- To enable reintegration into the community by providing therapy and management for children and young people after their discharge from acute care
- To restore children's former quality of life or to establish an alternative life plan that is acceptable to them.

It is important that everyone – children, their families and the rehabilitation team – acknowledge that, although rehabilitation can assist in achieving the above aims, it is unable to make the trauma and its effects completely disappear (Mazaux & Richer 1998).

REHABILITATION

Rehabilitation needs to be delivered by a multidisciplinary team who are able to make the process a 24-hour-a-day experience. The team provides nursing and care, physiotherapy, speech and language therapy, occupational therapy, educational psychology and psychiatry as well as recreational activities. Educational input can be provided by a dedicated teacher or by teachers provided by the home tuition service. The team needs to meet regularly to share their knowledge and goals and to enable everyone to have a greater understanding of a child. This enables the rehabilitation process to have continuity and to be effectively delivered over the 24-hour period.

There are different settings in which rehabilitation can take place and what is right for one child and family will not necessarily be right for another. There are very few residential rehabilitation centres in the country that are dedicated to acquired brain injury rehabilitation, so children and their families may have to be prepared to have some distance between themselves and home. These centres, however, are able to offer a holistic, continuous service. When a rehabilitation centre is not available or appropriate, rehabilitation can also take place in the acute hospital setting and once children have been discharged back into the community. If rehabilitation is taking place in the community setting, it is difficult for the team to provide an intensive rehabilitation programme as a child will be based at home and attending a centre for allotted therapy sessions.

The rehabilitation process can be broken down into two stages: an active rehabilitation stage and a reintegration stage.

The active rehabilitation stage

This is the stage when rapid change may occur and physiotherapy input needs to be at a high level to enable children to make good use of their returning gross motor skills. Physiotherapists need to be continually reassessing children to ascertain what weekly or even daily goals are realistic and achievable. Goal-setting plays an important part in acquired brain injury rehabilitation and is often very child-led, with the physiotherapist taking a guiding, supervising role.

Common gross motor problems

The gross motor problems experienced by children after brain injury can be similar to those of children born with cerebral palsy. There should, however, be a difference in approach and treatment as they are in a situation that is changing, possibly rapidly. They have also, depending on their age at the time of their injury, experienced normal movement; although this can be emotionally negative in that they are aware of what they have lost, it is positive in that some motor patterns may have been retained.

Spasticity

Spasticity is a common occurrence in the acute stage of acquired brain injury and it is often still present when children are medically stable and therefore ready to move on to rehabilitation (see Ch. 11). In the more severely affected children, decorticate posturing is commonly seen, with the upper limbs adopting a flexed position and the lower limbs held in extension (Griffith & Mayer 1990). Spasticity can quickly result in the loss of joint ranges and will greatly impinge on a child's ability to make good functional use of any returning active movement. The joints most at risk from contractures are the ankles, elbows, wrists and fingers.

The resolution of spasticity needs to be one of the primary aims of physiotherapy and, although this is not always possible, the effects of spasticity can hopefully be lessened.

Systemic muscle relaxants (Gormley 1999) such as baclofen (Meythaler et al 2004) and dantrolene will have been started in the acute stage and the multidisciplinary team need to make sure that these are at the optimum dose. Botulinum toxin can be used to target specific muscles and physiotherapists should be involved in the discussion as to which muscles need targeting.

Serial casting (Watkins 1999) is often necessary to regain a joint's full range of movement; if this is going to be the case, the sooner it is undertaken, the better the result is likely to be. A variety of splints can also be used; fixed polypropylene splints made by an orthotist can be used when the situation is stable but are expensive to supply if the children's needs are constantly changing. It is possible, however, to supply polypropylene splints with a ratchet joint so they can adjust to any changes in joint range. These can work well, especially on single-plane joints. Backslabs made from fibreglass splinting materials are also useful as they can be made quickly and changed frequently.

Passive stretching, performed slowly, can assist in reducing muscle tone (Zafonte et al 2004) and allows therapists to monitor the situation regularly. Parents can be taught to carry out a stretching programme: although it can have the benefit of giving them an active role in their children's rehabilitation as well as benefiting children, care must be taken that the movements are being performed in such a way as to encourage relaxation.

Careful positioning to try to avoid musculoskeletal changes is also important and the appropriate equipment should be used in lying, sitting and standing to reduce abnormal postural reactions (Jackson 2004).

Surgery may be necessary to correct contractures but this is a last resort and should not be carried out until the children's high muscle tone has stabilized and non-invasive changes in joint range are no longer possible (Anderson 1995).

Cerebellar ataxia

Cerebellar ataxia is the disruption of coordination of movement due to damage to the cerebellum. If there is unilateral damage, the symptoms will appear on the same side as the lesion (Bastian 1997). It may not be apparent in the early stages after a head injury and it may only come to light when a child starts to move; indeed, it often appears to be getting worse as movement increases.

Cerebellar ataxia is characterized by overshooting or undershooting of voluntary movement, tremor, hypotonia, disturbances of balance and gait and dysarthria. Children suffering from cerebellar ataxia may have generalized low muscle tone but it is the central low tone that tends to have the greatest effect on their functional gross motor ability.

Treatment should focus on increasing children's core stability to enable them to perform functional movements without the need to use their arms to provide a stable base from which to work. Lycra body suits can be a useful tool but children must be motivated and willing to wear the suit on a regular basis (Attard & Rithalia 2004). Wrist weights can be used to damp down the arm tremor and to improve hand function but these appear to have only a temporary effect; there tends to be very little carry-over once the weights are removed. Weighted boots are more practical, in that they can be worn for long periods of time and they can be effective in improving and retraining gait (Griffith & Mayer 1990). Children with cerebellar ataxia are generally willing to push their physical boundaries and need to be allowed to test their physical abilities and make mistakes whilst being kept safe.

Paralysis/weakness

If the motor cortex is damaged, it is unable to carry out its role fully in regulating the recruitment and frequency of motor neurone firing (Duncan 1990). This can result in a wide range of problems, from the paralysis of whole muscle groups to specific areas of muscle weakness.

There are many different means of trying to facilitate muscle contraction and, although a child may not be consciously activating the nervous system, it is hoped that, in time, it may lead to a voluntary contraction. The most common means of facilitating a muscle contraction include brushing, tapping and fast passive stretch (Jackson 2004). Electrical stimulation of muscles may be appropriate if a child is able to tolerate it and is sufficiently aware to be able to focus on and attempt to join in the movement.

Physiotherapists need to be aware that if a child has spent time immobilized in bed some muscle weakness is likely to be present. In this case, if there are no neurological signs, a graded muscle-strengthening programme and a gradual return to normal daily activities may be all that is necessary.

Initiation, planning and sequencing of movement

A substantial number of children who have suffered an acquired brain injury have difficulty initiating, planning or sequencing movement. Difficulty with initiating movement can be demonstrated by children who are unable to turn their heads voluntarily, but can spontaneously shake their head to give a no response. Physiotherapists can give manual prompts to assist with initiation difficulties.

Problems with planning and sequencing movement can result in children who are able to move from sit to stand, for instance, if the movement is spontaneous but find it very difficult to perform the task if the movement is not instant or if something happens to interrupt the manoeuvre. For these children tasks need to be broken down into a sequence of movements and the same verbal or manual prompts need to be given each time the task is practised. As these children improve, the prompts can be gradually reduced and withdrawn.

Neglect

Some degree of unilateral neglect is common in a child whose brain injury has resulted in hemiplegia. It can take the form of visual neglect when children may ignore writing on one side of the page, walk into objects on the affected side or leave food on one side of the plate untouched. It can result in the affected arm being ignored, even though it may have adequate movement to be functionally useful. Children need to be reminded that the arm exists by being presented with bilateral tasks and by the arm being positioned in sight, for instance, on the table rather than under it.

Constraint-induced movement therapy, which involves restricting the functioning of the unaffected arm, to encourage use of the affected arm (Karman et al 2003), may be appropriate for older children, who are able to understand and are willing to persevere. This is only necessary for upper-limb function as weight-bearing and lower-limb function tend to happen more spontaneously,

Orthopaedic

An appreciable number of children undergoing acquired brain injury rehabilitation will have sustained their injury in a road traffic accident. They may, therefore, have also sustained spinal or long-bone fractures and this will affect the way their treatment can be delivered.

Scoliosis is another orthopaedic problem which can occur over a period of time due to asymmetrical muscle tone in the spine; this needs to be monitored and the spine may need to be braced while the muscle tone stabilizes.

Heterotopic ossification is a possible complication after brain injury. New bone grows in the soft tissues and can cause pain, inflammation and loss of joint range (Jaffe et al 1990). Passive movements need to be carried out with care to avoid the possibility of stimulating ossification. The extra bone can be removed surgically when the situation has stabilized and if it is causing problems.

Regaining functional abilities

On admission to a rehabilitation service, most children and their families will declare their aims to be walking and talking. Most parents are anxious, understandably, to see quick results and will sometimes try to take a child forward too quickly or expect physiotherapists to do so as well. It is, however, the role of physiotherapists to guide children through the developmental stages at an appropriate rate and to explain to the parents the necessity for this approach.

Physiotherapy intervention is guided by accurate assessments of a child's deficits. Assessment must be ongoing and part of every treatment session, especially when a child's physical state is changing rapidly.

Normal patterns of movement have been established in a child who has suffered an acquired brain injury, unless the trauma occurred at a very early age. It therefore seems logical that normal movement is used as a model for therapy with these children. However, physiotherapists need to use a range of treatment techniques from neurodevelopmental to task-specific training (see Ch. 5). The approach will vary depending on the child's needs at the different stages of rehabilitation (Lennon 2004).

Lying

Positioning in lying is important until a child is actively moving around in bed. A good supported symmetrical lying position will help to minimize the development of deformities, reduce muscle tone and promote bilateral hand function. The amount of support needed will vary depending on the child; it may be that a T-roll under the knees in supine-lying is sufficient or the child may need a full lying support (see Ch. 10).

As lying is a totally supported position it is ideal for working on a wide variety of gross motor skills. Areas that can be worked on in this position include the following:

Gross motor movements of all four limbs

In supine-lying, assisted and manually resisted exercises can be carried out, encouraging control of flexion and extension of the hips and knees. In prone-lying hip extension and knee flexion can be encouraged and in side-lying hip abduction can be isolated. It is important to give accurate verbal feedback to a child without being negative if it is difficult to access a particular muscle group.

Play in supine-lying and side-lying can encourage gross motor activity of the upper limbs.

Head control

In supine-lying head-turning and lifting can be encouraged. If the therapist supports a child's head in his or her hands, assistance can be given when necessary and friction can be reduced. It is also a good position in which to facilitate activity in the neck extensors. In prone-lying a child can be assisted into a forearm prop position or placed over a wedge to work on head control: it may be necessary to use noisy toys to gain a small child's attention.

Rolling to side-lying and to prone

A child can be assisted to roll by manually rotating the pelvis and encouraging the child to turn the head and shoulders. In the early stages, a child might only be able to do this in small movements timed to an intake of breath so it is necessary to be patient and be aware of any change in a child's position.

Pelvic control and stability

Crook-lying is a good position in which to work on pelvic control. Bridging will encourage hip extension and lateral control and can be progressed by introducing single-leg bridging or the use of a physio ball under the feet.

Sitting

As soon as a child is able to tolerate a sitting position, it is important that a good position is achieved. This will help to prevent deformities occurring, reduce increased muscle tone and provide a stable base for the acquisition of head control and sitting balance. It also provides an optimum learning position and can encourage hand function. Ideally a range of chairs would be available to allow for children's individual needs; however, adaptations may be necessary. It is important to remember that a good sitting position will enhance a child's abilities but a poor sitting position will be detrimental. It is therefore necessary to avoid sitting until an acceptable position can be achieved (see Ch. 10).

If a child's head control is insufficient to maintain an up-right sitting position, it may be necessary to use a wheelchair with a tilt-in-space facility, a supportive collar or a head rest with a brow band to allow functional activity. A head rest with brow band can help achieve a good sitting position for eating and drinking and switch use.

It is important to provide a child with some form of independent mobility as soon as possible, as long as it is safe. A self-propelling wheelchair can be provided if there is sufficient hand function. If a powered wheelchair is a possible solution, this idea needs to be introduced sensitively as this can be seen as a prediction of a child's future abilities.

Once a child can be placed in a reasonably symmetrical sitting position, manually supported sitting can be used to work on head control, sitting balance and posture. Encouraging propping on both hands will also stimulate activity of the muscles around the shoulder girdle. A mirror is useful for a child to check his or her own posture and to correct it. Initially a child is likely to need verbal and visual feedback to achieve this; these aids can gradually be withdrawn as a child learns to self-correct. With older children a biofeedback machine can be used with pressure plates placed under the buttocks and a visual display showing the comparative weight-bearing loads.

Children can be gently moved to bring their trunk forwards, backwards and laterally over their base. Initially manual support the length of the trunk may be needed and this is best achieved by the therapist high-kneeling behind the child. As sitting balance improves, the level of support given can be lowered to pelvic level.

When static independent sitting balance has been achieved the task can be made more challenging by raising the plinth so a child's feet are not on the floor. Movement in sitting can be introduced by asking a child to reach outside his or her base in all directions or by introducing an activity such as throwing and catching a ball. Rhythmical stabilizations in sitting can be used to improve core stability but care must be taken to ensure that the child feels safe. Seating support can also be reduced, although it is necessary to be aware a child may fatigue quickly whilst practising a newly acquired skill. A Swiss ball can be used to work on sitting balance, starting with a child's feet wide apart to give a good base and the therapist giving some manual support. The exercise can be progressed by reducing the support and making the child's base smaller and less stable (Carriere 1998).

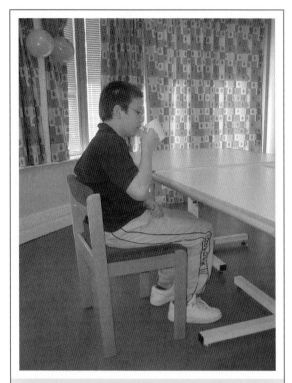

Figure 12.1 Poor posture on a standard dining chair. Posteriorly tilted pelvis and rounded spinal profile.

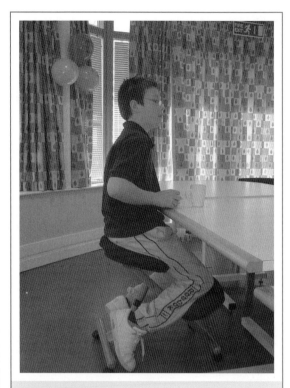

Figure 12.2 Corrected posture on kneeler chair.

When a child has achieved stable independent sitting balance, it is still necessary to be aware of posture and a kneeler chair can be a useful tool to gain a more upright position (Figures 12.1 and 12.2).

Kneeling

The majority of children who suffer a brain injury are of an age when it is not appropriate for them to be using crawling as a means of mobility. High-kneeling and four-point kneeling are, however, useful positions to work on pelvic control, balance and weight transference. In high-kneeling rhythmical stabilizations will work on a child's core stability and balance. Physiotherapists can also lift a child's feet off the surface in high-kneeling to challenge their balance further and develop their saving reactions.

Four-point kneeling can be used to encourage weight-bearing through the affected arm in a child with hemiplegia. Balance can be challenged by a child raising the opposite or same-side arm and leg off the supporting surface and maintaining that position for a few seconds. When a child has secure balance in high-kneeling, knee-walking can be introduced, forwards, backwards and sideways. Half-kneeling is a useful position in which to work, as it may enable children to learn to rise from the floor to standing.

Standing

Supported standing can be used to encourage activity of the antigravity muscles. If a child has very little head control a tilt table may need to be used initially. Care should be taken that the child feels safe, understands what is happening and is able to participate in the process. When bringing a child up into standing the first time using a tilt table, it is important to bring it up a few degrees at a time and to check that blood pressure remains within the normal limits. Standing is a good position for a child to work on head control as it tends to encourage a total extension pattern. Weight-bearing will also encourage a plantargrade position in the ankles and help to maintain the length of the plantarflexors.

When a child is able to weight-bear fully through the feet, the standing position can be used to work on trunk and pelvic control, weight transference, posture and balance. This can be done with the physiotherapist giving manual support and postural correction or with a child holding on to wall bars or a plinth at an appropriate height. A mirror should be used to enable a child to monitor posture and learn to self-correct. A feedback machine which gives the child accurate information about even weight-bearing and weight transference can be a useful tool.

When a child has achieved independent standing balance, it is necessary to continue to work on weight transference to achieve single-leg standing balance. As in sitting and high-kneeling, rhythmical stabilizations can be used to challenge balance and encourage saving reactions. When a child is secure in standing, balance can be challenged and hopefully improved by the use of a wobble board or trampoline (Figure 12.3). A step machine will encourage weight transference as well as being a muscle-strengthening activity. Activities such as kicking a football will encourage single-leg standing.

Independent sitting to standing can be started from a raised plinth so a child's feet can be on the floor whilst sitting on the edge of the plinth. As a child's ability to rise into standing and balance improves, the plinth can be lowered to make the exercise more challenging. If a child has weakness in one leg, the foot of the stronger leg can be placed on a box to encourage the weaker leg to do the majority of the work.

Mobility

As mentioned earlier, children and their families are anxious for them to walk again and as soon as possible. It is, however, necessary for physiotherapists to time the start of walking to give the best possible end result. If a child has poor balance, poor trunk control or is unable to transfer full weight from one foot to the other, it is probably too soon to attempt walking (Weston et al 1998). If these deficits are present, the stress of walking is likely to cause associated reactions and an excessive increase in postural tone (Rinehart 1990). The result of trying to walk at this stage may be a frightened and demoralized child. Early walking without control of the movement does not contribute any kind of useful information to a child's brain (Lynch & Grisogono 1991).

When the appropriate time has arrived, walking can start by encouraging cruising sideways using a high plinth, wall bars or parallel bars. A posture control walker can be used as long as a child has a good upright position in it, is fully weight-bearing and is just using the walker as a balance aid. For a child with ataxia, this may be the only way to get sufficient practice in an upright position to make unsupported walking a possibility. Manual assistance can be given via a chest strap held from behind, a handling belt round the waist, a pole held from in front or by a child placing the hands on the physiotherapist's shoulders. All of these methods can allow walking practice to be carried out safely when a child would not be safe walking alone.

It may be necessary for children to wear a helmet when mobilizing if they are in danger of falling. A child who has an incomplete skull due to a craniectomy or a fracture will need to wear a helmet until it is repaired (see Ch. 11) (Figure 12.4).

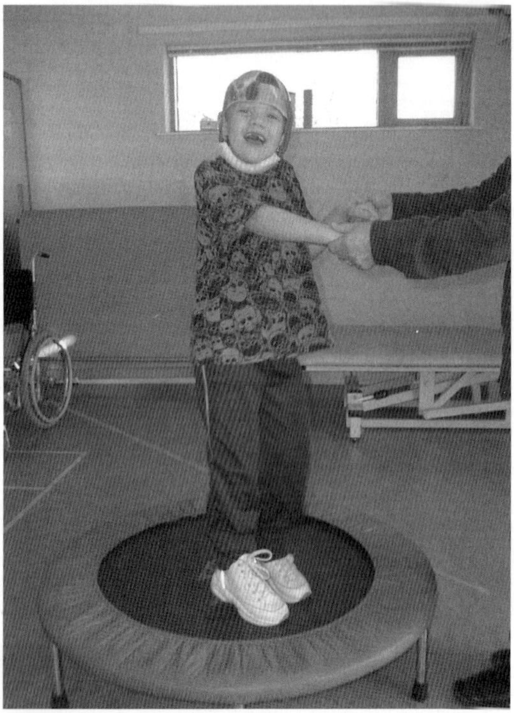

Figure 12.3 A trampoline can challenge balance and be fun.

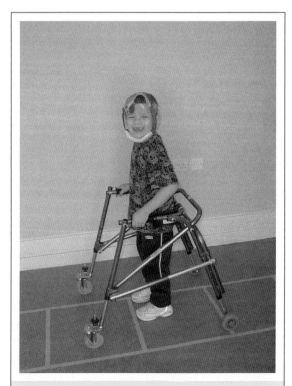

Figure 12.4 A hard helmet may be necessary when mobilizing to protect an incomplete skull.

When spasticity is present it will have an effect on a child's gait. It is important to identify the muscles that are causing the dysfunction and reduce the effects as far as possible. Gait laboratory analysis may be helpful at this stage (Esquenazi 2004) (see Ch. 4).

When a child has severe gross motor problems, at some stage during the rehabilitation process physiotherapists need to assess the likelihood of being able to walk again independently. If this is not going to be an option, then alternative methods of mobility need to be investigated. Occupational therapists will be involved in assessing a child for a powered or self-propelling wheelchair and physiotherapists may provide a walker that gives a lot of support but allows some mobility in an upright position.

Cycling may provide a child with independent mobility in some settings as well as providing a form of exercise. Tricycles can be adapted with a variety of supports to meet a child's needs.

KEY POINTS

Role of physiotherapist in the rehabilitation stage
- Regaining/maintaining joint ranges
- Provision of orthoses
- Facilitation of muscle contraction and muscle-strengthening
- Provision of postural management and other equipment
- Promoting postural ability in lying, sitting and standing
- Promotion of balance in sitting, kneeling and standing
- Encouraging mobility on the floor in sitting and walking

Measuring and recording physical ability

There are many different assessments which can be used for recording progress in acquired brain injury rehabilitation (see Ch. 3). Many of them will give a good overview of how a child is functioning but may not give a sufficiently indepth picture of a child's gross motor skills. The following can give useful information.

- The Movement Assessment Battery for Children is useful for children who have regained good motor function but may have some gross motor or dexterity problems (Henderson & Sugden 1992)
- The Gross Motor Function Measure assesses motor function in lying and rolling, sitting, crawling and kneeling, standing and walking, running and jumping, so is appropriate for a wide range of abilities (Russell et al 2002). It is appropriate for children with moderate to severe gross motor function deficits
- The Chailey Levels of Ability are observational scales which assess lying, sitting and standing abilities. They are especially useful to chart small changes at lower levels of ability (Pountney et al 2004)

- The Hawaii Early Learning Profile (HELP) covers all aspects of development in depth: sensory, cognitive, language, gross motor, fine motor, social–emotional and self-help (Parks 1999).

Other factors affecting gross motor ability

Information on the following areas will be provided by other disciplines within the team: speech and language therapists, occupational therapists and psychologists. It is important that physiotherapists are aware of all aspects of a child's difficulties. Many of these can affect the way in which treatment can be delivered and will alter the approach that is necessary. Joint sessions carried out with other disciplines can greatly enhance the physiotherapist's understanding of the overall effects of acquired brain injury.

Sensory

Damage to the sensory cortex can result in a disturbance or loss of sight, hearing, smell, taste or touch. Although the loss of smell or taste may not affect physiotherapy input, disruption of any of the other three senses needs to be taken into account.

It is fairly common for a child who has had an acquired brain injury to be hypersensitive to touch but may be unable to pinpoint the precise area that is painful. Proprioception is often disrupted and a child needs to be given manual, verbal and visual feedback to help monitor movement and minimize the effects of this loss (Giles & Clark-Wilson 1993).

Attention

Attention is the ability to focus on verbal and visual information. Problems with attention are common in children who have suffered an acquired brain injury and will affect their ability to progress physically (Dennis et al 1995). These children are easily distracted, and have difficulty blocking out irrelevant stimuli, concentrating and dividing their attention. A quiet working environment where outside stimuli are reduced to a minimum will help them attend to a task.

This problem is clearly demonstrated by children who are able to walk until someone speaks to them, whereupon they lose their balance or have to stand still to respond.

Memory

The hippocampus encodes a memory and relays it to different areas of the brain. The left and right temporal lobes are responsible for verbal and spatial memory respectively. The cerebellum is associated with motor skills and the frontal lobes are associated with future events and actions (Powell 2004). Problems with memory can be significant and will impact on a child's ability to make functional gains (Kerkering & Phillips 1994). Children forget, for instance, to carry out an exercise programme even if they are old enough, able and willing. They may over- or underestimate their motor abilities and therefore put themselves in danger or do not perform at their functional best.

The rehabilitation team needs to give a child verbal and written prompts throughout the day to help overcome these difficulties.

Language

The ability to produce speech may be affected and gaining a consistent yes and no is a priority (Middleton et al 1992). Even when a child can speak intelligibly, severe receptive and/or expressive language problems may be present. Physiotherapists need a basic understanding of these difficulties to enable them to communicate effectively during therapy sessions.

Receptive language deficits may result in an inability to follow instructions and these will need to be kept as simple and as brief as possible. Touching the appropriate limb or demonstrating a movement can help to overcome this block to therapy.

Expressive language deficits impair the ability to communicate with others. Word-finding difficulties frequently occur in children with acquired brain injury (McMahon 1998). This is frustrating for children; reading their body language and good guesswork can help ease the situation.

Speed of information-processing

A slowed speed of information-processing can occur following an acquired brain injury. It will, therefore, take a child longer to respond to a request. If a lot of information is given quickly, some of it will be lost so physiotherapists need to give brief instructions and wait for a response before repeating the request or giving hands-on assistance.

Emotional and behavioural problems

There are many emotional and behavioural problems that can arise following an acquired brain injury. These include disinhibition, irritability, frustration, insensitivity to others' feelings, anxiety, depression, eating disorders and verbal or physical aggression (Demellweek et al 1998). Physiotherapists need to be aware of these problems and adjust their approach accordingly.

A child entering the rehabilitation stage may be fearful, having probably undergone a considerable number of interventions in the acute stage; it is necessary for therapists to be sensitive to this and work hard to make therapy sessions a positive experience. A negative experience for a child will almost certainly produce a negative result whereas a positive experience may produce a positive gain.

The level of motivation after acquired brain injury can vary greatly. Some children push themselves to the extreme and it is sometimes necessary to try to limit their activities to avoid fatigue. At the other end of the scale, some children spend a considerable amount of time in denial, appearing to believe that they do not have a problem, or that tomorrow morning they will wake up and find that it was just a bad dream.

Fatigue

Fatigue can be a major problem, especially at the beginning of the rehabilitation stage. Many children are unable to recognize or acknowledge that they are tired; the rehabilitation team need to monitor this and adjust their timetable accordingly to allow for sufficient rest periods during the day.

Seizures

Although the majority of children and adults who have a head injury do not have seizures, it is the leading cause of epilepsy in young adults (Hudak et al 2004). These can take the form of tonic-clonic seizures or, more frequently, they will present as absences. Physiotherapists need to be able to monitor a child's seizure activity and feed back the information to the rehabilitation medical staff.

Reintegration stage

Discharge planning

Discharge planning needs to start as early as possible during the rehabilitation process, although this may be limited as a child's eventual needs may be difficult to predict. The local medical and therapy team need to be identified and involved. The community nurse team and social services are likely to be amongst the first to make contact with a child and family as they may be required when a child starts to visit home at weekends. A child's general practitioner will have been kept informed of that child's progress throughout rehabilitation. The community paediatrician will be contacted so that the child's ongoing care can be coordinated. Local therapy input will be provided by the community team or, if a child is not being reintegrated into mainstream schooling, it may be accessed at school.

Representatives of all the local services should be invited to a child's multidisciplinary reviews. Their attendance is especially important at the discharge review when a discharge date can be set and final checks, that the appropriate services are in place, can be made.

Reintegration

Reintegration back into home and school is possibly the most important part of the role of the rehabilitation team: it is the outcome of this process that has the greatest long-term impact on children and their families.

Home

Most children will have been visiting home, spending weekends there and making contact with old friends.

Unfortunately, friends often find it hard to adjust to a changed person and will themselves have changed and moved on in the intervening time. This can be very hard for injured children to understand and accept, and adjusting to their new situation and making new friends can be a lengthy process.

Within families, the position of a child may have changed. It is very difficult for teenagers, who have been independent, to accept new limitations to their freedom and the loss of their future plans. It is equally difficult for parents to come to terms with the changes in a child and to accept that their future will be very different from their former expectations.

The physiotherapist's role in reintegration back to home will depend on children's physical limitations. People can live with a bed in the lounge or a commode downstairs for a short period of time but decisions need to be made about home adaptations; the physiotherapist will become involved with assessing for equipment and predicting what will be necessary in the future.

School

Planning for a return to school needs to start as soon as it is clear what type of school is going to be appropriate. Most children and their families are keen for a return to the previous school if possible. Care needs to be taken that this is a realistic option as a failed reintegration is very disheartening for all concerned.

A gradual reintegration into mainstream schooling is more likely to be successful in that it allows a slow adjustment period for a child and school staff and will also help a child to build up stamina.

Although a child can move around and be safe in the quiet, controlled environment of a rehabilitation centre, a busy school is a very different proposition. Physiotherapists need to advise the school of a child's physical limitations and how to minimize their effects. The following areas need to be considered (Child Brain Injury Trust 2006):

- Moving around the school − a child may need extra time to move from one class to another so it may be necessary to leave the class early. Help may be needed to carry bags and the timetable organized to avoid long journeys
- Stairs − additional handrails may be necessary. The number of level changes a child undertakes needs to be minimized. Stairs need to be avoided or a lift installed
- In class − supportive seating may help to minimize physical effort and allow a child to concentrate on academic work. A child can be seated near to the door to make access easier
- Break times − close supervision may be necessary to ensure a child's safety. At lunchtime, extra time may be needed to get to the dining hall or to eat lunch. Help may also be needed to carry a tray
- Physical education lessons − activities may need to be adapted to allow a child to participate in physical education lessons. Alternatively, these lessons can be used as a catch-up session for classroom work or as an exercise programme session.

Since a child's brain is still maturing, the full impact of the injury may not become evident for many months or even years. A small number of children will need a lot of extra help at school and will need a statutory assessment of special educational needs for the child (see Ch. 2).

Table 12.1 Residual problem areas following acquired brain injury	
Physical and physiological problems	**Intellectual, educational and personality problems**
Mobility	Attention and memory
Coordination and balance	Speech and higher-level language skills
Intention tremor	Planning and organizing
Spasticity	Speed of information-processing
Hand–eye coordination	Impulsivity
Sight	Loss of initiative
Hearing	Disinhibition
Seizures	Lack of insight
Bladder control	Emotional difficulties
Weight increase	Social relationships

This document describes a child's needs and the support that is required to meet these needs. It is vital for the school and all other agencies involved to be aware of and recognize the short-term and long-term consequences of a child's head injury, both visible and invisible. If these consequences are not properly managed, wide-ranging and long-term problems may arise. It is also essential to highlight any additional problems that may arise during times of major transition such as moving on to secondary school.

Residual problem areas

There are many areas in which children may have long-term problems which could affect their successful reintegration into school and the community (Table 12.1).

Sport and leisure activities

Certain activities should be avoided in the months following an acquired brain injury as the result of a first injury can be compounded by a second one, even if it is minor. Activities that should be avoided are ones that may cause a direct blow to the head, such as contact sports or heading a football. High-velocity or pressure-shifting activities such as diving, trampolining or rollercoasters should also be avoided. Opinions as to how long after the injury these activities should be avoided vary between 6 months and a year (Child Development Centre 2006, Toronto Acquired Brain Injury Network 2006).

> **KEY POINTS**
>
> ### Role of physiotherapist in the reintegration stage
> - Advice for home adaptations
> - Input to statutory assessment of special educational needs
> - Early liaison with home therapy team – school and/or community
> - Handover meetings/visits to home and school
> - Advice to school staff

CASE STUDY 12.1

Sara's Story

When Sara was 12 years old, she went to school like any other day. In the morning, she had a science test in which, when it was later marked, she performed very well. At lunchtime she had what she later described as the worst headache imaginable. She went to the sick bay where she started vomiting. Her mother was called and she took her to the local Accident and Emergency department, where her Glasgow Coma Scale was recorded at 5. She was transferred to another local hospital and a computed tomography scan was performed; this showed a large collection of blood in the posterior fossa. At this point her intracranial pressure had risen to the extent that her brain was threatening to push through the foramen magnum. Dexamethasone and mannitol were administered to reduce her cerebral oedema. She was transferred to a London hospital where the clot was drained and she was intubated and ventilated. Her father, who had been following her trail, eventually caught up with her in London. A week later she was off the ventilator and being fed by nasogastric tube. Sara was making no purposeful movements. One month posttrauma she had a gastrostomy inserted. In the weeks that followed it was noted that as Sara's level of awareness rose, her level of cooperation deteriorated.

Three and a half months after her trauma, Sara, was transferred to the Children's Head Injury Service at Chailey Heritage Clinical Services for rehabilitation. Sara had some active movement of all four limbs. She was unwilling to sit in an upright position and spent most of the day in a reclined position with her knees drawn up defensively. She had no clear vocalization but could nod for 'yes' and shake her head for 'no'. At this moment in time Sara wailed continuously; she was angry, frustrated and frightened. She was aggressive and uncooperative. She would scratch, kick, pinch or pull hair to avoid what she saw as threatening contact. Sara had full range of movement in all joints apart from her left ankle which necessitated serial plastering over a period of 3 weeks, after which plantargrade was achieved. An ankle–foot orthosis was supplied to maintain the joint range. Sara was not keen to wear this; she would remove it and throw it across the room but managed a few hours every day.

Four and a half months posttrauma Sara was prescribed an antidepressant, sertraline. She was also starting to communicate using a word board. Sara was still frustrated and angry and repeatedly spelt out 'take me home, take me home *now*'.

Seven months posttrauma Sara was cooperative and very hard-working. She had severe cerebellar ataxia but had independent standing balance of a few seconds when placed. She was able to walk with a Kaye walker with some assistance to stabilize her at pelvic level. Sara's physiotherapy at this stage concentrated on the need to improve the muscle power and tone around her trunk and pelvis. She was willing to carry out an exercise programme and would work in sitting, high-kneeling, four-point kneeling and standing. She was, however, very focused on functional goals and would endlessly practise getting from sitting to standing, trying to find her

continued

standing balance and, of course, walking. Her central control slowly improved and Sara exchanged her Kaye walker for a pair of crutches 10 months after her trauma. She also started taking some unsupported steps. Sara would still work for periods on single-leg standing balance and independent position changes: she was still focused on walking and her therapy mainly consisted of very slow walks along a corridor with her physiotherapist giving her verbal feedback and acting as a catcher. The determination that Sara had initially used to avoid therapy

was doubled when working to achieve her goals. When Sara first returned to school 1 year and 4 months posttrauma she was refusing to use a wheelchair and walked with one crutch and some assistance.

Sara's physical ability progressed over the years and she is now, 7 years after her insult, able to walk without support. She has just finished her first year at university studying psychology and has a full social life and is enjoying herself. Extreme motivation can be challenging but it does get results!

REFERENCES

Anderson D 1995 Management of decreased ROM from overactive musculature or heterotopic ossification. In: Montgomery J (ed.) *Physical Therapy for Traumatic Brain Injury*. New York: Churchill Livingstone, pp. 79–97.

Attard J, Rithalia S 2004 A review of the use of Lycra pressure orthoses for children with cerebral palsy. *International Journal of Therapy and Rehabilitation* 11: 120–125.

Bastian A 1997 Mechanisms of ataxia. *Physical Therapy* 77: 672–675.

Carriere B 1998 *The Swiss Ball*. Berlin: Springer.

Child Brain Injury Trust 2006 Information for teachers. Available online a: www.cbituk.org.

Child Development Centre 2006 A guide for families of children with an acquired brain injury. Available online at: www.hoteldieu.com/cdcabi.pdf.

Demellweek C, O'Leary A 1998 The impact of brain injury on the family. In: Appleton R, Baldwin T (eds) *Management of Brain-Injured Children*. Oxford: Oxford Press, p. 207.

Demellweek C, O'Leary A, Baldwin T 1998 Emotional, behavioural and social difficulties. In: Appleton R, Baldwin T (eds) *Management of Brain-Injured Children*. Oxford: Oxford University Press, p. 167.

Dennis M, Wilkinson M, Koski L et al 1995 Attention deficits in the long term after childhood head injury. In: Broman SH, Michel ME (eds) *Traumatic Head Injury in Children*. Oxford: Oxford University Press, pp. 165–187.

Duncan P 1990 Physical therapy assessment. In: Rosenthal M, Griffith ER, Bond M et al (eds) *Rehabilitation of the Adult and Child with Traumatic Brain Injury*. Philadelphia, PA: Davis, pp. 264–283.

Esquenazi A 2004 Evaluation and management of spastic gait in patients with traumatic brain injury. *Journal of Head Trauma Rehabilitation* 19: 109–116.

Giles GM, Clark-Wilson J 1993 *Brain Injury Rehabilitation*. London: Chapman and Hall, p. 208.

Gormley M 1999 Management of spasticity in children. Part 2: oral medications and intrathecal baclofen. *Journal of Head Trauma Rehabilitation* 14: 207–209.

Griffith ER, Mayer NH 1990 Hypertonicity and movement disorders. In: Rosenthal M, Griffith E R, Bond M et al (eds) *Rehabilitation of the Adult and Child with Traumatic Brain Injury*. Philadelphia, PA: Davis, pp. 127–147.

Henderson SE, Sugden DA 1992 *Movement Assessment Battery for Children*. London: Psychological Corporation.

Hudak AM, Trivedi K, Harper CR et al 2004 Evaluation of seizure-like episodes in survivors of moderate and severe brain injury. *Journal of Head Trauma Rehabilitation* 19: 290–294.

Jackson J 2004 Specific treatment techniques. In: Stokes M (ed.) *Physical Management in Neurological Rehabilitation*. Edinburgh: Elsevier, pp. 393–411.

Jaffe KM, Brink JD, Hayes RM et al 1990 Specific problems associated with pediatric head injury. In: Rosenthal M, Griffith ER, Bond M et al (eds) *Rehabilitation of the Adult and Child with Traumatic Brain Injury*. Philadelphia, PA: Davis, pp. 539–555.

Karman N, Maryles J, Baker RW et al 2003 Constraint-induced movement therapy for hemiplegic children with acquired brain injuries. *Journal of Head Trauma Rehabilitation* 18: 259–267.

Kerkering GA, Phillips WE 1994 Brain injuries: traumatic brain injuries, near-drowning and brain tumors. In: Campbell SK, Vander Linder DW, Palisano RJ (eds) *Physical Therapy for Children*. Philadelphia, PA: WB Saunders, p. 604.

Lennon S 2004 The theoretical basis of neurological physiotherapy. In: Stokes M (ed.) *Physical Management in Neurological Rehabilitation*. Edinburgh: Elsevier, pp. 367–378.

Lynch M, Grisogono V 1991 *Strokes and Head Injuries*. London: John Murray, p. 116.

Mazaux JM, Richer E 1998 Rehabilitation after traumatic brain injury in adults. *Disability and Rehabilitation* 20: 435–447.

McMahon S 1998 Speech and language difficulties. In: Appleton R, Baldwin T (eds) *Management of Brain-Injured Children*. Oxford: Oxford University Press, p. 127.

Meythaler JM, Clayton W, Davis LK et al 2004 Orally delivered baclofen to control spastic hypertonia in acquired brain injury. *Journal of Head Trauma Rehabilitation* 19: 101–108.

Middleton J, Jones M, Moffat V et al 1992 Rehabilitation after acute neurological trauma. In: McCarthy GT (ed.) *Physical Disability in Childhood*. Edinburgh: Churchill Livingstone, pp. 249–268.

Parks S 1999 *Inside HELP and HELP for PreSchoolers*. Palo Alto, CA: VORT.

Pountney TE, Mulcahy CM, Clarke SM et al 2004 *The Chailey Approach to Postural Management*. North Chailey, East Sussex: Chailey Heritage Clinical Services.

Powell T 2004 *Head Injury: A Practical Guide*. Bicester: Speechmark, p. 75.

Rinehart MA 1990 Strategies for improving motor performance. In: Rosenthal M, Griffith ER, Bond MR et al (eds) *Rehabilitation of the Adult and Child with Traumatic Brain Injury*. Philadelphia, PA: Davis, pp. 331–348.

Russell DJ, Rosenbaum PL, Avery LM et al 2002 *Gross Motor Function Measure: User's Manual*. London: MacKeith Press.

Toronto Acquired Brain Injury Network 2006 Facts for physicians – mild acquired brain injury in children and youth. Available online at: www.abinetwork.ca.

Watkins C 1999 Mechanical and neurophysiological changes in spastic muscles. *Physiotherapy* 85: 603–609.

Weston J, Kinley E, Hughes B et al 1998 Physical (motor and functional) difficulties. In: Appleton R, Baldwin T (eds) *Management of Brain-Injured Children*. Oxford: Oxford University Press, pp. 71–105.

Zafonte R, Elovic EP, Lombard L 2004 Acute care management of post-TBI spasticity. *Journal of Head Trauma Rehabilitation* 19: 89–98.

Musculoskeletal

13 Orthopaedic conditions

Jeanne Hartley

INTRODUCTION

The term 'orthopaedic' originated with Nicolas André, a French physician who used the combination of two Greek words *orthos* (straight) and *paidi* (child). In 1741 his book, entitled *Orthopaedia: Or the Art of Correcting and Preventing Deformities in Children: By such Means, as may easily be put in Practice by Parents themselves, and all such as are Employed in Educating Children,* was published. At that time surgery was still primitive and limited to the correction of deformities by the use of crude apparatus, the reduction of fractures and dislocations by traction, and the amputation of limbs. Fortunately for us, orthopaedics evolved into a more 'scientific' speciality, concerned with the preservation and restoration of the musculoskeletal system, using sophisticated diagnostic, surgical and therapeutic aids.

An understanding of growth, both normal and abnormal, in a child is vital to our understanding of the paediatric orthopaedic problems. Bennet (2002) stated that over half the children seen in his orthopaedic clinic, referred by family practitioners, were within normal limits. Appreciation of what is 'normal' may also vary with

age and it is this understanding that is important in developing reasoning when counselling families seeking opinion regarding their concerns for their child and also to help us offer physiotherapy interventions appropriately.

This chapter will cover a variety of common paediatric orthopaedic conditions that may be referred to the physiotherapist for opinion and management, including club foot, flat foot, obstetrical brachial plexus injuries, Perthes disease, limb-length discrepancies, knee pain, torticollis and plagiocephaly. Also included is the orthopaedic assessment of infants and children. Normal variations in skeletal growth will also be discussed. Scoliosis has not been included in this chapter as the effectiveness of physiotherapy is unproven. The orthopaedic physiotherapist's role in the management of children with neurological conditions such as cerebral palsy has also not been included as local protocols and opinions vary (see Ch. 7).

GROWTH

Skeletal growth occurs by adding tissue to its outer surface:

- by intramembranous ossification on the surface of the cortex, as in the scapula and skull, or to increase circumference of long bones
- by enchondral ossification at the growth plates situated at either end of each long bone, increasing length.

In the first 18 months of life a baby undergoes the most rapid period of growth and development. At the age of 1 year, sitting height is 63% of a child's total height. The limbs are short in proportion. This disproportion in sitting height gradually reduces to 52% in males and 53% in females at skeletal maturity. From birth to cessation of growth at maturity, sitting height increases by 67%, whereas the legs increase in length by 145%. In infancy a child's spine lacks the normal adult curve. A long C-curve is replaced by the appearance of cervical lordosis at 3 months of age as the child develops head control and lumbar lordosis as the child develops sitting balance.

Skeletal growth is very rapid in infancy, slows down during childhood and increases again during the adolescent pubertal growth spurt. At the age of 2 years a child is approximately half adult height and three-quarters adult height by the age of 9. The ability to predict height at skeletal maturity is an important factor in the decision-making process for the orthopaedic management of some conditions such as congenital limb-length inequality. There are a variety of methods available to predict adult height, from percentile charts to the use of X-ray assessment of bone age to determine growth potential. The affects of underlying systemic, endocrine, nutritional and metabolic disorders, which may impact on skeletal growth, also need to be considered. Transverse growth arrest lines in a long bone (Harris lines) are often seen on X-ray following systemic illness. Hormones exert a powerful influence on growth plates. Growth hormone deficiency can cause premature closure of growth plates, resulting in short stature, whereas hypersecretion of the hormone results in widening of the growth plates and gigantism.

The growth of a single bone or several bones can be altered if damage has occurred to a growth plate from trauma, infection (neonatal sepsis, meningococcal meningitis) or iatrogenic causes (drip extravasation injury, irradiation).

During the final adolescent growth spurt, extending from puberty to skeletal maturity, certain orthopaedic problems may become apparent (such as scoliosis, slipped upper femoral epiphysis) or existing ones become more pressing as body image and psychosocial issues become more important for the young person. The thin calf and smaller foot resulting from a club foot become less tolerable when a teenage boy is facing a beach holiday with his friends. Accepting that working out in the gym will not build up the bulk in the calf can be very difficult to accept at this stage.

However, for most people, skeletal growth occurs without problems, ceasing at around 14 years in girls and 16 years in boys, on average. Growth plates close at differing times and also grow at differing rates. For example, 65% of all growth in the leg occurs at the knee, with 39% taking place at the lower femoral growth plate and 26% at the proximal tibial growth plate. Proportionally less growth takes place at the upper femoral and lower tibial growth plate. Information such as this can be important in calculating anticipated leg-length difference at skeletal maturity in a child with a congenital bone dysplasia.

ASSESSMENT

For physiotherapists the initial assessment of a child is the most essential step to plan appropriate management. A good understanding of child development is also valuable. Many children will experience pain and altered function due to trauma at some stage in their childhood. It is important to be mindful that a recent fall from a scooter or tumble in the garden may have been the reason the parents sought advice, but careful history-taking may uncover further information that indicates that the problem may

have been there previously and the injury may have been the catalyst for the consultation.

Assessment of a baby (under 24 months of age)

All babies should have a full and thorough assessment, including the following:

- Past history is essential and should include antenatal and birth history, family history and, if the baby is old enough, developmental history. Although all babies born in the UK are routinely screened for hip dysplasia in the neonatal period by medical staff, it is not uncommon in some tertiary referral centres to see older babies, toddlers and sometimes even older children with hip problems not noted in the neonatal checks.
- Undress the baby, even if the referral is for advice and management of a foot problem. Count the number of toes on each foot; check movement at the ankles, knees and hips. If the baby is very young (under 3 months), remember that physiological neonatal flexion contractures will be present in the hips and knees and there may be excessive dorsiflexion. Look for asymmetry in joint range of movement, limb lengths and girth as well as asymmetry of active movement.
- Turn the baby over and look at the spine. A baby's spine should be straight with a single curve. Scoliosis and sharp angulations require investigation. Look for skin changes such as birth marks, café-au-lait patches and skin dimples over the spine – these can be an indication of underlying spinal problems such as spina bifida occulta, spinal dysraphism or neurofibromatosis. Look for plagiocephaly (flattened appearance of the back or side of the skull) and asymmetry of neck range of movement.
- Examination of the upper limbs – look for asymmetry of active movement and joint ranges.
- Be aware that any baby with asymmetries due to intrauterine moulding, especially at the neck or feet, has an increased risk of hip dysplasia – as well as those where there is a family history of hip problems.

Assessment of a child (over the age of 2 years)

The assessment should include some or all of the following:

- Birth history, including antenatal history
- History of presenting condition
- Developmental milestones: did the child sit and walk at the right time?
- Family history of similar bone or joint problems: a surprising number of orthopaedic problems run in families
- Child/carer's concerns: listen to the mother if the child is young – her intuition is often very accurate. An older

child may be less concerned about leg-length discrepancy than their parents

- Joint range of movement (active and passive as appropriate)
- Muscle power: grading systems such as the Oxford rating scale
- Muscle length: such as the popliteal angle to assess hamstring length and Silfverskiold test to differentiate muscle tightness between gastrocnemius and soleus
- Bony rotational profiles (if appropriate) such as the thigh/foot angle to determine the presence of tibial torsion
- Deformity, e.g. scoliosis, club foot
- Limb lengths: traditionally measured from the anterior superior iliac spine (ASIS) to the medial malleolus. For congenital limb-length discrepancies, measurement may be from the ASIS to the base of the heel
- Limb girth: use a bony landmark and measure down from it to ensure consistency between assessment of girth of each limb, e.g. 7 cm below the tibial tubercle to measure calf girth
- Joint stability: such as the Ortolani and Barlow tests for hip instability; anterior draw test for knee joint stability
- Pain profile: see below
- Functional abilities.

Pain

The way a child perceives and expresses pain is age-dependent:

- An infant may fuss or cry or avoid moving the painful part. If the pain is severe, continuous crying is usual
- Children in pain may avoid using the affected part or will show altered function such as limping. They may also be able to voice their discomfort, although the description of the pain will be non-specific, e.g. 'I have a headache in my leg'
- Most adolescents have language and perception to describe their pain. An athletic boy may underreport his pain if there is a sporting event he is keen to take part in; conversely, a boy who hates sport may be exaggerating the problem.

Previous pain experiences and a family history of painful conditions should also be considered.

A parent's intuition needs to be given serious consideration. A diagnosis of pain of non-organic origin should only be entertained after all other possible causes have been discounted.

Consider using one of the many pain assessment tools that are appropriate to the age of the child to provide a baseline and outcome measure for your intervention (see Ch. 3).

Children with severe physical and cognitive disability need careful consideration and the use of tools such as the

Paediatric Pain Profile is an important adjunct to our understanding of the child and in planning interventions.

Assessment of children and babies with congenital orthopaedic conditions, which affect their functional potential or abilities, can be very challenging. It is important to include the family and child in all discussions at every stage so that aims of treatment and plans of management and everyone's expectations are realistic, achievable, pragmatic and, as far as possible, evidence-based.

Normal variants

Jones & Hill (2000) described the difficulty in counselling parents whose children's problems were due to normal variants of skeletal growth, such as bow leg, knock knee, in-toeing and flat feet. 'The five Ss' can be a helpful way of explaining to parents that treatment from a surgeon or a physiotherapist is unnecessary in some cases, whereas other cases may require intervention.

The five Ss

1. **Symmetry:** Does the problem under consideration affect both limbs equally? For example, if both lower limbs in a 3-year-old child are bowed, this is likely to be due to normal physiological bowing and it is safe to watch and wait. However, severe bowing, asymmetric bowing or bowing in only one lower limb is not normal and warrants further investigation.
2. **Symptoms:** Does the child have symptoms? If a child is running around happily and not complaining of pain or functional difficulties, then 'treatment' is not required, despite what the parent or the shoeshop assistant may say!
3. **Stiffness:** Is there a full range of movement in all a child's joints? Joint stiffness in a growing child is not normal and should be investigated further.
4. **Systemic:** Is the child well? It is important to remember that inflammatory conditions and metabolic problems can have an impact on skeletal growth. Conditions such as rickets can cause skeletal changes such as bow legs.
5. **Skeletal dysplasia:** Is a child of normal stature and proportion? Does the child have an unusual face?

Using this guidance a child who has marked but equal bowing of both lower limbs, with no pain or stiffness, and has no evidence of systemic disease or skeletal dysplasia, is normal. Using this guidance parents can be reassured that it is the passage of time that will be the best treatment and that shoe modifications and braces are ineffective, could make the child uncomfortable and self-conscious and impede play. Likewise physiotherapy exercises are unnecessary, time-consuming and ineffective. Time spent in careful explanation will be time well spent, along with the offer of further review if the parents have concerns in the future.

Conversely, a child with bowing of one lower limb has asymmetry and therefore warrants further investigation.

FEET

Children's shoes

Physiotherapists are frequently asked to give opinion and advice regarding suitable shoe wear for a child. Children's shoes are expensive and some companies recommend that a child's feet should be measured at 3-monthly intervals and new shoes provided (Bennet 2002). It has been suggested that if this is the case, children's shoes do not have to be expensive or long-lasting. There is little evidence to suggest that expensive 'good' shoes are in any way superior to a cheap pair of trainers. Although most children have straight feet, shoes are often shaped to fit a varus forefoot. Pressure and pain may ensue if the match in shape between the shoe and foot is markedly different.

Staheli (1991) stated that optimum foot development occurs in a barefoot environment and that the primary role of shoes is to protect the foot from injury and infection and that the provision of corrective (stiff and compressive) footwear may cause deformity, weakness and loss of mobility.

A prospective study to determine whether children with flexible flat feet needed treatment with orthotics or corrective 'orthopaedic' shoes was carried out with children randomly allocated to one of four groups, including a control group; the children underwent a minimum of 3 years' treatment. Final analysis demonstrated significant improvement in all groups, including the controls, with no significant difference between the controls and the intervention group. It was concluded that wearing corrective shoes or inserts does not influence the course of flexible flat foot in children (Wenger et al 1989).

Many high-street stores now carry an extensive range of children's shoes and are able to provide shoes with narrow to extra-wide fittings, high-top trainers and boots and many will even offer a service to provide shoes of differing sizes. The provision of prescription footwear is now primarily reserved for those children whose feet are particularly difficult to shoe or if there are considerations such as insensitivity or the need to maintain a corrected position after surgery. Orthotic supports such as ankle–foot orthoses do not need 'special footwear' in most circumstances and suitable shoe wear can be found in local high-street stores.

An important study reported on the effects of corrective shoe wear on the self-esteem and self-image of 46 adults who had been provided with corrective shoe wear as children. It suggested that common orthopaedic problems for which parents seek resolution, such as flat feet or in-toeing, may subject a child to unnecessary treatment and may have consequences in adulthood. In subjective reports participants in the study group vividly recalled being teased about their shoe wear and having their activities limited, as well as it being a negative experience during their childhood years. Furthermore, as adults they showed lower self-esteem than the control group. The study concluded that prescribed devices and corrective shoes do not alter physical conditions and are not a harmless placebo. Allowing childhood developmental variations to follow their natural courses is free, effective and harmless treatment (Driano et al 1998).

Flat foot (pes planus)

Flat foot simply means a foot with a large plantar contact area. Often the longitudinal arch is not visible and there may be some valgus of the heel. Flat foot can be flexible (physiological) or rigid (pathological).

Physiological flat foot

Physiological flat feet are very common, flexible, benign and a normal variant. Flexible flat foot can be divided into two types: developmental and static. Parents are often concerned that as their child starts to walk the feet appear to roll over. Until the age of 3–5 years, most children do not show a longitudinal arch when weight-bearing. Developmental flat foot is apparent when the child starts to walk and disappears spontaneously at around the age of 3–5 years. Asking the child to stand on tiptoe or using the great-toe extension test (Rose et al 1986) will demonstrate restoration of the medial arch to anxious parents.

Static flat feet are associated with generalized laxity and often other family members have flat feet.

Some children with ligamentous laxity due to conditions such as Down's syndrome or Marfan's syndrome may need orthotic support or high-top trainers to help them achieve stability for weight-bearing activity.

Flexible flat feet require no treatment. Advice regarding choice of shoe wear may be needed (high-top trainers, integral medial arch support, shock absorbence soles) and only occasionally is orthotic support indicated. The tendency for overtreatment of physiological flat feet by exercises, orthotics and special shoe wear is still observed, resulting in high-cost, ineffective treatment. Printed information can be very useful for the family to take home to share with anxious grandparents (Staheli 1998).

Pathological flat foot

Pathological flat foot shows some degree of stiffness, such as loss of subtalar movement or tightness of the Achilles tendon (less than 10° dorsiflexion). The deformities can be due to:

- Intrauterine crowding (talipes calcaneovalgus)
- Abnormal alignment of the tarsal bones (congenital vertical talus (CVT), tarsal coalition)
- A combination of Achilles tendon contracture with hypermobility.

Talipes calcaneovalgus

Talipes calcaneovalgus will resolve spontaneously but demonstration of passive stretches into plantarflexion and inversion, to be carried out regularly with nappy changes, may be helpful in supporting the parents. It is also important to look at the whole patient.

Congenital vertical talus

CVT is a severe foot deformity in which the head of the talus can be felt in the sole of the foot. Viewed from the side, the foot will have a rocker-bottom appearance with fixed equinus of the hindfoot and calcaneus and valgus of the forefoot. Surgical management is necessary to realign the talus.

Physiotherapy, although not necessary for the foot deformity, may be indicated as CVT is associated with neuromuscular problems and various syndromes as well as neural defects and spinal anomalies. Physiotherapy may help a child achieve developmental milestones as well as manage other joint and soft-tissue deformities that would be amenable to serial splintage, passive stretches, positioning advice, provision of aids and equipment.

Tarsal coalitions

Tarsal coalitions, also known as peroneal spastic flat foot, can be unilateral or bilateral. There may be a family history. The commonest sites are between the calcaneus and the navicular or the talus and calcaneus. The usual initial presentation is after a simple twist or sprain of the foot or ankle in a child over the age of 10 years. An abnormal fibrous band, present from birth, between the bones begins to ossify at around this age, causing stiffness and pain. At this stage a child may be referred for physiotherapy, as there may be difficulties in walking and running, as well as pain. However if the symptoms persist a child may be viewed as exaggerating the symptoms, if peroneal spasm is not recognized. At this stage the foot will be held in valgus and passive inversion causes pain, usually over the lateral border of the foot. The medial arch is not restored when the child attempts to stand on tiptoe. Immobilization of the foot and ankle in a plaster cast will relieve symptoms, which commonly relapse when the cast is removed. Surgical resection of the bar can be successful in relieving symptoms.

Physiotherapy may be needed to restore range of movement and re-educate gait after the postoperative plaster has been removed.

Hypermobile flat foot with a tight Achilles tendon

This combination will alter foot mechanics as well as producing obligatory heel valgus (valgus ab equinus), which may cause discomfort and in the long term lead to pain and arthritis. Contracture of the heel cord is apparent on assessment. Flat foot is present on standing but the medial arch is restored when standing on tiptoe. Dorsiflexion is usually absent beyond neutral.

A programme of weight-bearing stretching exercises may help in cases of mild contracture. However, application of below-knee plasters to maintain a sustained stretch is probably more beneficial. If pain recurs after plaster removal, surgery should be considered. Physiotherapy may be indicated if there are mobility problems following removal of plaster.

Neurogenic causes

Flat foot associated with neurological conditions, such as cerebral palsy and myelomingocele, results from valgus of the foot secondary to heel cord contractures. Management options will depend on the severity of the underlying condition and functional level. Serial casting and splintage may be successful in the management of mild contractures. Consideration may be given to the use of pharmacological agents to help decrease muscle spasm to facilitate treatment goals. Surgical lengthening of the Achilles tendon may be needed in extreme contracture with provision of appropriate supportive splintage to maintain position, particularly if there is imbalance of muscle power around the foot and ankle. Any splints provided, particularly for children with reduced skin sensation in their lower limb, should be closely monitored to prevent pressure sores.

Congenital talipes equinovarus

Congenital talipes equinovarus (CTEV), commonly known as club foot, is a common deformity in which the foot is pointing downwards and inwards. Its cause remains unknown and its treatment empirical (Catterall 2002).

Club foot can be broadly categorized into four types:

1. Positional – this is a normal foot, which was held in an abnormal position in utero. The bony anatomy of the foot is normal and the foot will usually correct spontaneously or with appropriate passive stretches carried out regularly by the carer
2. Teratogenic – this is club foot associated with neurological conditions such as spina bifida or sacral agenesis
3. Syndromic – syndromic club foot is associated with conditions such as arthrogryposis, Freeman–Sheldon syndrome and congenital myopathy
4. Congenital – there is abnormal bony anatomy which is not associated with a neuromuscular cause or syndrome.

Aetiology

The prevalence of CTEV is said to be 1–3 per 1000 live births in the UK. Worldwide there are marked variations in incidence, suggesting racial and genetic factors. In China and Japan the rate is 0.5/1000 whereas the incidence in the Pacific islands and the Maori race is of the order of 6–7/1000 live births. Some of this variation may be explained by the inclusion (or exclusion) of positional club foot and syndromic club foot in the reporting. Increasingly, club foot is being diagnosed antenatally by ultrasound (Tillet et al 2000).

Club foot is commoner in boys than girls, with an incidence of 2.5:1. Seasonal variations in incidence have also been reported (Pryor et al 1991, Barker & Macnicol 2002). Effects of intrauterine moulding and environmental factors such as first pregnancy, oligohydraminos and twin pregnancy may be contributory factors to the deformity but do not explain the marked calf muscle wasting.

The high incidence of familial club foot suggests an inherited abnormality, which could be of neurological or vascular origin. A number of studies have established that the foot in utero develops in an equinovarus position, moving into a calcaneovalgus position as the pregnancy progresses. It has been postulated that an incident at around the 10–13-week gestational stage prevents the foot position from progressing. It has also been observed that the blood supply to the limb is changing from primordial to secondary at this stage. Failure of this change has been linked to cessation of growth of the foot and development of the deformity (Hootnick et al 1982). Underlying neurological causes such as spinal dysraphism may explain the muscle imbalance, calf wasting and small foot and are now considered to be a major factor in the high recurrence rate of the deformity with growth in some cases. Differences in muscle fibre type have been identified with a high proportion of type 1 fibres, increased fibrosis and reduced excursion in the lower-limb muscles of club foot, as well as changes in the structure of ligaments, particularly on the medial side of the foot compared to the norm (Handelsman & Badalamente 1981, Zimny et al 1985, Macnicol et al 1992).

Pathology

Bony changes

As well as fixed joint deformities throughout the foot and ankle, many bones in the foot are of abnormal shape and size. Disturbances in the growth of the bones of the whole affected limb may become apparent later, resulting in a limb-length discrepancy, which is more common in girls with club foot than boys.

Joint deformities

In the ankle joint the head of the talus points downwards and medially and there may be anterior subluxation in severe deformities. Fixed deformity will also be present in the talonavicular and calcaneocuboid joints with possible subluxations. There will be cavus deformity at the tarsometatarsal joints caused by shortening of the plantar fascia and long and short plantar ligaments.

Muscle changes

The most obvious change is calf muscle wasting. The amount of wasting appears to be directly related to the severity and stiffness of the foot deformity. Individual muscle fibre size is decreased but not decreased in amount, particularly in the peronei. There are more type 1 fibres and increased fibrosis in the muscles themselves, especially in the calf muscles and tibialis posterior, and less so in the long-toe flexors. Muscle imbalance is particularly noticed between the peronei, elongated and weaker because of the foot position, and tibialis anterior, which is tight and apparently stronger because of reduced excursion of the foot.

Effects of growth

The foot doubles in size in the first year of life. As the soft tissues must grow at the same rate, the underlying abnormal changes inherent in these structure, as well as disturbances in bony and cartilaginous growth, explain the recurrence of deformity at times of rapid growth.

Dynamic concept of the foot

The bones making up the medial and lateral rays of the foot are linked together by interosseous ligaments and various plantar ligaments. Movement of the foot at the ankle and subtalar joint is restricted by the elasticity of these tethers as well as joint capsules, ligaments and the insertion of tibialis anterior. In club foot deformity the movement is further restricted by abnormalities in the composition of these structures (Figure 13.1).

Management

The aim of club foot management should be to correct the foot position carefully, without injuring the soft cartilaginous structures of the foot, and retain mobility. The foot should be plantargrade, have a normal load-bearing area and fit into normal shoes. Surgical division of inelastic structures should be looked on as a protective incident during continuing therapy. Flattening of the dome of the talus as well as damage to the lower tibial growth plate have been attributed to aggressive conservative treatments, such as forced dorsiflexion of the hindfoot before correction of the forefoot deformity using, for example, adhesive strapping (Lloyd-Roberts 1964, Dobbs et al 2004).

It is generally accepted that initial treatment for club foot should be some form of serial splintage, traditionally carried out under the supervision of a physiotherapist, and started soon after birth. There are varied opinions regarding the method of conservative management use.

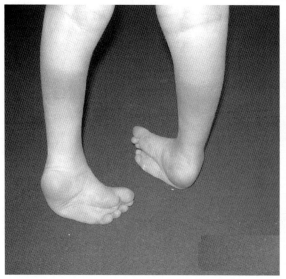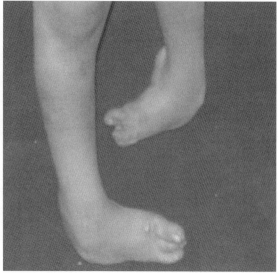

Figure 13.1 A 6-year-old boy with untreated bilateral club feet, surprisingly able to walk, run and play football. (a) Back view;

In recent times the Ponseti method (carefully applied serial full-leg plaster casts, early Achilles tendon tenotomy and the use of boots and bar to maintain the corrected position) following an exacting and defined regime has gained popularity. Contemporary reports state that feet treated with this regime have improved long-term outcomes compared to feet treated by more traditional means (Herzenberg et al 2002, Ippolito et al 2003, Dobbs et al 2004).

There are many assessment tools used to evaluate club foot deformity by the physiotherapist but the resurgence of the Ponseti method in the last decade has resulted in the adoption of the Pirani scale as a valid outcome tool to determine the effects of the serial casting (Patel & Herzenberg 2005). Prior to this, most assessment tools were descriptive of the deformity but were not sensitive enough to detect effects of therapy (Harrold & Walker 1983, Catterall 1991).

The Pirani scale records the salient features of the deformity as follows:

Hindfoot deformity

- The rigidity of the equinus deformity
- The depth of the posterior crease
- The ability to palpate the calcaneus at the posterior aspect of the heel.

Midfoot deformity

- The depth of the medial crease
- The position of the head of the talus
- The curvature of the lateral border of the foot.

These six items are each scored from 1 (most severe) through 0.5 to zero for full correction of each item. A score of 6 denotes a foot with severe deformity.

Reappraisal of the foot position with every plaster change, using the scale, will give an objective score for each element of the deformity as well as charting progress in the midfoot and hindfoot, with a total score for the whole foot.

At some stage surgical release of the Achilles tendon will be required for some patients. Careful full-leg plasters are applied immediately afterwards with the foot in dorsiflexion of 20° and everted to at least 50°. Approximately 3 weeks later the plaster is removed and boots attached to a bar, keeping the feet in 70° eversion and 20° dorsiflexion, are applied. Ponseti recommends that these are worn full-time for the first 3 months, apart from when bathing, and then at nighttime until the child is 4 years of age (Figure 13.2).

Although the popularity of the Ponseti method is spreading, other methods of serial splintage, such as application of adhesive strapping, are still in use. Whatever the method used, much care should be taken, as excessive compressive pressure on the soft cartilage can result in permanent damage. Remember that the feet you are treating are very young – they have to last a full lifetime!

Once the deformity has been corrected, the opinion of physiotherapists regarding ongoing input or review seems to be divided. There is the propensity for club foot to recur with growth and many therapists view it as important that a child who had club foot is monitored. Further serial casting or soft-tissue surgery may be needed and therapy input following procedures will be to reduce joint stiffness, re-educate gait patterns and, in the case of muscle transfer, encourage and strengthen the muscle in its new action.

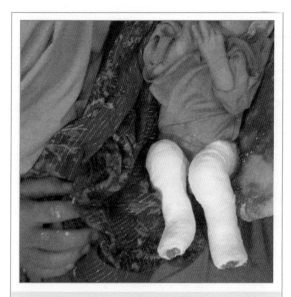

Figure 13.2 Ponseti treatment for a 4-week-old child with bilateral club feet in Afghanistan.

Children with stiffness at the ankle and subtalar joint often complain of problems with balance and still find standing difficult. Although they are able to run, they are often much slower than their peers. Advice may be needed regarding appropriate activities in which the child can partake on equal terms, such as swimming and cycling.

Severe recurrent deformities, as the child gets older, will need corrective bony surgery, either carried out conventionally or with the use of external fixators such as the Ilizarov frame. Physiotherapy input will again be needed.

KNEES

Anterior knee pain

Overuse injuries causing aching or pain around one or both knees are relatively common complaints, particularly in young people who engage in sport. Traction injuries tend to occur wherever powerful muscles, such as the quadriceps, attach to bone, particularly during periods of rapid skeletal growth.

Osgood–Schlatter's disease

Osgood–Schlatter's disease is a stress-related partial avulsion of the tibial tubercle apophysis. Pain, swelling and tenderness are located over the tibial tubercle and may be very troublesome during the inflammatory stage. Young people are often advised to restrict their activity, rest the affected part and take analgesia. In cases of severe pain the limb may

be immobilized in a plaster cast. As this is a self-limiting condition, which may be problematic for varying periods until skeletal maturity, many young people find it frustrating to have activity levels restricted and some may also find little sympathy from the PE teacher. Liaison with the school may be necessary so that the young person can be excused from physical activity during painful episodes (see Ch. 16).

The following physiotherapy interventions can be useful in managing the symptoms:

- Ice applied to the part may relieve pain and reduce swelling.
- Strapping to relieve the pull of the quadriceps tendon on the tibial tubercle can be very effective and allows the young person to walk with reduced or no pain. Visual analogue scales can be used to assess the effectiveness of the strapping and, if strapping is seen to be effective, the young person can be trained to apply the strapping when there is pain or before partaking in activities that may cause symptoms.
- Hamstring-stretching exercises. Many young people with Osgood–Schlatter's disease have tight hamstrings and may also have accompanying tightness of the Achilles tendon. Hamstring-stretching exercises will give more length to the muscle, thereby decreasing the mild flexor tightness at the knee when weight-bearing, allowing less tension to be placed on to the quadriceps insertion. A combination of appropriate muscle-stretching exercises and patella tendon strapping can be very effective in reducing symptoms. Quadriceps stretching may be indicated but may not be tolerated whilst there is severe pain.

Osteochondritis dissecans

Osteochondritis dissecans is probably due to repetitive trauma to segments of bone with a marginal blood supply, usually the lateral border of the medial femoral condyle. A piece of articular cartilage, with or without the subchondral bone, becomes unstable or may become detached, forming a loose body. A child will complain of knee pain, with tenderness located over the lesion, and effusion may also be present. If a loose body occurs there may be locking of the joint.

The cause is uncertain but there may be a positive family history in some patients, patellar instability, knee malalignment or discoid meniscus in others. Juvenile boys are affected twice as frequently as girls (Macnicol & Jackson 2002).

A child may be advised to rest the joint initially and icing can be used to reduce pain and swelling. Static quadriceps exercises can be started to prevent muscle-wasting, followed by a programme of progressive exercise to regain range of motion, strength, power, endurance and coordination. Advice may be needed regarding the gradual resumption of appropriate sporting activities. Symptoms should gradually settle.

Troublesome loose bodies will require surgical removal. Physiotherapy will then focus on preventing muscle weakness, restoring range of movement, re-educating gait and return to activity.

HIPS

Perthes disease

Perthes disease is also known as Legg–Calvé–Perthes disease, Waldenström's disease or cox plana. Perthes disease is an idiopathic juvenile necrosis of the femoral head and remains poorly understood. The head of the femur undergoes early-stage infarction, followed by collapse and fragmentation of the femoral head and then gradual healing. The whole process may take 3–4 years to complete.

Perthes disease is more common in boys and typically occurs between the age of 3 and 12 years. There may be a family history of Perthes and the boy is often on the lower percentiles for height. It can be bilateral but with an interval between onset on each side. A painful limp which comes and goes or aching or pain around the knee or thigh is usually the first sign and may have been present for several months before advice is sought. Loss of hip movement may follow, with loss of medial rotation at first, and then abduction.

During the disease process it is now generally accepted that the hip should be kept as mobile as possible with the aim of preventing a flexion/adduction contracture and encouraging the hip to remodel as a congruent joint (Jones & Hill 2000). Although the use of crutches may be advised to rest the joint, these should only be used for short periods of time as relying on crutches encourages the limb to develop a flexed adducted posture. Exercise programmes aimed at maintaining hip abduction range and hip extension by stretches, prone-lying and active exercise are very useful. Hydrotherapy is an excellent medium to increase range of movement and allows a child to exercise without undue stress on the joint. Activities which stress the joint such as trampolining or contact sports are generally discouraged.

Some children may need surgery to achieve containment of the femoral head. Physiotherapy will be needed to mobilize and strengthen the limb as well as re-educate gait once weight-bearing is permitted.

Most children with Perthes have a good prognosis for function in the long term. Young children and those with partial femoral head involvement do better than older children.

LIMB-LENGTH DISCREPANCY

Opinions vary on the adverse effects of limb-length discrepancy and causal effects such as the development of low-back pain, scoliosis and hip and knee problems in adulthood are unproven.

Broadly, the causes of limb-length discrepancies can be divided into those of congenital origin and those that have been acquired.

Congenital

Congenital causes vary from mild deficiency to complete absence. Features associated with congenital deficiency are:

- Skin dimpling
- Abnormality and instability in adjacent joints (anterior cruciate deficiency or complete absence; ball-and-socket ankle joint may be present)
- Shortening elsewhere in the limb, e.g. although the shortening may be most obvious in the fibula, there will also be some shortening in the femur and foot as well as possible absence of rays in the foot
- Abnormal soft tissues with increased fibrosis, which do not like to stretch and therefore will challenge the physiotherapist if surgical lengthening is undertaken
- Curvature or other deformity in the involved bone.

Acquired

Infection

Damage to growth plates may occur following septicaemia, with resulting loss of linear growth (and deformity if the growth plate has been affected asymmetrically). Septic arthritis, especially in the hip joint, can cause avascular necrosis and growth plate damage. Osteomyelitis may result in bone necrosis and loss.

Vascular

Growth plates are very vascular structures. Drip extravasation injuries, radiation and burns may damage the blood supply to the growth plate, leading to temporary or permanent cessation of growth. Hyperaemia (increased vascularization) around the growth plate will likewise cause increased growth in the bone (juvenile arthritis, vascular malformation).

Neurological

Abormalities affecting the spine, such as spinal dysraphism and spina bifida, resulting in more weakness in one limb than the other, will result in a limb-length discrepancy on that side. The mild limb-length discrepancy seen in hemiplegia can be advantageous in allowing foot clearance during swing phase. Polio is a major cause of limb-length discrepancy worldwide.

Trauma

Fractures in children may result in initial overgrowth of the limb but usually need no treatment. Fractures through a growth plate will lead to premature closure and cessation of bone growth and have much more serious implications. If the closure is not complete then the consequential asymmetrical growth will lead to deformity as well as shortening. The younger the child at the time of injury, the greater the loss of bone growth potential and the greater the deformity. For example, an injury resulting in complete closure of the lower femoral growth plate in an 8-year-old girl could result in an 8–9-cm leg-length discrepancy at skeletal maturity.

Other causes

Other causes include conditions such as Ollier's disease, in which there are masses of hyaline cartilage in the metaphyses of long bones, commonly the leg. The severity of involvement, usually asymmetric, can lead to marked deformity as well as shortening in the more severely involved limb.

Irradiation injuries to growth plates following bone tumour treatment, as well as resection of tumours, will require management of the resultant discrepancy.

Measuring limb-length discrepancy

The accepted method of measuring limb lengths, apart from radiologically, is to use a tape measure placed on the ASIS and the medial malleolus of the limb. In cases of congenital causes for the difference in limb length, there may be associated problems with growth in the foot. It is usual in centres advising on limb-length problems to measure from the ASIS to the base of the heel with the foot in a plantargrade position – the functional leg-length discrepancy. A more sensitive method is for children to stand with blocks under the short limb, looking to see if the iliac crests are level, the knees equally extended and, most importantly, asking them whether they feel balanced and adjusting the height of the blocks until they do feel so.

Management options (Hill & Tucker 1997, Jackson et al 2002)

The amount of shortening, predicted skeletal majority and the stability of adjacent joints are used to decide which management option would be the best for a child.

The options can broadly be categorized as follows:

- Under 3 cm: treatment is not necessary unless children have a limp which is bothering them. In such cases a shoe raise can be offered – 1 cm can be placed inside the shoe. Such a small raise is unseen and therefore more acceptable to a fashion-conscious teenager.
- 3–5 cm: a shoe raise is used: this can be split, with 1 cm inside the shoe and the rest outside. Nowadays

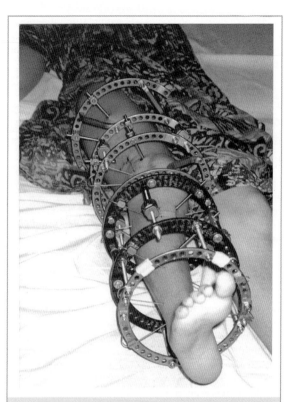

Figure 13.3 The Ilizarov frame being used for femoral and tibial lengthening for a girl with a 12-cm leg-length discrepancy.

shoe raises can be integrated into most shoe soles and are not so obvious to casual observers. However, providing a raised shoe for a child who will not wear one is expensive and unnecessary treatment *or*

- Epiphysiodesis: slowing down the growth of the longer leg by drilling out a growth plate or plates around the knee at an appropriate time, giving the shorter leg time to catch up, achieving equality at cessation of growth.
- 5–15 cm: lengthening of the short leg (see below) *or*
- Combination of lengthening the short leg and epiphysiodesis for the long leg
- More than 15 cm: lengthening and shortening may be considered
- Use of an extension prosthesis
- Amputation and provision of a prosthesis – probably a better long-term functional outcome compared to a child who has undergone 2–3 lengthening procedures to achieve equal leg lengths at skeletal maturity.

Limb-lengthening

The choice of an external fixator to carry out bone lengthening is between a circular frame such as the Ilizarov (Figure 13.3) or Taylor spatial (Figure 13.4) or a

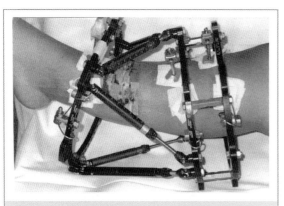

Figure 13.4 Taylor spatial frame for deformity correction of Blount's disease (severe tibia vara).

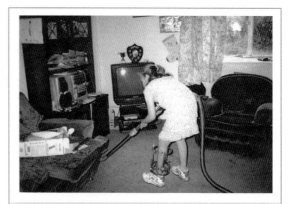

Figure 13.5 Helping with the housework!

monolateral fixator such as the Orthofix. Although there are advantages and disadvantages for each, circular frames tend to be used with increasing frequency as they are stable, versatile, adjustable during the lengthening and allow weight-bearing.

Surgery to lengthen a bone involves the application of an external fixator, cutting the bone, a wait of a few days to allow bone healing to commence and then gradually and slowly separating the healing bone. As the gap between the bone ends widens, new bone forms in the gap. Bone lengthening is usually carried out four times a day when the fixator is adjusted to allow a widening of the gap by 0.25 mm, giving a total increase in bone length of 1 mm a day Therefore a 7-cm lengthening will take 75 days to achieve. Adjustment of the fixator is quickly taken over by the family.

Once the bone is out to length, the distraction stops and the bone is allowed to harden off. This equates to approximately 30–35 days per centimetre gained in the frame.

Physiotherapy for children undergoing limb-lengthening and limb reconstruction procedures

The physiotherapist is an essential member of the multidisciplinary team managing children undergoing procedures to achieve limb-length equalization and should be involved at every stage to provide advice and therapy.

Hill & Tucker (1997) suggested that preparation beforehand is very important to ensure that a child and family are fully informed about the length of time the treatment will take and have realistic expectations, as there will be much disruption to school and home life. Preadmission clinics are a useful forum for such discussion and allow the team to plan for wheelchair provision, a reducible shoe raise if needed, make contact with the local physiotherapy team to arrange ongoing therapy once the child has returned home as well as making sure that any issues that may compromise the treatment are dealt with before a child is admitted.

Aims of physiotherapy:

- Maintain joint range of movement
- Maintain muscle length and strength
- Encourage functional weight-bearing activity
- Anticipate (and deal with) problems!

Preoperative assessment of joint range of movement, stability and muscle length and strength are necessary to pre-empt the development of problems during the bone-lengthening phase. Simple splints to maintain the foot in a plantargrade position during tibial lengthening should be made preoperatively and applied soon after a child has returned to the ward.

No child should be expected to perform exercises or weight-bear in the postoperative period without adequate analgesia given in plenty of time to be effective during physiotherapy sessions. Functional weight-bearing exercises and mobility are to be encouraged for those children in circular frames (Ilizarov, Taylor spatial frame), whereas those with monolateral fixators should not weight-bear during the callus distraction phase and will be allowed to take weight progressively during the bone consolidation phase, on the surgeon's advice. Discharge home should be planned when a child is mobile on crutches, is able to go up and down stairs and perform transfers (from chair to bed, from chair to floor and back) independently or with minimal help. Home exercise programmes are useful whilst a child awaits input from the local community physiotherapy team.

As children increase in confidence, they should be encouraged to be as active as possible in their circular frames (Figure 13.5). Many children manage to be very active in their frames and ride bikes, use climbing frames,

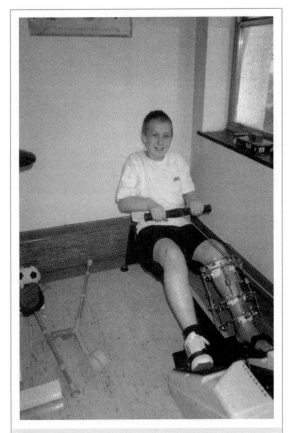

Figure 13.6 Working out in the gym. Return to normal life is to be encouraged.

play tennis and swim (Figure 13.6). Hydrotherapy is an excellent medium to encourage activity and is usually much enjoyed.

Managing problems (Eldridge & Bell 1991)

Joint range of movement may decrease during the callus distraction phase, not only because movement may be restricted by the fixator itself, but also as the soft tissues come under tension as the bone length increases. At this time it may be prudent to increase therapy input to regain lost range, using specific stretches, exercises and serial casting. Once the lengthening has finished there will be time to regain lost range of movement. Contractures are particularly likely to occur when lengthening congenitally short bones and the potential for knee joint subluxation during femoral lengthening is a major concern.

Pin site infections are painful and a child will tend to hold the joint nearest the inflamed pin site in a flexed position. A course of antibiotics and analgesia are often needed and the child will need much encouragement to stretch out the flexed joint. Very occasionally, if there is

persistent infection at a pin site a child may be admitted for the wire to be re-sited under general anaesthetic.

Poor new bone formation may be due to the underlying pathology, particularly when there is a congenital bone problem, but more commonly it is because a child is not taking weight through the limb. Many children become very adept at hopping around on their crutches. Circular frames are very strong and full weight-bearing is possible from the start. Although many children need crutches to help with balance, very young children and children with upper-limb as well as lower-limb deficiency tend to get up and walk without hand-held aids.

Psychosocial issues also need to be taken into account. The fixator will be attached to a child's limb for several months. After the initial excitement it all gets very boring. If children are not able to get to school or meet their friends they become very isolated. Issues around body image, particularly in adolescence, can further compound matters. Many children may experience times of low mood or anger during their treatment, which may challenge their physiotherapy sessions.

Once the bone is assessed as being sufficiently strong to bear weight without the support of the fixator, the apparatus is removed. A child then gradually increases the amount of weight taken through the limb over a period of 4–6 weeks, progressing from partial to full weight-bearing. Plaster casts are used very occasionally, only if there are concerns about strength of the bone when the fixator is removed. Physiotherapy may need to be continued to regain lost range of movement, increase muscle strength and re-educate gait. However it is important to be aware that a congenital short limb, although now a longer limb, will still have abnormalities in adjacent joints. A ball-and-socket ankle joint, as a result of fibular deficiency, remains as such. Now the child no longer walks on tiptoe but with the foot flat, the previously unnoticed valgus at the ankle is suddenly apparent.

Many children with congenital bone deficiencies will require repeat lengthening procedures to achieve limb-length equality at skeletal maturity. Although limb-lengthening is demanding and time-consuming for therapists, careful attention to detail can produce successful results. Young adults who underwent limb-lengthening as children reported high levels of satisfaction and few physical, occupational or psychosocial problems (Hartley et al 2003).

OBSTETRICAL BRACHIAL PLEXUS PALSY (OBPP)

This unfortunate birth injury is always due to a tearing force on the cervical nerve roots caused by extreme traction of the head from the shoulder girdle during delivery (Boome & Kaye 1988, Geutjens et al 1996).

Gilbert (2002) describes two basic types of lesion:

1. Overweight babies (more than 4 kg) in a vertex presentation and with shoulder dystocia (the shoulders

becoming stuck in the birth canal) whose delivery requires excess force by traction, usually with forceps or ventouse extraction, resulting in injury to the upper nerve roots (C5, C6 and occasionally C7) but never the lower nerve roots.

2. Breech presentation, usually of small babies (less than 3 kg) requiring excessive extension of the head and, often, manipulation of the hand and arm in such a fashion that exerts traction on both the upper and lower roots, causing rupture or avulsion of any, or occasionally all, of the roots.

Other risk factors are prolonged second stage of labour (over 60 minutes), a previous child with OBPP, as well as multiple parity.

The initial diagnosis is apparent at birth, as the upper limb is flail and dangling. Examination of the other limbs is important to exclude neonatal quadriplegia. Fractures of the humerus or clavicle can be associated with this injury and occasionally bilateral OBPP has been reported.

Classification of the lesion should be undertaken no earlier than 48 hours after delivery, when a more accurate examination and muscle testing can be undertaken and will allow the patterns of paresis to be differentiated:

1. Erb–Duchenne: paralysis of the upper nerve roots. The arm is held in internal rotation and pronation. The elbow may be held in extension (C5–6) or slight flexion (C5–7). There is flexion of the fingers and thumb but no extension. Pectoralis major is usually unaffected, giving an appearance of forward flexion at the shoulder. There are no vasomotor changes, nor marked sensory loss in the hand.

2. Dejerine–Klumpke: complete paralysis. The entire arm is flail and the hand fisted. Vasomotor impairment gives the limb a pale or marbled appearance and sensation is diminished. Horner's sign (constriction of the pupil, drooping of the eyelid and lack of sweating on the affected side of the face and neck) may be present.

In between these two types are injuries involving primarily C7 and sometimes C8 and T1, as well as injury involving C8 and T1.

Prognosis

Most children with OBPP achieve full recovery from their birth injury, with reported rates varying between 75% and 95% (Narakas 1987, Eng et al 1996, Gilbert 2002).

Guidelines for recovery give an indication of outcome:

- Complete or close to complete recovery if biceps and deltoid activity is present by the end of the first month and normal contraction by the end of the second month.

- Poorer results will be found in those infants who have neither deltoid nor biceps contraction by the third month. As testing of deltoid is difficult in small babies, assessment of biceps, looking for any active contraction, is the most reliable indicator for operative intervention. However, if recovery is reached by 3½ months, there will still be satisfactory function.

- Referral should be made to a specialist centre if there is no recovery in biceps by 3 months of age to consider surgery. Nerve grafting may be carried out and postoperative recovery will begin by 6–10 months and continue for 2 years in upper nerve root lesions for 3–4 years in complete lesions (Gilbert et al 1988, Duclos & Gilbert 1995).

Physiotherapy

Evidence-based guidelines (Association of Paediatric Chartered Physiotherapists 2002) have been published to aid the management of babies who have sustained OBPP.

Early intervention (birth–6 months)

The clinical position will change rapidly, and although muscle charting and assessment may be carried out not less than 48 hours after birth, a full range of passive movement of the hand, wrist, forearm and elbow can begin immediately.

Movement of the shoulder should preferably be started at 5 days of age.

Both limbs should be compared when assessing active movement and regular reassessment of muscle power will show whether there is recovery in the limb.

Continuing physiotherapy should concentrate on educating the parent/carer on:

- Correct positioning and handling of the limb
- Passive stretches to prevent muscle and joint contractures (Figures 13.7 and 13.8)
- Tactile stimulation
- Weight-bearing exercises through the affected limb, when indicated.

Physiotherapy is important to maintain a full and equal range of movement in all the joints of the limb whilst awaiting recovery. Parents are instructed to carry out stretches regularly throughout the day, e.g. at nappy changes. Of particular importance is maintaining range of movement at the shoulder joint to prevent contracture of the subscapularis, teres major and latissimus dorsi and deformation of the humeral head in the long term. Specific stretches should also be aimed at maintaining lateral rotation, abduction and elevation of the shoulder as well as scapulohumeral movement. It is advisable that regular contact is maintained by the physiotherapist during the first 3 months so that judicious referral to a specialist centre is made for surgical opinion regarding nerve grafting.

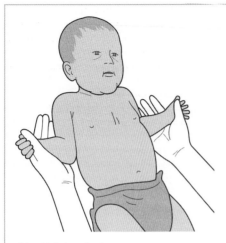

(a) Lie baby on back.

Bend both elbows and keep elbows tucked into side of body.

Roll arms outward and down towards surface.

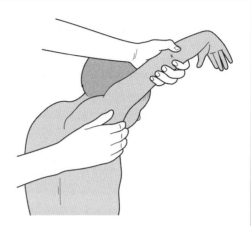

(b) Lie baby on unaffected side.

Hold shoulder blade down firmly against chest wall with thumb and palm.

Lift arm out to side and stretch up towards head.

Keep shoulder blade throughout the stretch.

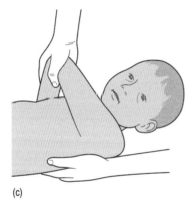

Lie baby on back.

Hold shoulder blade firmly to chest wall and gently stretch arm across to the opposite shoulder.

Keep the elbow at shoulder level.

(c)

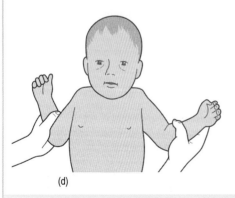

Lie baby on back.

Hold elbows bent by sides.

Slide arms up to head.

Keep arms as near to bed as possible.

(d)

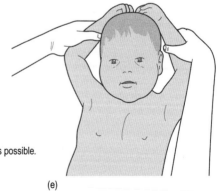

(e)

Figure 13.7 Parental information to prevent contractures at the shoulder. Reproduced by kind permission of Association of Paediatric Chartered Physiotherapists.

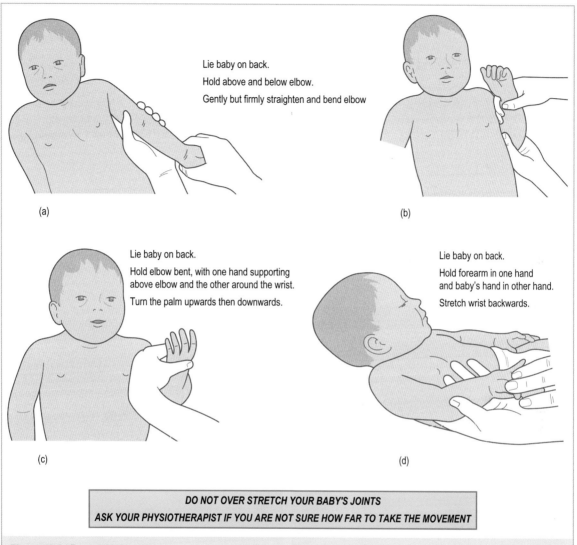

(a) Lie baby on back.
Hold above and below elbow.
Gently but firmly straighten and bend elbow

(b)

(c) Lie baby on back.
Hold elbow bent, with one hand supporting above elbow and the other around the wrist.
Turn the palm upwards then downwards.

(d) Lie baby on back.
Hold forearm in one hand and baby's hand in other hand.
Stretch wrist backwards.

DO NOT OVER STRETCH YOUR BABY'S JOINTS
ASK YOUR PHYSIOTHERAPIST IF YOU ARE NOT SURE HOW FAR TO TAKE THE MOVEMENT

Figure 13.8 Parental information to prevent contractures at elbow and wrist. Reproduced by kind permission of Association of Paediatric Chartered Physiotherapists.

After 6 months of age advice may be needed to encourage awareness and use of the affected limb, as well as ideas to help the child with physical development if there is slow recovery.

Advice for older children (nursery to adolescence)

Following early intervention, many children with OBPP no longer receive physiotherapy but evidence suggests that review throughout growth is desirable as problems may emerge or become more apparent over time. Problems such as progressive loss of external rotation at the shoulder or scapular winging may become more apparent as a child becomes functionally independent. As children get older they should be encouraged to take responsibility for the exercise and stretching programme, using age-appropriate activities. The physiotherapist may be asked to advise the school on appropriate activities but children with OBPP should be encouraged to take part in all activities at school, as they are able. Extra time may be needed to complete tasks and advice from an occupational therapist may be useful to provide equipment to help them achieve their full potential. Occupational therapy may be needed to help with fine motor skills.

Physiotherapy following surgery

Surgical intervention may be needed to increase range of movement in joints to facilitate function, such as sub-scapular release to improve lateral rotation at the shoulder or osteotomy to place an arc of movement into a more useful position. Physiotherapy to maintain the range of movement gained by the soft-tissue releases and to encourage functional use of the arm is needed to maximize any opportunity given by the surgery.

TORTICOLLIS

Torticollis, from the Latin *tortus* (twisted) and *collis* (column), is a descriptive term of abnormal posture in which the head and neck are held in side flexion towards the affected side, with rotation of the head to the opposite side. Ballock & Song (1996) stated that in the literature there are more than 80 causes for torticollis. They suggested an algorithm to determine differential diagnoses, which can be summarized thus:

- Muscular: contracture of the sternomastoid muscle on one side, noted in the early months of life. Although the cause may be undetermined, it is thought that it may have been some sort of trauma during delivery
- Trauma: fractures of the upper humerus, clavical, C1–2 subluxation (Figure 13.9)
- Congenital: abnormal formation of the cervical spine resulting in bony deformity
- Infection: viral infections causing inflammation of the cervical glands, retropharyngeal abscesses
- Occular problems: squint, visual field defects
- Neurological: such as dystonia, posterior fossa tumours, Sandifer's syndrome
- Pain: bone tumours such as osteoid osteoma, Ewing's sarcoma
- Idiopathic: no obvious organic cause.

Congenital muscular torticollis (CMT)

CMT may not be noticed initially but at around the age 4 months or so, the parent may notice a lump in the muscle (sternomastoid tumour), level with the angle of the jaw, which is apparent when the baby cries. There may be accompanying plagiocephaly and on assessment it is obvious that there is restriction of movement at the

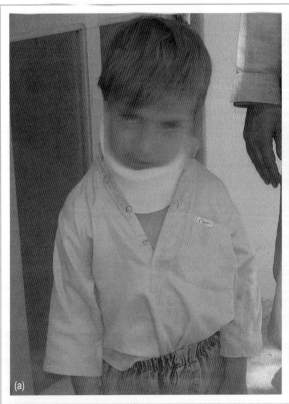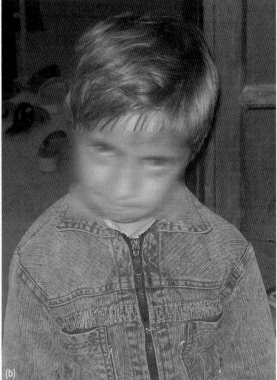

Figure 13.9 (a) A 5-year-old boy with Down's syndrome who acquired a torticollis after a fall. (b) Neck supported in a collar.

neck on that side. Tightness of the sternocleidomastoid muscle may not be accompanied by a tumour.

At this stage the baby may be referred for physiotherapy. Traditionally physiotherapy has consisted of passive stretches to the neck carried out by two people, one to stabilize the shoulder girdle whilst the other stretches the neck by exerting traction using the baby's head. Although it is generally agreed that muscle stretching should not be painful, the literature seems to have little consensus on the frequency or the number of stretches needed (Emery 1994, Staheli 1998, Cheng et al 2000). Usually the family are taught the stretches and advised to carry out them out several times a day. The physiotherapist then leaves the family to carry out the stretches in between appointments. The baby quickly learns that being placed on its back may spell trouble, the hands come down from above and the baby tenses and cries as soon as it is touched, leaving the family fraught and tired by the time of their next appointment.

Many physiotherapists involved in the management of babies with torticollis have ceased passive stretches in this fashion and use positioning to improve the head position and muscle length, as well as encouraging active movement to address the muscle imbalance, and are finding similar success in this more 'gentle approach' (Taylor & Stammos Norton 1997). Parents are encouraged to be creative during their therapy sessions with their baby and therefore feel empowered in their baby's recovery. Strengthening the overstretched muscles on the other side of the neck can be achieved through the use of postural reactions as the baby gains head control, such as the neck-righting reflex. The parents are encouraged to hold, carry and play with the infant in positions that will encourage the desired active and passive movements.

At this age torticollis usually resolves without long-term effects. Surgical release may be necessary if there is restriction of movement by more than 20° by the age of 1 year.

Juvenile muscular torticollis

It is uncertain whether juvenile torticollis has been present but not recognized since infancy or if onset has occurred during late infancy or early childhood. Careful assessment is needed to exclude significant pathologies and a child should be referred back if there are any concerns that this is not a muscular torticollis. A child may have developed facial asymmetry and review of family photographs will show that a child's head may have always been tilted to one side. Both heads of the muscle will be contracted and require surgical release. Physiotherapy cannot overcome this contracture.

Physiotherapy following surgical release

Following surgical release of the sternomastoid muscle it will be necessary to carry out passive stretches to maintain the length achieved during the operation. Timing of postoperative physiotherapy is usually dependent on surgeon's preference but may begin as early as 24 hours. In any case it is advisable to teach the parents how to do the stretches before a child goes for surgery.

No physiotherapy should be carried out without analgesia given in good time to be effective before stretching is started. A child may also have been given a soft collar to wear for support and comfort and in the first few weeks this should only be removed for physiotherapy, washing and meals.

Stretches to the neck need to be carried out with a child lying supine with the shoulder girdle stabilized, so that the neck can be moved throughout a full range of side flexion to the opposite side and rotation to the same side as well as full extension. Gentle traction should be applied throughout and slowly released at the end of the stretch. There appears to be little in the literature about postoperative physiotherapy but generally parents seem to be advised to carry out the stretches twice a day, doing each stretch 5 times with a hold of 10–20 seconds (Emery 1994).

Active exercise is important to address the muscle imbalance resulting not only because the tight muscle is now longer and needs strengthening, but also to address the 'overlong' muscle on the opposite side. It is important to use mirror work as the child may have no concept of having the head in a central position and will need visual prompts to correct the head position between each exercise. There may also be some short-term visual disturbance until the eyes accommodate to the improved head position. Advice regarding positioning to encourage head-turning when watching TV or looking at the blackboard may be needed before the child goes home. Therapy supervision should continue until the child is habitually holding the head in the corrected position.

POSITIONAL PLAGIOCEPHALY

Flattening of the skull in babies, due to intrauterine moulding, is commonly associated with torticollis as the head tends to be turned towards the flattened side. It has been noted that the incidence of positional plagiocephaly appears to have increased since parents were advised to lay their babies on their backs to sleep to reduce the risk of sudden infant death syndrome (SIDS). Although some of these babies may have tightness of their sternomastoid muscle, many, on assessment, do not. They have a full range of passive movement but not active movement. This results in muscle imbalance which can be improved by positioning the baby to encourage it to turn its head into the desired direction, using toys and mobiles and ensuring frequent position changes so that pressure is not always on to the flattened area of the skull. In the first few months of life, supervised tummy time is important, not only to take pressure off the flattened area but also as part of the baby's general motor development, encouraging limb girdle stability, weight-bearing through the upper limbs, extension and preparation for crawling (Davis & Moon 1998, Hutchison et al 2004).

The majority of heads recover their shape as babies grow and spend less time lying on their backs. However there is increasing interest amongst anxious parents about the use of helmets to reshape their babies' heads. At the present time the medical profession remains unconvinced as to the efficacy of their use in a condition that will usually correct itself in due course.

This chapter has attempted to discuss some of the common and less common but important orthopaedic conditions that may be seen by paediatric physiotherapists in acute and community settings. The importance of careful history-taking has been discussed and the associated conditions that need to be considered during assessment identified. This is by no means an exhaustive exploration of the physiotherapist's role in the management of children with orthopaedic conditions but should be viewed as a pragmatic approach from which to build up knowledge and experience.

CASE STUDY 13.1

A 12-year-old boy with a 6-cm leg-length discrepancy due to congenital femoral deficiency underwent lengthening using an Ilizarov frame. It was apparent preoperatively that he was at risk of knee joint subluxation during the lengthening as he was anterior cruciate-deficient (increased anterior draw test and confirmed on magnetic resonance imaging). The frame was therefore extended to his upper tibial to prevent subluxation. Hinges allowed the tibial and lower femoral ring to be unlocked to permit knee flexion under the supervision of the physiotherapist. Postoperatively the boy did very well and was able to walk, initially with the help of crutches and eventually

without. Apart from one painful pin site infection, which made knee flexion exercises painful, there were no major problems apart from knee flexion being limited by the frame. He achieved his lengthening goal of 5 cm. His knee was stiff following the removal of the fixator but responded to physiotherapy over several months. He achieved full knee flexion after approximately 1 year. Eight years later the boy took part in an outcome survey following limb-lengthening. He was working as a builder, having no problems going up and down ladders, carrying loads despite his known knee instability. He played football in his spare time and stated that he had no physical limitations.

CASE STUDY 13.2

A 5-year-old boy was brought to a physiotherapy clinic in Afghanistan, following a fall 1 month before, after which he persistently held his head tilted to the left. The physiotherapist noted that he also had Down's syndrome and remembered that there was an increased risk of atlantoaxial instability in children with Down's. On examination it was not possible to for the boy to correct his head tilt. Weakness was noted in both

upper limbs. X-rays showed that there was subluxation of C1 and C2. He was referred to an American surgeon working in the clinic who recommended supporting the head and neck with a soft collar. His family were advised to take him to Pakistan for a surgical opinion. If this child had lived in a First-World country he would have been immediately referred to a neurosurgeon to have the lesion surgically stabilized.

CASE STUDY 13.3

A 6-year-old girl fell from a climbing frame. She landed awkwardly and the next day her parents noticed that she was holding her head on one side. She was seen in the local Accident and Emergency Department where an X-ray showed there was no injury to her cervical spine. She was referred for physiotherapy. On examination the physiotherapist found there was tightness of the girl's right sternomastoid, with limited neck rotation to the right and side flexion to the left. There was no spasm in the muscle and no pain on movement. The physiotherapist

also noted that there was some facial asymmetry. A photograph in the father's wallet showed the girl aged 4 years with her head tipped to the right, indicating that she probably had a congenital muscular torticollis. Further family photographs confirmed this. The child was referred to an orthopaedic surgeon for opinion and surgery was carried out to lengthen the tight muscle, accompanied by physiotherapy to maintain the improved range of movement achieved by the surgery and to address muscle imbalance and posture.

CASE STUDY 13.4

A 15-year-old boy with back pain was taken by his mother to a physiotherapist for advice regarding his posture. His mother suggested that his poor posture was due to the large weight of books he had to carry to and from school, along with his sports kit. A careful history was taken. There was obvious truncal asymmetry with significant muscle spasm and some weakness in the lower limbs. The physiotherapist referred the boy to the local hospital for an opinion. Further investigations diagnosed a spinal cord glioma, which was successfully treated by the neurosurgeons.

CASE STUDY 13.5

An 8-year-old boy was very quiet and withdrawn during his visit to the clinic. Eventually he told us, when asked if anything was bothering him, that he was worried about being 'put to sleep'. Despite reassurance, he could not be pacified. The psychologist in the clinic offered the family appointments to discuss the boy's worries and discovered that his fears centred on the fact that a few months previously the family dog had been taken to the vet and 'put to sleep'. The psychologist spent time working with the boy, his admission for surgery was unremarkable and he went on to manage his treatment successfully.

REFERENCES

Association of Paediatric Chartered Physiotherapists 2002 *Obstetric Brachial Plexus Palsy. A Guide to Physiotherapy Management.*

Ballock RT, Song KM 1996 The prevalence of non-muscular causes for torticollis in children. *Journal of Pediatric Orthopaedics* 16: 500–504.

Barker SL, Macnicol MF 2002 Seasonal distribution of idiopathic congenital talipes equinovarus in Scotland. *Journal of Pediatric Orthopaedics B* 11: 129–133.

Bennet GC 2002 Growth and its variants. In: Benson MKD, Fixsen JA, Macnicol MF, Parsch K (eds) *Children's Orthopaedic and Fractures*, 2nd edn. London: Churchill Livingstone, pp. 11–27.

Boome RS, Kaye JC 1988 Obstetric traction injuries of the brachial plexus: natural history, indications for surgical repair and results. *Journal of Bone and Joint Surgery* 70B: 571–576.

Catterall A 1991 A method of assessment of the club foot deformity. *Clinical Orthopaedics and Related Research* 264: 48–53.

Catterall A 2002 Early assessment and management of club foot. In: Benson MKD, Fixsen JA, Macnicol MF, Parsch K (eds) *Children's Orthopaedics and Fractures*, 2nd edn. London: Churchill Livingstone, pp. 464–477.

Cheng JCY, Tang SP, Chen TMK et al 2000 The clinical presentation and outcome of treatment of congenital muscular torticollis in infants. A study of 1086 cases. *Journal of Pediatric Surgery* 35: 1091–1096.

Davis BE, Moon R 1998 Effects of sleep position on infant motor development. *Pediatrics* 102: 1135–1141.

Dobbs MB, Rudski JR, Purcell DB, Walton T, Porter KR, Gurnett MD 2004 Outcome of the use of the Ponseti method for the treatment of idiopathic club foot. *Journal of Bone and Joint Surgery* 86A: 20–27.

Driano AN, Staheli L, Staheli LT 1998 Psychosocial development and corrective shoe wear use in children. *Journal of Pediatric Orthopaedics* 18: 346–349.

Duclos L, Gilbert A 1995 Obstetric palsy – early treatment, secondary procedures. *Annals of the American Academy of Medicine* 24: 851–855.

Eldridge JC, Bell DF 1991 Problems with substantial limb lengthening. *Orthopaedic Clinics of North America* 22: 625–631.

Emery C 1994 Determinants of treatment duration for congenital muscular torticollis. *Physical Therapy* 74: 921–929.

Eng GD, Binder H, Getson P et al 1996 Obstetrical brachial plexus palsy outcome with conservative management. *Muscle and Nerve* July 884–891.

Geutjens G, Gilbert A, Helsen K 1996 Obstetrical brachial plexus palsy associated with breech delivery: a different pattern of injury. *Journal of Bone and Joint Surgery* 78B: 303–306.

Gilbert A 2002 Obstetrical brachial plexus injuries. In: Benson MKD, Fixsen JA, Macnicol MF, Parsch K (eds) *Children's Orthopaedic and Fractures.* London: Churchill Livingstone, pp. 321–327.

Gilbert A, Razaboni R, Amar-Khodja S 1988 Indications and results of brachial plexus surgery in obstetrical brachial palsy. *Orthopaedic Clinics of North America* 19: 91–93.

Handelsman JE, Badalamente MA 1981 Neuromuscular studies in club foot. *Journal of Pediatric Orthopaedics* 1: 23–32.

Harrold AJ, Walker CJ 1983 Treatment and prognosis in congenital club foot. *Journal of Bone and Joint Surgery* 65B: 8–11.

Hartley J, Hill R, Coutts F 2003 The physical, occupational and psychosocial function of young adults who underwent Ilizarov procedures as children. Conference presentation, European Paediatric Orthopaedic Society 22nd Annual Meeting, London, 2–5 April.

Herzenberg JE, Radler C, Box N 2002 Ponseti versus traditional methods of casting for idiopathich club foot. *Journal of Pediatric Orthopaedics* 22: 517–521.

Hill RA, Tucker SK 1997 Leg lengthening and bone transport in children. *British Journal of Hospital Medicine* 57: 399–404.

Hootnick DR, Levinsohn EM, Crider RJ et al 1982 Congenital arterial malformations associated with club foot. A report of two cases. *Clinical Orthopaedics* 167: 160–163.

Hutchison BL, Hutchison LAD, Thompson JMD, Mitchell EA 2004 Plagiocephaly and brachycephaly in the first two years of life: a prospective cohort study. *Pediatrics* 114: 970–980.

Ippolito E, Farsetti P, Caterini R et al 2003 Long term comparative results in patients with congenital club foot treated with two different protocols. *Journal of Bone and Joint Surgery* 85A: 1286–1294.

Jackson AM, Macnicol MF, Saleh M 2002 Leg length discrepancy. In: Benson MKD, Fixsen JA, Macnicol MF, Parsch K (eds) *Children's Orthopaedic and Fractures.* Churchill Livingstone, pp. 427–447.

Jones DHA, Hill RA 2000 Children's orthopaedics: diseases of the growing skeleton. In: Russell RCG, Williams NS, Bulstrode CJK (eds) *Bailey and Love's Short Practice of Surgery,* 23rd edn. London: Hodden Arnold, pp. 441–462.

Lloyd-Roberts GC 1964 Congenital club foot. *Journal of Bone and Joint Surgery* 46B: 369.

Macnicol MF, Jackson AM 2002 The knee. In: Benson MKD, Fixsen JA, Macnicol MF, Parsch K (eds) *Children's*

Orthopaedic and Fractures. London: Churchill Livingstone, pp. 409–426.

Macnicol MF, Nadeem RD, Maffuli N et al 1992 Histochemistry of the triceps surae muscle in idiopathic congenital club foot. *Journal of Foot and Ankle Surgery* 13: 80–84.

Narakas AO 1987 Obstetrical brachial plexus injuries. In: Lamb DW (ed.) *The Paralysed Hand.* London: Churchill Livingstone, pp. 116–135.

Patel M, Herzenberg J 2005 Clubfoot. www.emedicine.com/orthoped/topic598.

Pryor GA, Villar RN, Ronen A et al 1991 Seasonal variation in the incidence of congenital talipes equinovarus. *Journal of Bone and Joint Surgery* 73-B: 632–634.

Rose GK, Welton CA, Marshall T 1986 The diagnosis of flat foot in the child. *Journal of Bone and Joint Surgery* 67B: 71–78.

Staheli LT 1991 Shoes for children: a review. *Pediatrics* 88: 371–375.

Staheli LT 1998 *Fundamentals of Pediatric Orthopaedics,* 2nd edn. Philadelphia: Lippincott-Raven.

Taylor JL, Stammos Norton E 1997 Developmental muscular torticollis: outcomes in young children treated by physical therapy. *Pediatric Physical Therapy* 9: 173–178.

Tillet RL, Fisk NM, Murphy K et al 2000 Clinical outcome of congenital talipes equinovarus diagnosed antenatally by ultrasound. *Journal of Bone and Joint Surgery (British)* 82-B: 876–880.

Wenger DR, Mauldin D, Morgan D et al 1989 Corrective shoes and inserts for flexible flat foot in children. *Journal of Bone and Joint Surgery (American)* 71: 800–810.

Zimny ML, Willig SJ, Roberts JM et al 1985 An electron microscopic study of the fascia from the medial and lateral sides of club foot. *Journal of Pediatric Orthopaedics* 5: 577–581.

14 Rheumatology

Susan Maillard

INTRODUCTION

Paediatric rheumatology is a relatively new specialist area within paediatrics and its case load encompasses a variety of different conditions. These conditions can generally be divided into two categories, inflammatory disease and non-inflammatory disease, but the commonality between them is that all the conditions have features of pain and loss of function within the musculoskeletal system, specifically the muscles and the joints. The difference between inflammatory disease and non-inflammatory disease, however, is that inflammatory disease is an autoimmune disease and is driven by the immune system of the body and this can only be modified by the control of the immune system by medication as well as physical means. Non-inflammatory disease is driven by biomechanical abnormalities, it is not immune response-mediated and it does not resolve with medication, only by the correct realignment of the biomechanical functioning of the body – usually through physiotherapy (Figure 14.1). Table 14.1 lists the most common conditions seen in a rheumatology department and classifies these according to whether they are inflammatory or non-inflammatory. The following section will describe these conditions.

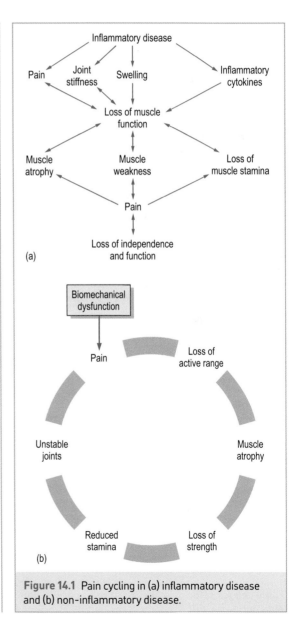

Figure 14.1 Pain cycling in (a) inflammatory disease and (b) non-inflammatory disease.

Table 14.1 The most common conditions seen and managed within a rheumatology department

Inflammatory disease	Non-inflammatory disease
Juvenile idiopathic arthritis	Hypermobility syndromes, e.g. benign joint hypermobility syndrome, Ehlers–Danlos syndrome, Marfan syndrome
Juvenile dermatomyositis Scleroderma	Chronic pain syndromes, e.g. reflex sympathetic dystrophy, complex regional and diffuse pain syndromes
Systemic lupus erythematosus	Chondromalacia patellae
Vasculitis	Generalized musculoskeletal pains
Chronic recurrent multifocal osteomyelitis (CRMO)	
Chronic infantile neurological cutaneous and articular syndrome (CINCA)	

INFLAMMATORY DISEASES

Juvenile idiopathic arthritis

Juvenile idiopathic arthritis (JIA) is an autoimmune inflammatory condition of childhood. Arthritis is defined as swelling within a joint or limitation of range of joint movement with joint pain or tenderness that persists for more than 6 weeks and is not due to a primary biomechanical dysfunction. There are however no specific tests to diagnose JIA and it therefore remains a diagnosis of exclusion. Previously it was named 'Still's disease' and 'juvenile chronic arthritis' or 'juvenile rheumatoid arthritis', but the classifications have been redefined and there are now eight different subgroups, which are described below.

Systemic-onset juvenile idiopathic arthritis

Ten per cent of children with JIA have severe systemic involvement and overt arthritis. The diagnosis of systemic-onset JIA is dependent on the onset of a systemic illness and the presence of active arthritis. The typical systemic presentation is of high spiking fevers (temperature spikes occur 1–2 times a day, with a rapid return to baseline or below baseline temperature) and a discrete erythematous macular rash, often described as salmon-pink in colour. The rash commonly occurs on the trunk and proximal extremities and usually appears with the fever (Figure 14.2). The associated arthritis is often in many or all joints and, though the systemic features often resolve after a few months, the joint disease can persist for many years.

Polyarticular juvenile idiopathic arthritis

This is defined as the presence of arthritis in five or more joints during the first 6 months of the disease. The disease

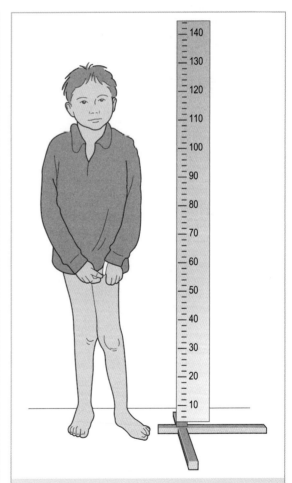

Figure 14.2 Young boy with systemic-onset juvenile idiopathic arthritis, showing many swollen joints and that he is generally unwell and unable to get out of bed easily.

often follows a pattern of flare and remission and tends to be symmetrical and involve large joints such as knees, elbows, hips and ankles (Figure 14.3).

Rheumatoid factor-negative polyarticular juvenile idiopathic arthritis

This is the main presentation for polyarticular JIA and occurs mainly in younger girls and, although many joints may be initially involved, with good management the outcome is positive. Arthritis in finger and toe joints often occurs after the initial onset and is associated with a slightly less favourable outcome.

Rheumatoid factor-positive polyarticular juvenile idiopathic arthritis

This is a small subgroup of the polyarticular JIA group: it mainly affects girls during late childhood or early adolescence and who are rheumatoid factor-seropositive. This pattern of arthritis is more like that of adult rheumatoid arthritis, with nodules and early-onset erosive disease and less symmetrical joint involvement. This form of arthritis requires early and aggressive treatment to minimize the long-term damage.

Oligoarticular juvenile idiopathic arthritis

This is the most common presentation of arthritis in children (60% of all children with JIA) and causes inflammation in four joints or fewer in the first 6 months of the disease course. These children are not systemically unwell and, except for chronic uveitis (inflammation in the eye), extra-articular manifestations are rare. The arthritis mainly affects the lower limbs: the knees are invariably the main joint involved, followed by ankles and wrists (Figure 14.4). Hips are rarely involved. In half of these children only one

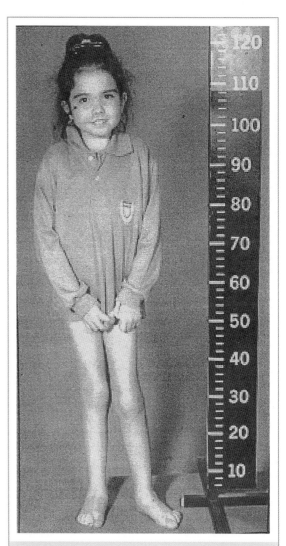

Figure 14.4 Young girl with extended oligoarticular juvenile idiopathic arthritis, showing evidence of swollen knees, leg-length discrepancy and tibial torsion abnormal foot position. She is also wearing a wrist splint, indicating wrist disease.

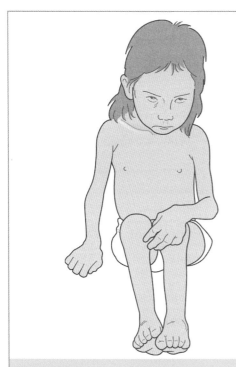

Figure 14.3 Young girl with polyarticular juvenile idiopathic arthritis showing involvement of all joints, including neck.

joint will be affected (monoarthritis) and this is usually the knee. Uveitis affects about 20% of these children and is more likely to occur in young girls with a positive anti-nuclear antibody result. Uveitis is an inflammation that does not produce many symptoms initially and therefore needs to be examined for routinely using a slit-lamp test. This is extremely important, as untreated uveitis causes permanent blindness. However the outcome for this group is excellent and this disease is most likely to be inactive at the end of childhood.

Extended oligoarticular juvenile idiopathic arthritis

A small percentage of children with oligoarticular JIA will develop a polyarticular course after 6–12 months. This subgroup often continues to have more aggressive disease which may be active for many years; however they usually have less joint involvement than the polyarticular JIA group.

Psoriatic juvenile idiopathic arthritis

About 5% of children with JIA have a diagnosis of psoriatic JIA and the diagnosis is easy if the young person started with arthritis before the age of 16 and has psoriasis. However the occurrence of the psoriasis may not occur until later and this makes diagnosis difficult. Therefore diagnosis requires arthritis and either psoriasis in the young person, a first-degree relative with psoriasis, dactylitis (swelling of a digital joint and periarticular tissues, extending beyond the joint margin, often giving a typical 'sausage joint') and nail-pitting. The age of onset is around 10 years and the condition affects more girls than boys. The joint distribution is asymmetrical, with the knee being the most commonly affected joint; however the small joints of the hands and feet are also most commonly affected with this form of arthritis.

Enthesitis-related juvenile idiopathic arthritis

This form of arthritis was previously called 'juvenile spondyloarthropathy' and this was the juvenile form of ankylosing spondylitis. Enthesitis-related JIA is defined as arthritis with enthesitis (inflammation at the enthesis, sites of tendon and ligament attachment to bone, particularly at heel or knee) or arthritis/enthesitis with at least two of the following:

- Sacroiliac joint tenderness
- Presence of the genetic marker human leukocyte antigen (HLA) B27
- Family history of HLA B27-related disease
- Anterior uveitis
- Onset of arthritis in a boy over the age of 8.

Other juvenile idiopathic arthritis

This category includes conditions that do not meet the criteria for any other criteria or meet the criteria for more than one group.

Common presenting features of JIA

The most common presenting feature for all groups of JIA is early-morning stiffness in the affected joints. The affected joints must also have active inflammation (swelling, pain and stiffness/loss of movement) for at least 6 weeks (compared to swelling lasting for a few days in biomechanical disorders). Children with JIA also experience significant muscle weakness and atrophy (Table 14.2) and the stamina

Table 14.2 Reasons for muscle weakness and muscle atrophy in children with juvenile idiopathic arthritis

Cause	Muscle response
Pain in joint	Inhibits function of muscles that control that joint
Stiffness/loss of movement of specific joint	Muscles working with specific joints are unable to function through full range and therefore the muscles weaken within the range not used
Joint swelling	Inhibits function of muscles that control the joint
Systemic illness	Causes generalized loss of muscle strength and endurance
Deranged cytokines	The cytokines that promote active disease also affect muscle function and cause a non-specific myositis, muscle weakness and loss of endurance
Decreased physical function due to pain and fatigue	Less physical activity causes global loss of strength and endurance

of specific muscles is reduced as well as the general fitness of each child. Pain is a variable feature in this condition and is due not only to active inflammation but also to the resulting abnormal biomechanics which cause muscle imbalance and abnormal stability around joints. Therefore it is important always to assess a child carefully to distinguish between inflammatory pain (requiring medical as well as physical intervention) and pain from abnormal biomechanics (requiring a physical intervention only). Bony abnormalities and overgrowth also need to be considered, as JIA is an extremely common cause of leg-length discrepancies, especially in the oligoarticular group, and medial-epicondyl overgrowth, causing valgus deformities at the knees (Petty & Cassidy 2001).

Juvenile dermatomyositis (JDM)

JDM is a multisystem disease of uncertain aetiology that results in inflammation of striated muscle, skin and the gastrointestinal tract. JDM often presents with a combination of malaise, easy fatigue, proximal muscle weakness and rash (Figure 14.5). Joint and muscle pain is often present and the muscle weakness can also involve respiratory and swallowing muscles. The rash is distributed over the extensor surfaces of the small joints of the hands, the elbows, knees and around the eyes. Children often experience severe irritability and mood changes and report that they are unable to lift their heads off the pillow, get up from lying down or climb the stairs. Loss of movement in joints is common and caused by a combination of shortened muscle length, due to the inflammation in the muscles, and contractures due to the presence of

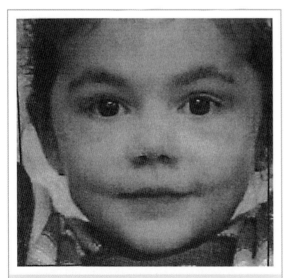

Figure 14.5 Young girl with juvenile dermatomyositis, showing typical rash around eyes and face.

arthritis. Movement can be lost due to inflammation in the skin causing a scleroderma-like (tight, thin, shiny skin) appearance. Independent mobility is affected at the beginning of the disease and these children often require hospital admission in order to initiate medical and physical treatment and ensure a good initial recovery.

More severe cases present with a vasculitic rash and skin ulceration, especially around the hands and eyes, and this is an indication for more aggressive medical management. The most significant complication in JDM is thought to be calcinosis (deposition of calcium in other tissues around the body) and is due to long-term and inadequately treated disease, though this has still to be proven.

Long-term outcome has improved considerably over the years and the mortality has dropped considerably. With aggressive medical and therapeutic intervention, full health and function are possible.

Physiotherapy management of this condition has changed and it has been shown that exercise during active disease is no longer contraindicated. Therefore physiotherapy should be started at the same time as the medication and progressed as the child is able. The ultimate goal will still be full strength and stamina (Cassidy & Petty 2001a, Maillard et al 2004b, 2005).

Scleroderma

The word 'scleroderma' means 'hard skin' but the diseases in this group have a great many more features than this. Scleroderma is simply classified into localized or systemic scleroderma. The underlying disease process is an abnormal accumulation of collagen in the tissues.

Systemic scleroderma often presents with skin-tightening (mainly around the face and hands), Raynaud's phenomenon, joint contractures, arthralgia, muscle weakness and pain and cutaneous telangiectases (swollen red capillaries). There is often a delay in diagnosis due to the slow and subtle presentation of symptoms; however the underlying systemic disease, mainly visceral involvement, is extremely serious and may lead to death. Initially the skin presents with oedema, followed by induration and sclerosis, resulting in marked skin-tightening and contracture, resulting in atrophy.

Localized scleroderma is generally benign and self-limiting and confined to the skin and subdermal tissues (Figure 14.6). The term *morphea* is often used in reference to the appearance of the skin lesions. There are a variety of subtypes of localized scleroderma and the most common is *morphea en plaque*; this is characterized by the insidious onset of an oval or round defined area of induration with a waxy, ivory colour in the centre surrounded by a violaceous halo. It resolves into a hypo- or hyperpigmented area and is mainly focused on the trunk. *Linear scleroderma* is the second most common presentation and is characterized by one or more linear streaks that typically involve a limb and are usually unilateral. Often the lesion

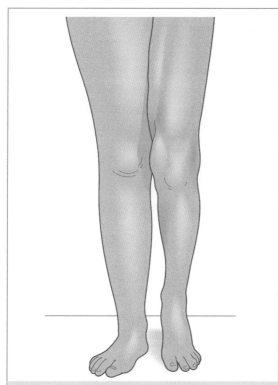

Figure 14.6 Young girl showing linear scleroderma affecting the left leg.

crosses a joint and growth deformities and contractures develop. Very rarely, *generalized morphea* occurs and this term is applied when many areas of the body are affected by these lesions (Nelson 2001).

Systemic lupus erythematosus (SLE)

This is an episodic multisystem disease characterized by widespread inflammation in the blood vessels and connective tissue. The clinical manifestations are extremely variable and its natural history is very unpredictable. Diagnosis is specific and there are 11 diagnostic criteria that have been developed (Box 14.1).

The physiotherapy management will depend upon the clinical presentation of the young person with SLE. However, fatigue is often a feature for all these children so a programme to build general strength and stamina is often extremely helpful (Cassidy & Petty 2001b).

Vasculitis

There is no easy classification of this condition, and in fact many of the other inflammatory conditions also have elements of vasculitis as part of their clinical presentation and pathology. The main feature is evidence of inflammation of blood vessels and therefore many systems can be involved. The most common vasculitis in childhood is polyarteritis nodosa and this is identified by the pathological features of necrotizing arteritis with the formation of nodules along the walls of small and medium-sized muscular arteries.

Physiotherapy requirements will vary depending upon symptoms; however muscle weakness and fatigue are common features and require a progressive programme to improve the symptoms (Figure 14.7: Bagga & Dillon 2001).

NON-INFLAMMATORY DISEASES

Benign joint hypermobility syndrome

Benign joint hypermobility syndrome is a diagnosis given to children who are assessed as having hypermobile joints and who become symptomatic with pain or fatigue and mild loss of coordination. A hypermobile joint is one in which the range of movement significantly exceeds the expected range for that individual, taking into consideration age, sex and ethnic background. There have been many scoring systems devised for measuring and defining hypermobility. The most commonly used measure is the Beighton score (Beighton 1988).

Joint hypermobility has been reported in 6.7–57% of children, depending upon age, ethnicity and criteria for assessing hypermobility. The prevalence is higher in females – 7.1–57% compared to 6.0–35% of boys – and is more prevalent among Asians (57%) than Africans (45%)

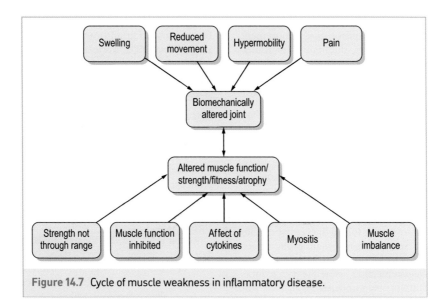

Figure 14.7 Cycle of muscle weakness in inflammatory disease.

and Caucasians (6–10%). It appears that hypermobility decreases with age, and that far fewer adults are hypermobile compared to the number of hypermobile children.

Joint hypermobility is understood to result from either genetic defects or variations in connective tissue matrix proteins which result in more elastic tissues. Within this group are disorders such as Ehlers–Danlos syndrome, Marfan's syndrome and osteogenesis imperfecta. All these genetic collagen disorders have hypermobility as a feature, but since hypermobility is also relatively common within the general population, this may be a result of more common genetic variations rather than mutations.

Many children have hypermobile joints; however, only a percentage of those will suffer from symptoms, and if they follow a chronic pattern these children will be diagnosed as having benign joint hypermobility syndrome (Grahame 1999). The symptoms and severity may vary from child to child, and can occur at any age. Symptoms generally include muscle and joint pain, particularly after activity, towards the end of the day and at night time (growing pains). Occasionally a joint can become swollen but this lasts for hours to days, and not weeks, as in JIA. On examination either all or some of the joints can be hypermobile and there is an associated loss of muscle strength, particularly in the lower limbs. The knee is often the main area of pain, followed by the ankle (Figure 14.8).

The muscle weakness follows a specific pattern, usually involving inner-range quadriceps, hip abductors and extensors as well as plantarflexors. The only management for this condition is physiotherapy to improve the strength and function of the muscles in order to control the hypermobile joints (Jessee et al 1980, Beighton 1988, Murray & Woo 2001, Sherry & Malleson 2001, Maillard & Murray 2003, Maillard et al 2004c).

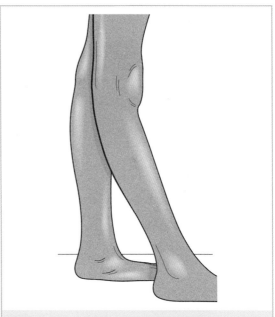

Figure 14.8 Young boy with hypermobility in knees and feet.

Chronic pain syndrome

This is a condition that tends to affect older children (>10 years) and young people and is often associated with hypermobility. The initial presentation of this condition is usually a fairly minor trauma but from this a severe level of pain is experienced. The level of pain and disability in this condition is out of proportion to the physical abnormalities present or the stimulus that causes the pain. Often normal sensations of touch, movement, heat and cold are understood by the brain as pain messages and therefore the smallest activity can often cause the greatest pain. These conditions are often differentiated into two different terms: complex regional pain syndrome and complex diffuse pain syndrome.

Complex regional pain syndrome

This is applied to a pain syndrome localized to one area of the body. *Reflex sympathetic dystrophy* is a condition that takes these symptoms to the extreme, resulting in a blue, cold, hypersensitive, swollen and immobile limb – usually the foot or the hand. The young person will often refuse to move the limb or to have it touched, even by clothes. The most important aspect of management is physiotherapy, which is required to be done regularly throughout the day in order to regain function before the pain reduces. It is vital that the young person understands that the pain will not resolve until the function has completely returned and nothing will remove the pain until normal function is regained (Maillard et al 2004a).

Complex diffuse pain syndrome

In this condition the pain affects many areas or all of the body, resulting in severe pain and fatigue and a large loss of function, often resulting in poor school attendance and loss of social activities.

Medication, such as strong pain relief, often does not help with these conditions and the best results are gained with intensive physiotherapy with the aims of regaining movement, strength and function as fast as possible before there is resolution of the pain (Sherry & Malleson 2001).

OSTEOPOROSIS

Immobilization causes increased bone reabsorption and decreased bone formation and it is believed that bone density loss due to immobilization may be as high as 5% per month for the first 6 months; the rate of loss then slows but does continue. Evidence shows that children who exercise regularly have stronger bones and that it is vital that children exercise regularly, especially during puberty, in order to maximize bone density for adulthood. It is estimated that 90% of bone mineral density is accumulated by the end of adolescence. However, differences in bone mineral density are 75% genetic, with the other variations due to level of calcium uptake, disease activity and up to 17% of the variation due to the amount of weight-bearing activity being performed. Therefore for children with inflammatory disease who have medication which often causes bone loss (such as steroids) combined with the actual disease process and the immobility and loss of function as a result of the disease, osteoporosis is a very real concern. Impact exercise

is the most effective way to lay down bone and should be encouraged at all times (Bachrach 2001, McDonagh 2001, Cimaz 2002, Tortolani et al 2002, Davies et al 2005).

MEDICAL MANAGEMENT

The inflammatory diseases require aggressive medical management in order to control the disease so that physiotherapy can then be at its most effective. The non-steroidal anti-inflammatory drugs (NSAIDs) are used routinely to control the symptoms of pain and stiffness but they do not reduce the inflammation. Steroids are the main initial treatment and these can be given orally, though this is used to a minimum to avoid the side-effects that are dose- and duration-linked. Commonly steroids are injected directly into a swollen joint and this successfully controls the disease in that joint. Steroids can also be given as an intravenous infusion of methylprednisone for children who have many joints involved or who also have systemic illness. Other drugs, called disease-modifying antirheumatic drugs (DMARDs), are also commonly used: methotrexate is the most common and the most effective with few side-effects. This is given once a week either as an oral preparation or as a subcutaneous injection. The injection has a much better effect and is less likely to produce side-effects. Other medications such as 'biologics' are also being used now. The most commonly used now are the antitumor necrosis factor-α (TNF-α) therapies such as infliximab and Enbrel. Other medications are also being developed within this group.

The biomechanical pain conditions do not usually respond very well to medication (analgesic or NSAID) and therefore use of these drugs is discouraged.

PHYSIOTHERAPY MANAGEMENT

The physiotherapy approach for all the rheumatology conditions described follows similar principles and will be described generally initially, with specifics described in more detail as appropriate.

Assessment

All assessments include subjective and objective aspects and the rheumatology assessment is no different. The assessment below is based on work done within an expert consensus in the management of rheumatological conditions and can be found in more detail through the British Society of Paediatric and Adolescent Rheumatology (BSPAR: www.BSPAR.org).

In order to plan effective management of children with a rheumatological condition, an assessment will need to encompass the physical, psychological and social impact of the disease on a child and family. This section includes a comprehensive list of topics that could be covered in the

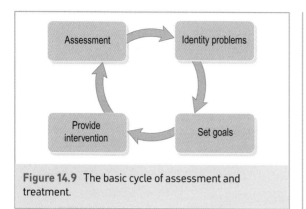

Figure 14.9 The basic cycle of assessment and treatment.

the treatments that have already been provided are discussed in order to establish what treatments have been given from the onset, including alternative therapies and response to them.

Presenting problems and symptoms

There is a need to establish when the changes occurred during the progression of the disease, because the longer the condition has been present, the greater the clinical changes. However, the main current problems need to be established within a relevant timescale, i.e. in the last 1–2 weeks. Allow a child, young person or family the time to tell you what they are experiencing now and then focus your questioning upon the following areas.

Pain

Gain a good description of the areas affected, type, severity and intensity of the pain, how long it lasts, when the pain is experienced (periodic, constant) and what are the relieving and exacerbating factors. This will gives a clear picture of the biggest concern for the child and indicate what treatment is most appropriate where. A pain scale is often very useful and provides a slightly more objective outcome measure (e.g. pain visual analogue scale (VAS) 0–10).

General functioning (in the context of the appropriate developmental milestones)

Establish what activities a child is able to do now compared to previously and what activities the child has difficulty with, particularly in functional tasks, walking distance and stairs. Fatigue is an issue for many children with these conditions and provides a clear picture of function and problems experienced now.

Early-morning stiffness

Early-morning stiffness particularly affects children with JIA and it is useful to know how severe the stiffness is, how long it lasts, what areas of the body are affected and whether there is stiffness at any other time in the day. Early-morning stiffness is an indication of the severity and degree of activity of inflammatory disease. Stiffness at other times of the day may indicate other issues, i.e. in the evening stiffness is often an indication of muscle fatigue due to biomechanical abnormalities and hypermobility. It can be experienced with inflammatory and non-inflammatory

assessment, both subjectively and objectively, and their relevance to the information gathered. This information can be used at the initial assessment and at reassessment to ensure that a comprehensive treatment programme is established (Figure 14.9).

Relevant age-appropriate milestones should be considered at all times during the assessment to ensure that the correct inferences are made from all the information.

Subjective assessment

History of present condition

Take a history of the symptoms and their progression and any important factors that precipitated them, including systemic features such as:

- Spiking fever
- Rash
- Mouth ulcers
- Headaches
- Sore throats
- Trauma
- Viral/bacterial infection
- Travel abroad
- Vaccinations received.

This information helps to differentiate between diseases and gives an indication of severity and speed of onset of disease, length of time of symptoms and possible precipitating factors.

Previous experiences of hospitals, which different professionals families have seen and diagnosis given are helpful in order to gain a clear history and identify any underlying issues such as pain amplification. It is recommended that previous hospital admissions and investigations are recorded chronologically to ensure that a clear picture is gained as to the investigations and treatments already provided.

It is useful to identify how the diagnosis was arrived at if the disease has been untreated for a significant period of time. During the assessment it is recommended that conditions alike, but evening stiffness is due to fatigue and not inflammation.

Child's and parents' main concerns

Ask what they are most worried about, and what they think can be done about it. This ensures that everyone is aware of the issues, their main concerns are considered within the treatment programme and that everyone is focused upon the same goals.

Past medical history

Birth and delivery

Were there any difficulties or issues perinatally? This will indicate whether any other pathology is occurring.

Developmental history

Check when developmental milestones were achieved and those of any siblings. Often children with hypermobility will be slightly slower in reaching their milestones and will often not crawl at all.

Immunizations and vaccinations

Check whether these are up to date in order to determine a child's immunity to infectious diseases. This is especially pertinent if group treatment sessions are established or DMARD treatment is indicated.

Other medical problems

Are they seeing a doctor for any other reason? Have there been any admissions to hospital for other reasons? Other conditions will be relevant to the provision of treatment and diagnosis of rheumatological/musculoskeletal condition. Enquire about any operations that a child has had previously or has planned for the future and whether there have been any other injuries such as fractures, sprains or dislocations. This will give an indication about previous hospital and pain experiences. Ask about all the investigations that the child has received, for this condition or other conditions.

Medication

Ask about all medication taken previously, including dosage, dates started and finished, so that it is clear about the drugs taken, e.g. steroids, their effect on the disease and any potential side-effects. Take a complete list of current medication and doses prescribed, including homeopathic medicines, to be aware of all drugs taken and their potential effect on treatment.

Social history and family history

Drawing a tree of the relationships in the immediate family, including ages of other children, provides a clear picture of who is present in a child's life. It is also necessary to ask who actually lives at home as this may well be different from the family tree.

Ask about the parents' occupations as this will give some indications about the pressures on the family, both as regards time and financially.

Identify the primary carer(s) of a child so that relevant carers can be included in the provision of a home treatment plan.

Ask about any diseases or illness within the family, i.e. diabetes, rheumatoid arthritis, thyroid conditions, psoriasis, gastrointestinal tract problems, chronic pain or other conditions, noting who are blood relatives. The family's experience of illness will have an impact upon a child's coping mechanisms and the perception of his or her condition.

Accommodation

Ask about type of accommodation, ownership, stairs, general access and accessibility of bathroom. This will indicate whether mobility is an issue and if adaptations are needed to the house.

Benefits

Check with the family whether they are aware of any benefits they are entitled to and how to claim them to ensure the appropriate support is provided.

Activities of daily living/function: home and school

Hygiene

Record information on mobility in and out of the bath/shower; whether the child can wash him/herself and hair independently, whether the child can use the toilet independently, i.e. getting on and off or flushing the toilet, undressing, wiping bottom. The level of age-appropriate independent functioning needs to be established to guide the treatment programme to independent function. Establish if any specific equipment is required for any of these tasks.

Dressing and grooming

Can a child dress independently, including buttons, shoes and laces, socks, trousers and pullovers, teeth-brushing and hair-brushing? Are any aids used or extra time required? This will determine further difficulties in activities of daily living.

Walking distance and mobility

- How far can the child walk before a rest is required?
- Can the child continue after a period of rest (note the time of rest required)
- Can the child keep up with peers or family?
- Does the child need any mobility aids and if so, why, when and for how long?
- Stairs: can they be completed fully using one leg after another or has the technique been adapted? How many steps can the child complete?
- Can the child get on and off a chair/bed and on and off a bus/car/train?

This information will give a good baseline assessment that can be used as an outcome measure.

Eating and food preparation

- Can the child cut up food independently?
- Does the child need any specific aids to help with eating?
- Can the child prepare food, e.g. cutting food, opening jars, turning taps and lifting kettles/pans/cups?

Note any limiting factors for any of the above activities, including speed.

School

As it is a legal requirement to gain permission from parents before contacting a school about their child, agreement needs to sought. Signing the assessment form or devising a specific form for this may be appropriate.

- Does the child attend school regularly? If not, explore the reasons why the child has missed school
- What time does the child start and finish the school day?
- How many times has the child changed school?
- How does the child get to and from school? How far away is the school?
- If the child walks, how is he or she affected by the time he or she gets to school?
- How does the child move around at school?
- Are stairs and distance around school problematic?
- Does the child need help with carrying books?
- Is seating adequate?
- How long can the child write for?
- What are the limiting factors, e.g. pain, fatigue?
- Can the child join in PE lessons?
- Which activities can the child do?
- Which activities can the child not do?
- Does the child need a rest during the day and if so, is there access to a medical/rest room rather than being sent home?
- Does the child join in with playtime activities?
- Does he or she play with friends?
- Can the child use the school toilets independently?
- Does the child participate in trips/outings/extra-curricular activities in the same way as peers?
- Do any other school subjects cause problems, e.g. science, technology, home economics? Explore what the difficulties are.

A child may need a statement to provide additional help within the school environment (see Ch. **2**).

Other professional input

Physiotherapy

Has the child had physiotherapy before? What did it consist of? What effect did it have? It is important to know whether any other therapists are involved with the

---

> **Box 14.2** Different professionals who may be involved in the care of a child with a rheumatological condition
>
> Paediatric rheumatologist
> Orthopaedic surgeon
> Physiotherapist
> Occupational therapist
> District nurse
> Clinical nurse specialist
> Podiatrist
> Dietician
> Social worker
> Speech therapist
> Eye specialist
> Psychologist
> Voluntary organization (Children's Chronic Arthritis Association: info@ccaa.org.com)

child's care, i.e. at a specialist centre, as it is important that all professionals involved are providing consistent advice to the family (Box 14.2).

Specialist equipment

Splints and orthotics

List details of any splints/orthoses that have been provided, including whether they still fit and how often they are being used, who provided them, and their contact details.

Wheelchairs and crutches

Enquire whether any mobility aids have been provided, where from and who is responsible for providing them and repairing them.

Hobbies, interests and socialization

Knowledge of a child's interests can be useful when setting treatment goals or devising strategies to make interventions more relevant and fun.

- What hobbies and sporting activities does the child like to do, including any that have had to be stopped due to this illness?
- Can a child join in with family hobbies? Check whether the child can still participate or is unable to do so now due to this illness
- Does the child have stable friendship groups?
- Is the child feeling isolated by the condition?

Questions relating to drugs, alcohol and sexual activity need to asked sensitively and at an appropriate age.

Ethnic origin and cultural concerns

Religion

Some religions require strict worship and may be physically difficult to achieve, i.e. kneeling on a prayer mat, diet, dress and gender-appropriate activities. Check which is a child's and family's first language and whether an interpreter is required.

Objective assessment

Pain

Visual Analogue Scale (VAS) for pain completed by a child is a useful tool for the ongoing assessment of the level of pain the child is experiencing.

VAS global assessment of disease and function

VAS global assessment of disease and function, completed by the parents, provides one of the core outcome variables in the assessment of JIA (Box 14.3). A physician's VAS should also be completed, especially in the management of JIA (Rider et al 1997, Lovell et al 1999).

Assessment of each joint, including spinal movements

Active range of movement is important; however children will often not tolerate a very long assessment and therefore it is recommended to assess the passive range of movement as a priority. (Note the time of the assessment, as the findings will often differ depending on time of day, as children with arthritis are stiffer in the morning than the afternoon.)

Assess specific ranges using an accurate recording of joint angles and not just to know that the joint is restricted. Many of the interventions will be designed to increase range in the joints restricted due to pain, stiffness, muscle-shortening or true joint contracture. This will then determine the treatment plan.

- Fluidity of movement will provide information as to the causes of the loss of movement and whether there is any muscle spasm protecting the joint. Hypermobility

---

Box 14.3 Core-outcome measurements for the assessment of juvenile idiopathic arthritis (Giannini et al 1997, Ruperto et al 1999)

Number of joints with active inflammation
Number of joints with limited movement
Parental visual analogue scale
Physician's visual analogue scale
Childhood Health Assessment Questionnaire (CHAQ)
Erythrocyte sedimentation rate (ESR: blood test)

---

is as important a finding as a restricted joint. All joints and deformities need assessment as the parents or a child will often miss important changes which affect the prescribed programme
- Note colour and temperature around the joint and any pain associated with the movement or palpation and observe any bony overgrowth affecting a joint.

Palpation

Note the following:

- End-feel of a joint
- Stability of a joint, including evidence of subluxation or dislocation
- Swelling of joint (effusion), soft tissues or tendons
- Muscle spasm, which is often evident around the neck and spine.

Muscle strength and function

Many scales are used in the assessment of muscle strength. They all have a slightly different focus and give different information. The most common testing system used is the Medical Research Council scale of 0–5 and this is widely accepted despite its limitations (Medical Research Council 1943, McDonald et al 1986, Burnett et al 1990, Barr et al 1991, Florence et al 1992, Young & Wright 1995).

Muscle testing is an extremely important outcome measure for effectiveness of treatment and can be measured before and after intervention. It is vital to assess muscle function to ensure that the physiotherapy programme is prescribed specifically to address the muscle weakness experienced by each child.

Specific measures of muscle strength and function have been developed for the assessment of JDM. These include the Medical Research Council scale modified to a 0–10 scale, called the Kendal scale, and this is then applied to eight muscle groups to give a score of 80 (or 150 if used bilaterally).

The Childhood Myositis Assessment Scale (CMAS), which is a validated assessment tool of muscle function, is an accepted core outcome assessment tool for the management of JDM. This score is out of 52, with 52 indicating full function (Lovell et al 1999).

Muscle strength can be assessed in a more objective manner, such as using a hand-held myometer, and this will give measurements of force that can then be followed more accurately over time than the 0–5 scale. It does, however, have limitations as it only measures antigravity strength, but it is useful for research purposes (Miller et al 1988, Lennon & Ashburn 1993, Stratford & Balsor 1994).

Posture

Observe posture in standing and sitting, looking at the position of neck, shoulders, elbows, wrists, hand, spine, hips, knees and ankles. Note a familial tendency.

Gait

Observing gait provides a great deal of information about the function, independence, limitations and level of pain of the child, e.g. loss of big-toe extension limits the push-off phase; fixed flexion deformities of hips and knees often cause continual loss of strength in hip abductors and extensors and inner-range quadriceps, often resulting in the development of a positive Trendelenburg gait pattern. Valgus knees and ankles alter the correct muscle function and observing the heel/toe action highlights difficulties in the feet and ankles. Video may be a useful record of gait (see Ch. 4).

Observation of general movement and function

Look for any compensatory movements that may be performed both during the assessment and in movement from the waiting area to the examination room.

Functional questionnaires (or some form of validated disease function measure)

Questionnaires need to have been validated in the assessment of inflammatory disease in children. The ones that are most commonly used are the Childhood Health Assessment Questionnaire (CHAQ) (Huber et al 2001, Nugent et al 2001) and the Childhood Health Questionnaire (CHQ) (Nugent et al 2001, Ruperto et al 2001). In fact, the CHAQ is one of the core set outcome measures in both JIA and JDM.

Stamina

This is an important feature for all children with rheumatological conditions. However there are no routinely used objective assessments. The 6-minute walk test is a validated tool but is time-consuming and so is not usually used in a clinic setting (see Ch. 3). Therefore the most common assessment is just a subjective questioning of fatigue. This is not satisfactory and questionnaires regarding fatigue are being developed (Hamilton & Haennel 2000, Pankoff et al 2000, Takken et al 2002, 2003, 2003a, c, 2005a, b, Paap et al 2005).

Leg length

Children with both inflammatory and non-inflammatory disease develop transient differences which, if left unmanaged, can cause permanent deformities to the spine. All leg-length differences of greater than 1 cm should be treated with a complete shoe raise.

Muscle bulk

This is a useful measure, particularly when the condition only affects one side, as it can give an objective measure for change in muscle size. Measures are taken 10 cm above the knee joint line, at the knee joint line and 10 cm below the knee joint line to ensure this measure is consistent for each child.

Skin condition

Assess the condition of the skin and note any abnormalities or broken/vulnerable areas. In JDM you would expect to see a purple/red rash around a child's eyelids, across the knuckles and across the extensor surfaces of the knees and elbows. In SLE you would expect to see a red rash in a 'butterfly' distribution under the eyes and across the cheeks.

Also look for signs of scleroderma, as in mixed connective tissue disease several skin rashes can be present.

Following assessment, specific problems for each child are identified, i.e. what joints are restricted, which muscles are weak, how the balance is affected, so that the treatment programme can be planned. The treatment programme has to be prescribed specifically for each child and will need to be regularly reviewed and monitored.

Main goals of treatment

1. Full range of movement at each joint
2. Full muscle strength through the whole range, including hypermobile range
3. Stable joints
4. Excellent stamina:
   (a) specific muscles
   (b) general
5. Full physical function, independently of pain
6. Good balance and proprioception
7. Age-appropriate neuromuscular coordination
8. No pain
9. Independent function
10. Minimize loss of bone density
11. Educate family and child.

The programme may need to include many different techniques depending upon the specific problems. The main principles of each intervention will be described. These will include hydrotherapy, stretching, splinting, pain relief, pacing, balance and proprioception re-education, gait re-education and a muscle-strengthening programme.

Physiotherapy interventions

Hydrotherapy

Hydrotherapy has been a well-accepted technique for the management of paediatric rheumatology conditions for many years. However, research into its effectiveness has shown that it is not as effective as 'dry-land' treatment in regaining range of movement, increasing muscle strength or returning to full function; however, when asked, children preferred it as a treatment. Hydrotherapy is extremely effective when used in close conjunction with a land-based programme and when the hydrotherapy treatments are employed effectively. Unfortunately, it is sometimes too easy to put a child into hydrotherapy each week and not use the specific effects of buoyancy to target specific problems and make effective progress. Therefore hydrotherapy should be provided with specific goals in mind, combined with a land-based home treatment programme.

When hydrotherapy is being provided the effect of buoyancy needs to be remembered at all times as this dramatically affects the muscle function used. Young children find it difficult to understand initially what is required and unless closely supervised may in fact not complete the exercises correctly. The physiotherapist and child need to remember that moving through the water is much easier than walking on land, due to buoyancy, and that this technique will not make up for the work they do on land (Takken et al 2003b, Epps et al 2005).

Effects of hydrotherapy

These are gained with the combined effect of the warmth from the water, the effect of buoyancy supporting the body and the fun element to the treatment programme. Hydrotherapy aims to:

- Reduce pain and muscle spasm
- Increase joint range of movement and muscle strength by using buoyancy to stretch
- Reduce joint stiffness – allowing more comfortable movement, especially first thing in the morning, encouraging joints to move through range and therefore improving circulation and reducing swelling
- Increase muscle strength – when movement is completed against buoyancy and turbulence
- Increase aerobic capacity by encouraging swimming and fast action games.

Stretching

Stretching is an integral part of the treatment programme, both for reducing contractures and preventing them and also for lengthening shortened muscles. In inflammatory disease the joints become swollen and the synovial fluid becomes thinner but full of inflammatory cells. These cells alter the effectiveness of the synovial fluid in its role as a lubricant and change the structure of the capsule and other soft tissues. These soft tissues lose elasticity and become stiffer and in children this then causes rapid development of contractures. Often children with inflammatory disease experience stiffness in the joints first thing in the morning and after periods of immobilization such as sitting in a classroom or after a car journey. This is caused by a lack of

movement of the joint resulting in poor circulation around the joint and build-up of fluid. The capsule becomes tighter, limiting range at both ends, i.e. full flexion and full extension. Pain is also produced by this process both in and around the joint and in the surrounding muscles.

Joints need to be stretched out first thing in the morning to regain full range of movement as soon as possible to prevent the development of contractures and to reduce the pain and stiffness. If a child has particularly active disease with many swollen joints then initially you will need to discuss with the medical team whether there is adequate medical control of the disease and whether the stretches may be more effectively completed in a warm bath or hydrotherapy pool.

Role of stretching

1. To reduce pain
2. To reduce stiffness
3. To maintain or increase joint range of movement in order to prevent contractures or to resolve them if necessary
4. To increase muscle length.

Stretching stiff joints is one of the few techniques used in the management of these conditions that should not be completed by the young person as it is extremely difficult to do this effectively by oneself. However muscle-length stretches can be completed by themselves.

Important rules for stretching joints

1. Only stretch one joint at a time
2. Initially apply slight traction in order to reduce any muscle spasm and to ensure the joint is in good alignment
3. The stretch needs to be completed gently but firmly to ensure that it is effective
4. The stretch should be uncomfortable (not painful) and into a new range that a child is not able to do actively
5. Most stretches are into extension, as that is the end of range that is most often lost and muscles become weaker and find it difficult to maintain the range against gravity. Exceptions are the fingers and elbows and plantar and dorsiflexion which range into flexion. Some joints will also need rotational stretches completed.

KEY POINT

Stretches must be completed when the joint is inflamed as this is the time when the most movement is lost. However, if a joint is swollen then it will probably require an alteration in the medical management in order to reduce the swelling effectively and limit the damage

Stretching shortened muscles

Muscles are very likely to shorten in conditions such as JDM due to the inflammatory nature of the muscle disease and in children with hypermobility and pain syndromes. The muscles most commonly affected are gastrocnemius, hamstrings and the long flexors of the arm, preventing full extension of all joints in the upper limbs. However, muscle tightening can also occur, as well as joint contractures, and these will need to be assessed.

Stretch and cast

In some cases the contracture may be very severe and will not be able to be stretched on a daily basis and progress maintained. These types of contracture are often associated with active disease and are most common in the knees. It would then be recommended to take a child to the operating theatre. Under general anaesthetic the joint would be injected by the medical team and then the physiotherapist can stretch very slowly into full extension and a full cast can then be applied. This cast should remain on for only a few days and then it should be removed and intensive physiotherapy provided. The cast should not be kept on for too long – 5 days maximum – in order to prevent stiffness into extension instead of flexion. While the cast is on the child must perform static quadriceps contractions in order to start the process of gaining adequate inner-range quadriceps strength so as to maintain full range and to prevent the contracture returning.

When the cast is removed intensive physiotherapy – twice a day minimum – is indicated. The main focus of the programme should be to regain full strength, particularly in inner-range quadriceps, but also hip abductors and extensors and plantarflexors, which also become very weak.

Splinting

Splinting in the management of juvenile arthritis was one of the main treatments in years gone by. However, with new and more effective medical management, splints are rarely required now. The main splints now required are active wrist support splints that support the wrist into extension but allow full function of the fingers. These are mainly used during activities such as writing to prevent fatigue and pain and to maintain a good functional position.

Very rarely leg splints are now made to keep the knee into extension and the ankle into dorsiflexion. These would be used when the disease was refractory or was responding poorly to medical management.

This type of splinting is mainly used in inflammatory disease and should not be encouraged in biomechanical problems such as hypermobility, as the splints encourage muscle weakness which then increases pain.

Splinting is completely contraindicated in pain syndromes such as reflex sympathetic dystrophy as immobilization always makes these conditions worse.

Pain relief

Techniques such as ice and heat are useful in the management of pain in all these conditions and both ice and heat can be used. The best judge of which is most effective is the child. However, when reflex sympathetic dystrophy is present, then cold is contraindicated as it makes the condition worse.

Other techniques such as wax can be useful in all these conditions and will not only help with pain but can also be used as exercise.

Self-massage is a useful technique to teach to a young person. Massage is useful as a desensitization technique for the management of the pain syndromes and for the reduction of muscle spasm to help improve circulation around an inflamed joint.

The main approach for reducing pain in all these conditions is to regain normal movement and full muscle strength and for the joint, limb and body to be used normally. This applies to all the conditions, but especially the pain syndromes. Waiting for the pain to go before physiotherapy is started will mean that it is never started (Maillard et al 2004a).

> **KEY POINT**
>
> Exercising and stretching are the most effective methods of reducing pain and keeping it away

Pacing activities

Children and young people naturally have lots of energy and want to keep going all day and then still keep going. However, with these types of inflammatory and non-inflammatory conditions often the pain and symptoms are made worse by doing too much on one day, which results in pain and stiffness at night or the next day. A child and family need to be taught about pacing and energy conservation. Simple techniques can include proper planning for a task to ensure that children have everything they need before they start, to avoid many individual trips to get the items needed during the task. It is useful to advise patients to plan activities throughout a week, so that each day has similar challenges, and to avoid doing more on one day than another, which often results in less activity for the next few days.

After a flare in the condition, a gradual return to activity is recommended to ensure that energy is conserved and that there is a paced approach back to full function. This may include reducing some activities initially so that the young person can manage school first and as that becomes easier gradually add in more activities around that. When progressing back to full function, the tasks need to be achievable, whether it is a good day or a bad day, and if it is a good day the young person should not do more than the programme requires. This is important to avoid activity cycling and the 'rollercoaster' effect.

Balance and proprioception

Balance and proprioception are altered by joint swelling, joint pain, muscle weakness and inactivity. However without adequate balance or proprioception it is very difficult to complete some tasks safely and the risk of injury is increased. The most simple and effective exercise to improve lower-limb proprioception is just practising standing on one leg without wobbling, progressing to doing this with eyes closed and then progressing to adding in plantarflexion on one leg (i.e. going up and down on tiptoes). Other methods using equipment, such as a wobble board, are very useful and can be purchased for use at home (Mallik et al 1994, Hall et al 1995).

Gait re-education

In children it is not uncommon for the gait to be altered due to altered biomechanics, inflammation and muscle weakness; however, for some children correcting this is difficult as they have learnt a new gait pattern and that has become their normal walk. Practising walking and using mirrors are very useful. Marching can help with this process as it overcorrects most abnormal gaits and encourages good use of range and muscle strength. The use of supportive footwear, particularly around the heel, will help to ensure that normal gait is achieved. For children with unstable feet and ankles (hypermobile or inflamed joints), ankle boots with effective shock-absorbing soles are recommended.

Sporting activities

For all these conditions the aim of management is to give every child the chance of a normal and full life. In inflammatory disease medication and physiotherapy are required and in non-inflammatory disease only therapy is required. The principles for both are the same. Providing each muscle group is doing its job properly and children are fit and strong, they are encouraged to join in any sporting activity they want.

However, there are some sports for which they will need to be really strong. These include distance running, rugby and football. A trampoline should also be used with care as sometimes the lands and jumps can be unpredictable.

Muscle function

There are many reasons why children may have loss of muscle strength and stamina and these are listed below:

- *Pain inhibits muscle function:* pain in a muscle acting across the joint with which it is linked will reduce the strength and function of that muscle and atrophy of the muscle will occur very quickly
- *Inflammation:* inflammation or swelling in a joint will inhibit the functioning of the muscles around it and atrophy will occur within days of reduced function
- *Biomechanical:* joint function can change biomechanically for many reasons. If there is swelling then the position and movement of the joint will alter and this in turn will alter the muscle function around that joint. Equally, when the swelling has reduced, the ligaments and capsule are left overstretched and therefore render the joint unstable, also affecting muscle function.

In the case of non-inflammatory conditions, poor muscle control is not gained throughout the full range of the joint, especially into the hypermobile range, and this in turn causes misuse of the joint, resulting in pain. Then the pain inhibition cycle begins.

Loss of mobility

When a joint does not move fully, such as when there are contractures or a joint effusion, then the muscle is not able to move through full range and loses its function within the range not moved. This has a knock-on effect on the rest of the muscle and the whole muscle will gradually lose strength and function. In the case of hypermobility, the muscles are generally not functioning into the hypermobile range and therefore there is poor control into inner range, causing overstretching of the joints and pain.

Disease activity

In inflammatory disease the whole body is affected and causes a systemic response to varying degrees, depending on the nature and severity of the disease. This in turn affects the muscles as a child is not eating properly or maybe if the child is feeling unwell he or she will not be exercising and playing normally and this causes loss of muscle function. There are also small molecules called 'cytokines' which are important in the continuation of the inflammatory diseases that also have very significant roles in muscle function. This will be explained later.

Muscle imbalance

In all situations the body tries to compensate for difficulties and this also happens in the way the muscles function. For example, in the case of a child with a swollen knee, the knee flexes due to the swelling and therefore the inner-range quadriceps stops functioning. As the knee is flexed the hip flexes in compensation and the hip abductors and extensors – gluteus medius, minimus and maximus – also stop functioning. However other muscles start to compensate, such as psoas and mid-range quadriceps, which now do too much work but keep the body mobile. If this situation continues then the stronger muscles (psoas and mid-range quads) keep being used and get stronger and the other muscles just keep on getting weaker! This results in significant muscle weakness.

The role of cytokines in muscle function

Cytokines are small molecules produced by the body to send messages from one cell to another. Cytokines have become extremely important in our understanding of the nature of inflammatory disease and this knowledge has been used to produce a new group of medical therapies called the 'biologics'. Medicines such as etanercept and infliximab have been developed and these are anti-TNF-α drugs. Other important anticytokine drugs are also being developed, such as anti-interleukin (IL)-6 and anti-IL-1. However these cytokines also have an important normal role in the function of muscle and this may explain why children with inflammatory disease become so weak so quickly.

Cytokine function is extremely complex and each cytokine will have a different function depending on the cell it is communicating with, what other cytokines and how many there are around (Figure 14.10). Two of the most important cytokines in rheumatological conditions at the present time are TNF-α and IL-6. IL-1 is also an important cytokine and is important in the control of IL-6 and in pain sensation (Feghali & Wright 1997, Lundberg et al 1997, Ostrowski et al 1999, Scheett et al 1999, 2002, Pedersen 2000, Pedersen & Toft 2000, Lundberg 2001, Malm 2001, Nagaraju 2001a, b, Pedersen et al 2001a, b, Reid & Li 2001, De Bleecker et al 2002, Nemet et al 2002, Toft et al 2002).

TNF-α and IL-6 are homeostatic in their relationship. If the level of TNF-α reduces then the level of IL-6 is also reduced and because IL-6 has reduced, TNF-α production is then increased (Pachman et al 2001, Spencer et al 2000, Collins & Grounds 2001, Fedczyna et al 2001).

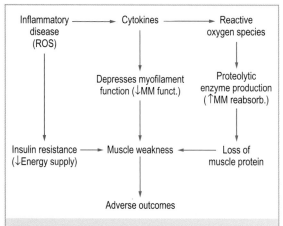

Figure 14.10 Diagram showing the simple relationship between cytokines and muscle function (Winkelman 2004). ROS, reactive oxygen species; MM, muscle.

TNF-α function and muscles

TNF-α has a very important role in the normal function of muscle and that is initially to increase the proliferation of new muscle cells and then secondly to facilitate the apoptosis of old muscle cells, therefore keeping the regeneration cycle active. However when the normal level of TNF-α is changed, then abnormal functioning of muscle occurs.

TNF-α inhibits muscle contractile function within hours of a raised TNF-α level by reducing the contractile force and blunting the muscle's response to calcium activation. It also causes muscle atrophy by increasing proteolysis, inhibiting the insulin effect on muscles and blocking the glycogen uptake by the muscles. A prolonged increase in TNF-α causes inhibition of skeletal muscle synthesis and skeletal muscle myopathy.

IL-6 function and muscles

This cytokine is vital for the normal function of healthy muscle but it is also understood to be a proinflammatory cytokine in the inflammatory diseases in childhood. IL-6 is vital for the homeostasis of muscle function and the provision of its food source – glycogen. The more IL-6 is produced, the more glycogen is made available for the muscles, either from using the available store in the blood or by lipolysis to create more supplies. IL-6 is therefore produced naturally by functioning muscles, not only to regulate the glycogen requirement but also within its role as a proinflammatory cytokine. In order to increase the strength and size of muscle, a small local inflammatory process is established, causing local damage which can therefore be repaired by the function of the satellite cells.

The amount of IL-6 produced naturally by the muscles is dependent on the type of exercise and its intensity. Eccentric muscle work produces more IL-6 than concentric, as does endurance work versus resisted work, and the longer and harder the exercise, the more IL-6 is produced. Therefore running a long distance downhill will produce the most IL-6! However in inflammatory disease there are increased levels of IL-6, promoting muscle inflammation beyond normal, resulting in loss of muscle function.

It has been shown however that the body's natural response to cytokine production can be altered by exercise and that muscles can become more efficient in their production of TNF-α and IL-6 by following a moderate progressive resisted exercise programme.

Muscle repair and growth

Satellite cells are extremely important in the process of muscle cell repair and growth. These cells are undifferentiated cells stored within the muscles which can then be stimulated either to replace damaged muscle cells or to add new muscle cells. These cells are stimulated by exercise and therefore muscles cannot gain strength, stamina or function without exercise. Daily exercise after damage encourages repair and is important in the healing process. There are a finite number of satellite cells: the body has

Box 14.4 Types of muscle work that should be included in a treatment programme

Concentric
Eccentric
Isometric
Isokinetic
Closed-chain
Open-chain

Table 14.3 Example of a home exercise programme for a child with a rheumatological condition

Muscle involved	Starting position
Inner-range quadriceps	**Lying supine** Static quadriceps contraction Straight-leg raise
Hip abductors	**Straight side-lying** Lift straight leg up, keeping body still and slightly tilted forwards
Hip extensors	**Prone-lying** Lift straight leg up, keeping hips still
Plantarflexors and balance	Standing on one leg going up and down slowly on to tiptoes

its maximum amount at birth and the number starts to decrease after about 9 years of age.

As muscles have such varied functions it is important to consider all of these in a training programme to regain full muscle function. Using concentric and eccentric muscle work is often the most effective and easier for children to manage (Box 14.4).

Training children's muscles

Research shows that to improve muscle strength and stamina, a programme of progressive resisted exercise using the principles of high repetitions and low weights is most effective. The exercise programme should be started slowly but constantly progressed until full strength and fitness are regained. Progressions on a daily or weekly basis are more effective than monthly progressions.

The following regime is recommended for muscle training:

- Increase repetitions to a minimum of 15 before weights are added
- Low weights are recommended, with increases of 0.5 kg to a maximum of 2.5 kg
- Most children can increase to 5 kg safely
- When there is full fitness of the muscles, 30 repetitions are recommended
- Regular exercise is recommended 4–5 times per week, minimum twice per week.

Remember that children can increase their strength and fitness beyond normal growth and maturation and this is a vital principle in the management of children with rheumatological conditions (Strong 1990, Purcell & Hergenroeder 1994, Faigenbaum et al 1999, 2001, 2002, 2003, Faigenbaum 2000, American Academy of Pediatrics Committee on Sports Medicine and Fitness 2001, Baquet et al 2001, Fowler et al 2001, Obert et al 2001, Helge & Kanstrup 2002, Klepper 2003).

Specific exercise programme

In developing a programme for any child with a rheumatological condition, the most important aspect will be regaining joint range of movement and muscle strength and fitness.

Children with these conditions often develop similar and specific muscle weakness patterns. These usually involve the hip abductors and extensors, inner-range quadriceps and plantarflexors. Therefore a home management programme should include a strengthening and stamina programme for these muscles. Muscles that are weak need to be isolated and have a specific strengthening programme so that they can then function fully in normal activities.

The child and family need to understand that, for any physiotherapy programme to be effective, it has to be completed regularly at home and that the role of the physiotherapist is to monitor the home programme and to facilitate its progression. If the exercises are not completed regularly at home then no progress can be made. It is vital that the child and family learn how to manage these conditions themselves.

For any specific prescribed exercise programme to be effective in the management of these conditions these principles need to be followed (and Table 14.3 and Box 14.5):

1. Muscle-strengthening and stamina of muscles are the most vital aspects of the programme. The specific muscles that are weak and unfit should be targeted and the programme should be regularly progressed until 30 repetitions and 2.5-kg weights can be used for each exercise. (These guides should be modified for the smaller or larger child)
2. If inflammatory disease is causing loss of joint movement, then a daily stretching programme should be included
3. Balance and proprioception activities should be included and can easily be included in a programme.

The exercises need to be easy to do at home

Minimal equipment should be used

Use progressive and resisted exercises that can be done on the floor

Ensure the programme is not too long

Make the programme specific to the muscle weakness found on assessment

Agree the programme with the child and family

SUMMARY

In the management of children with rheumatological conditions there are several principles to consider:

1. At the assessment there is often underestimation as to the muscle strength of children and so weakness is missed

2. With all the conditions involved, these children usually have less muscle strength than normal

3. Loss of strength and stamina is rapid, especially in inflammatory disease, and this is then exacerbated by:
   (a) lack of activity
   (b) pain
   (c) loss of range of movement

4. Muscle strength and stamina can only be regained by exercise

5. Muscles are the only dynamic control of joints and therefore need to be as strong and as fit as possible in order to protect the joints

6. Children with rheumatological conditions can regain full strength and function and then can be encouraged to join in with all activities as their peers would do.

So there are many reasons why children with rheumatological conditions are weak, but with a regular progressive and resisted exercise programme these children can be strong and fit and have an active and painfree life.

CASE STUDY 14.1

Chris is a 9-year-old boy who presents in clinic with a history of increasing pain in both knees which occurs at night time and often wakes him up. It is worse after activity and sport, so he has stopped all exercise, but the pain has continued to increase. His mother has noticed some swelling in his knees after exercise and this lasts for a few hours. Chris is also more tired than his friends; he cannot walk far before he complains of pain, he bruises easily and is very fidgety in class. He also trips over often and bumps into things.

On assessment he has no evidence of a swollen joint. (For it to be diagnosed as arthritis, there has to be a persistent swelling in the same joint for 6 weeks or more – transient swelling indicates a biomechanical condition.) All joints showed hypermobility and he has a Beighton score of 6/9 and knees that hyperextend to 20°. Muscle strength-testing shows that inner-range quads are grade 2/5 and he has a quadriceps lag of 30°, hip abductors and extensors are grade 3/5 and plantarflexors are 4/5. Abdominals are 3/5 and core stability is reduced. Other muscle groups have full strength. Balance on one leg is reduced to 5 seconds on each leg with eyes open and 2 seconds with eyes closed. His gait presents as flat feet with poor heel–toe action, flexed knees and flexed internally rotated hips. A diagnosis of benign joint hypermobility syndrome was made.

Treatment

A progressive resisted exercise programme was prescribed for completion at home. This included inner-range quads over a towel, straight-leg raises, hip abduction in side-lying, hip extension in prone-lying and tiptoes on one leg. Chris was advised to complete the exercises 5 times a week and to start for the first week with 5 repetitions for each exercise and then each week to increase by 5 repetitions until he was completing 30 repetitions of each exercise. He was advised to wear ankle boots in order to control the hypermobility around his ankles and support his flat feet.

Chris returned after completing the programme and reported a big reduction in the pain he was experiencing and that in fact he was only woken twice a week instead of seven times. He was also able to walk further and had played football without having a rest. On examination all muscle strengths had increased to 4/5 and balance was >10 seconds with eyes open and 7 seconds with eyes closed. The exercise programme was modified by adding resistance with the use of weights (adjustable ankle weights 0.5–2.5 kg) and these were started with all the exercises (except tiptoes) at 0.5 kg and increased by 0.5 kg every 2 weeks to a maximum of 2.5 kg.

continued

Chris returned after 3 months and he was completing 30 repetitions with 2.5-kg weights 5 times a week. He had no pain and was now able to do everything his friends did. On examination he had full strength in all muscle groups and balance was >20 seconds with eyes open and closed. He had had no episodes of joint swelling and was able to play football all day with no difficulties. He was advised to continue with the programme 2–3 times a week for a few months and then to stop and to observe what happened. If the pain returned then he should restart his exercises.

CASE STUDY 14.2

Elizabeth is a 5-year-old girl who woke one morning with a very swollen painful left knee. She was taken to the general practitioner who thought it was sprained and recommended rest. Over the next few weeks she developed swelling in her other knee and her left ankle. After 6 weeks of continually swollen joints she was diagnosed with oligoarticular juvenile idiopathic arthritis. She was given intra-articular steroid injections into both knees and the left ankle under general anaesthetic. She also had a slit-lamp eye test that showed that she had no uveitis. Elizabeth was referred to physiotherapy and on assessment she had a 10° fixed flexion deformity in the left knee. The right knee had full range of movement but the left ankle had lost movement at end of range in all directions and was still slightly swollen. Elizabeth had a leg-length discrepancy of 1 cm, with the left leg being longer than the right. Assessment of muscle strength indicated weak inner-range quadriceps, weak hip abductors and extensors and poor plantarflexors. Her balance was reduced, with the left side worse than the right side.

Treatment

Elizabeth was prescribed a progressive home exercise programme. Her mother was taught how to stretch her left knee into full extension and her ankle into dorsiflexion, inversion and eversion and these were to be completed 3 × 10 seconds twice a day. Elizabeth was given exercises to complete, including inner-range quads (over a towel and straight-leg raise), hip abductors in side-lying and hip extensors in prone-lying, mid-range quads over the side of the bed and tiptoes on one leg to improve plantarflexor strength and balance. She was advised to do these exercises every day, starting with 5 times each for the first week and then increasing by 5 times each week until she was doing 30 of each exercise.

Elizabeth returned after 6 weeks: she was completing her exercise programme and had improved. Both knees now had full range of movement, as did her left ankle. She was able to complete each exercise with good technique and 30 times each. On reassessment of leg length there was still a 1-cm difference and she walked with the left knee slightly bent. Elizabeth's programme was changed: the stretches were stopped but the exercises were increased with the use of weights, keeping 30 repetitions but adding 0.5 kg every 2 weeks to a maximum of 1.5 kg. She was advised to wear lace-up ankle books to support the previously involved ankle and to allow the insertion of three flat foam insoles into the right boot to start to correct the leg-length discrepancy.

After 3 months her knee became swollen again and was reinjected. Elizabeth was advised to continue with her exercises and only reduce the weight for the 2 days after the injection but then to continue with all other exercises as before.

Elizabeth continued to attend school and was encouraged to join in with as many PE activities as possible. She was advised to continue walking and to be encouraged in normal activities. She was however advised not to try trampoline as it is difficult to control landings and can cause damage to joints if the muscles around them are not adequately strong. Since she was so well she was placed on a review appointment system and seen every 6 months.

REFERENCES

American Academy of Pediatrics Committee on Sports Medicine and Fitness 2001 Strength training by children and adolescents. *Pediatrics* 107: 1470–1472.

Bachrach LK 2001 Acquisition of optimal bone mass in childhood and adolescence. *Trends in Endocrinology and Metabolism* 12: 22–28.

Bagga A, Dillon MJ 2001 Vasculitis and its classification. In: Cassidy JT, Petty RE (eds) *The Textbook of Paediatric Rheumatology*, 4th edn. Philadelphia, PA: WB Saunders, pp. 564–568.

Baquet G, Berthoin S, Gerbeaux M, Van Praagh E 2001 High-intensity aerobic training during a 10 week one-hour physical education cycle: effects on physical fitness of adolescents aged 11 to 16. *International Journal of Sports Medicine* 22: 295–300.

Barr AE, Diamond BE, Wade CK et al 1991 Reliability of testing measures in Duchenne or Becker muscular dystrophy. *Archives of Physical Medicine and Rehabilitation* 72: 315–319.

Beighton P 1988 Hypermobility scoring. *British Journal of Rheumatology* 27: 163.

Burnett CN, Betts EF, King WM 1990 Reliability of isokinetic measurements of hip muscle torque in young boys. *Physical Therapy* 70: 244–249.

Cassidy JT, Petty RE 2001a Juvenile dermatomyositis. In: Cassidy JT, Petty RE (eds) *The Textbook of Paediatric Rheumatology*, 4th edn. Philadelphia, PA: WB Saunders, pp. 465–504.

Cassidy JT, Petty RE 2001b Systemic lupus erythematosus. In: Cassidy JT, Petty RE (eds) *The Textbook of Paediatric Rheumatology*, 4th edn. Philadelphia, PA: WB Saunders, pp. 396–449.

Cimaz R 2002 Osteoporosis in childhood rheumatic diseases: prevention and therapy. *Best Practice Research in Clinical Rheumatology* vol. 16, no. 3, pp. 397–409.

Collins RA, Grounds MD 2001 The role of tumor necrosis factor-alpha (TNF-alpha) in skeletal muscle regeneration. Studies in TNF-alpha(–/–) and TNF-alpha(–/–)/LT-alpha(–/–) mice, *Journal of Histochemistry and Cytochemistry* 49: 989–1001.

Davies JH, Evans BA, Gregory JW 2005 Bone mass acquisition in healthy children. *Archives of Disease in Childhood* 90: 373–378.

De Bleecker JL, De Paepe B, Vanwalleghem IE, Schroder JM 2002 Differential expression of chemokines in inflammatory myopathies. *Neurology* 58: 1779–1785.

Epps H, Ginnelly L, Utley M et al 2005 Is hydrotherapy cost-effective? A randomised controlled trial of combined hydrotherapy programmes compared with physiotherapy land techniques in children with juvenile idiopathic arthritis. *Health Technology Assessment* 9: iii–x, 1.

Faigenbaum AD 2000 Strength training for children and adolescents. *Clinics in Sports Medicine* 19: 593–619.

Faigenbaum AD, Westcott WL, Loud RL, Long C 1999 The effects of different resistance training protocols on muscular strength and endurance development in children. *Pediatrics* 104: e5.

Faigenbaum AD, Loud RL, O'Connell J, Glover S, O'Connell J, Westcott WL 2001 Effects of different resistance training protocols on upper-body strength and endurance development in children. *Journal of Strength Conduction Research* 15: 459–465.

Faigenbaum AD, Milliken LA, Loud RL, Burak BT, Doherty CL, Westcott WL 2002 Comparison of 1 and 2 days per week of strength training in children. *Research into Quarterly Exercise and Sport* 73: 416–424.

Faigenbaum AD, Milliken LA, Westcott WL 2003 Maximal strength testing in healthy children. *Journal of Strength Conduction Research* 17: 162–166.

Fedczyna TO, Lutz J, Pachman LM 2001 Expression of TNF-alpha by muscle fibers in biopsies from children with untreated juvenile dermatomyositis: association with the TNF-alpha-308A allele. *Clinics in Immunology* 100: 236–239.

Feghali CA, Wright TM 1997 Cytokines in acute and chronic inflammation. *Front Bioscience* 2: d12–d26.

Florence JM, Pandya S, King WM et al 1992 Intrarater reliability of manual muscle test (Medical Research Council scale) grades in Duchenne's muscular dystrophy. *Physical Therapy* 72: 115–122.

Fowler EG, Ho TW, Nwigwe AI, Dorey FJ 2001 The effect of quadriceps femoris muscle-strengthening exercises on spasticity in children with cerebral palsy. *Physical Therapy* 81: 1215–1223.

Giannini EH, Ruperto N, Ravelli A, Lovell DJ, Felson DT, Martini A 1997 Preliminary definition of improvement in juvenile arthritis. *Arthritis and Rheumatism* 40: 1202–1209.

Grahame R 1999 Joint hypermobility and genetic collagen disorders: are they related? *Archives of Disease in Childhood* 80: 188–191.

Hall MG, Ferrell WR, Sturrock RD, Hamblen DL, Baxendale RH 1995 The effect of the hypermobility syndrome on knee joint proprioception. *British Journal of Rheumatology* 34: 121–125.

Hamilton DM, Haennel RG 2000 Validity and reliability of the 6-minute walk test in a cardiac rehabilitation population. *Journal of Cardiopulmonary Rehabilitation* 20: 156–164.

Helge EW, Kanstrup IL 2002 Bone density in female elite gymnasts: impact of muscle strength and sex hormones. *Medical Science and Sports Exercise* 34: 174–180.

Huber AM, Hicks JE, Lachenbruch PA et al 2001 Validation of the Childhood Health Assessment Questionnaire in the juvenile idiopathic myopathies. Juvenile Dermatomyositis Disease Activity Collaborative Study Group. *Journal of Rheumatology* 28: 1106–1111.

Jessee EF, Owen DS, Sagar KB 1980 The benign hypermobility joint syndrome. *Arthritis and Rheumatism* 23: 1053–1055.

Klepper SE 2003 Exercise and fitness in children with arthritis: evidence of benefits for exercise and physical activity. *Arthritis and Rheumatism* 49: 435–443.

Lennon SM, Ashburn A 1993 Use of myometry in the assessment of neuropathic weakness: testing for reliability in clinical practice. *Clinical Rehabilitation* 7: 125–133.

Lovell DJ, Lindsley CB, Rennebohm RM et al 1999 Development of validated disease activity and damage indices for the juvenile idiopathic inflammatory myopathies. II. The

Childhood Myositis Assessment Scale (CMAS): a quantitative tool for the evaluation of muscle function. The Juvenile Dermatomyositis Disease Activity Collaborative Study Group. *Arthritis and Rheumatism* 42: 2213–2219.

Lundberg IE 2001 The physiology of inflammatory myopathies: an overview. *Acta Physiologica Scandinavica* 171: 207–213.

Lundberg I, Ulfgren AK, Nyberg P, Andersson U, Klareskog L 1997 Cytokine production in muscle tissue of patients with idiopathic inflammatory myopathies. *Arthritis and Rheumatism* 40: 865–874.

Maillard SM, Murray K 2003 Hypermobility in children. In: Keer R, Grahame R (eds) *Hypermobility Syndrome – Recognition and Management for Physiotherapists.* Edinburgh: Butterworth Heinemann.

Maillard SM, Davies K, Khubchandani R, Woo PM, Murray KJ 2004a Reflex sympathetic dystrophy: a multidisciplinary approach. *Arthritis and Rheumatism* 51: 284–290.

Maillard SM, Jones R, Owens C et al 2004b Quantitative assessment of MRI T2 relaxation time of thigh muscles in juvenile dermatomyositis. *Rheumatology (Oxford)* 43: 603–608.

Maillard SM, Pilkington C, Hasson N 2004c Physiotherapy management of benign joint hypermobility syndrome. *Arthritis and Rheumatism* 50: 10.

Maillard SM, Jones R, Owens CM et al 2005 Quantitative assessments of the effects of a single exercise session on muscles in juvenile dermatomyositis. *Arthritis and Rheumatism* 53: 558–564.

Mallik AK, Ferrell WR, McDonald AG, Sturrock RD 1994 Impaired proprioceptive acuity at the proximal interphalangeal joint in patients with the hypermobility syndrome. *British Journal of Rheumatology* 33: 631–637.

Malm C 2001 Exercise-induced muscle damage and inflammation: fact or fiction? *Acta Physiologica Scandinavica* 171: 233–239.

McDonagh JE 2001 Osteoporosis in juvenile idiopathic arthritis. *Current Opinion in Rheumatology* 13: 399–404.

McDonald CM, Jaffe KM, Shurtleff DB 1986 Assessment of muscle strength in children with meningomyelocele: accuracy and stability of measurements over time. *Archives of Physical Medicine and Rehabilitation* 67: 855–861.

Medical Research Council 1943 *Aids to the Investigation of Peripheral Nerve Injuries.* War memorandum, revised 2nd edn. London: HMSO.

Miller LC, Michael AF, Baxter TL, Kim Y 1988 Quantitative muscle testing in childhood dermatomyositis. *Archives of Physical Medicine and Rehabilitation* 69: 610–613.

Murray KJ, Woo P 2001 Benign joint hypermobility in childhood. *Rheumatology* 40: 489–491.

Nagaraju K 2001a Immunological capabilities of skeletal muscle cells. *Acta Physiologica Scandinavica* 171: 215–223.

Nagaraju K 2001b Update on immunopathogenesis in inflammatory myopathies. *Current Opinion in Rheumatology* 13: 461–468.

Nelson AM 2001 Localised scleroderma. In: Cassidy JT, Petty RE (eds) *The Textbook of Paediatric Rheumatology*, 4th edn. Philadelphia, PA: WB Saunders, pp. 535–543.

Nemet D, Oh Y, Kim HS, Hill M, Cooper DM 2002 Effect of intense exercise on inflammatory cytokines and growth mediators in adolescent boys. *Pediatrics* 110: 681–689.

Nugent J, Ruperto N, Grainger J et al 2001 The British version of the Childhood Health Assessment Questionnaire (CHAQ) and the Child Health Questionnaire (CHQ). *Clinical Experiments in Rheumatology* 19 (Suppl. 23): S163–S167.

Obert P, Mandigout M, Vinet A, Courteix D 2001 Effect of a 13-week aerobic training programme on the maximal power developed during a force-velocity test in prepubertal boys and girls. *International Journal of Sports Medicine* 22: 442–446.

Ostrowski K, Rohde T, Asp S, Schjerling P, Pedersen BK 1999 Pro- and anti-inflammatory cytokine balance in strenuous exercise in humans. *Journal of Physiology* 515: 287–291.

Paap E, van der Net, J Helders PJ, Takken T 2005 Physiologic response of the six-minute walk test in children with juvenile idiopathic arthritis. *Arthritis and Rheumatism* 53: 351–356.

Pachman LM, Fedczyna TO, Lechman TS, Lutz J 2001 Juvenile dermatomyositis: the association of the TNF alpha-308A allele and disease chronicity. *Current Rheumatology Report* 3: 379–386.

Pankoff B, Overend T, Lucy D, White K 2000 Validity and responsiveness of the 6 minute walk test for people with fibromyalgia. *Journal of Rheumatology* 27: 2666–2670.

Pedersen BK 2000 Exercise and cytokines. *Immunology and Cell Biology* 78: 535.

Pedersen BK, Toft AD 2000 Effects of exercise on lymphocytes and cytokines. *British Journal of Sports Medicine* 34: 246–251.

Pedersen BK, Steensberg A, Fischer C, Keller C, Ostrowski K, Schjerling P 2001a Exercise and cytokines with particular focus on muscle-derived IL-6. *Exercise and Immunology Review* 7: 18–31.

Pedersen BK, Steensberg A, Schjerling P 2001b Exercise and interleukin-6. *Current Opinion in Hematology* 8: 137–141.

Petty RE, Cassidy JT 2001 The juvenile idiopathic arthritides. In: Cassidy JT, Petty RE (eds) *The Textbook of Paediatric Rheumatology*, 4th edn. Philadelphia, PA: WB Saunders, pp. 214–295.

Purcell JS, Hergenroeder AC 1994 Physical conditioning in adolescents. *Current Opinion in Pediatrics* 6: 373–378.

Reid MB, Li YP 2001 Cytokines and oxidative signalling in skeletal muscle. *Acta Physiologica Scandinavica* 171: 225–232.

Rider LG, Feldman BM, Perez MD et al 1997 Development of validated disease activity and damage indices for the juvenile idiopathic inflammatory myopathies: I. Physician, parent, and patient global assessments. Juvenile Dermatomyositis Disease Activity Collaborative Study Group. *Arthritis and Rheumatism* 40: 1976–1983.

Ruperto N, Ravelli A, Migliavacca D et al 1999 Responsiveness of clinical measures in children with oligoarticular juvenile chronic arthritis. *Journal of Rheumatology* 26: 1827–1830.

Ruperto N, Ravelli A, Pistorio A et al 2001 Cross-cultural adaptation and psychometric evaluation of the Childhood Health Assessment Questionnaire (CHAQ) and the Child Health Questionnaire (CHQ) in 32 countries. Review of the general methodology. *Clinical Experiments in Rheumatology* 19 (Suppl. 23): S1–S9.

Scheett TP, Mills PJ, Ziegler MG, Stoppani J, Cooper DM 1999 Effect of exercise on cytokines and growth mediators in prepubertal children. *Pediatric Research* 46: 429–434.

Scheett TP, Nemet D, Stoppani J, Maresh CM, Newcomb R, Cooper DM 2002 The effect of endurance-type exercise training on growth mediators and inflammatory cytokines in pre-pubertal and early pubertal males. *Pediatric Research* 52: 491–497.

Sherry DD, Malleson PN 2001 Nonrheumatic musculoskeletal pain. In: Cassidy JT, Petty RE (eds) *The Textbook of Paediatric Rheumatology*, 4th edn. Philadelphia, PA: WB Saunders, pp. 362–380.

Spencer MJ, Marino MW, Winckler WM 2000 Altered pathological progression of diaphragm and quadriceps muscle in TNF-deficient, dystrophin-deficient mice, *Neuromuscular Disorder* 10: 612–619.

Stratford PW, Balsor BE 1994 A comparison of make and break tests using a hand-held dynamometer and the Kin-Com. *Journal of Orthopaedic Sports and Physical Therapy* 19: 28–32.

Strong WB 1990 Physical activity and children. *Circulation* 81: 1697–1701.

Takken T, Hemel A, van der Net, J, Helders PJ 2002 Aerobic fitness in children with juvenile idiopathic arthritis: a systematic review. *Journal of Rheumatology* 29: 2643–2647.

Takken T, Spermon N, Helders PJ, Prakken AB, van der Net, J 2003a Aerobic exercise capacity in patients with juvenile dermatomyositis. *Journal of Rheumatology* 30: 1075–1080.

Takken T, van der Net, J, Kuis W, Helders PJ 2003b Aquatic fitness training for children with juvenile idiopathic arthritis. *Rheumatology (Oxford)* 42: 1408–1414.

Takken T, van der Net, J, Kuis W, Helders PJ 2003c Physical activity and health related physical fitness in children with juvenile idiopathic arthritis. *Annals of Rheumatic Disease* 62: 885–889.

Takken T, van der Net, J, Helders PJ 2003 Relationship between functional ability and physical fitness in juvenile idiopathic arthritis patients. *Scandinavian Journal of Rheumatology* 32: 174–178.

Takken T, van der Net, J, Helders PJ 2005a Anaerobic exercise capacity in patients with juvenile-onset idiopathic inflammatory myopathies. *Arthritis and Rheumatism* 53: 173–177.

Takken T, van der Net, J, Helders PJ 2005b The reliability of an aerobic and an anaerobic exercise tolerance test in patients with juvenile onset dermatomyositis. *Journal of Rheumatology* 32: 734–739.

Toft AD, Jensen LB, Bruunsgaard H et al 2002 Cytokine response to eccentric exercise in young and elderly humans. *American Journal of Physiology and Cell Physiology* 283: C289–C295.

Tortolani PJ, McCarthy EF, Sponseller PD 2002 Bone mineral density deficiency in children. *Journal of the American Academy of Orthopedic Surgery* 10: 57–66.

Winkelman C 2004 Inactivity and inflammation: selected cytokines as biologic mediators in muscle dysfunction during critical illness. *AACN Clinical Issues* 15: 74–82.

Young NL, Wright JG 1995 Measuring pediatric physical function. *Journal of Pediatric Orthopaedics* 15: 244–253.

15 Duchenne muscular dystrophy

Michelle Eagle

INTRODUCTION

Duchenne muscular dystrophy (DMD) was once thought of as an untreatable disease but over the last decade advances in management have delivered a range of therapies that significantly improve quality of life and life expectancy. Although a cure is still awaited, there is much that can be done to maintain muscle strength, functional ability, respiratory and cardiac status. DMD is the second most common inherited disease of childhood (Iannaccone 1992).

GENETICS

DMD follows a typical X-linked pattern of inheritance, i.e. a son has a 50% chance of inheriting the condition from a carrier mother and a daughter has a 50% chance of inheriting carrier status. However there is a high rate of mutation in the dystrophin gene, which is currently the largest identified gene, and approximately one in three cases is a result of a new mutation. Germline mosaicism may occur in mothers who are thought not to be carriers and in this case the mother has ova that carry the mutation but not in her somatic tissues. The exact risk to future children is unknown but thought to be around 10–20%.

Most commonly occurring mutations in the gene are deletions, which account for 65% of all mutations, duplications (6%) and point mutations, where there is only a single basepair change. These latter mutations are difficult to find and require complex analysis of DNA in specialist centres to determine the mutation.

There is some phenotypic variability within children who have DMD (McDonald et al 1995b). Traditionally DMD was clinically defined by loss of the ability to walk by the age of 13 years, children with intermediate DMD/Becker muscular dystrophy (BMD) lost the ability to walk between the ages of 13 and 16 and those with BMD lost ambulation after the age of 16 years. However, many individuals with BMD walk well into adult life and have a normal lifespan (McDonald et al 1995a). These traditional definitions of DMD are no longer appropriate because of treatment with glucocorticosteroids which may prolong walking until after this age and furthermore genetic advances, including mutation analysis and immunohistochemical techniques, have made the diagnosis more precise.

Dystrophin

The gene responsible for DMD is on the short arm of the X chromosome, in position 21. This is why dystrophinopathies that include Becker and DMD are sometimes described as Xp21 dystrophinopathies. This gene codes for dystrophin which is absent in DMD and reduced in BMD.

Dystrophin has a major role in the integrity of the cytoskeleton. It is located on the inner wall of the plasma membrane and makes up the dystrophin-associated glycoprotein complex (Figure 15.1) which causes tears and instability in the membrane when disrupted.

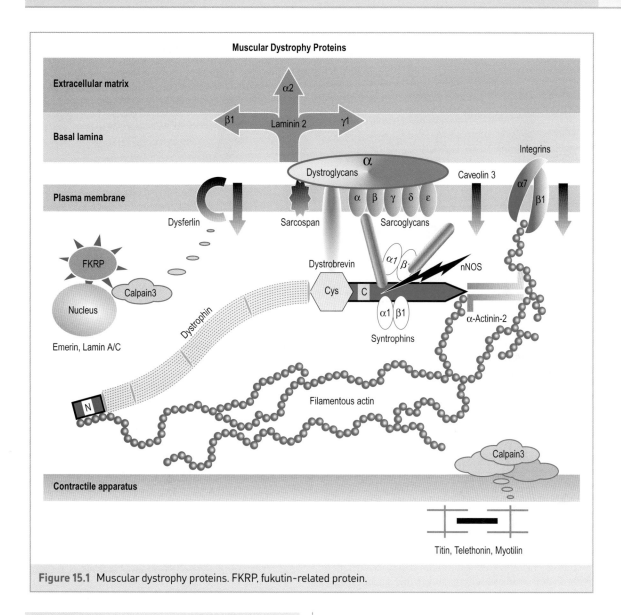

Muscular Dystrophy Proteins

Figure 15.1 Muscular dystrophy proteins. FKRP, fukutin-related protein.

DIAGNOSIS

If there is a known mutation in the family diagnosis can be made prenatally by chorionic villus sampling, amniocentesis or fetal muscle biopsy. Postnatal diagnosis may be suspected at any age by a massively raised creatine kinase level. A serum creatine kinase that is elevated 10–100 times normal is a non-specific test but it is always elevated in DMD. Analysis of DNA will elicit a diagnosis in about 70% of children. A muscle biopsy may not be required if a DNA diagnosis has been made but where the specific mutation has not been found, absence of dystrophin on a muscle biopsy will indicate DMD. Future therapies are likely to require specific DNA diagnosis which is also essential to provide accurate genetic counselling to potential carrier females.

The early clinical signs are most easily spotted by watching a child move (Gardner-Medwin et al 1978). One of the first noticeable physical manifestations is a 'Gowers' sign' (Figure 15.2).

A Gowers' sign on rising from the floor, a waddling run and observing the child jump may all indicate proximal muscle weakness. Large hypertrophied calves may add to the index of suspicion. Some children also have delayed speech and learning disabilities.

Males are mainly affected by DMD but rarely females can be affected and are known as manifesting carriers. This is thought to be caused by random inactivation in cells of the unaffected X chromosome. If this happens to a significant degree then the muscle cells will not produce enough dystrophin and weakness may occur.

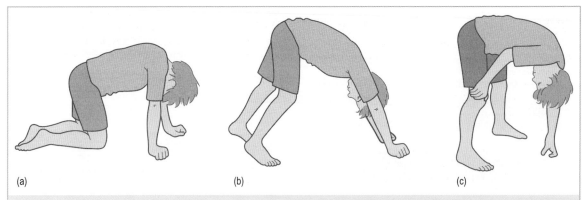

(a) (b) (c)

Figure 15.2 Gowers' manoeuvre. (a) The child turns towards the floor (generally into a four-point kneeling position) to place hands on the floor to assist rising, (b) walks the hands back in towards him then (c) uses arms to 'climb' up legs to achieve upright standing. A wide base of support is often assumed through the phases of rising from the floor. Reproduced from Gowers WR 1879 Clinical lecture on pseudohypertrophic muscular paralysis. *Lancet* ii: 73–75.

LEARNING AND LANGUAGE DIFFICULTIES IN DUCHENNE MUSCULAR DYSTROPHY

About 30% of boys with DMD have a learning problem (Bresolin et al 1994). Most boys will have an IQ that is within the normal range of 85–115 but on average the IQ is one standard deviation below the norm. The range of learning ability is very broad and yet there are specific features that are typical of DMD. For example, whatever the overall IQ, boys with DMD persistently score more highly on performance tests than on verbal tests on the Weschler Intelligence Scale for Children. Despite the progressive nature of the physical manifestations of DMD, there is no progression of the learning problems and over time they may even improve (Hendriksen & Vles 2006).

Hinton et al (2000, 2001a, b) have conducted detailed psychological profiles and concluded that all boys with DMD have a similar learning profile with specific strengths and weaknesses. For example, strengths include good vocabulary, rote learning and good general knowledge but weaknesses include difficulty in retaining sequentially presented material, such as a complex series of instructions, which may result in inattention. Hinton et al have shown that the ability of a child aged 6 years is more like that of a child of 4 years of age in ability to understand and follow verbal instructions, but also that by the age of 9 or 10 this improves.

THE COURSE OF DUCHENNE MUSCULAR DYSTROPHY IN UNTREATED BOYS

The natural history of untreated DMD is predictably bleak. After a short period of improvement between the ages of 3 and 6 years, motor deterioration is progressive.

Initially there will be more difficulty rising from the floor, the gait will become more laboured, then stairs will become impossible to climb and before the age of 12, though more usually 9, a child will be unable to walk (McDonald et al 1995c).

A progressive scoliosis will develop in 90% of children about 2 years after using a wheelchair full-time (Hsu 1983). In some children a severe and progressive cardiomyopathy will develop in early adolescence but a cardiomyopathy will be detectable in all by the late teens (Nigro et al 1990). Respiratory failure is the most common cause of death at an average age of 19 years (Rideau et al 1981).

Fortunately this picture is rarely seen where good health care is available and where health care professionals and families are aware of good practice. Guidelines for management are available for almost every aspect of care and management (Bushby et al 2003, Finder et al 2004, Moxley et al 2005, Bourke 2006, Muntoni et al 2006b).

INTERVENTIONS

Steroids

Treatment with glucocorticosteroids (prednisone/prednisolone/deflazacort) is now the gold standard for ambulant children with DMD (Bushby et al 2004). Randomized controlled trials show an improvement in strength (Brooke et al 1987, 1989a, b) and long-term cohort studies of daily deflazacort or prednisolone have demonstrated significantly prolonged walking ability to the mid-teens, vastly improved forced vital capacity (FVC), with reduction in the need for spinal surgery and improvement in cardiac functions (Biggar et al 2001, 2004, 2006, Silversides et al 2003, Alman et al 2004). Young boys with DMD are often able to ride a bike, jump and hop – all of which are unusual in boys not treated with steroids (Figure 15.3).

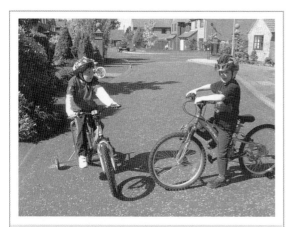

Figure 15.3 Young boy with Duchenne muscular dystrophy treated with steroids enjoying playing outside on his bike with his friend.

Side-effects are common in both intermittent and daily regimes but are probably less severe with intermittent use, though the benefits may not be so great. Side-effects include weight gain, osteoporosis, high blood pressure, behaviour problems, acne in teenagers, reduced growth and delayed puberty. Cataracts are more common with the use of deflazacort than prednisolone but are usually asymptomatic. A definitive long-term trial designed to elucidate practical information about the benefits versus the risks of steroid use is planned but for the moment children using steroids must be followed up by an experienced team (Bushby et al 2005).

Physiotherapy

Physiotherapy is part of the overall management from diagnosis into adulthood. There is no sound evidence to define the exact physiotherapeutic intervention, particularly now that the majority of ambulant children use steroids. What is clear, though, is that the pattern of progression is similar but at a slower rate; consequently, despite the use of steroids children will still develop contractures. Initially these develop at the ankle and hip but once children are non-ambulant, whether steroids have been used or not, contractures will become widespread and particular care should be taken to ensure that the upper limbs and hands remain functional.

In general, active exercise should be encouraged and resisted work discouraged because of the potential detrimental effect on the cell membrane (Eagle 2002). Hydrotherapy is beneficial at all stages of the condition. Active assisted, passive and respiratory physiotherapy can all be carried out in a pool. It is very important to ensure that the ambient air temperature is warm as these young people will get cold once out of the pool due to reduced muscle mass. Access to the pool and dressing arrangements need to be good as teenagers can be easily put off

hydrotherapy if the facilities are imperfect. In younger children hydrotherapy can encourage confidence and is fun and in the older child it may be the only way to achieve full range comfortably. The pleasure of movement in water can be enjoyed by all ages.

Regular stretching exercises incorporated into family routines are essential. In the early stages stretching is likely to be needed only to maintain the range of dorsiflexion at the ankle and at the hip where the iliotibial band becomes tight as the children adopt a wider base of support for stability. Expert opinion suggests that the appropriate stretches are carried out daily, in particular on the gastrocnemius–soleus complex which may be the only specific requirement in the early days. This should be introduced as soon as there is loss of range of dorsiflexion. Similarly, as soon as there is loss of the normal range of dorsi – flexion which may be at the time of diagnosis daily stretches should be done. Regular assessment will ensure that tightness can be detected before a fixed contracture develops. The physiotherapist must be careful not to overwhelm a family with a newly diagnosed young child with a prescription for lengthy sessions of numerous stretches. Of course prophylactic physiotherapy is important but careful evaluation will indicate when stretches are appropriate. Stretches for the gastrocnemius, hip flexors and iliotibial band are shown in Appendix 15.1.

Both night splints and stretches delay the progression of tightness of the gastrocnemius–soleus complex but a combination of the two is more effective. Two studies specifically evaluated the effect of orthoses on the development of contractures. Both concluded that the use of passive stretching and night splints was more effective than passive stretching alone at both delaying contracture development and prolonging independent ambulation (Scott et al 1981, Hyde et al 2000). Since gastrocnemius is a two-joint muscle, which crosses both the ankle and the knee, an effective stretch will be provided if both the foot is held at plantargrade or maximum dorsiflexion and the knee is held in extension. This type of night splint is not routinely supplied since anecdotally it is not well tolerated, interfering with sleep. Theoretically, an ankle–foot orthosis (AFO) crossing only the ankle joint could possibly increase knee contractures since the child may flex the knee to escape a stretch at the ankle. No information is available relating to this but clinical experience suggests this is not a major problem. AFOs worn during ambulation are usually unhelpful as they resist plantarflexion and so render gastrocnemius incapable of assisting knee extension.

Knee–ankle–foot orthoses (KAFOs) may be beneficial, particularly in prolonging walking and standing and therefore delaying the onset of contractures (Heckmatt et al 1985). Children with muscular dystrophy need ischial weight-bearing KAFOs such as those developed at the Hammersmith Hospital by John Florence. John Florence KAFOs should be supplied when the child is almost unable to walk as provision when walking is still functional will usually be unsuccessful. For KAFOs to be successful a child has to feel an improvement immediately. After casting,

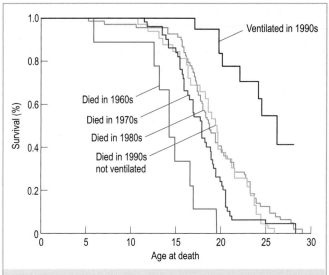

Figure 15.4 Improved survival over the decades in Duchenne muscular dystrophy. Better coordinated care and the use of antibiotics were probably responsible for the improvements in survival seen over the decades from the 1960s to the 1990s. The introduction of ventilation in the 1990s further increased survival.

supply must be rapid, usually within a week. They must fit perfectly or they will be rejected. For this reason it is vital to use experienced orthotists with knowledge of DMD to cast, supply and fit these orthoses.

It is known that prolongation of walking is associated with improved spinal posture and those who walk over the age of 11 years have a reduced rate of spinal fixation (Rodillo et al 1988). Lifting and handling regulations as well as the difficulties associated with therapeutic intervention in mainstream schools may make KAFOs a complicated treatment but it is worth a frank discussion with the family and child to see if KAFOs are worthwhile. It is possible that, with the increased use of steroids to prolong walking, KAFOs will be a rarer intervention. Similarly, standing frames and swivel walkers (Stallard et al 1992) may be used but have the same complications in their practical use.

The North Star project funded by the Muscular Dystrophy Campaign has developed an assessment protocol that will be used by all physiotherapists in the UK who work at a recognized muscle centre (Appendix 15.2). Regular assessment will enable specific treatment options to be determined and give objective evidence about the progression of the disease and impact of therapy (Scott & Mawson 2006).

Respiratory physiotherapy

Problems with secretion retention occur because of the inability to take a deep breath and the inability to cough effectively. Respiratory physiotherapy such as percussion and shaking or vibration is improved by the use of mechanical devices that increase the volume of inspired air. For example, a Bird ventilator or other means of mechanically inflating the lungs or an Ambu bag will increase the inspiratory volume and enable a more effective assisted cough to be given (Dohna-Schwake et al 2006a). Giving several inspiratory breaths without exhaling is called breath-stacking and is particularly helpful to achieve maximum inspiratory capacity. Assisted coughing should be taught to a family before coughing is inefficient and before the peak cough flow is below 160 l/min (Gomez-Merino & Bach 2002, Dohna-Schwake et al 2006b). The cough-assist machine is particularly helpful: not only does it increase the volume of air entering the lungs but it also increases the expiratory flow, enabling an efficient cough, especially when combined with an assisted cough (Kang et al 2005).

Glossopharyngeal breathing is a technique which can be taught or which develops spontaneously often in young adults who have been ventilated for several years and who resist daytime ventilation. The specific technique is quite individual in appearance but basically the aim is to open up the throat by moving the tracheal and laryngeal cartilages downwards and forcing air into the trachea, so the appearance is of 'air-swallowing'. This technique is often effective enough to enable hours of time off a ventilator in otherwise dependent young people and it can increase the volume of inspired air to enable a more effective cough, simply to take a deep breath or to raise the volume of the voice. An excellent video and DVD are available to demonstrate the use of this technique (Webber & Higgins 1999).

The ventilator should be used during physiotherapy for young people who are already ventilated. It is time-consuming, exhausting and frequently ineffective for a young person with a poor FVC to cooperate with chest physiotherapy. Using the ventilator, sufficient volumes of air will enter the chest at inspiration to enable more effective physiotherapy techniques during expiration and coughing than without.

Orthopaedic surgery

The most common orthopaedic procedure is lengthening of the tendo-achilles. Normally this should not be done in ambulant boys as the loss of the ability to plantarflex the foot in order to assist knee extension is likely to cause loss of ambulation. It is often performed in boys who are almost unable to walk so that they can be fitted immediately after surgery with ischial weight-bearing KAFOs. In Newcastle, casting is done in theatre after the surgical procedure to ensure that correctly fitting splints are available as soon as the plasters are removed. Once a child is wheelchair-dependent, tendo-achilles lengthening can be a simple procedure but if a fixed equinus has developed, then a more complex triple arthrodesis will be required to enable the foot to sit comfortably on the footplates, avoid pressure sores and enable normal footwear to be worn. AFOs must be worn even after triple arthro-desis to prevent further deformity.

Spinal surgery

Surgical fusion of the spine has been one of the most beneficial interventions for boys with a progressive scoliosis (Cervellati et al 2004). There is still debate about the precise timing of surgery but recent guidelines suggest that surgery should be performed when the curve has been proven to be progressive over a 6-month period, and that surgery is most successful when the curve does not exceed 20–40° (Sussman 1984, Muntoni et al 2006a). The presence of poor respiratory function is unlikely to prevent surgery, especially if it is done at an earlier stage, but a severe or progressive cardiomyopathy is a contraindication. Interestingly, young men who are treated with both spinal fusion and ventilation show an increased survival over those who have ventilation alone. Young people referred for spinal surgery are screened beforehand for the presence of cardiomyopathy and it is possible that survival is less in the non-operative group because of a higher incidence of early and more severe cardiomyopathy (unpublished data, M Eagle).

Spinal bracing is only an option to delay a curve progressing whilst surgery is awaited or in the case of a significant cardiomyopathy to provide postural support to enable continued comfortable sitting in a wheelchair.

Cardiac treatment

There have been significant advances in the treatment of cardiomyopathy. In the 1980s and early 1990s treatment for cardiomyopathy was only given in the presence of symptoms when the heart was already severely damaged. This did not lead to an increased lifespan, although there may have been a short-term improvement in well-being. Current research suggests that treatment with angiotensin-converting enzyme (ACE) inhibitors and then beta-blockers should be given when the echocardiograph demonstrates deterioration from the baseline assessment with or without the presence of symptoms (Duboc et al 2005, Bourke 2006). Trials are being conducted to determine whether even earlier prophylactic intervention between the ages of 6 and 10 will further improve cardiac function and outcomes.

Home ventilation

Improvements in respiratory management have been the most significant treatment for young adults with DMD and have increased survival from 19 years of age to the late 20s (Figure 15.4). The progressive deterioration in respiratory function is predictable and therefore manageable. At the Newcastle Muscle Centre young men with DMD are referred to the North East Assisted Ventilation Service. Treatment with non-invasive positive-pressure ventilation has increased the chance of survival to the late 20s to over 50% (Eagle et al 2002). In other countries where ventilation has been used for longer than in the UK, such as Denmark, invasive ventilation by tracheostomy has enabled patients in Denmark to survive well into their 30s (Jeppesen et al 2003). Non-invasive techniques seem to be preferred in the USA and in the UK and 24-hour ventilation is possible with non-invasive methods. The differences in management appear to be cultural. There are now significant numbers of young adults who survive into the fourth decade and, with the use of steroids and cardiac interventions, this should become the norm.

The key to successful non-invasive ventilation is preparation and assessment. In the late 1980s and early 1990s young men with severe symptoms tended to be ventilated when they were admitted to intensive-care facilities with severe respiratory failure. Many others died without ventilation being offered or chose to refuse treatment having already suffered years of ill health and repeated chest infections. Now assessment of respiratory function by spirometry, oximetry, clinical observation and sometimes blood gases will enable the timing of ventilation to be controlled and predicted. Predictive factors include the peak FVC and the age at which walking stops (Eagle 2003). A higher peak FVC and walking for longer than the average 9 years indicate a later-than-average requirement for ventilation. The average age of ventilation in the absence of treatment with steroids is between 17 and 19 years of age. Initially it will be used only at night but over the years dependence does increase and often over time the ventilator is needed during the day as well as overnight.

Symptoms of respiratory failure are the most important indicator of the need for ventilation. Symptoms of nocturnal hypoventilation will initially be mild and subtle but left untreated will develop into far more severe respiratory failure. Mild symptoms include frequent waking and unrefreshing sleep, feeling tired during the day, chest infections and weight loss. Severe or late symptoms include early-morning headaches, fear of going to sleep, anorexia, cyanosis and chest infections requiring hospital admission. At an early stage the provision of nighttime ventilation should be discussed with the family. This will give the family time to consider the options.

Prophylactic ventilation is not recommended following a French trial where more young people died in the treated group (Raphael et al 1994). The reasons for this are unclear but ventilation is not recommended in young people who have a normal carbon dioxide level. Once there is hypercapnia (elevated carbon dioxide levels) during the night, within a year or two this will develop into the more debilitating daytime hypercapnia (Ward et al 2005). Some young people do not complain of symptoms even despite a FVC below 20–40% or around 1 litre. Compliance in this situation may be difficult to achieve. Honest and open communication with the family and the young person about the implications of non-intervention with nocturnal ventilation is especially important in these circumstances as chest infections requiring hospital admission or even causing death are more likely with a deteriorating FVC below 1 litre. It is highly recommended that nocturnal ventilation is introduced before daytime carbon dioxide levels are abnormal. However most young people are accepting of the treatment where a clear benefit to their well-being is demonstrated by its use, for example by the alleviation of symptoms.

Emergency invasive ventilation is to be avoided as the weaning process is usually protracted; however the long-term outcome is good. There should be very few young people with DMD who end up on intensive care requiring emergency intubation. In Newcastle, before a system of regular assessment was introduced in the early 1990s, most young people who received ventilation did so after an emergency admission. In the last 10 years, only those who refused ventilation when it was offered as an elective treatment have subsequently been admitted to intensive care and required intubation before finally going home using nighttime ventilation.

The provision of safe home ventilation requires an experienced team with 24-hour back-up. Children and young people with a requirement for daytime ventilation should have battery back-up and those with a daytime dependence should have two ventilators in case of breakdown.

Other issues in Duchenne muscular dystrophy

Osteoporosis

Boys with DMD have low bone mineral density even before the loss of independent ambulation and even at diagnosis their bone mineral density is often below average (Bianchi et al 2003). It is unclear why this is the case but it may be due to relative immobility from a very early age in comparison to their peers. Traumatic fractures of the long bones are relatively common. In ambulant boys internal fixation may be required to ensure early remobilization as a lower-limb fracture may precipitate the loss of independent ambulation.

In the long term corticosteroid treatment reduces bone mineral density further, which may result in vertebral fractures in non-ambulant boys. Vertebral fractures can be treated with intravenous bisphosphonates (Bianchi 2005); however there is currently insufficient evidence to recommend the use of prophylactic oral bisphosphonates. Prophylaxis therefore relies on advice about calcium and vitamin D intake through diet and sunshine, with supplementation if necessary, to reach an intake of 1000 mg/day of calcium and 400 units of vitamin D (Quinlivan et al 2005).

Nutrition and gastrointestinal issues

The issue of weight control in DMD is taxing. Some boys tend to stay thin throughout their lives whereas others struggle with obesity. Sometimes weight increases as mobility decreases and as respiratory failure develops, loss of appetite is a frequent symptom and may be accompanied by weight loss. Weight gain is the most common complication associated with use of steroids and support from a dietician is recommended before steroids are introduced. In later stages of the disease there can be difficulty swallowing and where this leads to aspiration and/or undernutrition, discussion of feeding by nasogastric tube or gastrostomy is indicated. Detailed nutritional support should be provided to give advice on weight control, sodium restriction and calcium and vitamin D intake.

Urinary symptoms are not well described in the literature but may be a problem, especially in the transitional stage, when ambulation becomes increasingly difficult. Constipation is common and requires regular rather than episodic treatment, especially in older boys. A combination of senna and docusate may be helpful.

Anaesthetic issues

Volatile anaesthetic agents and depolarizing relaxants should be avoided due to an increased risk of hyperkalaemia, malignant hyperthermia-like crises and rhabdomyolysis in dystrophic muscle (Allen 1993, Breucking et al 2000). A thorough preoperative assessment is recommended and for children and young people with declining respiratory function it may be prudent to introduce non-invasive ventilation preoperatively. Current opinion would suggest that stable cardiac function on treatment might not be an absolute contraindication to surgery, but that rapid deterioration of cardiac function would be. It is important that airway protection is considered in young people who are at risk of respiratory problems or who are already ventilated even for procedures that require sedation or a local anaesthetic only. Ventilated patients should always take their ventilator with them when undergoing any medical treatment.

Wheelchair provision

When walking long distances is difficult a light-weight manual chair is adequate but regular self-propulsion is demanding and overtiring. Prior to this when a child is at nursery a buggy may suffice but is not recommended for older school age children.

When a child is unable to walk safely or comfortably then a high-quality powered wheelchair will be needed. Given the progressive nature of DMD, many wheelchair services will be prepared to issue a powered chair when walking is difficult but before a child is unable to walk, and this is to be recommended.

A powered wheelchair should be supplied with advance consideration for the potential complications. The back rest should support the normal spinal curves and extend to the spine of the scapula. Lateral support to the pelvis and trunk should be provided to promote good posture and resist leaning. The seat should not be too wide and caution must be taken not to supply a chair with too much 'room for growth' as excessive width will encourage leaning to one side or forwards to gain support from the thighs. The cushion needs to be firm but with pressure-relieving properties and enable good contact with the thighs and buttocks so that weight can be evenly distributed through them. The arm rests should be removable, adjustable in height and ideally also in width. They should be wide enough to enable weight to be taken comfortably through them.

Tilt-in-space and recline facilities should be provided routinely with the first powered chair. A child should be encouraged to change position regularly. A slightly tilted position is helpful to take the weight off the upright spine and therefore may delay the progression of a scoliosis. Reclining and tilting wheelchairs ease positioning of a child and may be used comfortably for recreational activities. Reclining when tired avoids the need to go to bed to rest, which can be isolating. A head rest should always be given and must be used when transporting and when tilting or reclining. Without a head rest boys will adopt a forward-leaning posture, which encourages posterior neck contractures. As these progress, sitting back in the chair is uncomfortable and becomes impossible; vision is obscured unless the forward-leaning posture is adopted, which in turn leads to further hip flexion contractures (see Ch.).

Specialist technological support

High-quality assistive devices significantly enhance the quality of life for families, children and young people with DMD. Specialist powered beds, environmental control systems, access to the internet and computers are all essential to enable as independent a life as possible (Soutter et al 2004). Details can be obtained through the Muscular Dystrophy Care Advisor network (see Ch. 10).

RESEARCH AND THE FUTURE OF DUCHENNE MUSCULAR DYSTROPHY

Several international collaborations are currently investigating the potential for disease-modifying drugs. At present glucocorticosteroids are the gold standard for boys with DMD and further research is required to understand better the benefits versus the side-effects in different regimes and different types of steroid.

There are a number of potential therapies for DMD (Kapsa et al 2003, Brockington & Muntoni 2005, Hirst et al 2005). Many aim to induce the production of dystrophin or a shortened version of it. The most appropriate treatment for each individual child may well be determined by the nature of the mutation. For boys who have a premature stop codon ,the aim is to 'read through' the premature stop and induce a full-length dystrophin (Scheuenbrandt 2004, 2005). Gentamicin and PCT124 are compounds that cause the RNA translation mechanism in the ribosomes to ignore such a premature stop codon, i.e. to read through it. The read-through technique has variable efficiency at the moment but if it can be developed to a Duchenne therapy, the new dystrophin will practically have the normal structure. However, only 5–10% of patients with DMD have a premature stop codon and because read-through occurs during protein synthesis in the ribosomes, treatment will have to be repeated periodically.

Exon skipping

The exon-skipping technique tries to change a Duchenne mutation into a Becker mutation. If a deletion or a point mutation disturbs the reading frame and thus causes Duchenne dystrophy, the reading frame can be restored by artificially removing one or more exons directly before or after the deletion or point mutation from the mRNA by using antisense oligoribonucleotides (Wilton & Fletcher 2005). As the mRNA is shorter than normal, the dystrophin protein is also shorter; it contains fewer amino acids. If the missing amino acids are part of the central region of the dystrophin, they are often not essential, and the resulting shorter protein can still perform its stabilizing role of the muscle cell membrane. The result would be the change of the severe Duchenne symptoms into the much milder symptoms of BMD. As the dystrophin gene itself will not be altered, the effect of the antisense treatment will not be permanent, so it will have to be repeated at intervals still to be determined. The sequence of the basepairs of the entire dystrophin gene is known in detail, so one can predict which exon or exons would have to be skipped to restore the reading frame of an individual patient. However, it is not certain whether the experimental results now being obtained in cell culture or in mice will be the same in Duchenne boys, and whether the shortened dystrophin will really lead to the clinical symptoms of a BMD. At this time, such predictions can only be purely theoretical. Phase I trials of antisense oligonucleotides have already started and the hope is for therapeutic trials to begin in the next 2–5 years (Muntoni et al 2005).

LOOKING FORWARD TO ADULT LIFE

Most young men with DMD in the UK live at home and very few have paid employment or attend university. This is not the situation in other countries such as Denmark (Rahbek et al 2005). There independent living is expected with full personal attendant care 24 hours a day. Of course, social service systems vary, but so do expectations. It should no longer be the norm for a young man with DMD to die before he reaches adulthood. There are many studies that demonstrate the high quality of life that is possible for adults with DMD (Miller et al 1990, Bach et al 1991, Kohler et al 2005). We therefore have to view DMD in a different way because it is no longer a disease of childhood but one that extends into adulthood. Given this, children with DMD have to be prepared for adult life. Social and health services must be developed and extended to provide for them. Better intervention is required in the early years to ensure full potential for education is reached and high-quality adaptations and aids are needed to ensure the maximum potential for independence is reached.

CASE STUDY 15.1

John was born in 1970. He was the first of two sons to be born with Duchenne muscular dystrophy (DMD). His mother had two brothers, also with DMD, who lived in residential care until they died aged 16 and 17 years of age. John was slow to talk and walk and his mother was sure that there was something wrong. She had not been offered any genetic counselling during or before her pregnancy. John was 5 years old when a creatine kinase test was done. The highly elevated levels and the family history confirmed a diagnosis of DMD. John's mother was pregnant at the time of the diagnosis. A blood test soon after the baby was born in 1976 confirmed her worst fears, that Peter was also affected.

John used a wheelchair full-time when he was 8 years old. John went to a special school where he received daily physiotherapy, including stretches and hydrotherapy. He developed a very progressive scoliosis at the age of 11, which was treated with a spinal brace. The local Muscular Dystrophy Group raised money to buy him a powered wheelchair, which he loved. John was an active member of the wheelchair hockey team and played with the other boys who also had DMD. At 15, John started to develop frequent chest infections and was often admitted to hospital where he was treated with physiotherapy and antibiotics. John had regular chest physiotherapy in school and at home, which was time-consuming and tiring. By the time he was 17, John was thin, had pressure sores, was uncomfortable in his wheelchair and spent much of his time in bed. He began to fear going to sleep and woke in the mornings with headaches and nausea. He was fatigued during the day. John developed a severe chest infection and was admitted to hospital but he arrested in the casualty department and it was decided not to attempt resuscitation. John was 18 when he died.

Peter was nearly 12 when John died. He had lost independent ambulation at 9 years of age but walked using knee–ankle–foot orthoses (KAFOs) for another 18 months. He also went to a special school where he received daily therapy. Once he was unable to walk in KAFOs he used a swivel walker to stand for an additional year. He developed a scoliosis when he was 14 years old and it was decided that he would benefit from a spinal fusion. Peter recovered well following the surgery. His physiotherapy continued with daily stretches and hydrotherapy whilst in school. When he was 18 years old, he began to wake frequently through the night and used to fall asleep on the bus on the way home from school. He felt generally off-colour but there were no specific signs. It was noted at his routine follow-up appointment that his forced vital capacity was less than 1 litre so overnight pulse oximetry and echocardiography were arranged. The tests revealed significant oxygen desaturation so Peter was given a ventilator to use overnight. The echocardiograph was normal but he was slightly tachycardic. The symptoms of nocturnal hypoventilation and tachycardia resolved shortly after nocturnal ventilation was established. Two years later, at his routine cardiac follow-up, it was noticed that one of the measures to document the efficiency of the heart (the ejection fraction) had fallen from its previous level, although it remained in a low-normal range. Angiotensin-converting enzyme (ACE) inhibition and beta-blockers were started and the cardiomyopathy remained stable but slightly progressive over the years.

continued

Peter, aged 30, still lives at home with his mum. He went to college after leaving school but left after 6 months as the facilities were not suitable. Peter found it almost impossible to get regular physiotherapy once he left school. His mum does passive movements most days as Peter finds this helps to ease his joints. He rarely sees a physiotherapist except on the rare occasions that he requires chest physiotherapy. Peter has learnt that using his ventilator during chest physiotherapy is more effective than without. Most days he uses the ventilator for a couple of hours during the day but more so if he has a chest infection. Peter spends most of his time at home with family. His leisure activities include shopping, playing games on his computer, going to football matches and watching television. He collects model cars which he buys and sells on E-Bay. He would dearly love a girlfriend.

CASE STUDY 15.2

Jack was born in 1997. There was no family history of Duchenne muscular dystrophy (DMD) but subsequent genetic testing showed that his mum was a carrier of DMD. Jack was diagnosed aged 4 after the health visitor noticed that he was not running smoothly and struggled to get off the floor. DNA testing showed that Ian had a mutation of exons 51–53 on chromosome 21.

Jack started steroids when he was nearly 5 years old. After 3 months on treatment he was jumping and running and had much more energy. Jack goes to his local primary school where he joined the after-school football club. His physiotherapist worked with the school to include Jack in PE sessions and after-school clubs.

When Jack was 8, his parents noticed that he was struggling to walk long distances, for example on school trips, so a light-weight manual wheelchair was supplied from wheelchair services. Jack is 9 now and still able to get up from the floor and climb stairs. He is currently independent in activities of daily living, including dressing. Jack's mum does stretches every evening after his bath. She finds that routine is helpful. Initially, after diagnosis Jack only required stretches of the tendo-achilles; however, as his gait became more lordotic and wider-based, hip flexor and iliotibial band stretches were introduced. He also has night splints which, after some persuasion, he wears nightly during sleep. These were supplied once there was loss of full passive range of dorsiflexion.

His parents are hopeful that a disease-modifying treatment will be developed whilst he is still ambulant.

REFERENCES

Allen GC 1993 Malignant hyperthermia and associated disorders. *Current Opinion in Rheumatology* 5: 719–724.

Alman BA, Raza SN, Biggar WD 2004 Steroid treatment and the development of scoliosis in males with Duchenne muscular dystrophy. *Journal of Bone and Joint Surgery of America* 86-A: 519–524.

Bach JR, Campagnolo DI, Hoeman S 1991 Life satisfaction of individuals with Duchenne muscular dystrophy using long-term mechanical ventilatory support. *American Journal of Physical Medicine and Rehabilitation* 70: 129–135.

Bianchi ML 2005 How to manage osteoporosis in children. *Best Practice Research in Clinical Rheumatology* 19: 991–1005.

Bianchi ML, Mazzanti A, Galbiati E et al 2003 Bone mineral density and bone metabolism in Duchenne muscular dystrophy. *Osteoporos International* 14: 761–767.

Biggar WD, Gingras M, Fehlings DL, Harris VA, Steele CA 2001 Deflazacort treatment of Duchenne muscular dystrophy. *Journal of Pediatrics* 138: 45–50.

Biggar WD, Politano L, Harris VA et al 2004 Deflazacort in Duchenne muscular dystrophy: a comparison of two different protocols. *Neuromuscular Disorders* 14: 476–482.

Biggar WD, Harris VA, Eliasoph L, Alman B 2006 Long-term benefits of deflazacort treatment for boys with Duchenne muscular dystrophy in their second decade. *Neuromuscular Disorders* 16: 249–255.

Bourke JP 2006 Cardiac monitoring and treatment for children and adolescents with neuromuscular disorders. *Developmental Medicine and Child Neurology* 48: 164.

Bresolin N, Castelli E, Comi GP et al 1994 Cognitive impairment in Duchenne muscular dystrophy. *Neuromuscular Disorders* 4: 359–369.

Breucking E, Reimnitz P, Schara U, Mortier W 2000 [Anesthetic complications. The incidence of severe anesthetic complications in patients and families with progressive muscular dystrophy of the Duchenne and Becker types.] *Anaesthesist* 49: 187–195.

Brockington M, Muntoni F 2005 The modulation of skeletal muscle glycosylation as a potential therapeutic intervention in muscular dystrophies. *Acta Myologica* 24: 217–221.

Brooke MH, Fenichel GM, Griggs RC et al 1987 Clinical investigation of Duchenne muscular dystrophy. Interesting results in a trial of prednisone. *Archives of Neurology* 44: 812–817.

Brooke MH, Fenichel GM, Griggs RC et al 1989 Duchenne muscular dystrophy: patterns of clinical progression and effects of supportive therapy. *Neurology* 39: 475–481.

Bushby K, Muntoni F, Bourke JP 2003 107th ENMC international workshop: the management of cardiac involvement in muscular dystrophy and myotonic dystrophy. 7th–9th June 2002, Naarden, the Netherlands, *Neuromuscular Disorders* 13: 166–172.

Bushby K, Muntoni F, Urtizberea A, Hughes R, Griggs R 2004 Report on the 124th ENMC International Workshop. Treatment of Duchenne muscular dystrophy; defining the gold standards of management in the use of corticosteroids. 2–4 April 2004, Naarden, The Netherlands. *Neuromuscular Disorders* 14: 526–534.

Bushby K, Bourke J, Bullock R, Eagle M, Gibson M, Quinby J 2005 The multidisciplinary management of Duchenne muscular dystrophy. *Current Paediatrics* 15: 292–300.

Cervellati S, Bettini N, Moscato M, Gusella A, Dema E, Maresi R 2004 Surgical treatment of spinal deformities in Duchenne muscular dystrophy: a long term follow-up study. *European Spine Journal* 13: 441–448.

Dohna-Schwake C, Ragette R, Teschler H, Voit T, Mellies U 2006a IPPB-assisted coughing in neuromuscular disorders. *Pediatric Pulmonology* 41: 551–557.

Dohna-Schwake C, Ragette R, Teschler H, Voit T, Mellies U 2006b Predictors of severe chest infections in pediatric neuromuscular disorders. *Neuromuscular Disorders* 16: 325–328.

Duboc D, Meune C, Lerebours G, Devaux JY, Vaksmann G, Becane HM 2005 Effect of perindopril on the onset and progression of left ventricular dysfunction in Duchenne muscular dystrophy. *Journal of the American College of Cardiology* 45: 855–857.

Eagle M 2002 Report on the muscular dystrophy campaign workshop: exercise in neuromuscular diseases Newcastle, January 2002. *Neuromuscular Disorders* 12: 975–983.

Eagle M 2003 *The Impact of Nocturnal Ventilation in Duchenne Muscular Dystrophy.* PhD thesis. Newcastle: University of Northumbria at Newcastle.

Eagle M, Baudouin SV, Chandler C, Giddings DR, Bullock R, Bushby K 2002 Survival in Duchenne muscular dystrophy: improvements in life expectancy since 1967 and the impact of home nocturnal ventilation. *Neuromuscular Disorders* 12: 926–929.

Finder JD, Birnkrant D, Carl J et al 2004 Respiratory care of the patient with Duchenne muscular dystrophy: ATS

consensus statement. *American Journal of Respiratory and Critical Care Medicine* 170: 456–465.

Gardner-Medwin D, Bundey S, Green S 1978 Early diagnosis of Duchenne muscular dystrophy. *Lancet* 1: 1102.

Gomez-Merino E, Bach JR 2002 Duchenne muscular dystrophy: prolongation of life by noninvasive ventilation and mechanically assisted coughing. *American Journal of Physical Medicine and Rehabilitation* 81: 411–415.

Heckmatt JZ, Dubowitz V, Hyde SA, Florence J, Gabain AC, Thompson N 1985 Prolongation of walking in Duchenne muscular dystrophy with lightweight orthoses: review of 57 cases. *Developmental Medicine and Child Neurology* 27: 149–154.

Hendriksen JG, Vles JS 2006 Are males with Duchenne muscular dystrophy at risk for reading disabilities? *Pediatric Neurology* 34: 296–300.

Hinton VJ, De Vivo DC, Nereo NE, Goldstein E, Stern Y 2000 Poor verbal working memory across intellectual level in boys with Duchenne dystrophy. *Neurology* 54: 2127–2132.

Hinton VJ, De Vivo DC, Nereo NE, Goldstein E, Stern Y 2001a Selective deficits in verbal working memory associated with a known genetic etiology: the neuropsychological profile of Duchenne muscular dystrophy. *Journal of the International Neuropsychological Society* 7: 45–54.

Hinton VJ, De Vivo DC, Nereo NE, Goldstein E, Stern Y 2001b Selective deficits in verbal working memory associated with a known genetic etiology: the neuropsychological profile of Duchenne muscular dystrophy. *Journal of the International Neuropsychological Society* 7: 45–54.

Hirst RC, McCullagh KJ, Davies KE 2005 Utrophin upregulation in Duchenne muscular dystrophy. *Acta Myologica* 24: 209–216.

Hsu JD 1983 The natural history of spine curvature progression in the nonambulatory Duchenne muscular dystrophy patient. *Spine* 8: 771–775.

Hyde SA, Filytrup I, Glent S et al 2000 A randomized comparative study of two methods for controlling tendo Achilles contracture in Duchenne muscular dystrophy. *Neuromuscular Disorders* 10: 257–263.

Iannaccone ST 1992 Current status of Duchenne muscular dystrophy. *Pediatric Clinics of .North America* 39: 879–894.

Jeppesen J, Green A, Steffensen BF, Rahbek J 2003 The Duchenne muscular dystrophy population in Denmark, 1977–2001: prevalence, incidence and survival in relation to the introduction of ventilator use. *Neuromuscular Disorders* 13: 804–812.

Kang SW, Kang YS, Moon JH, Yoo TW 2005 Assisted cough and pulmonary compliance in patients with Duchenne muscular dystrophy. *Yonsei Medical Journal* 46: 233–238.

Kapsa R, Kornberg AJ, Byrne E 2003 Novel therapies for Duchenne muscular dystrophy. *Lancet Neurology* 2: 299–310.

Kohler M, Clarenbach CF, Boni L, Brack T, Russi EW, Bloch KE 2005 Quality of life, physical disability, and respiratory impairment in Duchenne muscular dystrophy. *American Journal of Respiratory and Critical Care Medicine* 172: 1032–1036.

McDonald CM, Abresch RT, Carter GT, Fowler WM Jr, Johnson ER, Kilmer DD 1995a Profiles of neuromuscular diseases. Becker's muscular dystrophy. *American Journal of Physical Medicine and Rehabilitation* 74 (Suppl.): S93–S103.

McDonald CM, Abresch RT, Carter GT et al 1995b Profiles of neuromuscular diseases. Duchenne muscular dystrophy. *American Journal of Physical Medicine and Rehabilitation* 74 (Suppl.): S70–S92.

McDonald CM, Abresch RT, Carter GT et al 1995c Profiles of neuromuscular diseases. Duchenne muscular dystrophy. *American Journal of Physical Medicine and Rehabilitation* 74 (Suppl.): S70–S92.

Miller JR, Colbert AP, Osberg JS 1990 Ventilator dependency: decision-making, daily functioning and quality of life for patients with Duchenne muscular dystrophy. *Developmental Medicine and Child Neurology* 32: 1078–1086.

Moxley RT III, Ashwal S, Pandya S et al 2005 Practice parameter: corticosteroid treatment of Duchenne dystrophy: report of the Quality Standards Subcommittee of the American Academy of Neurology and the Practice Committee of the Child Neurology Society. *Neurology* 64: 13–20.

Muntoni F, Bushby K, van Ommen G 2005 128th ENMC International workshop on Preclinical optimization and phase i/ii clinical trials using antisense oligonucleotides in Duchenne muscular dystrophy 22–24 October 2004, Naarden, The Netherlands. *Neuromuscular Disorders* 15: 450–457.

Muntoni F, Bushby K, Manzur AY 2006 Muscular Dystrophy Campaign funded workshop on management of scoliosis in Duchenne muscular dystrophy 24 January 2005, London, UK. *Neuromuscular Disorders* 16: 210–219.

Nigro G, Comi LI, Politano L, Bain RJ 1990 The incidence and evolution of cardiomyopathy in Duchenne muscular dystrophy. *International Journal of Cardiology* 26: 271–277.

Quinlivan R, Roper H, Davie M, Shaw NJ, McDonagh J, Bushby K 2005 Report of a Muscular Dystrophy Campaign funded workshop Birmingham, UK, January 16th 2004. Osteoporosis in Duchenne muscular dystrophy; its prevalence, treatment and prevention, *Neuromuscular Disorders* 15: 72–79.

Rahbek J, Werge B, Madsen A, Marquardt J, Steffensen BF, Jeppesen J 2005 Adult life with Duchenne muscular dystrophy: observations among an emerging and unforeseen patient population. *Pediatric Rehabilitation* 8: 17–28.

Raphael JC, Chevret S, Chastang C, Bouvet F 1994 Randomised trial of preventive nasal ventilation in Duchenne muscular dystrophy. French Multicentre Cooperative Group on Home Mechanical Ventilation Assistance in Duchenne de Boulogne Muscular Dystrophy. *Lancet* 343: 1600–1604.

Rideau Y, Jankowski LW, Grellet J 1981 Respiratory function in the muscular dystrophies. *Muscle Nerve* 4: 155–164.

Rodillo EB, Fernandez-Bermejo E, Heckmatt JZ, Dubowitz V 1988 Prevention of rapidly progressive scoliosis in Duchenne muscular dystrophy by prolongation of walking with orthoses. *Journal of Child Neurology* 3: 269–274.

Scheuenbrandt G 2004 Report on a round table conference in Monaco on 17th and 18th January, 2004. *Acta Myologica* 23: 106–122.

Scheuenbrandt G 2005 Fourth round table conference in Monaco on 15 January 2005: regulation of muscle growth, a therapeutic issue for Duchenne muscular dystrophy? *Acta Myologica* 24: 25–35.

Scott E, Mawson SJ 2006 Measurement in Duchenne muscular dystrophy: considerations in the development of a neuromuscular assessment tool. *Developmental Medicine and Child Neurology* 48: 540–544.

Scott OM, Hyde SA, Goddard C, Dubowitz V 1981 Prevention of deformity in Duchenne muscular dystrophy. A prospective study of passive stretching and splintage. *Physiotherapy* 67: 177–180.

Silversides CK, Webb GD, Harris VA, Biggar DW 2003 Effects of deflazacort on left ventricular function in patients with Duchenne muscular dystrophy. *American Journal of Cardiology* 91: 769–772.

Soutter J, Hamilton N, Russell P et al 2004 The Golden Freeway: a preliminary evaluation of a pilot study advancing information technology as a social intervention for boys with Duchenne muscular dystrophy and their families. *Health and Social Care in the Community* 12: 25–33.

Stallard J, Henshaw JH, Lomas B, Poiner R 1992 The ORLAU VCG (variable centre of gravity) swivel walker for muscular dystrophy patients. *Prosthetics and Orthotics International* 16: 46–48.

Sussman MD 1984 Advantage of early spinal stabilization and fusion in patients with Duchenne muscular dystrophy. *Journal of Pediatrics and Orthopediatrics* 4: 532–537.

Ward S, Chatwin M, Heather S, Simonds AK 2005 Randomised controlled trial of non-invasive ventilation (NIV) for nocturnal hypoventilation in neuromuscular and chest wall disease patients with daytime normocapnia. *Thorax* 60: 1019–1024.

Webber B, Higgins J 1999 Barbara Webber and Jane Higgins in association with Aslan Studios Ltd. Video available from BA Webber, Sunnybank, The Platt, Amersham, Berks HP7 0HX.

Wilton SD, Fletcher S 2005 Antisense oligonucleotides in the treatment of Duchenne muscular dystrophy: where are we now? *Neuromuscular Disorders* 15: 399–402.

APPENDIX 15.1 EXAMPLES OF STRETCHING EXERCISES

Manual Achilles tendon stretch

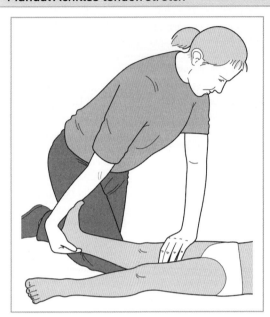

Position

- Child lying on back
- Cup heel in hand
- Rest sole of foot on forearm
- Stabilize above the knee with the other hand.

Stretch

- Pull down firmly on the heel while pushing the ball of the foot up. Keep knee straight
- Stretch is felt in calf

Special instructions

- If resistance to stretch is felt, bend the knee, stretch the ankle then straighten the knee while maintaining the ankle stretch. Place support under the knee to prevent hyperextension.

Hip flexor stretch (plus iliotibial tract)

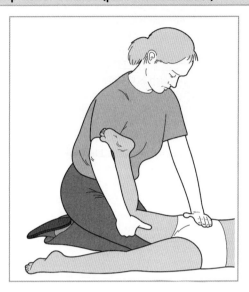

Position

- Child lies flat on tummy
- Cup bent knee in hand
- Ankle rests on elbow or upper arm
- Place other hand on bottom.

Stretch

- Pull knee up and **towards** the other leg while applying downward pressure on the bottom
- Stretch is felt in groin and outside of hip

Iliotibial tract (manual stretch in prone)

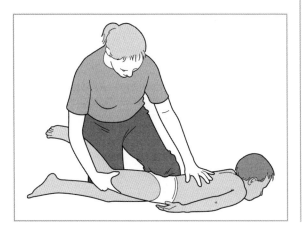

Position

- Child lies on tummy
- Grasp leg to be stretched at knee
- Stabilize and keep pelvis and trunk flat with knee and hand.

Stretch

- Lift leg up
- Pull leg across towards other leg
- Apply pressure on buttocks to keep pelvis flat
- Stretch is felt down outer thigh.

APPENDIX 15.2 NORTH STAR PHYSIOTHERAPY ASSESSMENTS

Patient: Assessed by: Date:

Steroids on day of assessment Y/N   State which day of cycle_____

	North Star Ambulatory Assessment (NSAA)	Score 2, 1, 0	Time (00.0s)	
1	Stand			
2	Walk (10 metres)			
3	Sit to stand from chair			
4	Stand on one leg – R			
5	Stand on one leg – L			
6	Climb step – R			
7	Climb step – L			
8	Descend step – R			
9	Descend step – L			
10	Get to sitting			
11	Rise from floor			
12	Lift head			
13	Stand on heels			
14	Jump			
15	Hop – R			
16	Hop – L			
17	Run			
	Total NSAA (out of 34)			

Joint range	R	L	Comments
Elbow extension			
Hip extension			
Knee extension			
Ankle dorsiflexion			
Iliotibial band tightness			

Forced vital capacity	Absolute value	% age predicted for height	Comments
Test 1			
Test 2			
Test 3			

(or attach spirometer printout)

Patient: Assessed by: Date:

Manual muscle testing (MMT)

Muscle group	Grade (0–5) R	L	Comments
Neck flexors			
Neck extensors			
Shoulder flexors			
Shoulder extensors			
Shoulder abductors			
Elbow flexors			
Elbow extensors			
Hip flexors			
Hip extensors			
Hip abductors			
Hip adductors			
Knee flexors			
Knee extensors			
Dorsiflexors			
Planterflexors			
Total score			
Muscle score (%)			

MMT not needed for North Star – Unit-specific

Muscle group	Grade (0–5) R	L	Comments

NORTH STAR PHYSIOTHERAPY ASSESSMENTS (*CONTINUED*)

Myometry: Dominant side: right/left (delete as appropriate)

Muscle group	Test results (N)	Best score (N)	Comments
Knee extensors	1		
	2		
	3		
Hip flexors	1		
	2		
	3		
Elbow flexors	1		
	2		
	3		
Shoulder abductors	1		
	2		
	3		
Grip	1		
	2		
	3		

NORTH STAR PHYSIOTHERAPY ASSESSMENTS – SUPPLEMENTARY INFORMATION

Patient: Assessed by: Date:

Management of joint range (link to assessment of joint range)

Stretches	Summary of advice given and to whom. Include frequency and repetitions
Orthotics	e.g. foot orthoses, ankle—foot orthoses, knee—ankle—foot orthoses
Usage	e.g. night splints + estimated wear time and compliance
General advice given	e.g. hydrotherapy/swimming
Surgery (if any –specify)	
Comments	e.g. any problems with any of the above. Include compliance where possible

NORTH STAR PHYSIOTHERAPY ASSESSMENTS – SUPPLEMENTARY INFORMATION (*CONTINUED*)

Mobility equipment	
Wheelchair/buggy	Y/N
Model	
Wheelchair cushion	Y/N
Model	
Wheelchair services	
Contact	
Comments	

Gait analysis (brief description: include any aids used, frequency of falls)

Patient: Assessed by: Date:

General activity levels

Include extracurricular activities such as swimming, cycling, trampolining, horse-riding

---

Parent/carer perception of general health and well-being

Improvement/deterioration/no change

Comments:

Patient perception of general health and well-being

Improvement/deterioration/no change

Comments:

NORTH STAR PHYSIOTHERAPY ASSESSMENTS – SUPPLEMENTARY INFORMATION (*CONTINUED*)

Spinal posture

Sitting	Standing
Draw, describe	Draw, describe
Cobb angle (if known)	Rate of progression (if known)
Correctable: Y/N	

Comments (Include any action, spinal jacket – type and wear time, surgery)

16

Sports injuries

Julie Sparrow

INTRODUCTION

The success on the international stage of an increasing number of teenage athletes has provided motivation for many children to engage in organized sport. Children often come to sport with dreams of becoming a champion and, with increasing financial reward for sporting success, may begin formal training at an early age.

Sport offers a child the opportunity to develop body awareness through physical exploration and in the process to enhance coordination, balance and motor skill acquisition. Sport also plays an important part in social integration. The reduction in organized sport in schools has led to an increase in participation in organized competitive sport outside school, with many sports now developing youth academies. Training is however often designed and delivered by coaches who attempt to apply their experience of coaching adults directly to coaching children. This shift has led to an increased exposure of youngsters to more formal training and competition at an early age and with this increasing exposure comes an increasing risk of injury.

The effective management of children and adolescents participating in sport provides a major challenge for all involved, especially the parent, coach and medical support staff, of which the physiotherapist is a key member.

Children engage in sport for a variety of reasons and are influenced by many external factors. The physiotherapist working with children in sport should attempt to establish what motivates a child to participate, as this can then be utilized to establish compliance with the treatment programme to achieve a positive outcome.

The incidence of sports injury in children is not easily established as children and adolescents often present at clinic with non-specific pain and little in the way of objective signs, making it difficult to standardize the criteria used to classify injury across the research literature (Fuller et al 2006). Maffuli et al (2000), when considering epidemiology and injury, report that 30% of all injuries to children and adolescents are related to participation in sport, and that specific sports have specific patterns of injury. Recognition of injury patterns and early activity modification should therefore be part of the overall management of the young athlete (Kocher et al 2000). Many sports have now adopted regular screening programmes seeking to identify abnormalities that may result in injury (Gerbino & Micheli 1996) so that preventive measures can be initiated.

COMPONENTS OF PHYSICAL PERFORMANCE

Success in sport demands the effective integration of three major body systems: the musculoskeletal, neural and cardiorespiratory systems. Each sport has its identifiable skill performance signature derived from the specific optimum mobility demands of the sport. The physiotherapist working with young athletes needs an appreciation of the individual specific sport skill demands and the relative contribution of each component of optimum mobility (Figure 16.1). This is essential in the design of a treatment programme that will not only treat the symptoms but will also prevent recurrence by eliminating causative factors.

Individual athletes bring to this model their individual genetic endowment, anatomical architecture and tissue load history. It is also important to include in this model the influence of the psychological components of confidence, personality and competitive nature of the individual.

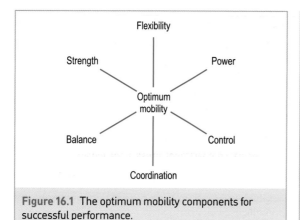

Figure 16.1 The optimum mobility components for successful performance.

Table 16.1 Overuse injuries associated with situations of increased pronation	
Situations associated with increased pronation	**Overuse injuries related to prolonged pronation**
● Pes planus	● Medial tibial stress syndrome
● Forefoot varus	● Tibialis posterior tendonitis/apophysitis of the navicular
● Weakness of the gastrocnemius	● Achillies tendinitis/ Severs disease
● Tightness of triceps surae	● Plantar fasciitis
● Ankle joint equinus	● Patellofemoral pain syndrome
● Leg-length discrepancy	● Iliotibial band friction syndrome

COMPONENTS OF SPORTS PERFORMANCE

Sports performance is based on a combination of activities that can be considered under four general headings:

1. Weight-bearing
2. Take-off/landing
3. Flight
4. Propelling.

Each of the skills of weight-bearing, take-off/landing and propelling can be either by the upper-limb or the lower-limb dominant activities. Evaluation of the individual athlete's sequencing of the skill elements is an essential component of successful prehabilitation and rehabilitation design.

Weight-bearing

Weight-bearing can be static, as in the balance activities seen in gymnastics, where weight-bearing can be through either the upper or the lower limbs, or dynamic, as in running and jumping activities.

Dynamic lower-limb weight-bearing is usually considered in relation to the gait cycle in which variation in speed, inclination, surface and direction of motion are factors to be considered in athlete assessment and management.

Weight-bearing function is also influenced by the posture and alignment of the individual, both of which will alter in response to growth (McConnell 2001, pp. 204–218).

At initial foot contact in the gait cycle the foot is in supination. The impact force is absorbed by approximately 10–15° of knee flexion and the ability of the subtalar joint to move rapidly into pronation. Failure of these mechanisms of shock absorption will require the

next level of the kinetic chain to absorb the impact, making it vulnerable to injury (see Ch. 4).

During the mid-stance phase the subtalar joint is returned to a neutral position. Stability in mid-stance requires the synergistic integration of peroneus longus and tibialis posterior. Disturbance of this mechanism will result in instability, requiring adaptation of the more proximal segments to produce a stable platform for weight transference.

In order to facilitate the toe-off phase it is necessary to invert the calcaneus in order to resupinate the foot to provide a rigid lever for propulsion. This mechanism is facilitated by pelvic rotation producing external rotation via the kinetic linkage of the weight-bearing limb.

An excessive or prolonged pronation phase of gait has been associated with a number of overuse injuries of the lower limb as altered rotational forces are compensated along the kinetic chain (Table 16.1).

A pronated foot posture is a common feature seen in young children; however, this tends to resolve with skeletal maturity and alteration in more proximal alignment (Hawkins & Metheny 2001). Use of orthotic devices to manage overpronation in growing athletes should therefore be undertaken with caution and if supplied should reviewed regularly.

Take-off and landing

Some sports are jump-specific, e.g. long jump and triple jump, whereas others are jump-intensive, for example,

Box 16.1 Injuries commonly associated with jumping sports in children and adolescents

- Osgood–Schlatter's disease – traction apophysitis at the tibial tubercle
- Sinding–Larsen–Johansson syndrome – traction apophysitis at the inferior pole of the patella
- Severs disease – traction apophysitis at the calcaneus
- Patellofemoral pain syndrome
- Anterior fat pad irritation at the knee
- Plantar fasciitis

Box 16.2 Common upper-limb injury associated with upper-limb load-bearing in gymnastics

Shoulder

- Rotator cuff tear
- Glenohumeral impingement

Elbow

- Medial compartment stress at the elbow
- Osterochondral defect of the capitellum of the humerus

Wrist

- Compression of the distal radial epiphysis
- Tearing of the triangular fibrocartilage
- Osteochondritis of the lunate (Kienbock's disease)

basket ball and volley ball. Other sports are jump-incidental, where jumping occurs only occasionally, for example heading the ball in soccer.

Take-off can be considered in two phases: the preset phase and the acceleration phase. In order to generate optimal force for take-off, the preset phase engages the stretch-shortening mechanism. By applying a prestretch to the quadriceps, gastrocnemius and gluteus maximus through preparatory flexion at the hip and knee and dorsi-flexion at the ankle, the stretch reflex is stimulated (Marieb 2004, p. 523), enhancing the concentric contraction of the same muscles during the acceleration phase.

The athlete must have sufficient range at the ankle, knee and hip joints and sufficient soft-tissue length to allow the two joint quadriceps muscle, rectus femoris and gastrocnemius to stretch. Growth-related alteration in the length of soft tissue can result in a temporary shortening of the muscle, producing an increase in the tensile load at the apophysis, leading to traction apophysitis (Dalton 1992). This is a common cause of Osgood–Schlatter's disease at the knee and Severs disease at the calcaneum (Box 16.1). Assessment of these ranges should be part of any sport prehabilitation athlete profiling.

During the acceleration phase of take-off, the athlete must have the capacity for rapid and full toe-off and plantar flexion of the ankle and extension of the knee, hip and trunk. Loss of range at any one of these sites will increase the load on another part of the kinetic chain, increasing the risk of injury.

The stresses of landing are influenced by the aerial directional changes. Safe landing is dependent on the rapid deceleration and dissipation of force. To achieve effective safe landing, an athlete requires the functional integrity of the articular supporting structures at the hip, knee and ankle and the eccentric control of the antigravity muscles of the trunk and lower limbs. In progressive rehabilitation of the jumping athlete there therefore needs to be a carefully monitored progression of the rehabilitation demand from low-load bilateral activities,

e.g. bilateral squat and bilateral low-level drop landing, through to high-load unilateral activity, e.g. hopping and single-leg land and balance activities.

In the sport of gymnastics it is important to remember that weight-bearing and take-off and landing through the upper limb are major features of the sport that bring with them their own unique potential for injury (Box 16.2). The loads applied to the upper limbs are both compressive and distractive. The swing, e.g. high bar, and support components, e.g. handstand, of gymnastic skills are particularly stressful, combining strength, flexibility and speed which together impart high impact load, rotation stress and compression force to the tissues (Sparrow 2001). As a consequence the shoulder complex, elbow and wrist are all vulnerable to overuse injury in the young gymnast.

Flight

Flight occurs when the body is moving in free space and is the time between take-off and landing. An athlete has to be able to manage changes of direction in flight and then accommodate changes in orientation in landing. All flight activities are in open kinetic chain whole-body activities. Management of the body in space requires well-developed spatial awareness generated by integrated input from the visual and vestibular mechanisms and proprioceptive awareness through receptors throughout the neuromuscu-lokeletal system. Efficient movement and control of the body in flight are dependent on sound trunk and girdle stability. Re-education of the flight components of sports skill should take place in the final stages of rehabilitation when necessary joint ranges, muscle strength, proprioception, motor control and core stability have been fully restored.

Propelling

Propulsive force is a feature of a great many sports, e.g. kicking a football, throwing a javelin or hitting a shuttlecock. There are sports that require propulsion of an object with the feet, e.g. football, and others where an implement is required, e.g. hockey, tennis. Others require the propulsion of the whole person or the movement of an external vehicle, e.g. swimming, rowing. Each will place its own pattern of stress on the developing neuromusculoskeletal system. The sports physiotherapist needs to become skilled in movement observation and analysis in order to evaluate the individual athlete's response to the multisegmental demands of propelling activities.

Efficient use of the upper body to produce a propulsion in throwing, racket sport or swimming activities requires the coordinated transmission via the trunk energy generated from the lower extremity and the ground. The range of motion, muscle power and timing of all components of the involved kinetic chain must be assessed to ensure movement efficiency. For example, when managing shoulder pain in the overhead athlete the physiotherapist must evaluate not only the range and stability of the shoulder girdle, but must also include the range and stability of the trunk along with the range and power of the lower limbs. Growth-related alteration in the lever arms and changes in the trunk-to-limb ratio can lead to alteration in force production, resulting in an alteration in timing increasing the risk of injury.

Swimming places perhaps the highest repetitive load on the neuromusculoskeletal system of the upper body, applying particular stress to the shoulder complex and the spine. It has been recognized that the skeletal system of a child is capable of pronounced adaptive response to intensive training (Maffuli & Baxter-Jones 1995); however, Gerrard (1993) reports that the immature musculoskeletal system of a young athlete is less able to cope with repetitive biomechanical stress and is therefore more vulnerable to injury. The physiotherapist must therefore aim to establish the training load on injured young athletes in order to manage their rehabilitation and subsequent return to sport effectively.

Box 16.3 presents common injury patterns associated with upper-limb propelling sports.

THE ROLE OF THE TRUNK

The trunk can be considered as a force conversion zone responsible for transmitting forces between the pelvic and pectoral girdles via the linkage system of the motion segments of the spinal column and the large trunk muscles and fascial sheaths. Many of the skills of sport and functional activities of daily living require complex integration of the trunk musculature and the motion segments of the spinal column to produce and control motion, e.g. rotation and

---

Box 16.3 Common injuries associated with upper-limb propelling sports

Upper limb

- Stress fracture of the proximal humeral epiphysis
- Atraumatic instability of the glenohumeral joint
- Glenohumeral impingement (often secondary to the above)
- Traction injury to the medial complex of the elbow, resulting in a traction apophysitis of the medial epicondyle
- Ostrochondritis of the capitellum of the humerus

Trunk

- Spondylolysis (stress of the pars interarticularis)

---

counterrotation of the trunk in walking and running; diagonal transmission of force from the front foot to the opposite racket hand of the server in tennis and the extension rotation of the footballer ready to kick.

There is as yet limited understanding of the aetiology of low-back pain in young athletes (Jones & Macfarlane 2005). One of the most common low-back conditions found in young athletes is spondylolysis. Spondylolysis is associated with complex sporting activities involving extremes of lumbar flexion and extension combined with rotation, e.g. fast bowling, placing increased stress on the pars interarticularis of the vertebrae, resulting in stress fracture. As with all overuse injuries, in a young athlete symptoms are minimal, with local low-back discomfort in the absence of neurological signs and minimal loss of range being the main presenting features. Extension of the spine whilst in single-leg standing on the leg of the affected side is often enough to provoke the pain. Referral for confirmation via X-ray or bone scan is indicated.

The presence of radiological changes in an asymptomatic athlete should be viewed with caution. Several studies have identified radiological anomalies in the spine, especially in relation to the sports of gymnastics (McMeeken et al 2001), rowing (Harvey & Tanner 1991), golf and racket sports (Duggleby & Kumar 1997); however, the relationship between radiological changes and the reporting of low-back pain has yet to be clearly established.

It has been hypothesized that low-back pain and spondylolysis in a young athlete may be as a result of a differential growth rate between the bony structures of the motion segment and the surrounding soft tissues. Feldman et al (2001) report that the onset of low-back pain in young athletes corresponds to the adolescent growth spurt, and that those with a high growth spurt may be more at risk. The physiotherapist working with a young athlete should therefore try to establish the phase of growth and where possible to encourage the responsible adult and/or the coach of the young athlete to monitor growth through regular measurement.

THE CHALLENGE OF GROWTH

As can be seen from the preceding section, the pattern of growth of the musculoskeletal system and the development and maturation of the nervous system play a significant part in the aetiology of non-traumatic injury seen in the adolescent and preadolescent athlete.

Young athletes presenting at the sports injury clinic display a wide variation in size, physique and body composition, reflecting the variation seen in growth and physical maturity within and between genders (Malina et al 2004). The range of variation makes generalization on injury,

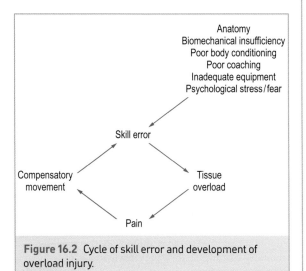

Figure 16.2 Cycle of skill error and development of overload injury.

aetiology and subsequent management in the developing athlete challenging, requiring from all involved individualized assessment and intervention planning.

Adolescence is characterized by a growth spurt and changes in body shape as a response to sexual maturation and hormonal stimulus. The changes in height, weight and size in response to growth and maturation may significantly alter the biomechanics of sports skills. Changes in the line of gravity, alteration in lever arm and increased muscle strength production place increasing stress on the developing immature skeleton and challenge the central nervous system motor patterns. These changes result in a challenge to sports skill, contributing to skill error (Figure 16.2), resulting in an increased potential for injury.

COMMON INJURIES IN CHILDHOOD AND ADOLESCENCE

Sport skills will apply the same stress to the musculoskeletal system for both a child and an adult. It is the body's response and adaptation to the stress that produce the difference in the injury seen. The young athlete is more likely to suffer an injury to the vulnerable growth plates of the immature bone and the articular cartilage rather than the ligamentous injuries seen in the adult.

Forces of sport skills acting on the tissues are:

- Compression
- Shear
- Tensile load
- Bend
- Torsion.

Each has a major influence on the growing skeleton.

Figure 16.3 shows a diagrammatic representation of a growing long bone.

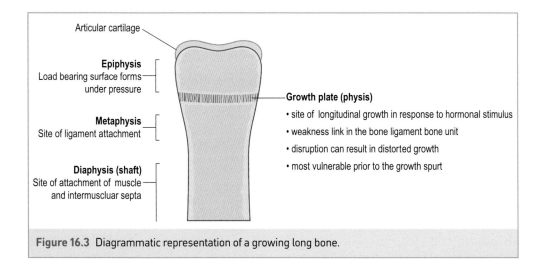

Figure 16.3 Diagrammatic representation of a growing long bone.

Table 16.2 Features of musculoskeletal growth

Feature	Clinical relevance
Articular cartilage	The articular cartilage of a growing child is thicker than that found in a mature bone. The articular cartilage in growing bone is able to remodel itself.
Epiphyseal (growth) plate	The epiphyseal plate is vulnerable to disruption, especially in relation to shearing and compression forces. Disruption of the growth plate is concerning as it may result in interruption of the growth process.
Metaphysis (shaft)	The shaft of long bones in children and adolescents is more elastic than adult bone and is therefore able to withstand greater deformation without complete fracture. Vulnerable to excessive sudden or progressive bending and torsion.
Osseous versus soft-tissue growth	During periods of high-velocity growth the bone lengthens first. The stretch applied to the soft tissue by the increase in bone length provides the stimulus for soft-tissue lengthening. During periods of high-velocity growth, the soft tissues may be under greater stress, which may result in muscle imbalance or soft-tissue injury. Vulnerable to tensile loading.
Tendon attachment	The sites of tendon attachment are called apophyses. They are cartilaginous plates that provide a relatively weak cartilaginous attachment. Sport skills that place sudden loading or repeated traction (tensile loading) on these sites can result in traction apophysitis or avulsion injuries.

Growth-related features of musculoskeletal system are summarized in Table 16.2.

Acute injury

Acute injury may be as a result of direct trauma, e.g. a fracture of the clavicle following a fall on an outstretched arm, or as a consequence of indirect trauma, e.g. avulsion of the conjoint tendon on the hamstrings in the adolescent sprinter.

Acute bony injuries in the young athlete fall into three categories and are summarized in Table 16.3.

Common features of all acute injury

All acute injury to the neuromusculoskeletal system responds in a similar predictable pattern:

- Response phase
- Regeneration phase
- Remodelling phase.

Response phase

The initial response is bleeding, resulting in swelling, redness and warmth. At this stage the principal aim of treatment is to stop the bleeding and minimize the extent of the trauma. The course of action is to follow the PRICE (protect, rest, ice, compression and elevation) guidelines, protecting the area, minimizing movement, cooling the area and applying compression and elevation to slow the blood flow (Chartered Society of Physiotherapy 1998). This minimizes the swelling and facilitates clotting at the ruptured blood vessels. Unless the physiotherapist is working pitchside, the immediate first aid will be applied by others. It is important in the subjective assessment of the athlete following a traumatic injury to establish the immediate first aid and subsequent management as this will help in establishing the status of tissue repair.

Regeneration phase

During this phase new collagen is laid down to produce the repair. In the growing athlete the tissue is repaired with like-for-like tissue. To ensure that the repair is strong the new collagen must be progressively stressed in the direction it is needed for optimal function. Early restoration of movement patterning and progressive load-bearing is essential during this phase to maximize the strength of the collagen repair. It must be remembered that during the development of the collagen repair the new collagen goes through a period of vulnerability, usually between 14 and 21 days postinjury. At this time the new tissue must be protected from overstress to prevent reinjury.

Table 16.3 Acute skeletal injury in the adolescent

Type of fracture	Feature
Metaphyseal fracture	• Common in the long bones of the arm and leg. Usually incomplete 'greenstick' fracture • Usually treated with simple immobilization • If angular or rotational deformity is present, internal fixation may be required
Growth plate fracture	• Classified according to Salter Harris (Brukner & Khan 2001, p. 654) • Types i and ii are disruption through the growth plate • Type iii and iv fractures involve the articular surface as well as the growth plate • Type v, often missed at the time of injury, involves compressive closure of the growth plate • Types iii–v present a high risk for long-term complications if poorly managed

Avulsion fracture	• Sudden and excessive shearing force can result in avulsion fracture at ligamentous attachments. Especially vulnerable is the anterior cruciate ligament (ACL) at the knee. All knee injuries in children and adolescents with a suspected haemarthrosis should be X-rayed to exclude an avulsion fracture
	• High-velocity muscle contraction can result in an avulsion fracture at the apophyseal attachment of the tendon
	• Common sites are:
	  ○ Sartorius at the anterior superior iliac spine
	  ○ Rectus femoris at the anterior inferior iliac spine
	  ○ Hamstrings at the ischial tuberosity
	  ○ Iliopsoas at the lesser trochanter

Remodelling phase

This is the longest phase of repair, leading to the restoration of full function of the injured tissue. During this phase the physiotherapist must plan carefully the progressive application of normal strain and stress. In order to do this effectively the physiotherapist must have a complete understanding of the specific sport skill stresses to which the tissue will be exposed.

Overuse injury

Overuse injuries can be considered as an injury to normal tissue as a result of cumulative, repetitive submaximal microtrauma with an associated lack of adequate recovery between stress episodes (Krivickas 1997). This resulting microtrauma may lead to an alteration in the tissue matrix which in turn makes the tissue vulnerable to further overload (Curwen & Stanish 1984). O'Neill & Micheli (1988) report that repetitive overload may result in subtle neurovascular injury, There are, however, no longitudinal studies that consider the impact of these responses on growing tissue or their potential long-term consequences for future injury.

No work has specifically quantified the impact of growth on overuse injury but an association can be assumed as growth itself produces changes in muscle balance and anatomical alignment (Dalton 1992). This is supported by Mackova et al (1989), who identified the occurrence of muscle imbalance during the adolescent growth period.

The complex integration of the whole-body kinetic chain in sport skill activities makes it very difficult to establish a direct causal relationship between posture alignment and activity. The cause of overuse injuries must therefore be viewed as multifactorial, involving both intrinsic and extrinsic factors. Figure 16.4 presents the intrinsic factors that should be evaluated in the effective management of the young athlete.

Extrinsic factors relate to training error. This is usually as a result of inappropriate training, too much too soon, inadequate or unsuitable equipment and adverse environmental factors. Careful subjective history-taking is essential if the impact of these factors on the aetiology of the injury in the young athlete is to be established.

Clinical features of overuse injuries are often unspectacular, presenting as a slow insidious onset of symptoms following a progressive pattern with few objective findings. The common pattern of onset is:

- Pain after activity
- Pain during activity
- Pain inhibiting activity
- Pain preventing activity.

The progressive nature of overuse injury is indicative of a subthreshold range of structural change within the affected tissues (Leadbetter 1992). The pain response resulting from these changes can in turn lead to pain avoidance strategies and the development of compensatory mechanisms. These

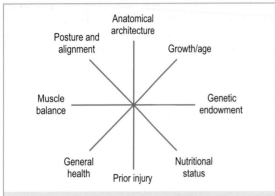

Figure 16.4 Intrinsic factors contributing to overuse injury.

compensatory mechanisms can themselves produce skill errors which, left unchecked, lead to further tissue overload and the development of a spiral of tissue dysfunction. Figure 16.4 presents a model of skill error and overuse injury.

PHYSIOTHERAPY MANAGEMENT

Conventional treatment approaches used in the management of adults are not always appropriate in the management of young athletes. Research into management and treatment of young athletes is limited due to ethical constraints. Effective management and treatment must therefore be based on the development of a clinical hypothesis derived from a comprehensive assessment of the athlete and an appreciation of the impact of the physical demands of the sport on the neuromusculoskeletal system.

Effective rehabilitation is dependent on the young athlete's adherence to treatment. It is therefore essential to involve an athlete in the treatment-planning and goal-setting from the outset and to establish excellent communication with both the athlete and the responsible adult to ensure that they are fully informed and engaged in the treatment process throughout.

The first priority in effective management is careful and systematic assessment to determine the sensitivity of the structures in the immediate vicinity of the problem. Levels of compensatory hypomobility and hypermobility in the associated neural, fascial and muscular tissue should then be identified.

Once the problem list has been fully established treatment can be commenced. The goals of treatment are to minimize/resolve the presenting symptoms, achieve optimal loading of the target joint, and achieve dynamic control of hypermobile segments and enhanced flexibility of hypomobile structures. Throughout the rehabilitation programme activity to maintain cardiovascular fitness should be encouraged.

Active physiotherapy treatment can be loosely divided into several overlapping phases:

- Protected posture
- Protected early motion
- Increasing movement boundaries
- Progressive movement challenges
- Staged return to sport and competition.

Protected posture

During this phase management of painful symptoms is the priority. In the majority of injuries affecting adolescent athletes, pain is managed by avoidance of the pain-provoking activity and relative rest. For example, a footballer with an acute onset of Severs disease may be engaged in kicking skill activities while sitting, initially on the stable base of a stool, progressing to the unstable base of a physio ball. This will eliminate full weight-bearing and repeated impact, which are the main pain-provoking activities in Severs disease. This will allow the athlete to work on core balance, ankle proprioception and ball skills while at the same time resting from the aggravating activities. The creative sports physiotherapist can devise activities with an increasingly competitive element to keep the athlete motivated during the period of rest needed for pain resolution. Conventional electrophysical modalities for pain relief are considered inappropriate in the management of the growing athlete and should be avoided (Kitchen 2002).

Protected early motion

Once the pain has resolved, activities can be introduced to develop dynamic stability. Active range of motion is reintroduced during this phase of treatment. As far as is possible the young athlete should again be engaged in sport-related activity. Motivation and compliance can be achieved if there are measurable targets incorporated into the rehabilitation planning. At this level normal painfree range is the goal of the intervention. Our youngster with Severs disease would now be working on ensuring the full extensibility of the soft tissue of the lower limb with specific emphasis on stretching of the calf and Achilles tendon of the affected limb along with strengthening exercises. Full weight-bearing activities could be progressively reintroduced, building on sitting activities on the physio ball and progressing to standing. Running and jumping activities would still be restricted at this stage. Activities that may be incorporated at this stage are balance and stepping games to encourage dynamic stretch in multiple directions whilst minimizing impact.

Increasing movement boundaries

At this stage sport skill re-education becomes the focus of attention. Full range of motion and controlling muscle strength of the target tissue should be achieved before progression to this stage. Skill-based neuromuscular re-education, including core stability and girdle stability activities, should be incorporated into the programme at this stage. For our young footballer this may involve footwork drills, getting used to moving in all directions, and ball skill activities within a limited space performed at low speed with the emphasis on skill accuracy.

Progressive movement challenge

When full range, muscle strength and power have been achieved in the target tissue and the associated kinetic chain, progressively more complex movements can be incorporated. Sport-specific activities should move progressively towards multiplanar and multilevel motion utilizing increasing load and unstable surfaces. Sport-specific conditioning of major muscle groups should be part of treatment at this stage in the older adolescent. Here we would see our young footballer able to run at varying paces with increasing directional changes. Ball skills would now progressively involve kicking, dribbling, running, collecting and passing activities. Jumping and landing activities would be reintroduced bilaterally at first, progressing to unilateral hopping activities as strength and control increased. At the end of this phase the young athlete should be able to perform all of the necessary sport-specific skills with good technique and be painfree. All compensatory mechanisms must be resolved. This is often the point of discharge for our young athlete but there is still work to be done.

Staged return to sport and competition

If at all possible this stage should be planned and implemented in partnership with the athlete, the responsible adult, the coach and physiotherapist. Sports skills must now be returned to the context of the competitive sport. This phase moves from the rehabilitation gym to the field of play. At the end of this phase all skills must be restored at full pace and with optimal mobility. Here our young footballer will need to be able to run at a range of pace up to all-out sprint, cope with sudden stops and starts and changes of direction at speed, be able to take off and land with full power, control as well as kick effectively with both the dominant and non-dominant foot and be happy to commit to a tackle. Only at this point will the young athlete be ready to return to competition.

KEY POINTS

- Growth-related alterations in posture and alignment make the young athlete vulnerable to musculoskeletal injury
- The inherent adaptability of the growing body makes prehabilitation of injury in the young athlete challenging for the physiotherapist
- Effective physiotherapy must be based on a thorough careful subjective and objective clinical assessment, including static alignment and dynamic functional activities to establish a working clinical hypothesis for treatment
- The cause of injury in the young athlete is multifactorial. Effective management must also be multifactorial, based on a comprehensive assessment of the athlete and sound clinical reasoning
- Treatment should focus on minimizing pain, restoring hypomobile ranges, stabilizing hypermobile ranges and re-establishing sport-specific skills
- The young athlete, the responsible adult and the coach should all be included in the rehabilitation planning
- Physiotherapeutic management of the athlete requires creative thinking to keep the young athlete motivated and engaged while nature takes care of the tissue repair process.

CASE STUDY 16.1

Dominic, a 15-year-old county-standard tennis-player, presented at the clinic with a 3-month history of anterior knee pain aggravated by tennis, especially shots low to the net. The pain has been progressively worsening since onset and Dominic is now not able to play. There is no history of trauma.

Differential diagnoses to consider:
- Chondromalacia patellae
- Osteochondritis diseccans
- Osgood–Schlatter disease
- Sinding–Larsen–Johansson syndrome
- Patellofemoral pain syndrome

- Plica syndrome
- Fat pad irritation
- Patella subluxation.

Subjective assessment

- Behaviour of the discomfort: onset duration and location of the discomfort
- Provoking activities – sport activity and skill-specific
- Provoking activities – others, including hobbies and interests
- Previous history
- Growth history

continued

- Training history – what is new, what is different?
- Competition history – preseason, midseason, end-season level
- Other sports
- General health

Objective assessment

- Sport-specific skill analysis if appropriate (liaise with coach if possible for advice on technique)
- Posture evaluation
- Low-limb alignment – static and dynamic
- Foot type and foot posture
- Core stability
- Skill-specific stability evaluation, respecting discomfort. This may include the following
  - Single-leg balance
  - Bilateral squat
  - Single-leg squat
  - Side lunge
- Low-limb muscle length and balance
- Patella mobility
- Palpation of the patella margins, tibiofemoral joint and supporting structures.

Treatment

Based on a working clinical hypothesis derived from the assessment findings:

- Work with the coach and athlete to modify training and competition schedule to allow for relative rest, avoiding the provoking activities
- Correct as far as is reasonably practicable any posture and alignment anomalies
- Stretch out and mobilize shortened or tight structures
- Strengthen stabilizing muscle groups at the pelvis and knee to enhance the dynamic stability of the affected lower limb
- Gradually reintroduce tennis-specific skills, building progressively to re-establish the provoking activity. For example, starting with simple squat activities, progressing to stepping activities, before developing footwork drills working laterally initially before progressing finally to activities involving forward lunge, the original provoking mechanism.

REFERENCES

Brukner P, Khan K 2001 *Clinical Sport Medicine*, 2nd edn. Sydney: McGraw Hill, p. 654.

Chartered Society of Physiotherapy 1998 PRICE Guidelines (ACPSM). London: Chartered Society of Physiotherapy.

Curwen S, Stanish WD 1984 *Tendinitis: Etiology and Treatment*. Lexington: Collamore Press.

Dalton SE 1992 Overuse injuries in adolescent athletes. *Sports Medicine* 13: 58–70.

Duggleby T, Kumar S 1997 Epidemiology of juvenile low-back pain: a review. *Disability Rehabilitation* 19: 505–512.

Feldman DE, Shrier I, Rossignol M 2001 Risk factors for the development of low-back pain in adolescence. *American Journal of Epidemiology* 154: 30–36.

Fuller CW, Ekstrand J, Junge A et al 2006 Consensus statement on injury definition and data collection procedures in studies of football (soccer) injuries. *Clinical Journal of Sports Medicine* 16: 97–106.

Gerbino PG, Micheli LJ 1996 Orthopaedic aspects of preparticipation screening in childhood. *Sports Exercise and Injury* 2: 126–135.

Gerrard DF 1993 Overuse and injury in growing bones: young athletes at risk. *British Journal of Sports Medicine* 27: 14–18.

Harvey J, Tanner S 1991 Low-back pain in young athletes. A practical approach. *Sports Medicine* 12: 394–406.

Hawkins D, Metheny J 2001 Overuse injuries in youth sports: biomechanical considerations. *Medicine and Science in Sport and Exercise* 33: 1701–1707.

Jones GT, Macfarlane GJ 2005 Epidemiology of low-back pain in children and adolescents. *Archives of Disease in Childhood* 90: 312–316.

Kitchen S 2002 *Electrotherapy. Evidence Based Practice*. Edinburgh: Churchill Livingstone.

Kocher MS, Water PM, Micheli LJ 2000 Upper extremity injuries in the paediatric athlete. *Sports Medicine* 30: 117–135.

Krivickas LS 1997 Anatomical factors associated with overuse sports injuries. *Sports Medicine* 24: 132–146.

Leadbetter WB 1992 Cell matrix response to tendon injury. *Clinical Sports Medicine* 11: 533–578.

Mackova J, Janda V, Macek M 1989 Impaired muscle function in children and muscle function. *Journal of Manual Therapy* 4: 157–160.

Maffuli N, Baxter-Jones AD 1995 Common skeletal injuries in young athletes. *Sports Medicine* 19: 137–149.

Maffuli N, Das D, Caine DJ 2000 Epidemiology of injury mechanisms in children sport. *Journal of Sports Traumatology and Related Research* 22: 100–122.

Malina RM, Bouchard C, Bar-Or O 2004 *Growth, Maturation and Physical Activity*, 2nd edn. Champaign, IL: Human Kinetics.

Marieb EN 2004 *Human Anatomy and Physiology*, 6th edn. San Francisco, CA: Pearson.

McConnell J 2001 Faulty alignment and posture perpetuating musculoskeletal problems. In: Maffulli N, Chang KM, MacDonald R, Malina R, Parker AW (eds) *Sports Medicine for Specific Ages and Abilities*. Edinburgh: Churchill Livingstone, pp. 204–218.

McMeeken J, Tully E, Stillman B 2001 The experience of back pain in young Australians. *Manual Therapy* 6: 213–220.

O'Neill DB, Micheli LJ 1988 Overuse in the young athlete. *Clinics in Sports Medicine* 7: 591–610.

Sparrow JM 2001 Overuse injuries in gymnastics. In: Maffulli N, Chang KM, MacDonald R, Malina R, Parker AW (eds) *Sports Medicine for Specific Ages and Abilities*. Edinburgh: Churchill Livingstone, pp. 119–130.

Cardiorespiratory

17

The anatomy and physiology of the immature respiratory system

Liz Hardy

INTRODUCTION

Children's respiratory systems cannot be treated as a 'mini-adult' system with 'scaled-down' characteristics. The respiratory system undergoes continual changes from conception through infancy and into adulthood, as it develops into a mature and fully functioning structure. The anatomical and physiological differences, as compared with the adult, are most marked in the preterm neonate, and although a change in one characteristic may influence the development of another, components mature at differing rates.

A clear understanding of this process and an awareness of its implications are fundamental to the paediatric respiratory physiotherapist who must consider all variations as part of clinical reasoning when identifying appropriate assessment or treatment strategies. Clearly a child of 3 years old with a respiratory illness has systems which will behave quite differently from an infant of 29 weeks' gestation or a 10-year-old – even if the pathological processes of the condition are the same – and the situation will be further complicated if the child requires ventilation.

PRENATAL DEVELOPMENT

Lung anatomy changes greatly during prenatal development (Inselman & Mellins 1981, Murray 1986), and can broadly be classified into four stages: embryonic, pseudoglandular, canalicular and saccular.

- *Embryonic*: endoderm and mesoderm are formed by the end of the third week following fertilization. These develop into the respiratory endothelium and the diaphragm respectively. Bronchial buds form at the end of the laryngotracheal groove during the next 2 weeks and separate from the foregut.
- *Pseudoglandular*: the bronchial buds grow and divide into lobar bronchi from week 5, subsequently dividing into terminal and respiratory bronchioles. All structures in the upper respiratory tract are recognizable by 12 weeks following fertilization and bronchial formation is complete by the 16th week. The pulmonary artery and vein develop from week 5, with bronchial arteries forming from week 9. The development of the airways and the blood vessels which supply them occurs in parallel, as does the development of alveoli and intra-acinar blood vessels. Tracheal cartilage appears from the 7th gestational week. Development of the lymphatic system and cilia begins in the 11th week, and that of goblet cells in the 13th.
- *Canalicular*: at 16 weeks, the lumen of the bronchial tree dilates and canalizes. The epithelial layer thins and gradually differentiates into flat type I pneumocytes for support and gas exchange, and rounded type II pneumocytes which produce and store surfactant from week 22.
- *Saccular*: by the 24th gestational week, primitive alveoli form, as terminal bronchioles differentiate into transitional ducts and terminal saccules. Further infiltration of the capillary network occurs and develops the potential to allow sufficient gas exchange to support life. Mature alveoli are present by the 36th week.

Fetal lungs produce pulmonary or luminal fluid, in volumes of approximately 30 ml/kg body weight, and also exhibit irregular respiratory movement. These factors appear to be important in the development of lung shape and volume (Avery et al 1981) and in lung growth (Harding & Hooper 1995). Some luminal fluid is expelled by the extrathoracic pressure exerted on the infant during delivery, whereas the rest is absorbed into the capillary and lymphatic systems.

POSTNATAL DEVELOPMENT OF THE TERM INFANT

After birth, it takes some time before the lungs are fully expanded and ventilated. Small amounts of air are retained in the lung during each early expiration, so preventing its collapse. As the pattern of breathing establishes, a functional residual capacity (FRC) is established and by 30 minutes of age this is approximately the same volume as the fetal lung fluid that was expelled (Avery et al 1981). Pulmonary artery pressure begins to drop after birth as the vessels reduce their musculature and, by 10 months, all are of adult thickness (Reid 1979). At birth, the pulmonary vascular resistance steadily falls, causing the blood flow to the lungs to increase, and this continues up to 6 weeks of age.

Growth and development of the lung follow a specific sequence. The airways are fully mature at birth, although they continue to broaden and lengthen. Alveoli increase in number from birth up to age 3 years, in both volume and number from age 3 to 8, and then in volume only until the chest wall stops growing in early adult life. At birth there are approximately 150 million alveoli, and by 4 years, the adult number of 300–400 million are present (Hislop et al 1986).

THE IMMATURE RESPIRATORY SYSTEM

The structural anatomy and functional physiology of the developing respiratory system predispose it to problems which do not affect the mature system of the adult. The following sections highlight the main areas of the developing system which differ from that of the adult.

- *Upper airway*: infants have a high larynx, allowing simultaneous breathing and swallowing. Their relatively large tongue produces a tendency to nose-breathing and may also contribute to obstruction of the upper airway. Purcell (1976) suggested that any narrowing of the nasal passage significantly increased the work of breathing. Infants who have nasogastric tubes in situ may be vulnerable to this. However a more recent study (Djupesland & Lodrup Carlsen 1998) found that even a 50% reduction in cross-sectional diameter of the nostril did not affect lung function.
- *Airway size*: the distal airways grow more slowly than those proximally positioned, causing high peripheral airway resistance. The average diameter of the infant trachea is 4–6 mm, compared with 15 mm in the adult. If this diameter is reduced, e.g. by oedema or mucus, the peripheral airway resistance rises further, increasing the work of breathing. In addition, narrow distal airways close at volumes above FRC, and are prone to blockage and atelectasis – this typical airway closure during ventilation may account for the normal PaO_2 being lower in infants than adults. The airway has a high proportion of mucus-producing glands in relation to its surface area, and therefore an increased likelihood of blockage with secretions (Table 17.1).
- *Alveolar diameter* is small in the infant, with most tidal volume breathing taking place at low lung volumes,

Table 17.1 Average diameter of respiratory structures

	Child	Adult
Trachea	4–6 mm	14–15 mm
Main bronchi	3.8–4.4 mm	11–14 mm
Bronchiole	0.1 mm	0.2 mm
Alveolus	0.05 mm	0.2 mm
Total surface area	2.8 m²	70 m²

predisposing alveoli to collapse easily. Low numbers of alveoli yield less surface area for gas exchange to take place.

- *Collateral ventilation*: little is known about the factors that influence the development of collateral ventilation, but it is thought that small but ineffective pores of Kohn and canals of Lambert may be present in the immature lung (Wohl & Mead 1990), predisposing them to the risk of atelectasis.
- *Supporting tissues*: the respiratory system's supporting structure is incomplete at birth, and bronchial wall cartilage continues to develop around the conducting airways throughout childhood (Sinclair-Smith et al 1976). The chest wall is cartilaginous, pliable and compliant. It is easily distorted, offers inadequate support to counteract the elastic recoil of the lung and provides little opposition to diaphragmatic contraction. In infancy, the chest wall is almost three times more compliant than the lung (which is relatively stiff) but by the second year of life the compliance of the chest wall and lung are almost equal, as in the adult (Papastamelos et al 1995).
- *Shape*: in the newborn infant, the thoracic cage is almost round. This immature shape influences the rib position to be horizontally aligned. The so-called bucket-handle mechanism for increasing the transverse and anteroposterior diameter of the chest cannot function, so limiting the extent to which lung volume can be increased. In addition, the angle of insertion of the diaphragm is horizontal, rather then oblique as in adults (Muller et al 1979), making its ability to contract less efficient, and producing inward distortion of the ribcage. In the healthy infant this alone causes the work of breathing to be 2–3 times that of adults (Hoffman 1995). The diaphragm is prone to fatigue in infants, since it contains only 25–30% of slow-twitch, high-oxidative type I fibres (fatigue-resistant), as compared with 55% in the adult (Muller et al 1979). It is thought that the more oval adult chest shape is influenced by gravity and begins to develop as the infant develops a more upright posture (Oppenshaw et al 1984). Children with developmental delay may retain some immature respiratory features.

- *Muscle tone*: during rapid-eye movement sleep, tone reduces in the intercostal muscles, effecting paradoxical movement of the compliant chest wall and therefore decreasing FRC. This results in an irregular breathing pattern, often with apnoeas, particularly in neonates. The immature vagally mediated Hering–Breuer reflexes may account for this (Hannam et al 1998).
- *Metabolic rate*: hypoxaemia can develop rapidly in acutely ill infants, as their metabolic rate, and therefore oxygen requirement, is relatively high. Hypoxia triggers pulmonary vasoconstriction leading to bradycardia, rather than tachycardia, as seen in adults. Bradycardia produces a reduction in cardiac output, due to the inability of the immature myocardium to increase stroke volume.
- *Distribution of ventilation*: infants and young children preferentially ventilate upper areas of lung, rather than dependent areas, as in adults. Additionally, the closing volume of alveoli occurs above FRC, especially in dependent areas. Perfusion is distributed preferentially to dependent areas, thereby causing a mismatch.

CONCLUSION

It is essential that the physiotherapist treating respiratory illness in neonates or young children has a thorough understanding of the anatomical and physiological factors which influence the mechanics of breathing. Only with this sound foundation will appropriate assessment and treatment techniques be selected.

REFERENCES

Avery ME, Fletcher BD, Williams RG 1981 *The Lung and its Disorders in the Newborn Infant*, 4th edn. Philadelphia, PA: WB Saunders, Chapter 1.

Djupesland PG, Lodrup Carlsen KC 1998 Nasal airway dimensions and lung function in awake, healthy neonates. *Paediatric Pulmonology* 25: 99–106.

Hannam S, Ingram DM, Milner AD 1998 A possible role for the Hering–Breuer deflation reflex in apnea of prematurity. *Journal of Pediatrics* 132: 35–39.

Harding R, Hooper SB 1995 Regulation of lung expansion and lung growth before birth. *Journal of Applied Physiology* 81: 209–224.

Hislop A, Wigglesworth JS, Desai R 1986 Alveolar development in the human fetus and infant. *Early Human Development* 13: 1–11.

Hoffman GM 1995 Airway complications of instrumentation. *Respiratory Care* 40: 97–107.

Inselman LS, Mellins RB 1981 Growth and development of the lung. *Journal of Pediatrics* 98: 1–15.

Muller N, Volgyesi G, Becker L et al 1979 Diaphragmatic muscle tone. *Journal of Applied Physiology* 95: 279–284.

Murray JF 1986 *The Normal Lung*, 2nd edn. Philadelphia: WB Saunders, pp. 1–21.

Oppenshaw P, Edwards S, Helms P et al 1984 Changes in ribcage geometry during childhood. *Thorax* 39: 624–627.

Papastamelos C, Panitch HB, England SE et al 1995 Developmental changes in chest wall compliance in infancy and early childhood. *Journal of Applied Physiology* 78: 179–184.

Purcell M 1976 Response in the newborn to raised upper airway resistance. *Archives of Disease in Childhood* 51: 602–607.

Reid LM 1979 The pulmonary circulation: remodelling in growth and disease. *American Review of Respiratory Disease* 119: 531–546.

Sinclair-Smith CC, Emery JL, Gadson D et al 1976 Cartilage in children's lungs: a quantitative assessment using the right middle lobe. *Thorax* 31: 40–43.

Wohl MEB, Mead J 1990 Age as a factor in respiratory disease. In: *Kendig's Disorders of the Respiratory Tract in Children*, 5th edn. Philadelphia, PA: WB Saunders, pp. 175–182.

18 Cardiorespiratory physiotherapy for the acutely ill, non-ventilated child

Liz Hardy

CHAPTER CONTENTS

INTRODUCTION

Paediatric respiratory illness is very different from that seen in the adult population. Children suffer from different conditions with different pathological processes, indicating different treatment applications. Respiratory illness may worsen and then rapidly improve, largely due to the age-specific anatomical and physiological factors observed in the immature respiratory system, and which influence the mechanics of breathing.

Respiratory illness may be seen as chronic disease, e.g. asthma or cystic fibrosis; or in association with neurological or neuromuscular disability; or in children who have previously required ventilation; or when there has been congenital abnormality of the respiratory or cardiac system. However, many previously well children will acquire acute chest infections or pneumonia, either in the community or following surgery.

Some of these conditions are self-limiting, or will not require physiotherapy input, but in some cases effective physiotherapy is a valuable intervention, and may be required to continue for prolonged periods or indeed throughout life. Often families will need to be taught appropriate techniques to manage their child's condition at home in the longer term.

Effective physiotherapy treatment for the non-ventilated child with a respiratory illness depends upon:

- knowledge of the pathological processes of common conditions
- a sound understanding of the anatomical and physiological factors affecting respiration at different stages of childhood
- ability to use a comprehensive range of age-appropriate assessment techniques
- an understanding of the normal values for vital signs and the application of their monitoring systems
- insight into lung function measurement (pulmonary function tests: PFT) and the ability to read chest X-rays (CXR)
- clinical reasoning and analysis of findings to identify whether or not treatment will be of benefit
- effective use of a variety of treatment techniques
- constant evaluation and reassessment, and the ability to recognize, minimize and manage problems which may arise during treatment
- excellent communication skills
- a sensitive approach to management of the sick child and carers and family.

This chapter aims to provide an introduction to the basic concepts that have an impact upon the assessment and treatment of respiratory illness in non-ventilated children and to offer strategies for treatment of common symptoms. The focus will be upon the infant and young child throughout – older children and adolescents can be assessed and treated in a similar manner to adults.

It is beyond the scope of the chapter to consider common paediatric respiratory conditions, but a list of some of these can be found in Box 18.1; see also Further reading.

ASSESSMENT

Carrying out a full respiratory assessment is vital to ensure that treatment is necessary and appropriate. Physiotherapists may also need to assess elements of neurological or musculoskeletal functioning as these will have an impact upon respiratory status in some children. A brief, informal appraisal of the child's cognitive and verbal skills will ensure

Box 18.1 Common respiratory conditions seen in children

- Asthma
- Bronchiectasis
- Bronchiolitis
- Bronchopulmonary dysplasia
- Chronic lung disease
- Cystic fibrosis
- Empyema
- Pneumonia – community- or hospital-acquired
- Primary ciliary dyskinesia
- Secondary to neurological, neuromuscular or cardiac conditions

that the physiotherapist's own communication is age-appropriate.

In order to decrease stress on the child and carers, much of the subjective assessment can be carried out away from the bedside. Nursing or medical staff will be able to provide the following information, which will influence the timing of assessment or treatment, and may indicate the level of intervention the child is likely to tolerate:

- *Does the child remain stable on handling?* Bradycardia, hypoxia and/or apnoea are common during any stressful activity, particularly in the youngest infants.
- *Is the child receiving feeds?* Children who are tolerating oral feeding are unlikely to have significant respiratory distress. If feeding has taken place recently, care must be taken not to induce reflux vomiting. It is always best to treat before feeds.
- *What are the short- and long-term plans for the child's current medical management?* It is especially useful to know about the delivery and requirement for supplementary oxygen therapy, nebulizers, requirement for suction or 'not for resuscitation' orders.
- *What information have carers been given about the child's illness?* The physiotherapist will be able to discuss treatment options and gain informed consent more easily if the parents have already received such information about the child's stability or prognosis from medical staff.

RESPIRATORY ASSESSMENT

Assessment will follow conventional lines but the following aspects are particularly important in the infant and young child.

Past medical history

- Prematurity, or previous medical conditions requiring long-term ventilation, can lead to the development of

chronic lung disease, which compounds the features of small airways. The infant may have alterations from the expected vital signs, appropriate to age group, even when well. The infant may normally be oxygen-dependent.

- Congenital cardiac problems causing inadequate or obstructed pulmonary blood flow may cause similar differences, particularly if they are uncorrected or if staged repair is carried out. Acceptable oxygen saturations may be at the low end of the expected range.
- Conditions which prevent normal development of the lung, e.g. congenital diaphragmatic hernia, may have long-term implications for the respiratory status of the child and may contribute to respiratory conditions persisting into adult life (Stick 2000).
- The child may have a long-standing respiratory condition, e.g. cystic fibrosis or asthma. In this situation it is likely that the parents will be highly knowledgeable about the condition and the possible treatment options.

Evaluation of baseline observations and their trends, chest X-ray, pulmonary function tests and blood gas analysis

The values of resting vital signs found in children differ from those of adults and alter throughout childhood (Table 18.1). Pain or anxiety as well as sepsis and respiratory distress can cause tachycardia and tachypnoea. Bradycardia is regarded as a heart rate below normal values. The child is considered to be hypoxic when the saturation of oxygen (SaO_2) falls below 93%. The use of oxygen therapy should be instituted to maintain SaO_2 at or above 95% (Poets 1998) and can be delivered in many ways. Children who do not tolerate the usual delivery systems should receive oxygen 'wafting' from a mask placed level with the sternum (Davies et al 2002). In the infant, erratic respiration or periods of apnoea can indicate the presence of secretions. Always consider the trend rather than taking factors in isolation.

CLINICAL TIPS

- When manually counting respiratory rate, do so for the whole assessment period (rather than for a few seconds and multiply up to get the rate per minute, as would be common practice in the assessment of adults). This counteracts the erratic respiratory pattern of the young child
- Always carry out assessment when the infant is awake and content

Plain CXRs in infants are usually the anteroposterior (AP) view, taken with the child lying on the CXR plate (Figure 18.1). In older children films are generally posteroanterior (PA) if the general condition of the child allows the erect posture. Structural abnormalities, horizontal ribs,

Table 18.1 Normal values for vital signs in children

Age	Heart rate (beats/min)	Respiratory rate (breaths/min)	Systolic blood pressure (mmHg)	Diastolic blood pressure (mmHg)
Preterm	120–200	40–80	38–80	25–57
Full-term	100–200	40–60	60–90	30–60
1 year	100–180	25–40	70–130	45–90
3 years	90–150	20–30	90–140	50–80
10 years	70–120	16–24	90–140	50–80
Adolescent	60–100	12–18	90–140	50–80

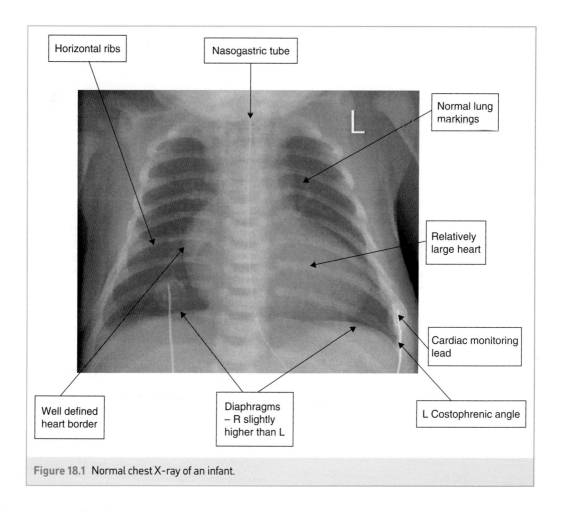

Figure 18.1 Normal chest X-ray of an infant.

the relatively large heart and thymus observed in young infants will show clearly.

Pulmonary function tests

Pulmonary function tests give unreliable information in children aged below 5 years, as understanding of the requirements or the coordination to perform tests effectively is limited. Commonly used pulmonary function tests are as follows:

- Spirometry is the most reliable, valid and reproducible test used in children aged over 6 years measuring the rate of airflow and volume obtained during a maximum forced manoeuvre. The concave or convex appearance of the flow–volume curve or loop produced will indicate either obstructive or restrictive disease respectively. Specific measurement of forced expiratory volume in 1 second (FEV_1) and forced vital capacity (FVC), as well as other values, can be recorded (Table 18.2). The results are often expressed as a percentage of the predicted score related to the child's height and gender. Children must be instructed in the correct technique to be used, as the result is influenced by the amount of effort put in, as well as

by style. A maximal inhalation is followed by hard, long exhalation (Figure 18.2).

- A good seal around the mouthpiece is essential. Noises other than 'blowing' may indicate closure of the glottis, which reduces the volume of air exhaled.
- Peak expiratory flow rate (PEFR) can also be used consistently by children aged over 6 years to measure function in large airways. It is less reliable than spirometry, and the child can easily 'cheat'. The correct technique is maximal inhalation followed by hard and fast exhalation.
- R_{int} or airway resistance measured by the interruptor technique is gaining in popularity and use, as it offers reliable data, even in young children (McKenzie et al 2002).
- Exercise tolerance testing can sometimes provide a reflection of pulmonary function, and may in some conditions be a prognostic indicator. Physiotherapists must remember that poor exercise tolerance may also indicate other problems, e.g. cardiac, muscular weakness, pain, poor physical conditioning. A variety of tests are available to test exercise tolerance, e.g. 6-minute walk test, 3-minute step test, modified shuttle test, treadmill or cycle ergometry tests, some of which have been validated for use in children (Noonan & Dean 2000). Many children will enjoy performing the tests, but parents may be anxious about their child's participation and need reassurance and thorough explanation of the process. The test should be discontinued if the child complains of exercise-induced stress, e.g. lightheadedness, dizziness, headache, excessive breathlessness, chest pain, muscle cramps or reduced coordination. Children find it difficult to describe their perception of dyspnoea and the use of conventional visual analogue scales is unreliable. The Dalhousie dyspnoea scales (McGrath et al 2005) provide a child-friendly pictorial representation of breathlessness.

Table 18.2 Severity of dysfunction indicated by percentage of predicted forced expiratory volume in 1 second (FEV_1)

Level of dysfunction	FEV_1 (%)
Normal	80–100
Mild	60–79
Moderate	40–59
Severe	<40

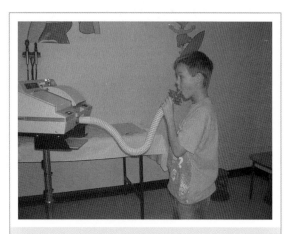

Figure 18.2 Testing of lung function using a *Vitalograph*.

Blood gas analysis

Blood gas analysis in paediatrics includes consideration of venous and capillary as well as arterial samples (Table 18.3). It is less invasive, particularly in the infant with low circulating blood volumes, to take capillary samples by heel or fingerprick, as very small amounts of blood are required. Capillary gases give an adequate indication of respiratory status, although partial pressure (PO_2) readings are always low when compared with arterial samples. Carbon dioxide measuring can be helpful in children with neuromuscular conditions where alveolar hypoventilation is a problem. There is less variation in blood gas analysis throughout childhood than seen in other vital signs.

Rate, depth and pattern of respiration

Significant changes in respiratory rhythm occur during the first year of life. Infants are unable to respond to respiratory distress by increasing the depth of respiration. This is due to the disparity between stiff lungs and compliant chest wall, and the angles of the ribs and diaphragm. Their only option is to increase rate, and as a consequence tachypnoea is a common feature of respiratory distress. It may also be an indicator of hypoxia.

CLINICAL TIPS

Respiratory distress can be identified by observation of the following:

- Tachypnoea – above 60 breaths/min in an infant
- Recession – subcostal, intercostal and sternal
- Tracheal tug – seen at the suprasternal fossa, may be accompanied by head-bobbing
- Nasal flaring – to reduce upper-airway resistance
- Expiratory grunt – the infant's attempt to maintain positive end-expiratory pressure (PEEP)
- Asynchronized breathing – the 'seesaw' paradoxical respiration caused when the negative pleural pressure required to inflate the lungs distorts the lower chest
- Periods of apnoea
- Cyanosis or pallor – infants have the ability to 'shut down' peripherally whilst optimizing oxygenation to major organs
- Irritability or altered level of consciousness – may indicate hypoxia

---

Auscultation

Chest auscultation of the neonate and infant is a refined skill, although it is easier in the older child. The trachea

---

Table 18.3 Normal blood gas analysis in children

Age	Arterial pH	PaO_2 (kPa)	$PaCO_2$ (kPa)
Preterm	7.30–7.40	7.3–12.0	4.6–6.0
Full-term	7.30–7.40	8.0–12.0	4.0–4.7
3 years	7.30–7.40	10.7–13.3	4.0–4.7
10 years	7.35–7.45	10.7–13.3	4.7–6.0
Adolescent	7.35–7.45	10.7–13.3	4.7–6.0

---

and bronchi are relatively large in comparison with the lung fields, and can pool secretions which transmit coarse sounds and may mask subtle changes to breath sounds. Heart sounds reverberate loudly, also making it difficult to hear breath and other adventitious sounds. It is essential that the correct size of stethoscope is used and that physiotherapists have a good knowledge of pulmonary anatomical landmarks in order to auscultate specific lobes. Palpation is often of equal value to auscultation.

CLINICAL TIPS

- Breath sounds should be equal on both sides, and quieter in the lower than the upper zones
- Wheeze is a common finding, due to the narrow airways in the immature respiratory system
- Dynamic compression of the relatively soft trachea during inspiration gives rise to stridor
- Expiratory grunt is caused by partial closure of the glottis, thus prolonging expiration and maintaining a high intra-alveolar pressure with increased lung volume in an attempt to prevent closure of small airways and alveoli. It is the spontaneous attempt of the infant with respiratory distress to generate PEEP

Cough and secretions

Children who have a chronic productive cough may manage their own secretions effectively without further physiotherapeutic intervention. It is helpful to consider whether the cough is moist, dry, chronic or associated with exercise or feeding. Small amounts of secretion are often present even when a cough sounds dry (Chang et al 2005), although dry coughs are more likely to resolve spontaneously. The quality of cough heard can indicate the pathology, e.g. cough associated with croup is often described as a 'bark' and may be heard with inspiratory stridor and hoarseness; pertussis (whooping cough) is characterized by prolonged paroxysms of coughing frequently associated with vomiting.

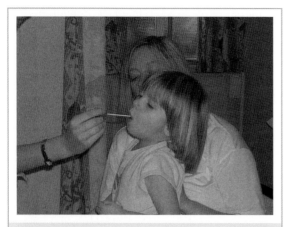

Figure 18.3 Cough swabs should be taken with care.

Physiotherapists may be asked to obtain specimens of the child's respiratory secretions. Many children are unable (or unwilling) to expectorate sputum. Young children may not have the coordination to do so or may not produce sufficient volumes of secretions to trigger the cough reflex. Induction of sputum could be considered, using 5 or 6% hypertonic saline via an ultrasonic nebulizer. Cough swabs should be taken by asking the child to cough on to a sterile swab positioned close to the child's throat. Care must be taken to avoid swabbing the throat or tongue (Figure 18.3). In order to minimize the risk of cross-infection, the physiotherapist should be positioned to the side of the child whenever possible. Hand hygiene before and after taking the swab is important.

The use of cough plates, where the child coughs on to a prepared Petri dish held in front of the mouth, is gaining increased favour as an alternative to the swab method, as it is a sensitive and non-invasive procedure (Maiya et al 2004). The use of nasopharyngeal suction to obtain secretions from the non-intubated child is a matter of some controversy. It is an unpleasant procedure, and should be carried out with care.

OTHER ASSESSMENT CONSIDERATIONS

Many children will require non-respiratory factors to be taken into consideration. The child who has sustained a recent head injury or undergone spinal or brain surgery will require a neurological assessment, careful monitoring and handling, and adaptation of some treatment options. Recent facial or abdominal surgery will restrict the positioning options for treatment, e.g. prone or head-down tip. Orthopaedic management, congenital or acquired deformity of the spine or limbs may also impact on the capacity for moving or repositioning the child, e.g. if scoliosis is present, or where there is a neuromuscular condition causing weakness.

CONTRAINDICATIONS TO CHEST PHYSIOTHERAPY

Carrying out inappropriate chest physiotherapy can adversely affect the condition of the child, so it should never be performed routinely. Following a careful and thorough assessment, the findings must be evaluated and the costs and benefits analysed by clinical reasoning.

Most contraindications to physiotherapy are the same as in adults. In a number of conditions, physiotherapy has been shown to be of minimal or no benefit. Physiotherapy does not alter the natural course of acute bronchiolitis (Webb et al 1985), unless complicated by concurrent infection (Perrotta et al 2005). Uncomplicated pertussis (whooping cough) will not be improved by physiotherapy intervention. It should be used with caution in any condition where there is narrowing of the respiratory tract, e.g. bronchospasm, and only after intubation in epiglottitis or croup. Chest physiotherapy is contraindicated before bronchoscopic removal of a foreign body (Phelan et al 1994). Some children may be too unstable to tolerate manual physiotherapy techniques, and it may only be possible to position appropriately.

TREATMENT STRATEGIES

In the spontaneously breathing child, treatment should usually be carried out when the child is awake, has adequate analgesic cover (if necessary) and has not been fed recently. Parents should receive full explanations of the likely process and expected outcome in order that they can give informed consent. Children should be involved in this process, with simple clinical information given in an age-appropriate manner. Often parents can be involved in treatment and taught to carry it out between the therapist's visits.

The purpose of carrying out chest physiotherapy in children is the same as in adults. It is a valuable adjunct to medical treatment, with the following clinical indications:

- retention of secretions
  - where there is chronic sputum production, e.g. cystic fibrosis, primary ciliary dyskinesia or bronchiectasis
  - when the child has an ineffective or depressed cough, e.g. in some postoperative patients, who may have inadequate analgesia
  - in some neurological and neuromuscular disorders
- decreased lung volume, e.g. as a result of acute lobar collapse due to mucus plugging
- if the child has increased work of breathing
- where there is inadequate ventilation/perfusion matching.

However, as in adults, these features are rarely seen in isolation, necessitating compromise or modification of treatment techniques. Many strategies can be useful in the treatment of several clinical indications. The physiotherapist must always consider the anatomical and physiological factors which affect the immature respiratory system, so that a therapeutically effective and cohesive plan can be devised and potential problems minimized.

Adherence to regular treatment can be a major issue for some children. The use of personalized star charts can be very helpful and many treatment modalities can be adapted to contain an element of fun.

MOBILIZING RETAINED SECRETIONS

The aim of treatment is to maintain a clear airway by mobilizing and clearing accumulated secretions from the respiratory tract (Figure 18.4). There are many modalities to consider:

- *The active cycle of breathing technique (ACBT)* is a well-established method of mobilizing secretions. It consists of periods of breathing control (relaxed abdominal breathing), deep breathing with inspiratory holds (thoracic expansion), mid to low lung volume huffs and coughs if required (Pryor & Webber 1979). It is often used in combination with postural drainage and with percussion applied during the phase of deep breathing.

- *Postural drainage* is the use of gravity-assisted positions to drain secretions into large airways. In the youngest children the upper lobes are vulnerable to secretion retention, but with maturity and more time spent in upright positions (sitting, standing), the focus changes to the lower lobes. The head-down position is contraindicated in neonates for several reasons: their great reliance on diaphragmatic function will be compromised, the position causes decreased SaO_2 (Thoreson et al 1988), it increases the risk of periventricular haemorrhage and it increases the possibility of gastro-oesophageal reflux. Postural drainage is often used in combination with manual techniques. Positions must be used accurately if treatment is to be effective.

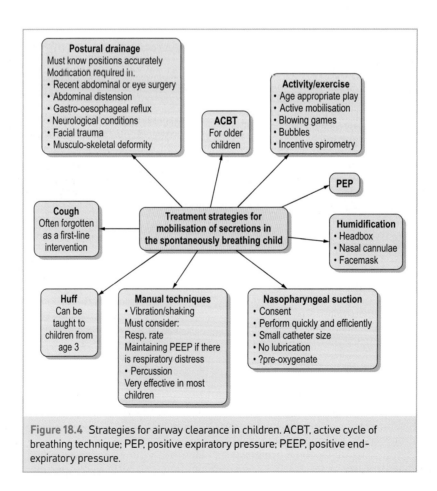

Figure 18.4 Strategies for airway clearance in children. ACBT, active cycle of breathing technique; PEP, positive expiratory pressure; PEEP, positive end-expiratory pressure.

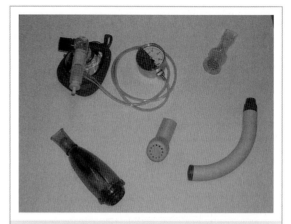

Figure 18.5 Positive expiratory pressure (PEP) devices. Clockwise from top left: Astra PEP mask with manometer, PARI PEP, RC Cornet, Flutter, Acapella.

Percussion is usually performed with a single hand over the appropriate area of the chest, using a towel to cushion the chest wall if preferred by the child. In small infants a soft facemask can be used, but, as this will decrease direct palpation, it is better to 'tent' the fingers to ensure maintenance of a cupped position. A slow rate is preferred, as firm or fast percussion can disturb airflow, causing local airway closure (Wollmer et al 1985). Timing which allows the infant to take a breath between each percussion reduces this risk.

Vibrations, performed during the expiratory phase of breathing, can be difficult to apply in infants with a high respiratory rate. They should be applied no more frequently than on alternate breaths, although greater spacing may be advantageous. If the infant is positive expiratory and pressure (PEEP)-dependent, care should be taken to stop vibration before the end of expiration, so that this is maintained during treatment. One hand may be required to stabilize the compliant chest wall.

Neither technique should be used in children with osteoporosis, clotting disorders or low platelet counts. Incision sites should be avoided. The head should be stabilized in infants, to prevent shaking injury.

- *Positive expiratory pressure* (PEP) helps to keep airways splinted open during exhalation by increasing intra-bronchial pressure in central and peripheral airways, thus increasing functional residual capacity (FRC). This modality is especially useful in children with unstable airways, chronic wheeze or tracheobronchial malacia. It can be delivered in several ways. All devices allow the resistance to be altered, and in some the expiratory pressures reached can be monitored. Acapella, Flutter and RC Cornet produce oscillating PEP and the vibrations may be palpated over the chest wall (Figure 18.5). PEP should not be used if the child is unable to tolerate increased work of breathing, has a raised intracranial pressure or is haemodynamically unstable.

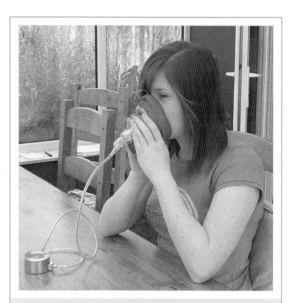

Figure 18.6 Airway clearance can be carried out independently using a positive expiratory pressure device.

Recent facial, oral, oesophageal or skull surgery would also contraindicate PEP treatment. The use of PEP devices enhances independent treatment, although many children will still require supervision and support to carry out treatment effectively (Figure 18.6).

CLINICAL TIPS

- Treatment should be carried out for 10–20 minutes depending upon clinical judgement
- Cycles of treatment consist of 8–10 breaths through the device, each having an inspiratory hold of 2–3 seconds. Slightly larger breaths than tidal volume are most effective
- Each cycle is followed by a short period of breathing control and completed with huffs and coughs to clear mobilized secretions
- The child should be encouraged to keep the cheeks flat, when blowing, to reduce the effects of pressure absorption
- High-pressure PEP modifies treatment by allowing forced expiratory technique (FET) through the device. Careful assessment is required using flow–volume curves to establish optimal pressure

Table 18.4 Suggested catheter size for nasopharyngeal suction in different age groups

Age	Catheter size (FG)
Neonate	5
6 months	6
1 year	8
2 years	10
6 years	12

- *Autogenic drainage* produces enhanced airflow in different generations of bronchi, so mobilizing secretions. It consists of three phases of breathing. Firstly, low lung volume breathing 'unsticks' secretions; these are then 'mobilized and collected' by utilizing tidal volume breathing with a slightly prolonged exhalation; high-volume breathing and coughing completes the technique by 'evacuating' secretions (Schöni 1989). Treatment often takes 45 minutes to complete and is most effectively carried out by older children and teenagers. However, if the technique is selected for use in young children, the physiotherapist can manually limit lung volume by applying pressure to the thorax.
- *Huffing*, or FET, from mid to low lung volume can be taught to children as young as 3 years, and is a very effective airway clearance technique (Pryor & Webber 1979). It is thought that huffing requires less energy expenditure than coughing. Some children find it hard to maintain an open glottis and this can be improved by placing a short tube in the mouth before performing the huff.
- *Coughing* may occur spontaneously as secretions are mobilized, but is often suppressed in the child with respiratory pathology because it causes pain, or because a single cough can quickly turn into a paroxysm of uncontrollable coughing, leaving the child desaturated and exhausted. Young children will rarely have sufficient coordination to expectorate, usually swallowing secretions. Gentle, brief compression of the trachea just below the level of the thyroid cartilage may stimulate the cough reflex, and can be a useful technique in neurologically impaired children. Tickling children to make them laugh can often stimulate coughing!
- *Nasopharyngeal suction*, in the non-intubated child, should only be carried out when secretions cannot be

cleared by any other means and when they are detrimental to the child's condition. Other treatment modalities should be used first to mobilize secretions so that they can be reached by the catheter. It is not a pleasant procedure and the child, and indeed the parents, should receive constant reassurance throughout. Suction must be performed quickly, with extreme care, using the smallest catheter that will remove secretions effectively, and using the lowest possible vacuum pressure to do so (Table 18.4).

The risk of damage to the sensitive bronchial mucosa is high. Kleiber et al (1988) described fibrosis and bronchial stenosis in airways which had required frequent suctioning. However, lubricating gel is not usually used as this tends to clog the airway and may contribute to airway narrowing. In rare cases, perforation of segmental bronchi has been reported (Vaughan et al 1978). The distance the catheter is inserted is crucial. One method of gauging this is by measuring the distance from the tip of the child's nose to the ear – this is roughly the same as the distance to the nasopharynx, although in many cases the physiotherapist may feel that deeper suction is indicated. Hypoxia during suction is well documented, particularly in neonates, but also in non-cyanosed, haemodynamically stable older children (Kerem at al 1990). Preoxygenation, for those children receiving supplementary oxygen, is recommended prior to suction in order to maintain SaO_2 at acceptable levels. Consensus opinion suggests that a 10% increase is usual, although higher levels can be used briefly, if indicated. Oropharyngeal suction is sometimes used as an alternative to nasopharyngeal suction, but can stimulate the gag reflex if not used cautiously and is often less well tolerated. Oral suction can be used to clear secretions which have been successfully expectorated if the child is unable to clear them independently. An airway should be inserted prior to suction in the child with a base-of-skull fracture with possible cerebrospinal fluid leakage.

- Infants and young children should be restrained from trying to handle the catheter, by wrapping them in a towel or blanket
- Side-lying position with neck slightly extended helps to facilitate introduction of the catheter and also prevents aspiration if vomiting occurs
- Catheters with graduated markings should be used whenever possible
- Wear a disposable glove to ensure clean technique
- Observe for adverse effects throughout the procedure

- *Mechanical in–exsufflation* or *CoughAssist* is mainly used for patients with ineffective coughing associated with neuromuscular weakness, but can offer benefits in other clinical situations. The machine is manually set to trigger a series of positive-pressure, lung-expanding breaths which are synchronized with the child's respiratory pattern. These are quickly followed by setting a negative-pressure exhalation which mobilizes secretions (Miske et al 2004).
- *Intrapulmonary percussive ventilation*, known as Percussionaire, mobilizes secretions by directing bursts of air at high frequency (up to 300/minute) into the airways via a mask or mouthpiece (Toussaint et al 2003).
- *Humidification* should be considered as an adjunct to treatment when secretions are thick or resistant to mobilization, in infants whose airways are prone to blockage, or in oxygen-dependent children, using flow rates above 4 l/min. Cold water 'bubble-through' humidifiers or heated humidifiers use sterile water and produce large droplets of vapour which will only reach the upper respiratory tract in non-intubated children. Aerosol from both can be delivered to small infants via headboxes made from clear plastic or to older children using a mouthpiece or facemask. Conventional jet or Venturi nebulizers, powered by compressed air or oxygen, produce smaller droplets which are able to reach the airways and will offer short-term benefits when used before physiotherapy. Ultrasonic nebulizers produce dense clouds of aerosol and can overhydrate, whereas Active Venturi nebulizers e.g. Ventstream, Pari LC plus, offer enhanced deposition of aerosol during inspiration.

- Ensuring the child has appropriate fluid intake is the simplest method of providing hydration
- Green bubble tubing or nasal cannulae are unsuitable for humidification, due to the small diameter of the tube
- A Venturi mask will entrain room air and so deliver lower levels of humidity
- Water bath humidifiers should be kept below the level of the child to minimize the risk of scalding

Mobilization offers many respiratory benefits and should be commenced early. Tidal volume and therefore minute ventilation are improved, as are inspiratory and expiratory flow rates (Dull & Dull 1983). Children can be encouraged to get out of bed to play actively for a short time, even when unwell. In bed, many young children will join in with activities such as action songs but ensure suggestions are age-appropriate. Observation is required as exercise will increase respiratory rate and the demand for oxygen. Specific shoulder, trunk and postural exercises may be indicated postoperatively, particularly if the child has had a thoracotomy or chest drain. Passive exercises can be carried out for children unable to mobilize independently.

INCREASING LUNG VOLUME

Maintaining and improving lung volume is a challenge for the physiotherapist, due to the tendency towards airway closure seen in immature lungs. The aim of treatment is to re-expand collapsed segments of the lung and prevent secondary complications occurring. Children with advanced neuromuscular disease may persistently breathe at low lung volumes, and demonstrate chronic hypoventilation. Scoliosis will further compound this.

Positioning of the child should always be the first consideration in maximizing respiratory function. A child who is being nursed in bed will usually be found in a slumped position, compressing the diaphragm and lower-lung zones. Improving the child's position will improve the breathing pattern. It may also encourage the child to play or take an interest in surrounding activities.

- Use cuddly toys as positioning equipment
- Sitting on a parent's lap will encourage upright posture
- Use neck or lumbar rolls to support a child with low tone

- *Breathing exercises* carried out formally lack interest for children and are difficult to encourage in the absence of the therapist. Young children, however, enjoy blowing games, e.g. blowing windmills or bubbles, noisy toys, blow football or simply blowing a parent's fingers (Figure 18.7). They do not realize the benefit of the spontaneous deep inspiration prior to the blow, which causes expanding alveoli to exert pressure on adjacent collapsed ones. In older children this, coupled with an inspiratory hold, encourages airflow through collateral channels.
- *ACBT*, whilst being an excellent method of mobilizing secretions, is also a useful method of systematically achieving increased lung volume. Children feel comfortable with the repetitive nature of the technique, and parents will easily continue with its use.

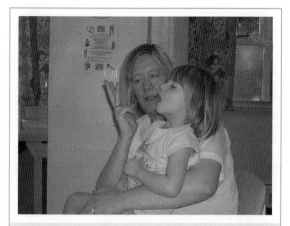

Figure 18.7 Blowing games are a fun and simple way of increasing lung volume.

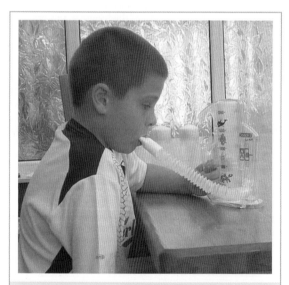

Figure 18.8 Incentive spirometry gives the child a target to achieve.

- *Postural drainage and manual techniques*, as described above to promote reinflation of areas of lobar collapse due to mucus plugging, are well documented.
- *Incentive spirometry* will enhance motivation to take deep breaths, by providing visual reinforcement, a target to achieve and an indication of success (Figure 18.8). For best effect use a device that encourages slow, controlled inspiration.
- *Continuous positive airway pressure (CPAP) or non-invasive ventilation (NIV)* using nasal prongs or a facemask are valuable adjuncts to treatment and are becoming increasingly commonly used in paediatric practice. Both offer pressure support to increase recruitment of poorly

ventilating alveoli. Whilst CPAP delivers throughout both inspiration and expiration, NIV delivers a positive pressure breath to a pre-set limit, synchronized to the child's own breathing pattern and triggered by active inspiration. Both can be used in association with physiotherapy treatment.

DECREASING THE WORK OF BREATHING

Increased work of breathing indicates respiratory distress, but can also be caused by fear, crying and general stress. Children exhibiting this symptom should not be allowed to become overexcited and should receive constant reassurance during interventions. A consistent approach, including being regularly treated by the same physiotherapist, is helpful.

- *Positioning in prone-lying* with the head of the bed elevated stabilizes the anterior chest wall, limiting inward collapse of the ribcage. Improved respiratory rhythm and tidal volume are achieved and a 25% increase in SaO_2 is possible (Hussey 1992). This position should not be used in patients with abdominal distension.

> ### CLINICAL TIPS
>
> - It is essential that infants nursed in the prone position should be closely monitored and supervised, as this position is implicated in sudden infant death syndrome
> - Always advise parents that infants must not be left in this position at home
> - *Positioning in side-lying* removes abdominal loading on the diaphragm, so producing increased diaphragmatic movement and basal lung expansion
> - *Sitting* upright increases the lung volume by allowing improved diaphragmatic excursion and increasing FRC
> - *Limiting treatment time* by constantly evaluating the child's response to treatment will prevent breathing from becoming unduly laboured (Figure 18.9).

IMPROVING VENTILATION/PERFUSION RATIO

The physiological characteristics of the immature respiratory system influence an inability to match ventilated areas of lung tissue with perfused areas. It is important to try and counteract this imbalance in order to improve perfusion of the tissues, by optimizing conditions for gaseous exchange within the lungs. In infants and young children, the distribution of ventilation is preferentially directed to upper regions since the dependent lung is relatively poorly ventilated. This phenomenon occurs because airway closure takes place before FRC is reached as a result of the incomplete airway supporting system

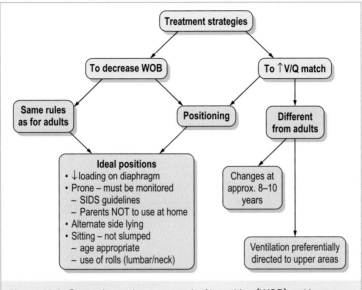

Figure 18.9 Strategies to decrease work of breathing (WOB) and improve ventilation/perfusion (*V/Q*) matching in children. SIDS, sudden infant death syndrome.

and highly compliant chest wall seen in early life. In contrast, the dependent lung always has enhanced perfusion compared with the upper lung, as in adults.

Consequently, the principles which apply when positioning to improve gas exchange are opposite to those expected in adults, e.g. the infant with right-sided pathology should be positioned lying on the affected side, thereby maximizing ventilation and minimizing the amount of mismatch. This feature is believed to be present until approximately age 10 (Davies et al 1990), although there is likely to be a period of transition to the adult pattern.

Many neonates and infants desaturate considerably when turned on to the unaffected side for postural drainage to be carried out. Discussions with parents or nursing staff and assessment should be carried out with the child in his/her preferred position, along with preparation of any equipment which may be required, e.g. suction equipment.

Such children should be preoxygenated, turned at the last possible moment and treated speedily but effectively, before being returned to the correct position to maintain adequate gas exchange.

SUMMARY

When assessing and treating a child with respiratory symptoms, an individualized approach must be adopted, taking into account all relevant factors. Treatment principles do not differ greatly from those applied in adults, but the reasons for their success, or failure, depend upon a sound understanding of the features of the immature respiratory system. Considerable skill and expertise are required to adapt and modify these principles in order to apply treatment safely and effectively.

CASE STUDY 18.1

History

A 13-year-old boy was admitted electively for laparoscopic fundoplication for management of severe gastro-oesophageal reflux leading to frequent chest infections and oesophagitis.

Past medical history

- Hypotonic quadriplegic cerebral palsy
- Severe kyphoscoliosis

- Epilepsy – last major seizure 4 months ago
- Recently confirmed as having severe oropharyngeal discoordination
- Insertion of percutaneous gastrostomy 4 years ago
- Recent fracture of the left tibial plateau – plaster of Paris removed 1 week ago
- Intermittent diarrhoea for last 6 months

Investigations planned

- Awaiting bone density scan

continued

Drug history

- Epilim
- Lioresal (baclofen)
- Diazepam
- Omeprazole
- Sucralfate
- Gaviscon
- Merbentyl
- Chloramphenicol

Social history

Lives with both parents. No siblings. Has a statement of special educational needs and attends a special school.

Preoperatively

Consent received from Mum. Physiotherapy assessment identified transmitted sounds in upper respiratory tract. Occasional coughing to clear secretions spontaneously – Mum reports this is 'normal for him'.

Postoperatively

Routine assessment 9 a.m. Supported half-lying in bed. Pain controlled. Apyrexial. Sao_2 96% in 4 litres humidified O_2 via facemask. Auscultation as pre-op.

11.30 a.m. Asked to review due to increased coughing but not clearing secretions. Sao_2 92% in 4 litres O_2. Auscultation unchanged. Treated in alternate side-lying with gentle percussion and vibrations. Weak cough, so large amount of secretions cleared with nasopharyngeal suction. Suo_2 increased to 98% after treatment.

During next 24 hours: Sao_2 up and down depending upon position. Physiotherapy continued, yielding large amounts of secretions on suction. Nurses suctioning between physiotherapy treatments. Oxygen increased to 8 litres but not maintaining Sao_2. Arterial blood gas (ABG) was within normal limits. Breath sounds decreased on left side. Chest X-ray (CXR) shows no focal signs. Becoming distressed and tone generally raised. Transferred to High-Dependency Unit (HDU).

Problems

- Retention of secretions
- Increased work of breathing
- Increased oxygen requirement
- Difficult to position due to kyphoscoliosis, recent fracture and hypotonia
- Possible osteoporosis
- Anxiety and agitation

4 days post-op: continued to deteriorate – Sao_2 92% in 90% O_2. Respiratory rate 55 breaths/min. Decreased breath sounds in right middle and lower lobes, consolidation on CXR. Blood gases show mild metabolic alkalosis. Agitated and not responding well to manual chest physiotherapy. Failed trial of continuous positive airway pressure – transferred to paediatric intensive care unit for intubation and ventilation.

Gradual improvement over next 3 days – tolerated physiotherapy well whilst ventilated. Extubated on 7th post-op day. Sao_2 90% in 2 litres O_2 via nasal cannulae. Respiratory rate 38 breaths/min. ABGs within normal limits. Ineffective spontaneous coughing so still requiring nasopharyngeal suction. Returned to HDU.

8th post-op day: increased work of breathing. ABGs – increased CO_2 and decreased pH indicate development of respiratory acidosis. Breath sounds now adequate in right side but decreased in left. Started on non-invasive ventilation (NIV) with facemask (inspiratory positive airway pressure (IPAP) = 11; expiratory positive airway pressure (EPAP) = 4, O_2 40%) Continuing to receive regular chest physiotherapy (IPAP increased to 12 during treatment). ABGs normal within 24 hours.

9th–11th post-op days: trial off NIV after physio treatment – managing 30 minutes initially, but 2 hours by next day. Weaning plan commenced – 2 hours on NIV and 2 hours off (with appropriate facemask O_2) alternately – plan to increase time off NIV as able. Frequently agitated and upset, leading to intermittent desaturations and periods of increased work of breathing requiring supplementary O_2 and NIV pressures to be increased and weaning delayed. Responding well to intermittent diazepam. Continuing to receive regular chest physiotherapy, 5–6 times over 24 hours, with positioning, gentle percussion, vibrations, cough stimulation and suction as required.

12th–21st post op days: transferred back to respiratory ward. Continuing with same physiotherapy treatment plan. Large amounts of secretion cleared at every treatment. Benefiting from regular diazepam to reduce agitation. Gradually increasing time off NIV until only required overnight. Discontinued on 19th post-op day. Still receiving intermittent and reducing concentrations of O_2. Frequency of treatment reducing and overnight/evening physiotherapy discontinued on 21st post-op day.

30th post-op day: Breath sounds consistent throughout (allowance made for scoliosis), no increase in work of breathing, CXR shows no focal signs. Sao_2 95% in air, respiratory rate 20 breaths/min. Chest physiotherapy not required for last 2 days. Monitoring continued.

36th post-op day: discharged from hospital.

Note: Passive movements and stretches were carried out regularly throughout, as long as indicated by general stability. Child enabled to sit out of bed in appropriate chair whenever possible.

REFERENCES

Chalumeau M, Foiz-l'Helias L, Scheinmann P et al 2002 Bloodless treatment of infants with haemolytic disease *Pediatric Radiology* 32: 644–647.

Chang AB, Gaffney JT, Eastburn MM et al 2005 Cough quality in children: a comparison of subjective vs. bronchoscopic findings. *Respiratory Research* 6: 3.

Davies H, Helms P, Gordon J 1990 The effect of posture on regional ventilation in children and adults. *Thorax* 45: 313–314.

Davies P, Cheng D, Fox A et al 2002 The efficacy of noncontact oxygen delivery methods. *Pediatrics* 110: 964–968.

Dull JL, Dull WL 1983 Are maximal inspiratory breathing exercises or incentive spirometry better than early mobilization after cardiopulmonary bypass? *Physical Therapy* 63: 655–659.

Hussey J 1992 Effects of chest physiotherapy for children in intensive care after surgery. *Physiotherapy* 78: 109–113.

Kerem E, Yatsiv I, Goitein KJ 1990 Effect of endotracheal suctioning on arterial blood gases in children. *Intensive Care Medicine* 19: 95–99.

Kleiber C, Krutzfield N, Rose EF 1988 Acute histological changes in the tracheobronchial tree associated with different suction catheter insertion techniques. *Heart Lung* 17: 10–14.

Maiya S, Desai M, Baruah A et al 2004 Cough plate versus cough swab in patients with cystic fibrosis; a pilot study. *Archives of Disease in Childhood* 89: 577–579.

McGrath PJ, Pianosi PT, Unruh AM et al 2005 Dalhousie dyspnea scales: construct and content validity of pictorial scales for measuring dyspnea. *BMC Pediatrics* 5:33.

McKenzie SA, Chan E, Dundas I et al 2002 Airway resistance measured by the interrupter technique: normative data for 2–10 year olds of three ethnicities. *Archives of Disease in Childhood* 87: 248–251.

Miske L J, Hickey E M, Kolb SM et al 2004 Use of the mechanical in-exsufflator in pediatric patients with neuromuscular disease and impaired cough. *Chest* 125: 1406–1413.

Noonan V, Dean E 2000 Submaximal exercise testing: clinical application and interpretation. *Physical Therapy* 80: 782–807.

Perrotta C, Ortiz Z, Roque M 2005 Chest physiotherapy for acute bronchiolitis in paediatric patients between 0 and 24 months old. *Cochrane Database of Systematic Reviews* (2): CD004873.

Phelan PD, Olinsky A, Robertson CF 1994 Pulmonary complications of inhalation. In: *Respiratory Illness in Children*, 4th edn. Oxford: Blackwell Scientific Publications, pp. 252–268.

Poets CF 1998 When do infants need additional inspired oxygen? A review of the current literature. *Paediatric Pulmonology* 26: 424–428.

Pryor JA, Webber BA 1979 An evaluation of the forced expiration technique as an adjunct to postural drainage. *Physiotherapy* 65: 304.

Schöni MH 1989 Autogenic drainage: a modern approach to physiotherapy in cystic fibrosis. *Journal of the Royal Society of Medicine* 82: 32–37.

Stick S 2000 The contribution of airway development to paediatric and adult lung disease. *Thorax* 55: 587–594.

Thoreson M, Cavan F, Whitelaw A 1988 Effect of tilting on oxygenation in newborn infants. *Archives of Disease in Childhood* 63: 315–317.

Toussaint M, De Win H, Steens M et al 2003 Effect of intrapulmonary percussive ventilation on mucus clearance in Duchenne muscular dystrophy patients: a preliminary report. *Respiratory Care* 48: 940–947.

Vaughan RS, Menke JA, Giacoia GP 1978 Pneumothorax: a complication of endotracheal tube suctioning. *Journal of Paediatrics* 92: 633–634.

Webb M, Martin JA, Cartlidge PHT et al 1985 Chest physiotherapy in acute bronchiolitis. *Archives of Disease in Childhood* 60: 1078–1079.

Wollmer P, Ursing K, Midgren B et al 1985 Inefficiency of chest percussion in the physical therapy of chronic bronchitis. *European Journal of Respiratory Disease* 66: 233–239.

FURTHER READING

Balfour-Lynn IM, Abrahamson E, Cohen G et al 2005 BTS guidelines for the management of pleural infection in children. *Thorax* 60: i1–i21.

Birnkrant D J 2002 The assessment and management of the respiratory complications of pediatric neuromuscular diseases. *Clinical Pediatrics* 41: 301–309.

Bush A, Cole P, Hariri M et al 1998 Primary ciliary dyskinesia: diagnosis and standards of care. *European Respiratory Journal* 12: 982–988.

Dinwiddie R 1997 *Diagnosis and Management of Paediatric Respiratory Disease*, 2nd edn. New York: Churchill Livingstone.

Doull IJM 2001 Recent advances in cystic fibrosis. *Archives of Disease in Childhood* 85: 62–66.

Hough A 2001 *Physiotherapy in Respiratory Care: An Evidence Based Approach to Respiratory and Cardiac Management*, 3rd edn. Cheltenham: Nelson Thornes.

Jobe AH, Bancalari, E 2001 Bronchopulmonary dysplasia. *American Journal of Respiratory Critical Care Medicine* 163: 1723–1729.

Lakhanpaul M, Atkinson M, Stephenson T 2004 Community acquired pneumonia in children: a clinical update. *Archives of Disease in Childhood Education and Practice* 89: ep29–ep34.

Martinez FD 2002 Development of wheezing disorders and asthma in preschool children. *Pediatrics* 109: 362–367.

Prasad SA, Hussey J 1995 *Paediatric Respiratory Care*. London: Chapman and Hall.

Seddon PC, Khan Y 2003 Respiratory problems in children with neurological impairment. *Archives of Disease in Childhood* 88: 75–78.

Spencer DA 2005 From hemp seed and porcupine quill to HRCT: advances in the diagnosis and epidemiology of bronchiectasis. *Archives of Disease in Childhood* 90: 601–607.

19

Paediatric intensive care

Jill Brownson, Helen Dewdney and Rebecca Biggs

CHAPTER CONTENTS

The role of physiotherapy in acute paediatric respiratory care is similar whether a child is intubated and ventilated on a paediatric intensive care unit (PICU), receiving non-invasive support on a paediatric high-dependency unit (PHDU) or self-ventilating on the wards. A thorough assessment will allow the physiotherapist to use clinical reasoning and formulate problem lists, treatment plans and goals. The role of treatment will be to promote secretion clearance and airway maintenance, normalize observations and blood gas values, reduce a child's work of breathing, reduce the amount of ventilation or oxygen support required and prevent intubation where appropriate and possible. Physiotherapists now take a much more advanced role in respiratory care in PICU. Examples of the physiotherapist's role include involvement in weaning from ventilation and the process of extubation, performing diagnostic procedures such as diagnostic bronchoalveolar lavage (BAL), bronchoscopy, taking blood gases, ordering investigations such as chest X-rays (CXR) and computed tomography (CT) and prescribing medications such as bronchodilators. It is important always to remember the additional roles of assessment and management of a child's neurological and orthopaedic function during an acute deterioration in respiratory status. This will often include

the assessment of and maintenance of range of movement, muscle length, muscle power and function. It requires a sound knowledge of normal development to be applied practically with the children on the PICU (Figure 19.1).

The role of physiotherapy within acute respiratory care is an important one, but it is essential to work closely with members of the multidisciplinary team (MDT). Effective treatment will rely on cooperation and assistance from the MDT, for example, nursing staff carrying out positioning, medical teams prescribing nebulizers, dieticians calculating calorie requirements (in order for children to have adequate energy for tolerating physiotherapy) and speech and language therapists undertaking a dye test to establish the integrity of the swallow reflex. A psychologist may be available to work with children and their families throughout this acute period and occupational therapists and play therapists can be invaluable throughout the rehabilitation period.

> ### KEY POINTS
>
> Acute respiratory care
>
> - Diagnostic procedures
> - Rehabilitation
> - Multidisciplinary working

All children must be assessed thoroughly before any physiotherapy techniques are performed. Intervention in acutely ill children needs to be beneficial – inappropriate treatment is at best ineffective and at worst detrimental.

PHYSIOTHERAPY ASSESSMENT ON THE PAEDIATRIC INTENSIVE CARE UNIT

Within many acute settings, working as an autonomous practitioner, the physiotherapist will assess children without a medical referral and use clinical reasoning skills to decide on appropriate physiotherapy management. Assessment provides detailed information on a child's main problems, looking at respiratory, cardiovascular, neurological and pharmacological factors. The SOAP (subjective, objective,

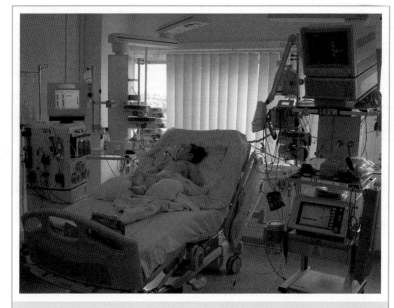

Figure 19.1 Paediatric intensive care unit environment.

analysis, plan) format of note-keeping encourages a structured process, leading to the formulation of a problem list, a treatment plan and SMART (specific, measurable, achievable, relevant, timed) short-term and long-term goals. This may incorporate standardized outcome measures, where available. There are numerous indications for physiotherapy assessment in the acute setting, including respiratory, orthopaedic, neurological and neuromuscular conditions. The following suggest the need for respiratory physiotherapy assessment:

- Intubation and ventilation
- Postanaesthesia, e.g. post Nissens fundoplication and gastrostomy or post cardiac surgery
- CXR changes, e.g. segmental, lobar or lung collapse or areas of consolidation
- Deterioration in respiratory status, i.e. changes in arterial blood gases or an increase in ventilatory requirements such as increased pressures or fraction of inspired oxygen (FiO_2) or the need for commencement of non-invasive ventilation.
- Increase in volume/viscosity of secretions as reported by medical or nursing staff
- Evidence of retained pulmonary secretions such as an increase in FiO_2 or partial pressure of carbon dioxide (PCO_2) or a reduction in tidal volumes
- Absent/ineffective cough either postsurgery or because of respiratory muscle weakness following a period of intubation or pre-existing neurological/neuromuscular disease

- Chronic respiratory disease, e.g. cystic fibrosis, where there will be chronic sputum problems or chronic lung disease due to prematurity, where there may be existing ventilatory requirements and an increased risk of developing infection
- Neurological and neuromuscular disorders, e.g. cerebral palsy, muscular dystrophy, myasthenia gravis, where there may be respiratory muscle weakness predisposing to hypoventilation, a weak or ineffective cough, the risk of retained secretions and the development of infection.

Physiotherapy is considered to be ineffective in the management of:

- Pulmonary oedema
- Pleural effusion
- Consolidated non-productive pneumonia
- Acute bronchiolitis (although a ventilated child will require assessment: Appendix 19.1).

Physiotherapy is contraindicated in the management of:

- Inhaled foreign body (preremoval)
- Pneumothorax (undrained)
- Severe bronchospasm.

Raised intracranial pressure (ICP: either suspected or confirmed) is a possible contraindication to treatment. The physiotherapy management of these children should be discussed with medical teams before implementation.

Table 19.1 Subjective assessment	
Present condition (PC)	Age of child Presenting complaint and diagnosis for this admission Current problem list
History of present condition (HPC)	History of current illness – timescale and features Relevant medical investigations and interventions
Past medical history: (PMH)	Is this a recurrent problem? Will any PMH affect physiotherapy interventions? Pre-existing conditions, e.g. neurodisability
Drug history (DH)	Information from medical notes or drug charts gives an indication of management of any chronic illness
Birth history (BH)	Gestation, mode of delivery, antenatal/perinatal/postnatal complications Birth weight Apgar scores
Developmental history (DVH)	Gross motor/fine motor/cognitive/behavioural skills and abilities Concerns from health professionals or family
Family and social history (FH/SH)	Note familial history of congenital disease Childhood illnesses/immunizations Main carer(s) Siblings and their general health (this may be presented as a family tree for easy reference)

SUBJECTIVE ASSESSMENT

See Table 19.1 and Figure 19.8.

OBJECTIVE ASSESSMENT

It is essential for physiotherapists to look at the observation trends over the 24 hours prior to assessment. Observations should not just be noted from the particular moment of being at a child's bedside; this can distort the true findings (Tables 19.2 and 19.3 and Figure 19.8).

Auscultation

Auscultation identifies and enables description of sounds; these can be separated into breath sounds and added sounds. Auscultation is routinely used by physiotherapists during a respiratory assessment. Critics of this technique question the reliability of the assessor to determine specific lung sounds consistently and accurately: the reliability of auscultation in children is questionable, but can improve with training (Brooks & Thomas 1995).

Auscultation of a baby or small infant is not easy and the correct-size stethoscope should be used. It is essential to compare auscultation of an area of the lung on one side with the corresponding area on the opposite side, including auscultation anteriorly and posteriorly.

Breath sounds

Auscultation will note the presence and quality of breath sounds. There is less lung tissue for the high-frequency sounds to be filtered in a baby or small infant, therefore the breath sounds tend to sound harsher than in an adult. It is also possible for normal breath sounds to be easily transmitted across an area of pathology. Bronchial breathing or marked reduced breath sounds will indicate a large area of consolidation or collapse.

Added sounds

Auscultation will also identify any added sounds. It is not always easy to determine whether the added sounds are pulmonary oedema or secretions. Generalized or widespread fine crackles usually indicate oedema (this may be fibrosis or respiratory distress syndrome). Localized fine crackles are likely to be resolving pneumonia or re-expanding lung tissue. Coarse crackles indicate either gross oedema or secretions. Loud transmitted sounds are either secretions sited

Table 19.2 Objective assessment

Observations	Temperature/heart rate and rhythm/blood pressure Self-ventilating or type of ventilatory support Respiratory rate
Ventilator settings	Mode of ventilation Rate set and actual rate Peak inspiratory pressure (PIP), positive end-expiratory pressure (PEEP), mean airway pressure (MAP) Tidal volume (TV) Fi_{O_2} O_2 saturations End-tidal carbon dioxide (ET_{CO_2})
Blood gases	Note whether venous, arterial, capillary
Chest X-ray	See text and Table 19.4
Position/work	Note and record chest movement Signs of respiratory distress (Table 19.3)
Cardiovascular status	Current accepted values of inotropic support/blood pressure/central venous pressure/fluid balance for that child
Neurological status:	Medication Sedatives, analgesics and paralyser agents Requirement for boluses of sedation prior to handling/physiotherapy treatment
Auscultation and palpation	See text

Table 19.3 Signs of respiratory distress

Mild	Moderate	Severe
Tachypnoea	Recession/retraction/indrawing	Head-bobbing
Tachycardia	Seesawing	Use of accessory muscles
Reduced activity	Nasal flaring Grunting Tracheal tug Inability to feed/talk in sentences	Bradycardia Sweating Pallor/grey/cyanosis Exhaustion Reduced consciousness

centrally or water in the ventilator tubing. Wheeze, if localized, is usually secretion-related. If it is monophonic, it could indicate an obstruction in the bronchus, e.g. a foreign body or very large plug of secretions. Generalized wheeze is representative of bronchospasm, but can occasionally indicate oedema. Stridor may be heard during auscultation. This is denoted by a high-pitched, harsh, vibratory noise caused by partial airway obstruction causing turbulent airflow. It is typically heard on inspiration, suggesting an upper-airway obstruction above the glottis. Expiratory stridor indicates an obstruction in the lower trachea.

Palpation

Palpation is the placement of hands on the chest either anteriorly or at the side of the chest wall to assess the symmetry and quality of chest movement and expansion. It also allows for any secretions in the central airways to be identified. It is important to be able to distinguish secretions from transmitted vibrations, for example water in the ventilator tubing or transmitted upper respiratory tract noises.

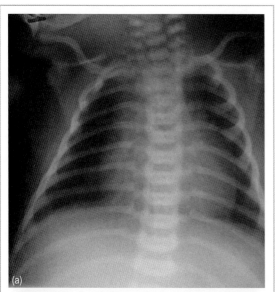

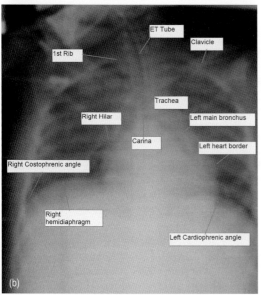

Figure 19.2 (a) A normal chest X-ray. (b) A normal chest X-ray with anatomical features marked.

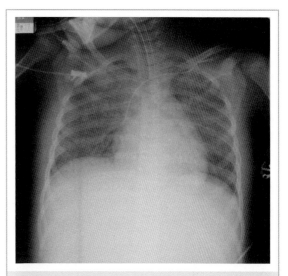

Figure 19.3 Chest X-ray showing acute respiratory distress syndrome.

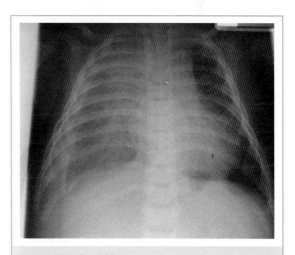

Figure 19.4 Chest X-ray showing pleural effusion.

Children with altered anatomy of the oropharynx, e.g. infants with Down's syndrome or cleft palate, may have pooling of upper respiratory tract secretions and these may be felt on palpation.

Paediatric chest X-ray

The reading of a paediatric CXR requires adaptation of the basic observational skills developed for reading adult X-rays. There are obvious differences in paediatric anatomy and physiology compared with that of an adult, which must be taken into consideration during analysis (Figures 19a and 19.2b). The CXR contributes to the assessment and analysis; together with other clinical signs treatment options can be determined (Table 19.4 and Figures 19.3 to 19.7).

Consolidation

Air can be replaced in the distal airways and alveoli by anything other than air, such as secretions, oedema, blood or fluid; these are denser than air and so the lung becomes

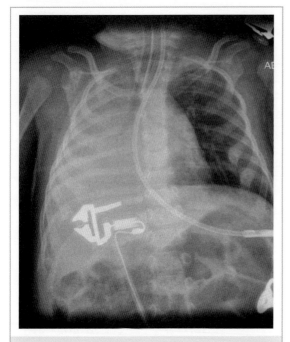

Figure 19.5 Chest X-ray showing right collapse and mediastinal shift.

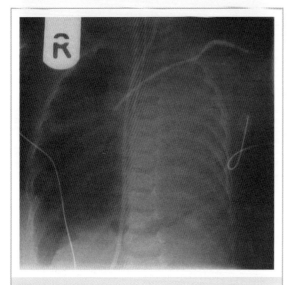

Figure 19.6 Chest X-ray showing endotracheal tube in right main bronchus.

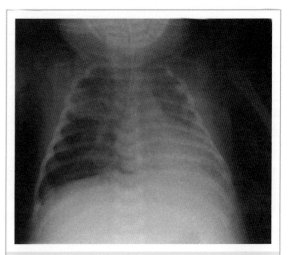

Figure 19.7 Chest X-ray showing right upper lobe and left lower lobe consolidation.

Collapse

There is a loss of lung volume affecting a lung, lobe or segment and the lung appears dense because all the air has been removed. This is usually due to airway obstruction from secretions or a foreign body or because of a mediastinal mass or pneumothorax. Signs of collapse include the shift of normal fissures, crowding of airways in the collapsed lung, a mediastinal shift *towards* the affected side, elevation of hemidiaphragm on the affected side (tenting), rib-crowding and at times compensatory hyperinflation of unaffected lobes.

Pleural effusion

Unilateral effusions are usually caused by infection. Bilateral effusions are often related to low albumin states. Classic signs on X-ray will depend on whether the X-ray was taken using an erect or supine posture. If a child is in an erect position at the time of X-ray, the fluid lies at the bases due to the effects of gravity, with resultant blunting of costophrenic angles. If it is a large effusion, the lateral border of the effusion will be higher laterally than medially. If a child is in supine when the X-ray is taken, the effusion will initially present as a uniform haziness throughout the hemisphere and then as a whitish line (soft-tissue density) between the chest wall and lungs (at the costal edge of the lung). Sometimes the fluid may collect around the lung apex: this is termed 'apical capping'.

Pneumothorax

There are absent lung markings beyond a visible lung edge with increased transradiancy (darker picture), except if the

consolidated. Classic signs of consolidation include increased opacity (areas of consolidation are irregular in shape, segmental or non-segmental), air bronchograms, loss of borders, e.g. the heart or diaphragm and the loss of either cardiophrenic or costophrenic angles. The volume of the affected lung segments remains unchanged.

Table 19.4 How to read a paediatric chest X-ray

Child's details	Name
	Date of birth
	Date and time of X-ray
	Hospital where X-ray was taken
View	Anteroposterior/posteroanterior/lateral: should be stated on the X-ray
	Supine/erect/prone: usually taken in supine in paediatrics
	Determine left from right: the hemidiaphragm on the right is higher than on the left due to the presence of the liver, the heart lies more to the left than the right, the cardiac apex, aortic arch, gas bubbles and nasogastric (NG)/nasojejunal (NJ) tubes may be apparent on the left side
	Quality/exposure: the vertebrae should be visible the whole length of the X-ray. If this is not possible, the exposure is not optimum for analysis. If the X-ray is too dark, it is overexposed and if it is too light, it is underexposed
	Inspiratory/expiratory: ideally the X-ray is taken towards the end of inspiration. This can be difficult with small children or those who are tachypnoeic or uncooperative. A good inspiratory film should have the anterior end of the fifth or sixth rib meeting the middle of the diaphragm. More than six anterior ribs shows hyperinflation and fewer than five indicates an underinflated or expiratory film
	Symmetry: check for rotation by looking at the position of the clavicles. A rotation to the left will leave the right clavicle higher than the left. The anterior ends of the ribs should be equal distance from the spine
	Rotation to the right makes the heart appear central; rotation to the left makes the heart appear large and can make the right heart border disappear
Non-anatomical structures	Endotracheal tube (ETT) position and length: The ETT should lie 1–2 cm above the carina and the ETT length may be documented on the X-ray. (It is not uncommon for it to slip down the right main bronchus.) Flexion of the neck will push the ETT further down and extension will pull it further out
	Tracheostomy
	NG/NJ tube
	Central lines
	Chest drains
	Artifacts, e.g. electrocardiogram (ECG) dots
	Extracorporeal membrane oxygenation (ECMO)
Anatomical structures	Clavicles: symmetry
	Vertebral column: exposure
	Ribs: hyperinflation/underinflation
	Trachea
	Heart: the ratio of the heart size relative to the diameter of the chest (the cardiothoracic ratio) measures approximately 50%. On a well-centred film, two-thirds of the heart is seen to the left and one-third to the right. Children with pulmonary oedema or cardiac pathology may have an enlarged heart
	Lung density: is either lung too lucent (black, usually due to air-trapping) or too opaque (white, usually due to collapse, consolidation, fluid or oedema)?
	Carina: situated at T3 in the neonate, T4/5 in the child and T6 in the adult

continued

Table 19.4 *continued*	
	Mediastinum: contains the structures between the lungs. It has superior, anterior, middle and posterior sections
	Hilus: bronchi, pulmonary vessels, lymphatic vessels and nerves enter and exit through this structure
	Costophrenic angle (between inner surface of the ribs and the dome of the diaphragm) and cardiophrenic angles (between the heart border and the diaphragm)
	Thymus gland: contained in the anterior mediastinum and appears largest at 2 years of age

pneumothorax is over the anterior basal segment. Classic signs on X-ray depend on a child's position. If the child was erect when the X-ray was taken, pleural air would collect at the apex. If the child was supine, pleural air would collect initially in the anterioinferior chest leading to subtle signs, including slivers of air at apex, heart, between lung and diaphragm and increased clarity of mediastinal borders. A lateral view may be useful for determining the evidence and position of a pneumothorax. There may be evidence of a mediastinal shift towards the contralateral side (unless a tension pneumothorax is present, in which case structures will be pulled towards the affected side).

Pulmonary oedema

The classic signs of pulmonary oedema on X-ray are a bilateral uniform haziness with no vascular markings evident. This is often described as having a 'ground-glass' appearance. There may be a loss of borders, e.g. heart or diaphragm, and a loss of the cardiophrenic or costophrenic angles. Cardiomegaly may result as part of the pathology of cardiac failure, resulting in pulmonary oedema.

Acute respiratory distress syndrome

The X-ray signs denoting this condition are similar in appearance to pulmonary oedema, with a bilateral uniform haziness and 'ground-glass' appearance. There will be no cardiomegaly because the respiratory distress syndrome leads to non-cardiogenic pulmonary oedema, with no cardiac pathology. There is no loss of heart or diaphragm borders and the costophrenic and cardiophrenic angles are also spared.

Lines and drains

During assessment, it is useful to make a mental note of lines and drains to avoid dislodging them during treatment. The presence of lines can give a good indication of the pathology and severity of the child's illness.

Some examples of the lines and drains used on a PICU include:

- *Central lines*: these may be jugular, supraclavicular or femoral. The central line is used to measure the central venous pressure and for drug administration and blood sampling.
- *Peripheral/arterial lines*: these are used for drug administration and blood sampling. A baby's blood volume is approximately 80–85 ml of blood per kilogram. A 3-kg baby has only 250 ml of blood in its entire circulation, therefore the accidental removal of an arterial line can lead to serious loss of blood volume. If a line is dislodged during handling the flow must be quickly stopped.
- *Urine catheters*: a baby or child may be catheterized or the nappy weighed to measure urine output.
- *Long line (e.g. Hickman or Broviac)*: this is used for administration of total parenteral nutrition (TPN: intravenous feeding) and chemotherapy drugs.
- *Nasogastric or nasojejunal tubes*: these are used for aspiration of stomach contents and feeding/oral drug administration.
- *Pleural, chest, mediastinal drains*: these drains are used after cardiac surgery; chest drains are used for draining pleural effusions and pneumothoraces.

PHYSIOTHERAPY TREATMENT ON THE PAEDIATRIC INTENSIVE CARE UNIT

A treatment programme on the PICU should be designed and implemented based on assessment findings, sound clinical reasoning and problem-solving skills. The intensive care environment creates factors that require consideration before treatment is implemented and may affect the treatment given. These factors may include a child's stability and ability to tolerate physiotherapy, service priorities on the unit (medical versus therapy priorities) and the use of rest periods for children when no medical or therapeutic interventions should take place.

The physiotherapist must maintain an awareness of the length of the treatment session and be wary of prolonging the treatment to the detriment of healing and

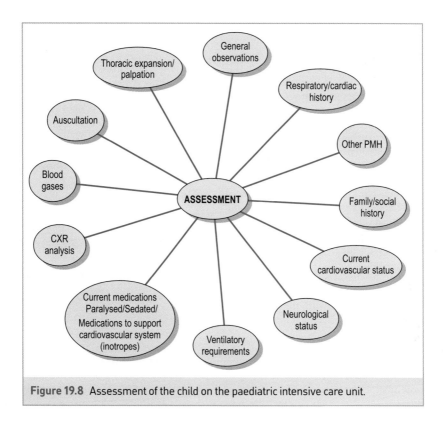

Figure 19.8 Assessment of the child on the paediatric intensive care unit.

recovery. Stable children may tolerate a substantial treatment session but interventions for less stable children must be carefully considered.

It is important to remember that treatment aims on the PICU not only involve respiratory techniques; developmental and/or neurological/orthopaedic interventions may be just as important for the child's recovery.

Once a child is extubated, it is sometimes difficult to ensure cooperation during treatment. Distraction and persuasion using games, television or books may prove beneficial and, for some children, rewards such as stickers can be of use. Involving parents, siblings or carers during treatment is essential for enhancing adherence, cooperation and understanding.

Aims of treatment

- Remove excess bronchopulmonary secretions
- Maintain alveolar expansion
- Re-inflate areas of atelectasis
- Achieve optimum ventilation/perfusion matching
- Maintain oxygenation
- Implement developmental/rehabilitation programmes.

Treatment techniques and indications for use

Secretion clearance techniques comprise positioning and postural drainage, manual ventilation/hyperinflation, manual techniques, saline instillation, suction and breathing exercises. There is limited evidence to support the use of chest physiotherapy in mechanically ventilated children (Krause & Hoehn 2000). Improvements in respiratory function, e.g. reduced respiratory resistance, and changes in arterial blood gases have been demonstrated when chest physiotherapy is compared with suction alone in ventilated infants and children (Main et al 2004). Further studies are required to investigate the effects of chest physiotherapy, both beneficial and deleterious, and for which children the greatest benefit can be anticipated. Judicious rather than routine application of respiratory physiotherapy techniques is advocated, with the clinician assessing the effects before, during and following each treatment.

Positioning and postural drainage

Careful consideration along with use of sound clinical reasoning skills is required when deciding on appropriate positioning for acutely unwell children. Positioning aims to redistribute ventilation. The young infant's response to gravitational forces differs substantially from that of an adult and therefore positioning strategies used by physiotherapists need to be modified (Oberwaldner 2000). Preferential ventilation is adopted by both infants and small children, meaning that they preferentially ventilate the uppermost non-dependent regions of the lungs, but they perfuse the dependent areas of their lungs, creating a ventilation/perfusion mismatch. Oxygenation of infants and small children therefore improves when the good lung is uppermost (Heaf et al 1983). This has implications for the use of side-lying in a child with unilateral lung disease and care should be taken when positioning these children with the affected lung uppermost because of the possible deterioration in their respiratory status (Davies et al 1985). Preferential ventilation has been shown to persist in young children up to the age of 27 months and possibly beyond, even as late as the second decade of life. It is important to note that newborn infants are optimally oxygenated with their head up: oxygenation can drop if they are placed flat or positioned head-down (Thoresen et al 1988).

Supine positioning has been shown to be the least effective position in which to place children to optimize respiratory function, although it is often used as the most convenient position in which to nurse a child.

Prone positioning is often used in special-care baby units and the PICU for children with acute respiratory distress syndrome to improve oxygenation. The benefits of prone positioning over supine in ventilated neonates and infants with acute respiratory distress include improved oxygenation, ventilation and chest wall stability (Wells et al 2005).

Advice should be given to parents not to use this position when babies are unattended at home because of the correlation between prone positioning and sudden infant death syndrome (SIDS). Constant cardiorespiratory monitoring should be used for all children placed in this position in hospital. (Wells et al 2005).

The American Association of Respiratory Care (AARC) produced an extensively referenced *Clinical Practice Guidelines on Postural Drainage Therapy* in 1991. This recommendation relates to older children and adults but acknowledges the use of postural drainage therapy for neonates, infants and children.

Postural drainage or gravity-assisted positioning, using knowledge of the bronchial tree anatomy, is used to mobilize and aid drainage of bronchial secretions, maximize ventilation/perfusion and aid re-expansion of atelectasis. By positioning lung segments above their respective bronchi, the effects of gravity will enable secretions to drain into more central airways, making them easier to clear (Zausmer 1968, Prasad & Hussey 1995, Berney et al 2004). Positioning is recommended for 3–15 minutes and even up to 30 minutes, allowing time for the secretions to move from one area to another. Success relies greatly on having a good technique. Postural drainage is rarely used in isolation.

It is more frequently combined with other physiotherapy techniques such as manual techniques (vibrations and percussion) and coughing and has been shown to be a cheap, practical and worthwhile modality for clearing secretions, particularly if they are copious but thin (Newhouse & Rossman 1984, Zhang & Zhang 1997, Fink 2001).

Postural drainage is used primarily for the treatment of conditions that produce a great deal of sputum, such as cystic fibrosis, but can have a place in the PICU where secretions are difficult to clear (Figure 19.9).

Contraindications. There should be careful consideration before employing postural drainage for children. The head-down tip position is contraindicated in:

- Preterm infants/neonates
- Abdominal distension

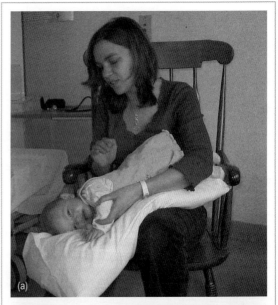

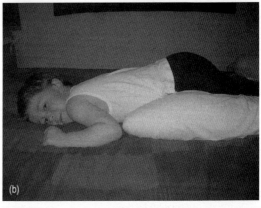

Figure 19.9 (a) Postural drainage for baby. (b) Postural drainage for child.

- Phrenic nerve palsy
- Raised ICP
- Postsurgery – abdominal surgery, neurosurgery and cardiac surgery
- Increased work of breathing.

A full layout of postural drainage positions can be found in Hough (1991).

Manual ventilation

Manual ventilation involves disconnecting the child from the ventilator and using a manual reservoir bag to maintain ventilation (Figure 19.10). This may be necessary when changing ventilator tubing, or when changing the child's position, such as from supine to prone. Manual ventilation can be useful for assessment purposes prior to extubation as it gives an indication of respiratory effort, lung compliance, expansion capacity and airway irritability. During manual ventilation, the pressures, volumes and rate given should remain the same as the ventilator settings; this can be ensured by placing a manometer into the circuit. When manually ventilating infants and small children, a 500-ml bag should be used; this often has an open end for controlling the volume of gas entering the bag and the positive end-expiratory pressure (PEEP) and for expelling excess pressure. The oxygen flow should be set at 8–10 litres. Older children will require a 1 or 2-litre bag which usually contains a valve for controlling the amount of PEEP being given; the flow of oxygen should be set at 10–15 litres. The size of the bag used relates to the child's lung volume.

Manual hyperinflation

Manual hyperinflation is frequently used as part of a physiotherapy treatment session. There is limited published research evaluating its use within the paediatric population and findings from adult studies have been extrapolated (Denehy 1999, Barker & Eales 2000). The technique is described within a number of respiratory therapy textbooks (Prasad & Hussey 1995, Prasad & Main 2002).

Manual hyperinflation aims to:

- increase tidal volumes
- recruit alveoli not expanded during tidal volume breaths, possibly through use of collateral ventilation
- reinflate areas of collapse
- increase expiratory flow rates and imitate a huff, assisting with the movement of secretions proximally.

It can also be used to preoxygenate prior to suctioning.

Technique for hyperinflation

When using hyperinflation as part of a physiotherapy treatment, the technique involves creating a long, slow inspiration with an inspiratory hold at the end. This is followed by quick release of the bag to expel the air rapidly, such as during a huff or a cough, in order to mobilize secretions. This technique is often used in a 'one in three' cycle, using vibrations to assist in the removal of bronchial secretions. During this cycle, two breaths mimicking the pressures and rate set by the ventilator are given, followed by a hyperinflated breath. The vibrations are applied on this third breath and the cycle continues until coughing starts or the secretions are felt when palpating the chest, indicating that they have moved centrally and will be easier to remove.

A technique known as 'jet bagging' is another form of manual hyperinflation. Its aims are the same as in simple manual hyperinflation, with a greater emphasis on secretion clearance. The technique is different: the inspiration volume is slowly increased to a high peak inspiratory pressure, introducing small tidal volumes at a very rapid rate. A rapid expiration phase mimics a huff and cough, assisting the mobilization of secretions. Vibrations may be used during this expiratory phase. There are currently no published data on this technique.

Precautions to hyperinflation

As a general rule, manual hyperinflation pressures should not exceed 20% above the peak inspiratory pressure because of risk of barotraumas (Prasad & Hussey 1995). If manual hyperinflation is indicated as a physiotherapy technique for a child whose CXR shows hyperinflation, care must be taken because of the increased risk of barotrauma and pneumothorax. If a child is receiving nitric oxide, then during both manual ventilation and manual hyperinflation the nitric oxide must be entrained into the circuit. Physiotherapists treating children with cardiac conditions must take into account their normal oxygen saturations. Children with cardiac conditions may deteriorate and the shunting of their blood may increase if too much oxygen is given and their oxygen saturations are allowed to rise too high. Children with cardiac conditions

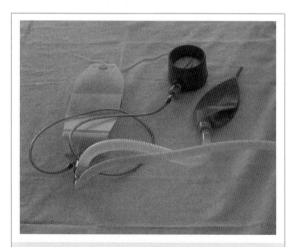

Figure 19.10 Manual ventilation circuit.

may therefore require manual ventilation and hyperinflation to be administered using an air/oxygen mix and only when absolutely indicated.

Other precautions with manual hyperinflation include:

- High levels of peak inspiratory pressure/PEEP (over $10\,cmH_2O$)
- Suspected or confirmed raised ICP
- Hyperinflation on CXR, i.e. in asthma and bronchiolitis
- Cardiovascular instability (particularly hypovolaemia, low cardiac output)
- Peritoneal dialysis – children undergoing peritoneal dialysis (haemofiltration) should be treated during the 'fluid out' phase of haemofiltration
- High-frequency oscillatory ventilation (HFOV)
- Preterm neonates less than 36/40 weeks' gestation.

Contraindications to hyperinflation

- Undrained pneumothorax
- Significant cardiovascular instability, including hypovolaemic shock, low cardiac output, cardiac arrhythmias
- Low/labile blood pressure
- Severe bronchospasm
- Emphysematous bullae, multiple cysts
- Unexplained haemoptysis
- Bronchial anastomoses, e.g. postlobectomy

Complications

- Pneumothorax – this should not occur if a manometer is in place and the physiotherapist is constantly monitoring the inspiratory pressures.
- Reduced/labile blood pressure – manual hyperinflation may compromise venous return, reducing stroke volume and dropping blood pressure. If blood pressure drops during treatment, smaller and slower tidal volumes should be given and the child reconnected to the ventilator if there is no improvement.
- Reduced oxygen saturations – this may occur because of sputum plugging, pneumothorax, bronchospasm or a ventilation/perfusion mismatch. If this does occur, the physiotherapist should reassess to establish the cause and put in place appropriate measures to rectify this as soon as possible.
- De-recruitment when returned to the ventilator – this may be due to the interruption of pressures during disconnection and reconnection to the ventilator. This can be minimized by increasing FiO_2 before and after treatment and increasing ventilator pressures briefly post-treatment. Children requiring high ventilator pressures will be most likely to de-recruit and therefore caution should be used when taking these children off the ventilator.
- Raised ICP – increased Pco_2 may lead to vasodilation and therefore increased cerebral blood flow.

- Reduced respiratory drive – if the child's Pco_2 reduces during treatment, this may lead to a reduced respiratory drive.

Manual techniques

The manual techniques used in paediatrics are the same as those used for adults. Chest physiotherapy techniques such as percussion and vibrations are widely used, but little is known about their effectiveness in children (McCarren et al 2003, Almeida-Celize et al 2005). Chest physiotherapy has been associated with the development of severe brain damage in very-low-birth-weight infants and potentially severe hypoxaemia in neonates (Fox et al 1978, Harding et al 1998). Rib fractures are a rare complication of manual physiotherapy techniques, with an estimated incidence of 1 in 1000 incidents of all rib fractures (Chalumeau et al 2002).

The aim of manual techniques is to facilitate the removal of secretions, which may be sticky, by moving them from peripheral to more central airways, making them easier to clear through coughing or suction (Schindler 2005). Research has shown that chest physiotherapy incorporating manual techniques can reduce respiratory resistance due to the removal of secretions and increase physiological dead space due to the opening of poorly perfused alveoli to ventilation (Argent & Morrow 2004). Chest physiotherapy should be performed before feeds or at least an hour afterwards to minimize the risk of vomiting and aspiration. The main difference between applying manual techniques to infants and young children compared to older children and adults is the compliance of the chest wall. Manual techniques should not cause pain, but can be upsetting for parents to watch; careful explanations should be given prior to commencement of treatment. Babies' heads should be supported to prevent head and neck movements during manual techniques. Manual techniques are rarely used in isolation; they are used in conjunction with positioning, postural drainage, manual hyperinflation, suction and active cycle of breathing technique in the extubated child.

Expiratory vibrations

This technique involves applying pressure in an inwards and upwards direction to the chest wall on expiration, creating an oscillatory movement and mimicking the direction in which the ribs and soft tissues move during expiration (Imle 1989, Prasad & Hussey 1995). It is said to move secretions from peripheral to central airways, making them easier to clear with coughing and/or suction.

Vibrations will only be effective if a child's respiratory rate is near normal. If it is faster than this, the expiratory phase will be too short for the vibrations to be effective. The pressure applied to the chest wall cannot be classified; it is dependent, to a large extent, on the therapist's beliefs and experience. The child's condition, cardiovascular stability, likelihood of bronchospasm, size and age are also taken into account. Current studies are investigating the amount of pressure different therapists exert on the chest wall during vibrations.

Vibrations seem to be most effective when there are thick, sticky secretions which are not palpable on the chest wall and are not cleared by coughing or suction. The oscillatory movements and vibrations will cause the secretions to become dislodged from the sides of the airways and the direction in which the pressure is applied will cause them to move towards the upper respiratory tract. Vibrations are often performed in conjunction with manual hyperinflation when a child is ventilated. A cycle of two breaths mimicking the pressures and rate set by the ventilator are given, followed by a hyperinflated breath. Vibrations are applied during the expiration phase of this third breath and the cycle continues until either spontaneous coughing begins or secretions are felt when palpating the chest, indicating that they have moved centrally and will be easier to remove by suction. In a self-ventilating child, the vibration should be performed on expiration and preferably after a deep breath has been taken. For this reason and for comfort, vibrations should not be performed after each expiration, but instead on every third breath, allowing the child time to recover from the action. In the absence of spontaneous coughing, suctioning can be performed.

Percussion

Percussion is rhythmic clapping over specific lung segments or lobes affected by pathology; it is performed alongside the normal respiratory cycle. The aim is to loosen bronchial secretions from the bronchial walls through the production of an energy wave, which is transmitted through the chest wall to the affected airways. The secretions move from the bronchial walls to peripheral and then central airways before clearance by coughing or suction. Percussion is usually well tolerated in children; babies and young infants will often be soothed and fall asleep.

In paediatrics, percussion usually uses a one-handed technique: a cupped hand creates a hollow sound as an 'air cushion' is created on impact with the chest wall. A rate has been recommended of approximately 40/minute for 3–5 minutes. A slower rate of percussion may be better tolerated by children at risk of developing bronchospasm or by children who are critically ill or cardiovascularly unstable.

Some physiotherapists use the three-fingered 'tenting' technique, with the middle finger raised to overlap the third and first fingers or small anaesthetic masks with the open end occluded to help create a vacuum.

Percussion should not cause pain and should not create a 'slapping' noise or leave red marks on the skin. Most therapists use a thin layer of clothing, towel or pillowcase over the skin. The use of percussion is indicated when there are added sounds on auscultation, not palpable and not cleared by coughing or suction, or if nursing

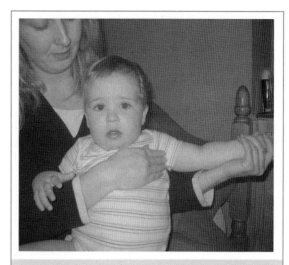

Figure 19.11 Percussion for a baby.

staff report the presence of thick secretions. Percussion may be of benefit in the younger age group who may not be able to coordinate taking a deep breath when carrying out vibrations (Figure 19.11).

Precautions in percussion and vibrations

- Pain
- Coagulopathy/abnormal clotting (manual techniques should be applied with caution if platelets are less than 50)
- Known history of bronchospasm (the use of bronchodilatory therapy prior to administering manual techniques may reduce the incidence or severity of bronchospasm)
- Cardiovascular instability
- Premature babies.

Contraindications to percussion and vibrations

- Coagulopathy/abnormal clotting (manual techniques are not indicated if platelets are less than 20 because of the risk of petechiae, bruising and bleeding)
- Acute pulmonary haemorrhage
- Rib fractures
- Osteoporosis/bone mineral deficiency (e.g. children with long-term loss of independent mobility)
- Severe bronchospasm
- Open sternum.

Suction

Suction is used to clear retained thick and tenacious secretions. It is used in the intubated child who is prevented from coughing effectively, to maintain tube patency and for the self-ventilating child who has a weak and ineffective cough, Suction may be via the endotracheal or tracheostomy tube if a child is ventilated and nasopharyngeal or oropharyngeal if a child is self-ventilating. The size of the suction catheter should be carefully considered in order to be able to clear secretions but minimize trauma; in the intubated child the size will bear a direct relationship to the size of the endotracheal tube, e.g. a size 10 catheter can be used with a size 5 endotracheal tube. In a non-intubated child who is self-ventilating, the catheter size will be at the discretion of the therapist, in consideration of the size of the child's nostrils. Suction is extremely unpleasant for the non-intubated child. An infant or young child may need to be swaddled and the head held to prevent unnecessary soft-tissue trauma. As with all treatment techniques, parents and carers should be given adequate explanation regarding the reasons for suctioning and the technique in order to give informed consent.

Suction technique

The AARC compiled comprehensive guidelines regarding the application of nasotracheal suction in 2004 (Bennion 2004). The use of universal precautions will follow local departmental guidelines. Some units recommend that physiotherapists use eye shields and masks when suctioning all children; others restrict the use to the treatment of children with infectious diseases. The use of either sterile or clean technique is variable. A bolus of sedation may be required prior to suctioning for children who are alert, have pulmonary hypertension or raised ICP. Aquagel may be used when suctioning a non-intubated child if the nasal passage appears dry; it can be effective for preventing mechanical trauma. It is unlikely to be necessary in children aged under 2 years whose nasal passages tend to be well lubricated and its use may block the nasal passages. One suction catheter should be used on each occasion of endotracheal or tracheostomy suction, although during nasopharyngeal suction it may be appropriate to reinsert the catheter before complete withdrawal in order to minimize trauma to the nose. There are few published data to indicate the appropriate depth of suction. Mechanical trauma may be reduced by passing the suction catheter no more than 1 cm beyond the end of the endotracheal or tracheostomy tube. Alternatively, pass it until resistance is felt then withdraw slightly before applying suction (Swartz et al 1996).

Deep suction (defined as passing the suction catheter more than 1 cm beyond the end of the endotracheal or tracheostomy tube) has been associated with collapse of the right upper lobe. This is thought to be due to trauma around the right main bronchus and de-aeration of the right upper lobe. These factors need to be balanced against the need to stimulate a cough when deciding on the depth to pass the suction catheter. Suction should not be applied during the insertion of the suction catheter but it is applied continuously when withdrawing the catheter. The use of intermittent pressure or rotation of the catheter on withdrawal increases the risk of barotrauma (Young

1984a, b, 1988). The recommended pressures for suctioning children are 60–170 mmHg. The suctioning process should take only 10–15 seconds. Nasopharyngeal and oropharyngeal suction is used following endotracheal or tracheostomy suctioning, to prevent aspiration of secretions past the uncuffed endotracheal or tracheostomy tube. Used catheters must be discarded appropriately according to hospital infection control policies. Auscultation and evaluation of observations following suction will allow for any side-effects to be recorded.

Precautions to suction

- Cleft palate repair
- Tracheo-oesophageal fistula repair (TOF) – a TOF catheter must be used
- Evidence of stridor
- Adenotonsillectomy
- Abnormal clotting (platelets less than 50)
- Pulmonary haemorrhage (if the child is at risk of this, the catheter should not be inserted more than 1 cm beyond the end of the endotracheal tube).

Contraindications to suction

- Severe cardiovascular instability
- Abnormal clotting (platelets less than 20)
- Frank haemoptysis
- Severe bronchospasm
- Undrained pneumothorax
- No nasopharangeal suction on children with basal skull or facial fractures.

The side-effects of suction have been well documented. Side-effects include hypoxaemia, barotrauma, introduction of infection, apnoea, bronchospasm, pneumothorax, atelectasis, increase in ICP, cardiac arrhythmias, particularly bradycardia because of a vasovagal response, and, on very rare occasions, even death (Stone & Turner 1989, Clark et al 1990, Kerem et al 1990, Czarnik et al 1991, Jaw et al 1991, Shah et al 1992, Singer et al 1994, Wood 1998, Clarke et al 1999). Much remains unknown about the interaction between catheter size, suction pressures, intrapulmonary airflow and effective secretion clearance (Morrow et al 2004).

These side-effects can be reduced through:

- Preoxygenation of the child prior to suction, either via the ventilator or manual inflation (Kerem et al 1990). Care should be taken not to overoxygenate preterm infants as this has shown to be associated with retinopathy of prematurity (Robertson 1996)
- Selection of an appropriately designed suction catheter (Shah et al 2005)
- Using the minimum suction pressure to clear secretions effectively (Argent & Morrow 2004)
- Suctioning to an appropriate depth. Graduated suction catheters are available which allow the depth of suction to be measured and related to the length of

the endotracheal or tracheostomy tube. This is particularly relevant if there are concerns regarding trauma through suction or if a child has low platelets or signs of active bleeding

- Extra care being taken when suction is required for a recently extubated child to avoid precipitating laryngospasm
- The use of in-line suction: many intensive care units now use in-line suction (closed suction): a suction catheter is passed through a sheath, preventing the need for disconnection from the ventilator circuit. This is usually changed every 24 hours. The rationale for use is the reduction of cross-infection, uninterrupted nitric oxide flow (when in use), maintenance of PEEP and prevention of lung collapse, and minimization of oxygen desaturation during suctioning, which is of particular pertinence in children requiring high ventilator pressures. There is some disagreement over the use of closed suction, with some studies showing that children are more stable with regard to their heart rate and oxygen saturation. Others have indicated that closed suction shows no clinical benefit over open suction in terms of arterial oxygenation and may actually cause more marked swings in alveolar pressures and potential loss of lung volume (Cereda et al 2001, Choong et al 2003, Tan et al 2005). Bronchial perforation after closed endotracheal suction has also been reported (Thakur et al 2000, Garcia-Aparicio et al 2002).

Saline

Instillation of normal, isotonic saline 0.9% NaCl into a child's artificial airway prior to suction or as a component of physiotherapy is widely practised, yet remains controversial. It is proposed that saline instillation enhances the clearance of tenacious secretions, stimulates a cough and reduces the rate of airway occlusion. However there are few published studies to support this in critically ill children (Blackwood 1999). Volumes between 0.5 and 2 ml per instillation are suggested, depending upon the size of the child (Schwenker et al 1998). Although the frequency of use and maximum volume are not reported, clinical reasoning should assess its efficacy within a given clinical situation. Saline instillation may cause a reduction in oxygen saturations and its routine use is not advocated (Ridling et al 2003). Other mucolytics are occasionally instilled in the presence of thick secretions, e.g. *N*-acetylecysteine.

Surfactant

Synthetic and combined natural and synthetic preparations of surfactant are used to increase arterial oxygen tension (PaO_2), thought to be caused by an improved match between ventilation and perfusion (Fanaroff & Martin 1992). The use of surfactant has been routine in the management of respiratory distress syndrome of prematurity;

in the PICU it is used in the medical management of respiratory failure, e.g. near-drowning.

Breathing exercises

Traditional breathing exercises, such as the active cycle of breathing technique, are often difficult and even impossible to use with young children, particularly those under 5 years of age, and effectiveness in this age group is unknown. Laughing and crying are often very effective means of gaining lung expansion in infants. In mobile children, playing can also be effective. Children over the age of 2 years old can be encouraged to take deep breaths through the use of games such as blowing bubbles and through the use of incentive spirometry and positive expiratory pressure masks once they reach the age of 5–6 years. It is also very difficult to persuade a child who is unwell to cough on command and near impossible in those under 2 years of age, so appropriate positioning, stimulation of a cough through suctioning and reliance on techniques such as blowing games to produce a spontaneous cough are required.

Incentive spirometry

Incentive spirometry is commonly used in the PHDU setting in the prevention of acute chest syndrome of sickle-cell disease. It also has a role in the postoperative management of surgical procedures where mobilizing is not permitted, for example spinal surgery. It is thought to be able to reduce the incidence of respiratory complications and lessen admissions to PICU.

Incentive spirometry is designed to encourage deep breathing; it measures the inspiratory capacity of the lungs. The deep inspiratory efforts performed encourage good expansion of the alveoli, reducing mismatch of regional ventilation and perfusion, and can prevent the development of atelectasis. The spirometer provides children with a visual feedback on their performance; the consideration is that the use of a tangible object may influence an increase in volume and produce a more controlled flow. It is a programme that needs to be implemented throughout the day and waking hours at night; it can be implemented within nursing care plans (Bellet et al 1995, Yale et al 2000, Salzman 2002, Hsu et al 2005, Ong et al 2005; Figure 19.12).

Diagnostic non-bronchoscopic bronchoalveolar lavage (BAL)

Non-bronchoscopic BAL involves the instillation of a high volume of 0.9% NaCl via a BAL catheter inserted into the endotracheal tube while the child is manually inflated. Suction is carried out while manual techniques are applied. This procedure may be undertaken by physiotherapists as an aid to the diagnosis of opportunistic lung disease, e.g. viral and fungal infections and pulmonary

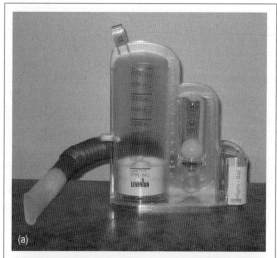

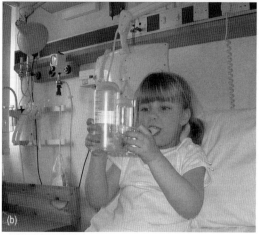

Figure 19.12 (a) Incentive spirometer. (b) Incentive spirometer in use.

pathology unresponsive to drug therapy. These may include *Aspergillus*, pulmonary tuberculosis, cytomegalovirus and *Pneumocystis jiroveci* pneumonia. The procedure requires careful preparation and is a skilled technique which should only be undertaken by experienced physiotherapists and with senior medical staff present. The diagnostic yield of the procedure has been reported as 69% (Morrow & Argent 2002).

Procedure

- Children are either electively intubated, or already intubated and ventilated on PICU. They should have dependable venous access and either be well sedated or have been administered a paralysing agent to prevent them coughing.

- Consent must be obtained for this procedure. Written consent is required when a child is electively intubated; parents must be fully informed of the risk of a child remaining ventilated post procedure.

- Protocols define the preparation, precautions and stages of the procedure (Morrow et al 2006). Current evidence recommends that 1 ml 0.9% NaCl per 1 kg of child's weight is instilled per specimen. Four or five specimens can be taken and sent for virology, cytology, histology, bacterial and fungal screen.

REHABILITATION

Physiotherapists working in the PICU setting must have a working knowledge of normal development and the influences of acute and long-term illness upon a developing child. The use of positioning, passive movements and splinting may form part of the early management of the acutely ill child on PICU.

Neurological and orthopaedic assessment tools, used at the appropriate time, will be relevant for the management of head injuries, orthopaedic surgery, trauma or prolonged stays on PICU/PHDU (see Ch. 11).

Care should be taken to ensure that neurological assessment takes into account the effects of the withdrawal of opiates on the neurological state, e.g. jittery movements and/or hallucinations. Appropriate physical management programmes should be implemented at the earliest opportunity to optimize muscle tone and function, encourage appropriate developmental positioning and minimize loss of range of movement. Parents/carers will generally be grateful for the opportunity to contribute to the care and rehabilitation of their child; a multidisciplinary approach will enable a physical management programme to be implemented throughout the day and night. Positioning charts or tick boxes are useful as a visual prompt. Many units have access to a paediatric occupational therapist or play therapist who will contribute to the plan. Splinting, passive movements, positioning, tilt tables, standing frames, appropriate seating, rolls, wedges and T-rolls all have a place in the rehabilitation of children on PICU and their transition to a PHDU or ward setting (Figure 19.13).

VENTILATION

Children are usually ventilated on pressure-cycled modes of ventilation in an attempt to prevent barotrauma, but babies who are difficult to ventilate on pressure-cycling may sometimes require volume-cycled ventilation.

Children aged less than 10–12 years are usually intubated with uncuffed endotracheal tubes using the subglottic region as the cuff. There should be a very small leak around the tube to prevent damage to the mucosa. (If a child is in, or at risk from, pulmonary oedema a cuffed tube may be

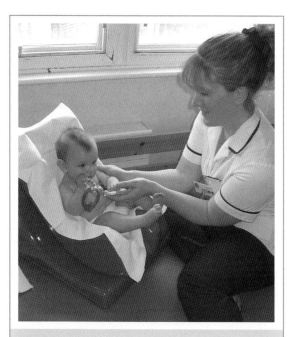

Figure 19.13 Physiotherapy for a baby following a PICU admission.

used in anticipation of the high ventilatory pressures that will be needed to control the pulmonary oedema.)

Nasal intubation is most frequently used. The tube needs to be firmly secured to prevent damage to the subglottic region and accidental extubation: endotracheal tubes are secured either by strapping or a tunstall connector. Oral tubes are often precarious and care is needed when treating and turning the child. All babies and young children are ventilated with some PEEP to maintain small-airway patency during expiration, as there is a loss of intrinsic PEEP during intubation. This ensures that the child's closing volume is outside the tidal volume, thereby increasing functional residual capacity to help prevent atelectasis. The exception to this is children with traumatic brain injury or those with potentially raised ICP (Tables 19.5 and 19.6; Figures 19.14 and 19.15).

Heliox

Heliox is a helium–oxygen gas mixture containing 79% helium and 21% oxygen. Its efficacy has been noted in relieving dyspnoea and upper-airway obstruction. It is an inert gas, lighter and less dense than air, and can therefore pass through airways into the more distal airways more easily,

Table 19.5 Ventilation of intubated children	
Bi-level positive airways pressure (BiPAP)	Pressure-cycled modes of ventilation are most commonly, but not exclusively, used in paediatrics. Tidal volume varies according to the pressures set. Tidal volumes are determined by the child and measured through a ventilator. Positive inspiratory pressure (PIP) is set between 12 and 30 cmH$_2$0. Positive end-expiratory pressure (PEEP) is set between 2 and 12 cmH$_2$0. Patient-triggered breaths are supported by assisted spontaneous breaths (ASB)
Physiotherapy considerations	If airway resistance is reduced, airway compliance is increased and atelectic areas re-expanded by the removal of secretions during physiotherapy; the child's tidal volumes will be greater for a set inspiratory pressure and it may be possible to reduce ventilator pressures following discussion with medical teams
Continuous positive airway pressure (CPAP)	A set continuous PEEP is given throughout the respiratory cycle to splint open the airways and improve ventilation and oxygenation. This form of ventilation reduces the work of breathing and opens up areas of atelectasis. CPAP can be administered through the ventilator via endotracheal tube, tracheostomy or nasal prong. CPAP is indicated in type 1 respiratory failure, when areas of atelectasis are present and during instances of increased work of breathing. Children may be weaned from invasive BiPAP on to CPAP through the ventilator prior to extubation
High-frequency oscillatory ventilation (HFOV)	An appropriate mean airway pressure (MAP) is set by the medical team. There is high-frequency movement of gas to the lungs around this MAP. The frequency is measured in hertz (Hz) and is usually set at 5–10 Hz. 1 Hz equals 60 breaths/minute. An amplitude is also set which describes the changes in pressure occurring around the MAP and is equal to the tidal volume in conventional ventilation. As amplitude is increased, the chest wall is seen to wobble/bounce. The amplitude is relatively small, hence the need for a

continued

Table 19.5 *continued*	
	high frequency to achieve adequate gaseous exchange. HFOV generates movement of gas to the alveoli by diffusion rather than the mass flow of conventional ventilation. HFOV is used in children requiring high ventilator pressures with the aim of recruiting alveoli, improving *V/Q* matching and minimizing barotraumas by avoiding the large cyclical distension that occurs with conventional ventilation
Physiotherapy considerations	When a child is receiving HFOV, auscultation is difficult but can still be useful for identifying gross changes. Disconnecting the child from HFOV for physiotherapy may cause alveolar collapse through loss of recruitment. The detrimental effect may outweigh the benefits of secretion clearance unless secretion retention is a major problem. Children should only be removed from HFOV for manual inflation/hyperinflation if they are stable and if assessment and discussion with medical teams have identified an absolute need. Some de-recruitment may be avoided by increasing the MAP and *Fi*O_2 pre- and post-physiotherapy. Closed suction circuits should be used for routine secretion clearance to reduce the risk of de-recruitment

Table 19.6 Non-invasive ventilation	
Continuous positive airways pressure (CPAP)	CPAP can be used as a form of non-invasive ventilation via a face mask, nasal mask or nasal cannulae. See Table 19.5 for a full description of CPAP
Bi-level positive airways pressure (BiPAP)	BiPAP can be delivered through a face or nasal mask. It is a pressure-cycled form of non-invasive ventilation. An inspiratory positive airway pressure (IPAP) and an expiratory positive airway pressure (EPAP) are set. Non-invasive BiPAP is indicated in type 2 respiratory failure and often in children requiring nocturnal ventilatory support for hypoventilation, e.g. children with Duchenne muscular dystrophy. Within the PICU/PHDU setting it may be used following extubation for children requiring short-term additional ventilatory support, e.g. a child with kyphoscoliosis secondary to cerebral palsy
Negative-pressure ventilation	RTX Medivent ventilator uses a cuirass jacket placed over the chest wall. It has three different settings, providing three different types of ventilation: 1. Continuous negative extrathoracic pressure (CNEP): a continuous negative end-expiratory pressure (NEEP) is applied to a spontaneously breathing child throughout the whole respiratory cycle to splint the airways open and improve ventilation and oxygenation. This form of ventilation reduces the work of breathing and opens up areas of atelectasis 2. Respiratory synchronized mode: a negative inspiratory pressure and a positive expiratory pressure are set and the ventilator synchronizes with the child's own respiratory rate. A back-up rate may be set in case a breath is not triggered. This mode may be used by children with neuromuscular disorders who require nocturnal ventilatory support because of hypoventilation 3. Secretion clearance mode: this mode produces a prolonged cycle of continuous vibrations followed by a cycle of increased negative, then positive, pressure which simulates a cough. The period of time for the vibration phase is set at twice as long as the coughing phase (i.e. 2 minutes vibration followed by 1 minute coughing). This mode may be used for children with muscle weakness who have secretion retention and an ineffective cough
Physiotherapy considerations	The cuirass jacket must be removed for auscultation and chest physiotherapy techniques. If the child is not able to tolerate this, then the secretion clearance mode can be a useful alternative in order to prevent secretion retention. Nursing staff can use this mode overnight to maintain adequate secretion clearance and prevent the need for physiotherapy call-outs. When using the secretion clearance mode, nasopharyngeal or oropharyngeal suction is used during the cough phase. If the cuirass jacket is removed for treatment, an increase in *Fi*O_2 or temporary use of non-invasive CPAP or BiPAP may be considered to maintain adequate observations and gaseous exchange
PICU, paediatric intensive care unit; PHDU, paediatric high-dependency unit.	

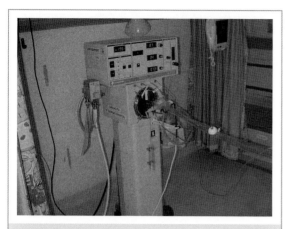

Figure 19.14 High-frequency oscillator.

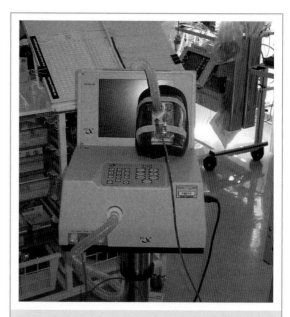

Figure 19.15 Medivent. Non-invasive, negative-pressure ventilator.

converting turbulent flow to laminar flow due to its viscosity; oxygen is delivered effectively with reduced respiratory effort. The effect lasts for as long as the gas is administered. It can be given via a facemask or through CPAP.

Several randomized controlled trials are currently underway, looking, for example, at the effects of heliox in bronchiolitis (BREATHE trial, St Mary's Hospital, London 2005–2006).

Nitric oxide

Nitric oxide can be entrained into the ventilator circuit; a normal dose is 2–5 parts per million (ppm), but can be as much as 80 ppm. Nitric oxide's main action is that of pulmonary vasodilation; it only vasodilates the alveoli that are perfused, improving ventilation/perfusion. It also acts as a bronchodilator, reducing albumin leakage into the alveolar spaces after lung injury, inhibits the aggregation of platelets and leukocytes and assists cytokine-activated macrophages in the destruction of tumour cells, fungi, bacteria and viruses. It is a neurotransmitter in both the peripheral and central nervous systems.

Nitric oxide works by rapidly diffusing across the muscle wall and combining with haemoglobin to form methylhaemoglobin. This is equivalent to reducing haemoglobin and so levels must be kept to a minimum: a safe level is below 1%.

Nitric oxide also combines with oxygen to make nitric dioxide and the levels are measured during administration. A safe level is said to be less than 5 ppm. Metabolites of nitric oxide are cleared from the body in 5–8 hours by the kidneys. It is used as a pulmonary vasodilator in the treatment of pulmonary hypertension and also pre and post cardiac surgery. It is particularly useful after open cardiac surgery when the normal

mechanisms of nitric oxide production are disrupted due to the damage to the endothelium which occurs during cardiopulmonary bypass. The full long-term effects of nitric oxide are unknown; it is therefore used with care. There are physiotherapy implications when treating children receiving nitric oxide: it must be entrained into a manual inflation/hyperinflation circuit because the effects wear off very quickly. It is important not to blow the nitric oxide into the face during manual inflation/hyperinflation and to ensure that nitric oxide attached to the bagging circuit is turned off immediately after use.

Emergency respiratory care

The provision of an 'out-of hours' emergency respiratory physiotherapy service requires well-defined criteria to ensure appropriate use and funding. Expert nursing care will implement appropriate positioning and suction into care plans; there will be some overlap of nursing and physiotherapy roles which may effectively manage respiratory care during the evening and night. Although it is not the role of the physiotherapist to supply an out-of hours service in order to provide simple secretion clearance, clinical assessment may be the only way to establish whether or not a treatment session is required (Table 19.7; Appendix 19.2).

Table 19.7 On-call criteria

Indication	Acute lobar collapse associated with drop in oxygen saturations (SaO$_2$) and/or sputum retention
	Sputum retention (i.e. unable to clear secretions effectively with positioning, bagging, saline, suction or coughing)
	Acute aspiration
	Any child whose condition will significantly deteriorate if not treated by a physiotherapist before the start of the next working day
No indication	Pulmonary oedema/pleural effusion
	Non-productive pneumonia
	Acute bronchiolitis (unless associated with focal changes on chest X-ray and/or sputum retention, Appendix 19.1)
	Inhaled foreign body (unless postbronchoscopy/removal of foreign body)
Prearranged treatments	The senior physiotherapist covering acute paediatrics during the day will arrange for a child to have evening/night treatment if it is clinically indicated. This will be discussed with the nursing and medical staff involved and documented in the shared-care records
Weekend treatments	The on-call physiotherapist working the weekend will treat any child who requires ongoing chest physiotherapy for an acute respiratory problem. Any new admissions with acute respiratory problems that require physiotherapy intervention must be referred to the weekend physiotherapist in accordance with the referral guidelines

CONCLUSION

The PICU environment is psychologically and emotionally draining. Staff can become highly involved with families and carers of children, particularly if the stay is lengthy. The balance of professionalism and empathy is at its most tested in this environment; senior physiotherapists soon learn to find and adopt their own strategies and support systems but need to be observant on behalf of their junior staff who may be confronting emergency situations and death for the first time. This particularly applies when a physiotherapy emergency duty rota utilizes staff from other service areas. Most units will debrief after a traumatic event and physiotherapists should take advantage of the opportunity to be included. This participation will allow staff to gain insight from the experiences of other team members. Conversely the environment and procedures undertaken in an intensive care unit will have a major impact on families and carers. A team-centred approach in a highly technological environment can be perceived as dehumanizing the situation and excluding the non-professional. For example, parents report being upset that eyes, mouth, nose and endotracheal tubes are not kept scrupulously clean while staff are observing a minimal handling regime for an extremely unstable child.

Parents are understandably hypersensitive about unrelated conversations taking place between staff members at the bedside. All staff must be vigilant with regard to their manner and behaviour in what is, to them, a familiar and comfortable environment. Senior staff should not underestimate their status as a role model. A high level of communication skills is vital: explanations should accompany all procedures. Factual information and discussion around alternative courses of action will empower carers to share in decision-making and accept outcomes. Many procedures undertaken in the critical care environment are performed 'in the child's best interests' (Children Act 1989). There will usually be the opportunity to explain and discuss physiotherapy interventions with parents/carers, enabling informed consent to be documented. Documentation of subjective and objective findings in the physiotherapy notes will give a clear indication of when physiotherapy was undertaken as an unplanned intervention, for example, emergency on-call. The acute setting is a very rewarding place to work; physiotherapists can take advantage of this environment to research, evaluate and share their practice alongside medical and nursing colleagues. There are many opportunities to learn, extend and teach new skills and contribute to the body of evidence for the physiotherapy role in intensive care.

Acknowledgement

We acknowledge the contribution of past and current staff of St Mary's Hospital Paediatric Physiotherapy Department.

CASE STUDY 19.1

MR was a 16-month-old girl who was admitted to hospital with meningococcal septicaemia and cardiogenic shock. She had been unwell for 24 hours with reduced appetite, diarrhoea, vomiting and fever. She had been taken to Accident & Emergency (A&E) and discharged, but presented a few hours later with a non-blanching rash, tachypnoea, tachycardia and a fluctuating Glasgow Coma Scale of 10–12/15. In A&E, she was given fluid resuscitation of 110 ml/kg, was electively intubated and ventilated and started on medications to support the cardiovascular system in the form of inotropes, then transferred to PICU. Her initial blood gases were recorded as pH 7.25, P_{CO_2} 3.9, HCO_3 13.4 and base excess −14 mmol/l.

MR's birth history had been uneventful. She was a twin pregnancy, born by spontaneous vaginal delivery at 37/40 weeks and twin number 2. There were no postnatal problems and no significant past medical history. Her immunizations were up to date. MR lived with her parents, twin sister and two other siblings within a very supportive family. There were no concerns regarding her development prior to admission; she was walking independently and although smaller than her twin, was said to be more sociable.

MR was intubated for 22 days and over this period was ventilated using bi-level intermittent positive airway pressure, high-frequency oscillatory ventilation and negative-pressure non-invasive ventilation. Throughout her admission she had many medical and psychosocial issues which affected her physiotherapy management. These included:

- Cardiorespiratory arrest – 1-minute cardiopulmonary resuscitation
- Low platelets (down to 22 with active bleeding from nose and mouth)
- Capillary leak syndrome/fluctuating whole-body oedema
- Pulmonary oedema
- Right pleural effusion
- Hypoxic–ischaemic myocardial damage with poor cardiac function
- Cardiovascular instability with large inotropic support requirement
- Enlarged kidneys and hyperechoiec on ultrasound
- Reduced range of movement bilaterally in upper & lower limbs
- Poor skin integrity – weepy, sloughy, fragile and blistering
- Necrosis developed bilaterally above knee and below elbow
- At risk of infection from necrosis
- Pain post extubation

- Withdrawal from opiates post extubation
- Normal neurological assessment
- Ischaemic four limbs, with decision made for conservative management and ongoing vascular and orthopaedic input to monitor blood flow and pulses
- Contractures of all necrotic fingers
- Indecision regarding level of amputation
- Reduced sitting balance
- Transferred to local hospital for amputations and further rehabilitation
- Psychosocial issues: parental relief at survival followed by grief at loss of limbs and disability
- MR's frustration, reduced motivation, fear of uniform and hospital environment.

Physiotherapy Management

For the 24 hours immediately after admission to PICU, MR's cardiovascular instability meant that physiotherapy assessment and treatment were contraindicated. Once stable, initial physiotherapy goals were to maintain adequate secretion clearance and optimize her ventilation and oxygenation while she was intubated and ventilated. Assessment and clinical reasoning indicated that manual hyperinflation, manual techniques, positioning, saline, suction and the use of bronchodilators were required. There was careful consideration of the type of ventilation she was receiving prior to each physiotherapy session, her platelet counts were noted and indications for physiotherapy were considered and discussed with her medical team. Ventilation was modified pre- and post-physiotherapy to help optimize her condition. Initial physiotherapy goals also included passive stretches, positioning and splinting of all her limbs. This was included in her care plan in liaison with the nursing staff, occupational therapists and the family; this management plan required a 24-hour approach in order for it to be effective.

A possible progression of the disease process of meningococcal septicaemia is ischaemic changes: MR's skin integrity declined within a few days, becoming fragile, sloughy and weepy, with blisters forming. This made it increasingly difficult to splint and stretch the limbs and multidisciplinary team working was essential, incorporating close liaison with the vascular and orthopaedic teams with regard to the likelihood of elective amputations, where the level of amputations was likely to be and therefore which joints needed to be splinted and stretched to maintain joint range of movement. At this time, many psychosocial issues emerged. The family's initial relief at MR's survival became both grief, over the likely loss of her limbs, and also fear and despair for what the future would hold for her and the family as a whole. These factors were

continued

always taken into consideration throughout treatment sessions and when therapy goals and management were discussed with the family.

When MR was extubated from mechanical ventilation (22 days after admission), she was placed on to non-invasive negative-pressure ventilation. Physiotherapy management continued to focus on respiratory care and adequate secretion clearance and ventilation. By this stage a decision had been made that bilateral above-knee amputations and bilateral forearm amputations would be required. This rendered lower-limb and lower-arm splinting unnecessary, but appropriate positioning of hips essential, to ensure that tightness in the iliotibial band did not occur (which would have hindered her future ability to stand).

Her parents were taught to position MR appropriately and a positioning chart was placed above her bed for nursing staff and family to use. MR was self-ventilating on room air after a couple of days and transferred to the ward. Physiotherapy assessment and intervention on the ward were initially very difficult; MR had developed a fear of uniform and of the hospital environment and was not motivated to play or interact; the physiotherapists decided not to wear uniform and began all contacts with informal play and talk. In this way her confidence was gained that those interventions would not be painful or upsetting. She was typically weak after a lengthy stay on PICU, unable to roll independently and did not have independent sitting balance. Physiotherapy sessions took place each day away from the ward in the paediatric physiotherapy department. In this environment gross motor activities could be facilitated through play; rolling and the use of the activity play ring to facilitate sitting balance. The change of environment was also very beneficial to MR psychologically and it was at this time that she became much more motivated and interactive with toys and people; she began smiling and laughing and occasionally babbled. Six weeks after admission, MR was transferred to her local hospital; she had full head control, was bringing her hands together and grasping objects using both hands, she was able to maintain

side-lying, roll left and right and had momentary independent sitting balance (Figure 19.16).

The planned amputations took place at her local hospital. Eight months later her family reported that she was progressing well with her prosthetic limbs, using her prosthetic hands functionally and was able to sit and stand independently.

Although MR did not stay in the acute setting for her rehabilitation, it was essential for her family that the multidisciplinary team were able to consider and predict the long-term issues. These included a lengthy rehabilitation process relearning her gross and fine motor skills and adjusting to a future which will include regular limb-fitting sessions as she grows. There will be financial implications for her family, long-term social and education issues and obviously psychological implications post amputation, with both grief and anger at the loss of the limbs.

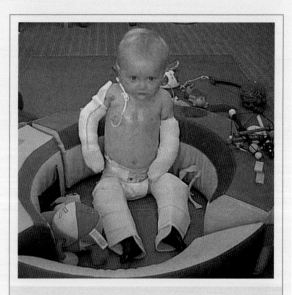

Figure 19.16 Early rehabilitation for MR.

REFERENCES

Almeida-Celize CB, Ribeiro-Jose D, Almeida-Junior-Armando A, Zeferino-Angelica MB 2005 Effect of expiratory flow techniques on pulmonary function of infants on mechanical ventilation. *Physiotherapy International* 10: 213–221.

American Association of Respiratory Care 1991 Clinical practice guidelines on postural drainage. *Respiratory Care* 36: 1418–1426.

Argent A, Morrow B 2004 What does chest physiotherapy do to sick infants and children? *Intensive Care Medicine* 30: 1014–1016.

Barker M, Eales CJ 2000 The effects of manual hyperinflation using self inflating manual resus bags on arterial oxygen tensions and lung compliance: a meta analysis of literature. *South African Journal of Physiotherapy* 56: 7–16.

Bellet PS, Kalinyak KA, Shukla R, Gelfand MJ, Rucknagel DL 1995 Incentive spirometry to prevent acute pulmonary complications in sickle cell diseases. *New England Journal of Medicine* 333: 699–703.

Bennion K 2004 American Association of Respiratory Care clinical practice guideline: nasotracheal suctioning. *Respiratory Care* 49: 1080–1084.

Bernard-Narbonne F, Daoud P, Castaing H, Rousset A 2003 Effectiveness of chest physiotherapy in ventilated children with acute bronchiolitis. *Archives de Pédiatrie* 10: 1043–1047.

Berney S, Denehy L, Pretto J 2004 Head down tilt and manual hyperinflation enhance sputum clearance in patients who are intubated and ventilated. *Australian Journal of Physiotherapy* 50: 9–14.

Blackwood B 1999 Normal saline instillation with endotracheal suctioning: primum non nocere (first do no harm). *Journal of Advanced Nursing* 29: 928–934.

Brooks D, Thomas J 1995 Interrater reliability of auscultation of breath sounds among physical therapists. *Physical Therapy* 75: 1082–1088.

Cereda M, Villa F, Colombo E, Greco G, Nacoti M, Pesenti A 2001 Closed system endotracheal suctioning maintains lung volume during volume-controlled mechanical ventilation. *Intensive Care Medicine* 27: 648–654.

Chalumeau M, Foix I, Helias L et al 2002 Rib fractures after chest physiotherapy for bronchiolitis or pneumonia in infants. *Paediatric Radiology* 32: 644–647.

Children Act 1989 Available online at: http://www.doh.gov.uk.

Choong K, Chatrkaw P, Fmdova H, Cox-PN 2003 Comparison of loss in lung volume with open versus in-line catheter endotracheal suctioning. *Pediatric Critical Care Medicine* 4: 69–73.

Clark AP, Winslow EH, Tyler DO, White KM 1990 Effects of endotracheal suctioning on mixed venous oxygen saturation and heart rate in critically ill adults. *Heart and Lung* 19: 552–557.

Clarke RC, Kelly BE, Convery PN, Fee JP 1999 Ventilatory characteristics in mechanically ventilated patients during manual hyperinflation for chest physiotherapy. *Anaesthesia* 54: 936–940.

Czarnik RE, Stone KS, Everhart CJ, Presseur BA 1991 Differential effects of continuous versus intermittent suction on tracheal tissue. *Heart and Lung* 20: 144–151,

Davies H, Litchman R, Gordon I, Helms P 1985 Regional ventilation in infancy. *New England Journal of Medicine* 313: 1626–1628.

Denehy L 1999 The use of manual hyperinflation in airway clearance. *European Respiratory Journal* 14: 958–965.

Fanaroff AA, Martin RJ (eds) 1992 *Neonatal-Perinatal Medicine*, 5th edn, vol. 2. St Louis, MO: Mosby, pp. 810–819.

Fink J 2001 Positioning versus postural drainage. *Respiratory Care* 47: 769–777.

Fox WW, Schwartz JG, Shaffer TH 1978 Pulmonary physiotherapy in neonates: physiological changes and respiratory management. *Journal of Paediatrics* 92: 977–981.

Garcia-Aparicio L, Castanon M, Tarrado X, Rodriguez L, Iriondo M, Morales L 2002 Bronchial complication of a closed tube endotracheal suction catheter. *Journal of Paediatric Surgery* 37: 1483–1484.

Harding JE, Becroft DMA, Allen BC, Knight DB 1998 Chest physiotherapy may be associated with brain damage in extremely premature infants. *Journal of Paediatrics* 132: 440–444.

Heaf D, Helms P, Gordon I, Turner H 1983 Postural effects on gas exchange in infants. *New England Journal of Medicine* 308: 1505–1508.

Hough A 1991 *Physiotherapy in Respiratory Care: A Problem-Solving Approach*. London: Chapman & Hall.

Hsu LL, Batts BK, Rau JL 2005 Positive expiratory device acceptance by hospitalized children with sickle cell disease is comparable to incentive spirometry. *Respiratory Care* 50: 624–627.

Imle PC 1989 Percussion and vibrations. In: Mackenzie CF, Imle PC, Ciesla N (eds) *Chest Physiotherapy in the Intensive Care Unit,* 2nd edn. Baltimore, MD: Williams & Wilkins, pp. 134–152.

Jaw MC, Soong WJ, Chen SJ, Hwang B 1991 Pneumothorax: a complication of deep endotracheal suction. Report of three cases. *Chinese Medical Journal* 48: 313–317.

Kerem E, Yatsiv I, Goitein KJ 1990 Effects of endotracheal suctioning on arterial blood gases in children. *Intensive Care Medicine* 16: 95–99.

Krause MF, Hoehn T 2000 Chest physiotherapy in mechanically ventilated children: a review. *Critical Care Medicine* 28: 1648–1651.

Main E, Castle R, Newham D, Stocks J 2004 Respiratory physiotherapy versus suction: the effects on respiratory function in ventilated infants and children. *Intensive Care Medicine* 30: 1144–1151.

McCarren B, Alison J, Lansbury G 2003 The use of vibration in public hospitals in Australia. *Physiotherapy Theory and Practice* 19: 87–98.

Morrow B, Argent A 2002 Risks and complications of non-bronchoscopic bronchoalveolar lavage in the paediatric intensive care unit. *Paediatric Pulmonology* 34: 87–88.

Morrow B, Futter M, Argent A 2004 Endotracheal suctioning: from principles to practice. *Intensive Care Medicine* 30: 1167–1174.

Morrow BM, Futter MJ, Argent AC (2006) Paediatric nonbronchoscopic bronchoalveolar lavage: overview and recommendations for clinical practice. *South African Journal of Physiotherapy* 62: 28–33.

Newhouse MT, Rossman CM 1984 Effects of chest physiotherapy on the removal of mucus in patients with cystic fibrosis. *American Review of Respiratory Disease* 127: 391.

Nicholas KJ, Dhouieb MO, Marshall TG, Edmunds AT, Grant MB 1999 An evaluation of chest physiotherapy in the management of acute bronchiolitis: changing clinical practice. *Physiotherapy* 85: 669–674.

Oberwaldner B 2000 Physiotherapy for airway clearance in paediatrics. *European Respiratory Journal* 15: 196–204.

Ong GL, Newell H, John Y, Ferguson K, Telfer P, Wilkey O 2005 Incentive spirometry for children with sickle cell disorder. *Nursing Times* 101: 55–57.

Perotta C, Ortiz Z, Roque M 2005 Chest physiotherapy for acute bronchiolitis in paediatric patients between 0 and 24 months old. *Cochrane Database of Systematic Reviews,* Issue 2.

Prasad SA, Hussey J 1995 *Paediatric Respiratory Care: A Guide for Physiotherapists and Health Professionals.* London: Chapman & Hall.

Prasad SA, Main E 2002 Paediatrics. In: Pryor JA, Prasad SA (eds) *Physiotherapy for Respiratory and Cardiac Problems: Adults and Paediatrics.* London: Churchill Livingstone.

Ridling DA, Martin LD, Bratton SL 2003 Endotracheal suctioning with or without instillation of isotonic sodium chloride solution in critically ill children. *American Journal of Critical Care* 12: 212–219.

Robertson NRC 1996 Intensive care. In: Greenhough A, Robertson NRC, Milner A (eds) *Neonatal Respiratory Disorders.* London: A Arnold, pp. 174–195.

Salzman SH 2002 Does splinting from thoracic bone ischaemia and infarction contribute to the acute chest syndrome in sickle cell disease? *Chest* 122: 6–9.

Schindler M 2005 Treatment of atelectasis: where is the evidence? *Critical Care* 9: 341–342.

Schwenker D, Ferrin M, Gift AG 1998 A survey of endotracheal suctioning with instillation of normal saline. *American Journal of Critical Care* 7: 255–260.

Shah AR, Kurth CD, Gwiazdowski SG, Chance B, Delivoria-Paladopoulous M 1992 Fluctuations in cerebral oxygenation and blood volume during endotracheal suctioning in premature infants. *Journal of Paediatrics* 120: 769–774.

Shah S, Fung K, Brim S, Rubin BK 2005 An in vitro evaluation of the effectiveness of endotracheal suction catheters. *Chest* 128: 3699–3704.

Singer M, Vermaat J, Hall G, Latter G, Patel M 1994 Haemodynamic effects of manual inflation in critically ill mechanically ventilated patients. *Chest* 106: 1182–1187.

Stone KS, Turner B 1989 Endotracheal suctioning. *Annual Review of Nursing Research* 7: 27–49.

Swartz K, Noonan DM, Edwards BJ 1996 A national survey of endotracheal suctioning techniques in the pediatric population. *Heart Lung* 25: 52–60.

Tan AM, Gomez JM, Paratz J, Matthews J, Williams M, Rajadbrai VS 2005 Closed versus partially ventilated endotracheal suction in extremely preterm neonates: physiologic consequences. *Journal of Intensive Care Nursing* 21: 234–242.

Thakur A, Buchmiller T, Atkinson J 2000 Bronchial perforation after closed tube endotracheal suction. *Journal of Paediatric Surgery* 35: 1353–1355.

Thoresen M, Cavan F, Whitelaw A 1988 Effect of tilting on oxygenation in newborn infants. *Archives of Disease in Childhood* 63: 315–317.

Webb MS, Martin JA, Cartlidge PH, Ng YK, Wright NA 1985 Chest physiotherapy in acute bronchiolitis. *Archives of Diseases in Childhood* 6011: 1078–1079.

Wells DA, Gillies D, Fitzgerald DA 2005 Positioning for acute respiratory distress in hospitalized infants and children. *The Cochrane Database of Systematic Reviews* Issue 1 article no.: CD003645. DOI: 10.1002/14651858.CD003645.pub2.

Wood CJ 1998 Endotracheal suctioning: a literature review. *Intensive Critical Care Nursing* 14: 124–136.

Yale SH, Nagib N, Guthrie T 2000 Acute chest syndrome in sickle cell disease. Crucial considerations in adolescents and adults. *Postgraduate Medicine* 107: 215–218, 221–222.

Young CS 1984a Recommended guidelines for suction. *Physiotherapy* 70: 106–108.

Young CS 1984b A review of the adverse effects of airway suction. *Physiotherapy* 70: 104–106.

Young CS 1988 Airway suctioning: a study of paediatric physiotherapy practice. *Physiotherapy* 74: 13–15.

Zausmer E 1968 Bronchial drainage, evidence supporting the procedures. *Physical Therapy* 48: 586–591.

Zhang LP, Zhang ZX 1997 Study of postural drainage of children with obstructive lung disease. *Chinese Medical Journal* 32: 559–561.

FURTHER READING

Campbell S (ed.) 1995 *Physical Therapy for Children.* Philadelphia, PA: WB Saunders, pp. 63–736.

Eckersley P (ed.) 1993 *Elements of Paediatric Physiotherapy.* Edinburgh: Churchill Livingstone, pp. 97–114, 357–360.

Pryor J, Prasad S (eds) 2002 *Physiotherapy for Respiratory and Cardiac Problems,* 3rd edn. Edinburgh: Churchill Livingstone.

Rogers M, Helfaer M (eds) 1999 *Handbook of Paediatric Intensive Care,* 3rd edn. Philadelphia, PA: Lippincott/Williams & Wilkins.

Schelvan C, Copeman A, Young J, Davis J (eds) 2002 *Paediatric Radiology.* London: Royal Society of Medicine Press.

Simonds A 2001 *Non-Invasive Respiratory Support: A Practical Handbook,* 2nd edn. London: A Arnold.

APPENDIX 19.1 GUIDELINE FOR THE PHYSIOTHERAPY MANAGEMENT OF CHILDREN WITH BRONCHIOLITIS

There is no indication for physiotherapy in a non-intubated child with bronchiolitis alone (Webb et al 1985, Nicholas et al 1999, Perotta et al 2005). However, where secondary pneumonia or lobar collapse occurs, physiotherapy assessment and treatment may be indicated by the presence of retained secretions.

There is some evidence to support the efficacy of chest physiotherapy in the intubated child with bronchiolitis (Bernard-Narbonne et al 2003). In the intubated and ventilated child physiotherapy treatment may be indicated by focal changes on chest X-ray, secretion retention or deteriorating arterial blood gases. Infants with bronchiolitis often have poor tolerance of handling and manual techniques. Adequate sedation and bronchodilators prior to treatment may assist physiotherapy management. Where treatment is detrimental to the infant, positioning to maximize ventilation and perfusion and minimal handling may be recommended by the physiotherapist.

APPENDIX 19.2 EXAMPLE OF ON-CALL GUIDELINE

Emergency physiotherapy is for children with respiratory problems whose condition will deteriorate if not seen until the following day.

Physiotherapists will leave instructions with the nursing staff at the end of the working day if a child will benefit from a specific intervention overnight, e.g. positioning, bagging or suction.

The on-call physiotherapist receives a detailed handover of all children with respiratory problems each evening from the senior paediatric physiotherapist on the paediatric intensive care unit (PICU).

A paediatrician who has personally assessed the child should make the referral. The only exception is within PICU where a senior member of nursing staff may call the physiotherapist.

The physiotherapist will ask for relevant information over the phone in order to establish the reason for referral and to ensure that any further interventions (e.g. chest X-ray, nebulizers, analgesia) which may be needed are given prior to assessment.

The physiotherapist will give an indication of when he/she expects to see a child. This will be within 45 minutes of telephone contact.

Following assessment and/or treatment the physiotherapist will liaise with nursing staff and referring doctor with regard to ongoing management, including documentation in the shared care records.

APPENDIX 19.3 PROFORMA FOR DOCUMENTATION

ST MARYS NHS TRUST — PICU PHYSIOTHERAPY DOCUMENTATION PROFORMA

Name: _____ Hospital No: _____ Date: _____ Time: _____

S:

O: CVS: HR: Rhythm: BP (I/IN):   Temp:

RENAL: Urine Output: Fluid Balance: Prev. Day Balance:

BLOODS: Platelets   Neuroprotected: Y / N   Comments:
        Hb:

**BLOOD
GASES:** Time: Art/Cap/Vein: pH: PCO_2: PO_2:   SBC: Beb:

ANALYSIS:

MEDS: Sedation/Analgesia: | **CXR ANALYSIS:**   DATE: TIME:
Paralytics:
Inotropes:
Diuretics:
Others:

INVASIVE VENTILATION: _
ETT/Tracheostomy (Delete as appropriate) Size: Depth at Lips/nose: cm   Cuffed/Uncuffed

---

BIPAP/CPAP ASB: _	**HFOV:** _	**INHALED NITRIC OXIDE:** _
PIP: FiO_2:	MAP: SaO_2:	Nitric Oxide (ppm):
		Nitric Dioxide (ppm):
PEEP: SaO_2:	DP: FiO_2:	**NEGATIVE PRESSURE NON-INVASIVE**
ASB: $ETCO_2$:	Hz:	**VENTILATION:** _
		CNEP/RESP SYNCHRONISED (delete):
RATE: TV:		Negative pressures:

NON INVASIVE VENT: _ | **SELF VENTILATING:** _
CPAP (facial/nasal)/BIPAP: _   IPAP: | Face mask/Nasal specs
Flow (O_2/L):   EPAP/PEEP: | Flow (O_2/L): SPO_2:
FiO_2: SpO_2: | RR:

AUSCULTATION/PALPITATION: | **CLINICAL REASONING:**

RX:

A:

P:

Signature   Name: Grade   Page No

Figure A19.1 Proforma for documentation.

Oncology and palliative care

20 Cancer in the child and young person

Victoria Mitchinson and Jan Davies

Although cancer in children and young people is relatively rare, it still remains one of the most common causes of death of this age group and is certainly one of the most feared diagnosis of parents and carers. In the UK there are approximately 134 new cases per million (0–14 years) and 214 new cases per million (15–24 years) annually (National Institute for Clinical Excellence 2005). The overall survival rate is high (currently 75% in the 0–14-year age group) but the disease-specific survival rates do vary (National Institute for Clinical Excellence 2005). The overall incidence of child and adolescent cancers has risen in the last 15 years; this apparent increase may be due to more sensitive diagnostic tools enabling easier identification (Gibson & Evans 1999).

The physiotherapist can play a vital role in the overall management of the child and young person with cancer. A child's parents and family are often devastated by the diagnosis and are naturally initially very protective of their child. It is vitally important to engage the family in a positive way so that they regard therapy as a helpful means of minimizing the effects not only of the disease but also of the side-effects of treatment. Parents spend prolonged periods of time with their children on the ward, and are often keen to be involved in therapy sessions or to supervise exercise programmes, particularly if they see this as a positive activity. Physiotherapy can include management and control of symptoms, prevention of secondary complications (e.g. respiratory infection), restoration and return to function following treatment (chemotherapy, surgery, radiotherapy), promotion of normal developmental progression in a younger child, minimizing neurological sequelae following central nervous system (CNS) treatments and emotional and psychological support to the child or young person and parents or carers.

The purpose of this chapter is to give an introduction to the incidence and management of cancer in children and young people. More specifically we will look at the impact of these treatments on a child or young person and the role the physiotherapist can play in the treatment process rather than give details of treatment regimes for individual cancers. Details of some common conditions requiring physiotherapy input will be given. Current research into physiotherapy with children and young people is very limited and therefore information is based on some research, best practice and clinical experience.

WHAT IS CANCER?

In its simplest form cancer is a disease affecting the cells of the body. These cancerous cells divide and reproduce without proper order or control and produce either a lump (a tumour) or too many white blood cells (leukaemia). Metastases occur when the cancerous cells break away and travel to other parts of the body via the blood stream.

In the UK when a child is diagnosed with cancer, care is offered in one of the 17 UK Children's Cancer Study Group (UK CCSG 1999)-registered centres. There are also eight Teenage Cancer Trust (TCT) units across the country that offer separate age-appropriate facilities and care for young people aged approximately 13–22 years. More TCT units are planned throughout the UK. The overall management of the child or young person with cancer is through a complex multidisciplinary team approach, the physiotherapist being part of that team, with the child or young person central to the team. Figure 20.1 illustrates the multidisciplinary team.

The medical management of a cancer is specific to the diagnosis and age of the child. There are three key modalities that are employed to treat cancer: radiotherapy, chemotherapy and surgery. Bone marrow transplantation (BMT) is commonly being added to this list. These modalities are not used in isolation and equally are not

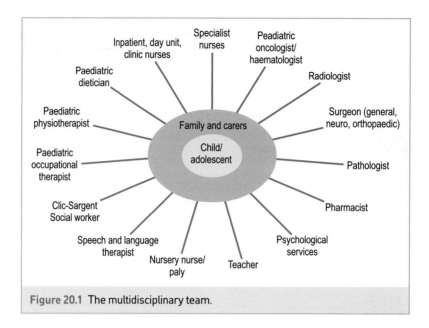

Figure 20.1 The multidisciplinary team.

always used with every diagnosis. This chapter will discuss the principles of these modalities and give details of their side-effects and how these can impact on the physiotherapy management. The general side-effects of surgery will not be discussed.

CHEMOTHERAPY

Chemotherapy refers to the use of cytotoxic agents to destroy cancer cells by stopping them from growing or multiplying at one or more points in their life cycle. These agents are most effective during the proliferation phase, i.e. when the cell is actively involved in reproduction (Gibson & Evans 1999). Chemotherapy drugs are classified according to the chemical within the drug; there are six major classifications. Along with minimal disruption to normal cell activities the main aims of chemotherapy are:

- Cure the cancer
- Prevent the cancer from spreading
- Kill metastases
- Relieve symptoms
- Slow the cancer growth.

Chemotherapy can be given via three routes: orally, intravenously (via a portacath or central venous catheter (CVC)/Hickman line) or intrathecally. Following insertion of a portacath but more commonly a CVC, many children present with neck and shoulder pain and stiffness, marked positional torticollis and poor posture. These symptoms are temporary but often need input from the physiotherapist for reassurance, positioning advice and exercises to improve range of movement. Younger

children often improve with distraction and involvement of the nursery nurse/play specialist may be required. Generally these symptoms will improve within a few days once the child/young person has adjusted to the CVC and returns to normal daily activities. The posture of these children should be monitored throughout their treatment to prevent future lumbar and thoracic problems.

Anticancer drugs affect cells which have a rapid mitotic rate. They are effective against malignant cells, but as they are not specific, they affect other 'normal' cells, such as haemopoietic cells of the bone marrow, the entire gastrointestinal mucosa and hair follicles, amongst others. Certain chemotherapy agents cause peripheral and central neurotoxicity and proximal myopathy. Other general side-effects, such as anorexia, nausea, vomiting and fatigue, may have multifactorial causes.

The short- and medium-term side-effects of chemotherapy can greatly affect the timing and extent of physiotherapy treatment that the child is able to tolerate and therapy sessions and goals are often reset to accommodate this. All of these side-effects combine to make physiotherapy treatment challenging, for both the child and the physiotherapist. It is important to be flexible and creative in managing these children, particularly in the younger age groups where formal exercise is not always appropriate. Developmentally appropriate activities targeting certain functional tasks are often successful. A multidisciplinary team approach (occupational therapists, teachers, play workers and nursery nurses) is invaluable.

Some of the general and specific side-effects and their causes, which can adversely affect physiotherapy treatment programmes, are discussed below and summarized in Figure 20.2 and Box 20.1.

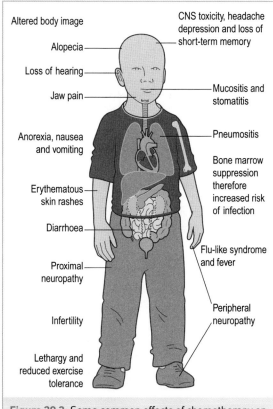

Altered body image

Alopecia

Loss of hearing

Jaw pain

Anorexia, nausea
and vomiting

Erythematous
skin rashes

Diarrhoea

Proximal
neuropathy

Infertility

Lethargy and
reduced exercise
tolerance

CNS toxicity, headache
depression and loss of
short-term memory

Mucositis and
stomatitis

Pneumositis

Bone marrow
suppression
therefore
increased risk
of infection

Flu-like syndrome
and fever

Peripheral
neuropathy

Figure 20.2 Some common effects of chemotherapy on the child and young adult. CNS, central nervous system.

Short-term side-effects

Anorexia, nausea and vomiting

These are all closely interlinked. Mucositis of the mouth and gastrointestinal tract can be very painful; as a result children find eating and drinking extremely difficult and may also suffer from stomach cramps and loose stools. Some chemotherapy agents cause vomiting through their direct effect on the vomiting centre found in the medulla oblongata. The vomiting centre is a convergence of numerous neuronal pathways which initiate the vomiting reflex. Stimulation of the vomiting centre can be caused by cytotoxic agents in the blood stream. Raised intracranial pressure (ICP), anxiety and pain also adversely affect the vomiting centre. Weight loss, muscle wasting, depression and low energy levels make physiotherapy activities difficult.

Short frequent treatment sessions and activities, with rewards for goals achieved, can often help overcome some of the problems.

Myelosuppression

One of the major side-effects of chemotherapy is myelosuppression, the reduction in production of red and white blood cells and platelets by the bone marrow, and this has a major effect on the delivery of physiotherapy. Anaemia may contribute to fatigue; low platelet levels may restrict physical activities due to the risk of bleeding. Low platelet levels (usually under $20 \times 10^9/l$) also limit the use of manual chest physiotherapy techniques to treat respiratory complications, as again there is an increased risk of bleeding. A reduced white cell count often heralds infections, which again affect a child's ability to start or continue with therapy programmes. Intravenous antibiotics and antifungal medication to treat the infections make physical activity more difficult as a child is often attached to intravenous drips for several days. A change in emphasis from active rehabilitation to monitoring respiratory function and bed exercises may have to be adopted during these debilitating episodes.

Neurotoxicity

The induction of peripheral neuropathy by chemotherapy agents is well recognized (Quasthoff & Hartung 2002). Depending on the drug, a pure painful sensory neuropathy or a mixed sensorimotor/autonomic neuropathy can occur. The effects depend on the total cumulative dose, although problems can sometimes emerge at the early stages of treatment. It is thought that the most challenging symptoms are seen in the youngest children (Harila-Saari et al 1998). Recovery depends on the ability of the peripheral nervous system to repair itself in the absence of the toxic substance and recovery can take a long time. Although effects are said to be reversible, in some cases recovery can be very slow and long-standing signs of motor disability have been documented (Harila-Saari et al 1998). It could be argued that if severe muscle wastage and tendo-achilles (TA) shortening have occurred then a full recovery is unlikely, unless the TA is lengthened. In some cases the neurotoxic effects of the drug can be enough to severely affect function and the dosage may be reduced.

In particular two drugs used in the treatment of cancer have neurotoxic effects.

Vincristine initially affects the sensory nerves of the hands and feet (typically in a stocking-glove distribution), pain and paraesthesia become apparent and tendon reflexes are diminished or absent. Vincristine is commonly used in the treatment of acute lymphoblastic leukaemia (ALL), Wilms tumours and some CNS tumours. As the toxicity progresses, peripheral muscle cramps occur; also motor weakness sufficient to affect hand function and gait become apparent. The help of the occupational therapist in providing functional advice, aids and activities is invaluable in this situation. Ankle splinting is often required as the child may develop a dropped foot and associated shortening of the TA if this is not addressed. Dynamic orthotics such as ankle–foot orthoses (AFO) enable an efficient gait pattern, and can prevent ankle inversion injury and falls (Gillis & Donovan 2001). Passive orthotics such as

---

Box 20.1 Summary of chemotherapy effects on physiotherapy

- Children have reduced exercise tolerance and fatigue quickly, therefore treatments need to be short and may need to be modified
- Check platelet count: if below $20 \times 10^9/l$, then omit use of manual chest techniques
- Monitor for signs of peripheral neuropathy and proximal myopathy and manage as indicated
- Monitor developmental progression in the younger child
- Insertion of a central venous catheter can induce neck pain and stiffness and affect posture: this will improve with gentle range of movement exercises and reassurance

---

Table 20.1 Signs of peripheral neuropathy

Hypersensitive feet or hands on examination	High stepping gait, wide based or foot slapping gait. Unable to heel walk
Reduced or loss of balance	Complaints of beuropathic pain, burning pains, tingling or pins and needles
Reduced fine and gross motor function	Jaw pain
Muscle wastage, particularly seen in the calf belly	Impaired short-term memory

---

below-knee night-resting splints support the joint and maintain TA length (Marchese et al 2004). Vincristine can also cause autonomic dysfunction, and symptoms such as constipation or paralytic ileus can occur.

Cisplatin and carboplatin are two closely related drugs that also have neurotoxic effects. Cisplatin tends to be more toxic than carboplatin. They affect sensory nerves more than motor nerves; the effects are paraesthesia of the hands and feet (typically stocking–glove distribution), loss of tendon reflexes, loss of vibration sense and joint proprioception and in severe cases can lead to ataxia. Massage and in some cases pressure stockings or bandages can help reduce hypersensitivity (Gillis & Donovan 2001).

Crucially, with these children side-effects can often go unnoticed until a child presents with severe mobility problems (Almadrones & Arcot 1999). The physiotherapist plays a vital role in the management and control of these symptoms and education of medical and nursing staff and parents of the signs of neurotoxicity so that interventions can be started early. Table 20.1 lists the signs of peripheral neuropathy that can be easily monitored by parents, children and medical and nursing staff. If these signs are noted a timely referral to the physiotherapist should be made.

Steroid-induced myopathy

Steroids are used in the treatment of some cancers, sometimes in high doses over relatively short periods, e.g. after surgery or radiotherapy (for CNS tumours) or more long-term use (leukaemia – for up to 3 years). In more prolonged use a pattern of muscle weakness evolves (Marchese et al 2004). The weakness tends to be proximal rather than distal and symmetrical rather than asymmetrical. The lower limbs tend to be more affected than the upper limbs. Functional problems such as stair-climbing and getting up from a chair or the floor become

apparent, and also the inability to walk moderate or short distances. There is some evidence that resisted exercise can reduce the effects of the myopathy, and a programme of strengthening and mobilizing activities can be provided, or incorporated into the patient's existing regime (Braith et al 1998).

RADIOTHERAPY

Radiotherapy is the use of high-energy X-rays to destroy cancer cells. It is normally used to treat one (local) area where the tumour was found. Radiotherapy is rarely the only treatment in children's cancers and is usually used in combination with chemotherapy or surgery (Pinkerton et al 1994). Although radiotherapy is no longer in use with some cancers (Wilms tumours, Hodgkin's disease) due to the advance of chemotherapy, it still plays a large role in the treatment of many other cancers, such as CNS tumours. Radiotherapy is carried out in specialist treatment centres. Planning and calculating the dose required and the method of administration is a complex and skilled process. Radiotherapy is normally given on weekdays for an extended period of approximately 6 weeks, although this can vary with individual children. Children are required to stay perfectly still and in the case of brain tumours masks are made of the head, which are then fixed to the radiotherapy table to ensure accuracy of the treatment. Great skill is required in getting young children to accept this restrictive method of treatment without the use of sedation or anaesthetic. Skilled nursing and play therapy staff are usually involved in this aspect of the planning process. It is a painless treatment.

The field of irradiation depends on the type of tumour, its site and the tendency to metastasize. Radiotherapy is a very effective treatment against cancer cells but it can cause some damage to healthy cells close to the area being treated. The immediate side-effects of radiation are usually very mild. The skin may become sore, as if it were sunburnt. As radiotherapy affects any normal tissue in its pathway there are some difficulties and therefore restrictions associated with its use. Some of these side-effects can impinge on physiotherapy treatment and management. Side-effects of radiotherapy depend upon the type, dose and frequency of the radiation, the area being treated, the child's maturation tolerance level and age (Pinkerton et al 1994).

Short- and medium-term side-effects

As radiotherapy affects the rapidly dividing cells, this is where most of the side-effects are seen. These include bone marrow suppression, skin reactions, alopecia, nausea, vomiting and lethargy (Pinkerton et al 1994). Loss of hair over the site of irradiation can occur, which may be temporary or permanent depending on the dose of radiotherapy and can be quite distressing to the child. The skin at the site of irradiation can also become red, inflamed and painful; this is temporary and will recover once treatment is over. It is recommended that children should avoid swimming or hydrotherapy for 6 weeks following completion of radiotherapy due to the effects on the skin. Craniospinal radiotherapy can also have more specific side-effects such as raised ICP due to cerebral oedema and inflammation (Berger 1992). This is normally treated with a short course of steroids, and can cause anxiety in a child and family as the effects may mimic the initial signs at the presentation of the tumour. Children may feel fatigue, nausea, have headaches and become anorexic. A period of somnolence can occur up to 2 months after craniospinal radiotherapy; this is due to temporary demyelination of the brain tissue.

Longer-term side-effects

Children are at risk of developing more long-term side-effects such as induction of secondary malignancies and abnormal growth and development. Children may suffer from hearing loss depending on the field of radiation. Around the age of 2–3 years the CNS has a rapid period of growth and development or myelination. This is said to be complete by age 5 (Pinkerton et al 1994); therefore craniospinal radiotherapy in the younger child will have more potentially irreversible effects on the CNS. These depend on the areas of the CNS that have been directly irradiated or involved in the field of radiation. Due to the adverse effect on cognition, cranial radiotherapy to some sites can be delayed in the under-5s by the use of chemotherapy in order to allow further cognitive and neurological maturation. Radiation to central areas of the brain such as the hypothalamus and the optic chiasm can result in endocrine dysfunction. These children may become obese, as they tend to eat obsessively and may require hormone support in future.

The late effects of radiotherapy are more important in terms of cognitive function, independent functioning and associated quality-of-life issues. Cranial irradiation has adverse long-term cognitive effects on the brain. The younger the child and the higher the dose, the worse the outcome is likely to be. These cognitive defects manifest themselves in poor short-term memory, attention deficits, poor verbal and non-verbal reasoning skills and result in an overall reduction in full-scale IQ. Combined with a hearing loss, this leaves the child very educationally vulnerable.

BONE MARROW TRANSPLANT

A BMT is the process of harvesting donor bone marrow and transfusing these cells into the recipient. It is used as standard treatment for children with poor-prognosis leukaemias and solid tumours (Pinkerton et al 1994). The aim of BMT is to destroy all cancerous cells, create space within the bone marrow and eliminate active host cells that would reject a transplant (Gillis & Donovan 2001). BMT, however, can also permit higher-dose chemo/radiotherapy to be used.

There are two main types of transplant used in children with cancer: stem-cell transplant and BMT. The former involves blood cells in the earliest form of development (stem cells) and the latter the more mature bone marrow cells. The grafting of bone marrow during a BMT can be autologous, allogenic or synergeneic:

- *Autologous*: cells are harvested from the child before the child receives high-dose chemotherapy or radiotherapy. On completion of the course of high-dose treatment the stem cells or bone marrow are given back via an infusion, allowing the body to be 'rescued'. Thus this allows higher doses of chemotherapy to be used with fewer effects on the body. This form of BMT is advantageous due to the lower risk of graft-versus-host disease (GvHD) and recovery is often quicker. There is a risk, however, of tumour cells being present in the marrow at harvest (Gibson & Evans 1999). The cells can go through a cleaning process to reduce the risk of cancer cell transfusion.
- *Allogenic*: cells are harvested from another person (related, unrelated, matched or unmatched). The ideal would be a matched related donor, i.e. sibling (Gibson & Evans 1999). Chemotherapy is first used to destroy the bone marrow before donor bone marrow is given. The recipient technically has 'healthy' bone marrow but there is a high risk of GvHD in which the donor cells react to the host cells. Allogenic BMT can have serious complications and therefore is only carried out in specialized centres.
- *Synergeneic*: cells are harvested from an identical twin. There is no risk of the recipient developing GvHD as the donor and recipient are matched in every way (Gibson & Evans 1999).

Short- and medium-term side-effects

Chemotherapy is the main agent used during BMT and therefore the effects are similar to or more severe than the results seen following routine chemotherapy, i.e. nausea, vomiting, anorexia, diarrhoea and neurotoxicity. This group of children all experience at some point a period of immobility following prolonged bed rest. Children develop markedly reduced cardiovascular fitness and muscle strength as the isolation restricts physical activity and motivation, due to periods of immobility and chemotherapy causing fatigue and muscle wastage. All of this combined means that the role of the physiotherapist is vital in maintaining a child's level of function. The physiotherapy programme needs to be very flexible and adapt to a child's condition. This may mean that an exercise bike can be taken into the cubicle to allow a high level of physical activity to be maintained or that physiotherapy is limited to bed exercises and monitoring of respiratory function. Passive or active assisted range of movement exercise may be required to maintain joint range (Gillis & Donovan 2001). Joint range of movement should be closely monitored and splinting used where appropriate. Postural exercises are required to prevent longer-term lumbar and thoracic problems.

As children are isolated for the duration of their BMT, this can cause many feelings of anxiety and depression for a child or young person. Children and their families need counselling before BMT to enable them to be fully prepared for the long periods of isolation and multiple procedures that follow. Restrictions on the number of visitors are employed to reduce the chances of exposure to infections. Involvement of the entire multidisciplinary team (occupational therapist, teacher, play specialist/nursery nurse) is essential to maintain a routine that is as 'normal' as possible.

Graft-versus-host disease

GvHD is a reaction of the donor cells to the host cells due to the cell incompatibility (Gibson & Evans 1999). GvHD is divided into acute (in the first 100 days post-BMT) and chronic (beyond 100 days posttransplant). This condition is serious and at times can be fatal. GvHD predominantly affects the rapidly dividing cells of the epithelium, gastrointestinal tract and liver (Gillis & Donovan 2001). This can present as skin rashes on the soles of the feet and palms of the hands, diarrhoea, nausea, jaundice and abdominal discomfort. Children with GvHD are thought to be at more risk of steroid myopathy as the main treatment for the condition is corticosteroids (Gillis & Donovan 2001).

Longer-term side-effects

Children are at risk of developing more long-term side-effects such as abnormal growth and development, infertility and secondary malignancies. The impact of isolation combined with the rigorous treatment, however, can affect a child or young person psychosocially, including cognitive effects, behavioural problems, impact on schooling due to prolonged periods of missed school, reintegration back to school, effect on family dynamics and reduced independence and self-confidence.

LEUKAEMIA

Leukaemia makes up approximately one-third of all childhood cancers, with approximately 450 new cases each year in the UK (UK CCSG 1999). Leukaemia is the malignant transformation of haemopoietic precursor cells in the bone marrow (Pinkerton et al 1994). In other words, it is an overproduction of immature malignant white blood cells as a result of a malformation of the bone marrow. Depending upon where in the stage this transformation occurs will determine the type of leukaemia. Leukaemia is classified according to the degree of cell maturity and the cell line that is affected. There are four classifications of leukaemia (treatment is dependent upon the type):

1. ALL: affecting the primitive lymphoblastic cells
2. Acute myeloblastic leukaemia (AML): affecting the primitive myelocytic cells
3. Chronic myeloid leukaemia (CML): affecting the mature myelocytic cells
4. Chronic lymphoblastic leukaemia (CLL): affecting the mature lymphoblastic cells.

ALL is the commonest form of leukaemia and current chemotherapy regimes cure at least 75% of all children with ALL (Hoelzer et al 2002). The chemotherapy regime is 3 years for boys and 2 years for girls. The cause of ALL is unknown. At diagnosis children will often have a history of lethargy, bruising and general aches and pains. Many younger children may have stopped weight-bearing and walking due to this pain.

It is well documented that treatment for ALL has long- and short-term effects on the musculoskeletal and neuromuscular systems (Marchese et al 2004), although there has been very little research looking at the impact on functional mobility. As discussed, children can experience symptoms early on in the treatment; Marchese et al (2004) note some of the long-term effects of vincristine chemotherapy used for children with ALL to be gross and fine motor delays and hypoextensibility of the gastrocnemius and soleus musculature, decreased energy expenditure, learning disabilities, avascular necrosis, osteopenia and osteoporosis. Marchese et al (2004) in their study demonstrated that specific stretching and strengthening exercise programmes rather than aerobic activity (swimming, dancing, bike-riding) significantly increased ankle dorsiflexion and knee extension. The authors advocate a physiotherapy assessment to look comprehensively at the neuromuscular and musculoskeletal systems of all children with ALL. As previously discussed, proximal myopathy is also common with this group of children due to the high doses of corticosteroids used during the treatment regime.

Physiotherapy for children and young people with ALL will often begin early in the chemotherapy treatment. Close monitoring of ankle range of movement, gait and functional ability is required. As indicated, a stretching and strengthening lower-limb exercise programme should commence (particularly during the intensification phase of treatment when the vincristine dose is prevalent). The posture of these children also needs to be closely monitored. As already noted, the insertion of a CVC or portacath can result in a very flexed posture with increased thoracic kyphosis and reduced lumbar lordosis and, when combined with a reduced gait pattern due to footdrop, reduced balance and reduced energy levels can render the child or young person quite debilitated. Through early identification of symptoms and timely implementation of physiotherapy, children can maintain a good functional level. Advice for children with impaired sensation may be necessary, such as massage to reduce hypersensitivity and appropriate footwear. A referral to occupational therapy may also be required for a hand-writing assessment for those children/young people with reduced fine motor control.

BONE TUMOURS

The incidence of bone cancer in young people is low – in the order of 150 new children in the UK each year. The disease tends to affect adolescents (10–20 years); boys are more affected than girls (National Institute for Clinical Excellence 2005). It appears that the rapid period of growth during adolescence is associated with the peak of incidence (Morland & Whelan 2004).

The two most commonly encountered bone tumours are osteosarcoma and Ewing's sarcoma of bone. Treatment of both tumours is complex and multimodal, involving different specialities and often different hospital sites. The development of active chemotherapy agents, reconstructive surgery, radiotherapy where appropriate and, more recently, aggressive removal of lung metastases has seen an increase in survival to over 50% of children (Morland & Whelan 2004).

Osteosarcoma

This is the most common primary bone tumour. The majority occur around the knee in either upper tibial or lower femoral areas. In the upper limb they tend to be proximal humeral in origin. Osteogenic sarcomas have a tendency to metastasize to the lung: approximately 15–20% of children will have them at presentation. Pathological fracture at the site of the tumour can occur in about 5–10% of children and carries a poorer prognosis.

The most common presentation is of pain, which is not necessarily mechanical and may disturb sleep. It is often brought to a child's notice by some minor trauma in the area. As the tumour continues to grow the pain increases and other features become more obvious, such as swelling and loss of function, particularly at a joint. It is unusual to see the symptoms of lung metastases at presentation.

Ewing's sarcoma of bone

The site of these tumours differs from osteosarcoma. The majority are found more axially, e.g. in the pelvis, ribs and vertebrae, rather than the long bones.

The initial features are of a more general malaise, such as fever and weight loss. Extensive soft-tissue involvement occurs in Ewing's sarcoma, leading to nerve root pain or neuropathy, depending on the site. It may be many months between presentation and diagnosis as the initial pain and discomfort can be dismissed as growing pains. Metastatic disease is found in 25% of children, mainly in the lungs.

Treatment

Treatment of bone sarcoma involves chemotherapy, surgery and possibly radiotherapy in the treatment of Ewing's sarcoma. Radiotherapy is rarely used to treat osteosarcomas, as they are not particularly radiosensitive. Local radiotherapy at high dose may be used for palliation or local recurrence.

Presurgical chemotherapy

The main aim is to shrink the tumour in order to facilitate surgical resection, and to provide systemic treatment of existing or potential metastases.

Surgery

The two main alternatives in distal disease are limb salvage surgery and amputation.

Complete surgical excision provides the best outcome, and ideally should be achieved with the least subsequent effect on function. The choice of surgery may depend on critical factors such as the position and the extent of soft-tissue involvement of the tumour.

Limb salvage surgery

A total of 85% of children with distal sarcoma have salvage surgery, which involves the excision of the affected part of the bone and replacement with an internal metallic prosthesis which usually incorporates the replacement of the adjacent joint, termed an endoprosthetic replacement.

Advantages

Body image is very important to this age group and the preservation of a limb will be very important. The ultimate prognosis of the child is unaffected by having salvage surgery. Generally, function of up to 90% is retained at best.

Disadvantages

Some 80% of children have some form of further surgery over the next 25 years. This involves minor surgery to adjust the length of the prosthesis. More recently, prostheses are lengthened, non-surgically, by the use of a strong magnetic field. There is an increased risk of local recurrence, which may lead to an amputation. Infection of the site of the prosthesis can occur and could result in an amputation. The prosthesis may fail as a result of wear and tear, or loosening due to the increase in intramedullary size as the child grows. Children often have poor function, particularly with upper-limb prostheses. Total femoral replacement is less functional than distal femoral replacement.

Physiotherapy in limb salvage surgery

- *Preoperative period:* a baseline physical assessment should be carried out, and an appropriate programme of therapy agreed. It is helpful to discuss with the child and family the rehabilitation required postsurgery, engaging them in the process as early as possible.

   Physiotherapy input can be more easily delivered in the physiotherapy department before and after each course of chemotherapy treatment, as the child is not attached to intravenous drips or lines. However, some exercises and activities are carried out during chemotherapy on or at the bedside on the ward. A referral to occupational therapy is required to assess the home environment for any adaptations and equipment needs. A wheelchair is often required for longer distances, and after surgery, as chemotherapy continues.
- *Postoperative period:* children start chemotherapy again 10–14 days postsurgery. Over the next 6 weeks children should begin to recover their range of movement and muscle strength. Progress may be slow as chemotherapy will continue for some time and it may take many months to gain the expected functional recovery. Children with lower-limb endoprostheses mobilize initially in partial weight-bearing and progress to normal gait as pain and range of movement improve. The knee prosthesis hyperextends, to provide stability in extension and facilitate early mobility with weak quadriceps. Problems unique to each prosthesis are described below.

Distal femoral prosthesis

Common problems are loss of range of flexion at the knee. Quadriceps lag and flexion deformity can be a problem, also patellar maltracking. A near-normal gait and a high level of function are expected ultimately.

Total femoral prosthesis

Total hip replacement precautions, for example, hip flexion limited to 90°, no hip adduction past midline and no hip rotation, should be enforced for 3 months. Functional outcome is poorer than for distal femoral replacement, due to difficulty in reattaching the muscles around the hip joint. Ultimately children mobilize with one stick or independently, but will have limited control of inner range of movement at the knee and poor stability and control of the hip.

Proximal tibial prosthesis

As the tibial tubercle is excised, the patellar tendon is sutured to the medial head of gastrocnemius that is mobilized and brought anteriorly. For the first 6 weeks passive knee flexion is limited to allow for healing of the tendon relocation. Static quadriceps contractions are allowed, and assisted calf stretches. Common problems are persistent quads lag, e.g. weakness in inner/outer quadriceps range, flexion deformity at the knee, tight gastrocnemius and temporary footdrop due to surgical nerve trauma. Independent mobility and functional flexion of the knee are expected.

Proximal humeral prosthesis

The humeral head and the greater and lesser tuberosities are excised, resulting in poor control of glenohumeral movement.

For the first 6 weeks the limb is supported with a sling and must not be allowed to hang dependently. Assisted movements of the shoulder girdle, elbow, wrist and hand are carried out. Assisted glenohumeral exercises are taught after 6 weeks. Children are taught trick movements at the shoulder girdle for function. Full range of movement should be possible at the wrist and hand with functional active range at the elbow.

General advice on long-term activities for children having endoprosthetic replacements

- No contact sports
- No high-impact activities
- No running or twisting (lower-limb prosthesis)
- No lifting of heavy weights (upper-limb prosthesis).

Amputation

In 15% of children with osteosarcoma an amputation is the only surgical option. The indicators for amputation are: an unresectable tumour involving the neurovascular bundle; large and extensive soft-tissue involvement, making functional reconstruction impossible; and pathological fracture.

Advantages

- The risk of recurrence is lower than that of salvage surgery
- The prognosis is no worse than that of salvage surgery
- Good functional outcome is possible, especially in below-knee amputation
- Fewer future surgical interventions will be necessary
- No restrictions as to contact sporting activities, e.g. football, providing the prosthetic supplied can be securely fitted and withstand the stresses.

Disadvantages

- Functional loss depends on the site of the amputation; upper-limb prostheses are generally less functional than lower-limb prostheses
- Psychological, emotional and social impact on the child
- Phantom-limb sensation can occur, when children are able to feel their amputated limb postsurgery. Itching or burning sensations are described alongside acute pain and pins and needles. The symptoms can be alleviated by the use of drugs, transcutaneous electrical nerve stimulation (TENS) and distraction/relaxation therapy
- Problems with the fitting and use of the prosthesis. Fluctuations in weight make early fitting of prosthesis difficult and use painful.

PHYSIOTHERAPY IN AMPUTATION

Preoperative physiotherapy

An initial assessment of a child is important for a baseline. Chemotherapy is administered in the same manner as for limb salvage surgery. An exercise programme to strengthen the remaining limb and to address the muscle imbalance of the affected limb postsurgery is started. A referral to the local occupational therapist and wheelchair services is made so that appropriate equipment and adaptations will be provided.

Amputation at any age is distressing. Young people or teenagers will have profound emotional needs and concerns, particularly about their appearance, acceptance by peers and independence. Children and families may ask to see types of prosthesis and meet with other children who have been through the same experience. Providing this is sensitively managed and with the right personality mix, it can be a positive experience for both parties.

Postoperative physiotherapy

Chemotherapy starts again 10–14 days postsurgery. Links with the local artificial limb centre or prosthetist need to be in place as children will be referred there for the supply and management of their prosthetic limb.

Above-knee amputation is the most common site of amputation for bone sarcoma. Therapy is aimed at improving the child's balance and gait, and functional activities such as stair-climbing and getting up from the floor. The stump can become flexed and abducted as a result of the imbalance in muscle control at the hip. A good range of hip extension and strong extensors are vital in controlling a prosthetic leg and knee joint. The physiotherapist needs to be aware of adaptive changes in posture, and correction may well be an issue in these children. A fixed knee prosthesis is sometimes used initially; children are progressed on to more technical and physically challenging prosthetic

limbs as they become more stable and stronger. Children are ultimately expected to mobilize independently.

Below-knee amputation poses less of a functional problem for a child and physiotherapist. The shorter and simpler prosthesis makes regaining function much easier than in an above-knee amputation. Physiotherapy is again aimed at improving the child's balance and gait and function. Children are expected to mobilize without any assistance and can take part in athletics and sport up to a high level.

Upper-limb amputation is seen less often. It may also involve the removal of the scapula. The physiotherapy input to these children is limited to advice on posture. Occupational therapists provide more input to these children, giving advice on adaptive functioning. The prostheses initially supplied are usually cosmetic.

CENTRAL NERVOUS SYSTEM TUMOURS

CNS tumours (comprising brain and spinal tumours) are the second largest group of solid tumours in children aged under 15 years, and comprise 20–25% of all paediatric cancers (Shaminski-Maher & Shields 1995). Certain types of CNS tumour are associated with inherited conditions, e.g. gliomas and neurofibromatosis (Estlin 2005).

The neurological presentation of the child is dictated by the site and type of tumour, making each child unique. An outline of the types of tumour and where they are commonly found is helpful to appreciate the challenges that the physiotherapist may encounter in treating their physical effects and managing the outcomes for these children. It is impossible to describe an exact treatment programme for types or sites of tumour; however, general principles of physiotherapy management in the different stages of recovery are highlighted here.

Sites of central nervous system brain tumours

Geographically the brain is divided into two sections by the tentorial membrane. This thick dural septum divides the cerebrum from the cerebellum. Supratentorial tumours occur in the cerebral region (40%) and tumours occurring below the tentorium (60%) are termed infratentorial. Tumours occurring in the cerebellum are often termed posterior fossa tumours as they lie in the posterior fossa of the skull (Wisoff & Epstein 1994). Different tumour types can occur in any of these areas. A further distinction can be made in tumours occurring centrally or in the midline of the brain.

Brainstem tumours

Different types of tumour occur in this important area of the brain. They can be high- or low-grade, diffuse or focal: the prognosis varies with these factors and their accessibility to surgical resection. The presenting features can be raised ICP, cranial nerve palsies, hemiparesis and ataxia.

Medical treatment involves primary surgery where possible, with radiotherapy for high-grade tumours. The role of chemotherapy is undefined in the treatment of brainstem tumours. New agents and combinations of radiotherapy with adjuvant chemotherapy are presently being studied in North America and Europe.

Midline tumours

This is a mixed group of tumours, including cranio-pharyngiomas, germ cell tumours, optic pathway, hypo-thalamic and pineal tumours. They are deep-seated and are therefore a challenge surgically. These tumours are mostly low-grade, but persistent.

The signs and symptoms are very variable, including cognitive impairment, memory loss, altered personality and endocrine dysfunction.

Medical treatment relies on surgery but due to their deep-seated position this is often impossible without significant neurological damage. Radiotherapy is commonly used; the role of chemotherapy for some of this group of tumours is being explored.

Types of brain central nervous system tumours

Primitive neuroectodermal tumour (PNET)

These types of tumour are the most common paediatric malignant primary brain tumour. The majority are found in the posterior fossa, originating from the cerebellum, and can involve the fourth ventricle and brainstem. These tumours are also termed medulloblastoma.

Children may present with signs of raised ICP: hydrocephalus, headache and vomiting. Ataxia, loss of balance, double vision, facial weakness and squint may also occur. These types of tumour have a tendency to recur and can metastasize to the spine (Geyer et al 1991). PNETs found in the supratentorial region can present with signs of raised ICP or epilepsy, depending on their exact site. Supratentorial PNETs have a poorer prognosis than infratentorial PNETs.

Medical treatment of theses tumours includes surgical resection, craniospinal radiotherapy and chemotherapy.

Astrocytoma

Approximately 40% of all paediatric brain tumours are astrocytomas; they are most commonly found in the supra-tentorium. The majority are low-grade and do not tend to metastasize or recur. They have a good prognosis following complete surgical resection. High-grade tumours have a poorer outcome. Signs and symptoms of these tumours are related to the site of the tumour, e.g. motor weakness epilepsy, visual disturbance or endocrine dysfunction.

Medical treatment of low-grade tumours may consist of surgery only with close monitoring and frequent scans. Radiotherapy for incomplete resection may be indicated. High-grade tumours are more aggressively managed postsurgery with radiotherapy and chemotherapy. Radiotherapy and chemotherapy are used as the mainstays of treatment if the site is considered inoperable. Chemotherapy treatment of these tumours is a relatively new adjunct to surgery and radiotherapy. There is increasing evidence of improved outcomes using multi-agent chemotherapy in this group (Finlay et al 1995).

Ependymoma

This tumour develops from the ependymomal cells lining the ventricles. The majority are found in the posterior fossa in the fourth ventricle, and they have a tendency for local recurrence. Signs and symptoms are of raised ICP. Tumours in the posterior fossa may also present with poor balance and ataxia and cranial nerve palsies.

Medical management of these tumours relies on total resection where possible followed by radiotherapy. The role of chemotherapy in this group is unclear. It can be used as a strategy to provide some treatment when radiotherapy is delayed in infants, or if the resection has been incomplete, or in disease recurrence (Duffner et al 1993, Grill et al 2001).

Investigations for central nervous system tumours

The appearance of individual brain tumours on scans is rarely specific. All tumours present as masses. The presence of haemorrhage, necrosis and calcification varies between different types of tumour, but can also vary within the same type of tumour. Generally, high-grade tumours are more likely to appear as heterogeneous masses with areas of necrosis, haemorrhage and oedema. Low-grade tumours are more likely to be homogeneous and without haemorrhage or oedema. Computed tomography (CT) and magnetic resonance imaging (MRI) are not used to give a precise histology of a tumour. They are used to give a diagnosis of a brain tumour and to differentiate it from other lesions such as infarcts and abscesses. MRI is used to localize the position of the tumour and its relationship to normal tissue and is necessary for planning surgical intervention. Scans are also used extensively in follow-up.

Surgical and medical management of brain tumours

The traditional mainstays of treatment for brain tumours have been primary surgery followed, when required, by radiotherapy. More recently there has been an increasing interest in using chemotherapy along with the traditional methods in order to improve survival rates (Ryan & Shaminski-Maher 1995).

Surgery

Surgical aims vary from biopsy to identify the histology of the tumour, management of complications, to intent to cure. However the morbidity associated with surgery must be considered and may limit the extent of the surgical intervention. This issue is particularly important when the tumour is found in a deep-seated area such as the hypothalamic region or in a critical area such as the brainstem. Complete surgical resection of a tumour does however offer the highest chance of cure.

The management of complications is usually related to raised ICP. The insertion of an external ventricular drain for temporary regulation postsurgery is not uncommon. If raised ICP becomes a longer-term problem, this is normally managed by the insertion of a ventriculoperitoneal shunt. These are not without problems, such as blockage and infection, and are not inserted without considering the benefits and difficulties associated with them. Raised ICP can sometimes be treated by performing a third ventriculostomy to improve the internal circulation of the cerebrospinal fluid. This is however not appropriate in all situations (MacArthur et al 2001).

Chemotherapy

The role and efficacy of chemotherapy in the treatment of CNS tumours are less well established than in the treatment of other solid tumours. This is a result of several factors, both intrinsic and extrinsic. The blood–brain barrier is uniquely effective in protecting the brain from many of the anticancer drugs commonly used. The type of tumour involved and the child's individual susceptibility to the chemotherapy agents are also important factors in the effectiveness of the agents.

Historically, children with a CNS tumour have not been treated within specialist paediatric neurosurgical and paediatric oncology centres. This has meant that their treatment and management have been carried out in a fragmented manner, and fewer children were registered in clinical trials. As a consequence the improvement in outcome and survival for other paediatric oncological conditions, seen over recent years, has not been seen in CNS tumours. There are few early robust clinical trials on which to build future treatment regimes. Chemotherapy has however been shown to be beneficial in certain tumours, such as medulloblastoma and high-grade glioma. At present rigorous trials are being undertaken in paediatrics and the outcomes of present-day person trials may help to inform future paediatric practice (Estlin 2005).

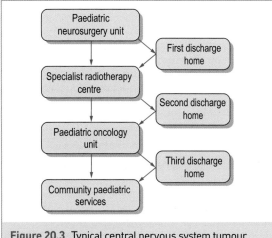

Figure 20.3 Typical central nervous system tumour patient pathway.

Physiotherapy intervention/management in central nervous system tumours

Introduction

The physiotherapists who are treating the child on a daily basis often form a close working relationship with the family. A peripatetic specialist oncology physiotherapist with the remit of providing continuity of care would be able to treat or manage children throughout their recovery, as they cross the boundaries of the different medical specialities and hospital sites. This model of therapy provision is adopted in some centres, with good effect.

The child pathway is complex (Figure 20.3). The family and child are exposed to many successive medical, nursing and allied health professions after being given a devastating diagnosis. They are likely to feel distressed and vulnerable, and will need support from all staff involved. The provision of a specialist clinical nurse to provide support, continuity and consistency of care across National Health Service (NHS) sites and stages of recovery is an invaluable asset to the multidisciplinary team.

Pre- and immediate postoperative period

Ideally the multidisciplinary team should carry out a preoperative assessment of the child. This is not always possible depending on how acute the child's presentation is, and how quickly neurosurgical intervention is needed.

A full assessment should be undertaken after consultation with medical and nursing staff as soon as possible postoperatively. The assessment should include respiratory function, a child's posture, muscle strength, tone, coordination and cranial nerve dysfunction. The initial assessment may take several sessions to complete. As children stabilize they can be mobilized to a chair, which will give an opportunity to assess functional activities such as sitting and standing balance, coordination and antigravity muscle activity. The initial postoperative physical findings may be a worsening of those found at presentation, due to local oedema from surgical intervention and resection of adjacent brain tissue.

Subacute recovery period

Further progression to walking and eventually stair-climbing, supervising and assisting activities such as eating, toileting and self-cares all give opportunities to assess functional abilities and will highlight any sensory/motor dysfunction, and dictate treatment and management strategies.

First discharge to community or transfer to other NHS site for continued chemo/radiotherapy

A lengthy discussion and possibly a home visit by the occupational therapist and physiotherapist to determine the need for any aids or adaptations should be undertaken before discharge. The provision of therapy equipment is usually undertaken by local social services or paediatric occupational therapists. Local therapists should be involved in the home assessment, particularly if they will be involved in providing therapy input in the future.

As the child recovers, the neurological sequelae generally resolve. The timescale involved can be days, weeks or months, and is very variable. Unfortunately, sometimes significant and long-term neurological damage is sustained. These children need to be followed closely over the weeks or months either by the community therapists or the therapist in the acute trust to continue appropriate therapy to maximize recovery. As a child returns to normal activities such as attending school, advice may be given to local education authorities alongside other allied health professions relating to appropriate levels and types of activities in school and recommendations for adaptations or aids required to enable access to the educational setting.

Follow-up

Children with a CNS tumour are followed up into adult life to monitor for any recurrences and the emergence of long-term sequelae. It is helpful to have a physiotherapist present at these clinics who has historical knowledge of a child to manage physical problems as they emerge, for example postural problems related to radiotherapy or visual defects, and obesity due to endocrine dysfunction.

CASE STUDY 20.1

Primitive Neuroectodermal tumour

Becky was a 10-year-old girl who was transferred to the specialist paediatric neurosurgical unit with a 5-month history of occasional morning vomiting and blurring of vision. Her symptoms had become more acute over the last week and she had presented at her local district general hospital and been transferred for a computed tomography (CT) scan and possible surgical management of a suspected space-occupying lesion.

A CT scan showed a midline cerebellar cystic lesion and an enlarged fourth ventricle.

Becky was taken to theatre the next day, where a total resection was carried out.

Her immediate postoperative progress was slow. After 24 hours she was not speaking, tending to dribble, had no upper-limb movement but exhibited spontaneous restless movements of her lower limbs. Histology confirmed an infratentorial primitive neuroectodermal tumour (PNET), also termed a medulloblastoma.

She was assessed in bed. She was unable to initiate rolling, had poor head control, no movement of her upper limbs and purposeless movements of her lower limbs. Her tone was low generally; she did not appear to be looking or focusing on anything. She was extremely agitated and unable to settle to sleep or rest. She was regularly positioned in alternate side-lying, passive movements were carried out to her upper limbs and assisted movements in pattern attempted on her lower limbs. Her respiratory status was monitored as she seemed unable to swallow her oral secretions effectively.

Over the next few days she became more settled, and she was assisted out into a chair at the side of her bed. She still required full support in attempting sitting; her head control was poor, tending to flop forwards on to her chest. Her seating had to be supportive and she was reclined to assist head control. No movements of her upper limbs were noted, she was still not speaking and she remained unsettled and troubled by constipation.

A few days later she was well enough to attend the physiotherapy department where three therapists were required to assist in sitting on a bench, whilst her arms were placed on a table to facilitate weight-bearing through them to increase tone in her trunk and

continued

upper limbs and stimulate head control. Becky was still mute and was struggling to fix and follow.

For a further 3 weeks she made very slow progress. She was facilitated in achieving sitting to stand with three therapists as her central tone and head control improved. She tended to hyperextend her knees and fixed her upper limbs into extension to provide some stability when standing as her trunk remained low in tone and did not provide her with the essential flexible stability she needed on which to stay still or to move.

A variety of treatment methods were used: sensory stimulation, vibration and weight-bearing through upper and lower limbs and longitudinal compression to normalize tone and encourage spontaneous movement of her upper limbs. She experienced episodic mood swings, giggling and crying almost simultaneously, and she tired very quickly. A wheelchair was ordered for her use.

Five weeks after her surgery spontaneous gross movements of her upper limbs were noted. Her trunk control was also improving; she was able to sit with the assistance of one therapist. She started to speak and attempted one or two steps with the assistance of three therapists. Her gait was very ataxic with poor grading of movement and placement of her feet. She required support at her pelvis, and through both upper limbs.

Her upper-limb function continued to improve and she was able to perform ataxic, antigravity movements. Becky began to initiate sitting to stand but tended to overuse flexion with little vertical movement to achieve the upright position.

Becky began to complain of headaches and was less able to cooperate in therapy. She suffered occasional vomiting and a swelling appeared over the wound. A CT scan was performed and a ventricular peritoneal shunt inserted the next day to treat her hydrocephalus. She made a good postoperative recovery and was able to perform assisted standing transfers and to manage stairs with close supervision either on her bottom or with the use of two hand rails. She was then transferred to the local radiotherapy treatment centre after a multidisciplinary discharge planning meeting.

The acute and local occupational therapy departments liaised closely and her home was equipped with appropriate moving and handling nursing equipment. The community physiotherapist was involved and agreed to take over her management after her radiotherapy until she commenced her chemotherapy. The physiotherapist working on the young oncology unit at the radiotherapy centre agreed to continue to monitor and manage Becky during her treatment there. Becky attended the radiotherapy centre daily for 6 weeks; she also attended the physiotherapy department to continue her rehab programme on a regular basis. On discharge from the radiotherapy centre, a joint home visit was made by the peripatetic physiotherapist from the acute oncology unit and the community physiotherapist to introduce the family to the community team, and to provide a seamless transfer of care.

Throughout her year of chemotherapy Becky made slow gradual improvements in her gross and fine motor function. She had a home tutor and attended her last year at junior school on an 'as and when' basis. She commenced the process of statement of educational needs, and the local occupational therapists ensured access was possible and educational and mobility aids were available for her. Becky required an adapted laptop and a scribe; she was able to use her wheelchair in school and walked short distances with a K-walker. She continued with hydrotherapy and enjoyed Pilates sessions with the community therapist amongst other treatment modalities. Postchemotherapy, Becky continued to be followed up every 3 months at the neuro-oncology clinic at the Young Oncology Unit. She is seen by her paediatric oncologist, her radiologist, the peripatetic specialist oncology physiotherapist and the specialist outreach oncology nurse.

Eighteen months after the initial surgery, Becky was still moderately ataxic; she was supported in mainstream high school, independently walking small distances, using an electric wheelchair for long distances in school and was independent in self-cares and activities of daily living. She attended and enjoyed a multiactivity holiday with a group of other oncology patients 3 years after her diagnosis.

Posterior fossa syndrome

It was felt that Becky was suffering from a rare complication of brain tumour surgery in the posterior fossa, called posterior fossa syndrome or akinetic mutism.

It is associated with resection of the vermis of the cerebellum, an area beneath which medulloblastomas are found. Its onset is usually 24–48 hours postoperatively and its features are global cerebellar dysfunction, e.g. ataxia, dysmetria, cranial nerve lesions, emotional instability, mutism, urinary retention, constipation and fluctuating control of homeostasis (Kirk et al 1995).

The cause is unknown.

Recovery can commence anywhere between 1 week to 6 months postsurgery and may not always be complete.

CASE STUDY 20.2

Leukaemia

Sarah (aged 9) was diagnosed with acute lymphoblastic leukaemia (ALL) following a 5-month history of bruising, pallor and lethargy. Blood tests showed a high white cell count and low platelets, confirming ALL. Bone marrow aspirate and lumbar puncture indicated clear cerebrospinal fluid and therefore Sarah was treated with the Medical Research Council 1997 (MRC '97) ALL protocol regimen B. This treatment consists of chemotherapy for 2 years: drugs used include weekly vincristine for the entire 2 years and regular dexamethasone (steroids). All children are assessed at day 8 for response to treatment; Sarah had a good response and therefore continued on the same treatment regime.

Six months into treatment Sarah was referred to physiotherapy due to reduced mobility, leg and foot pain and toe-walking. Physiotherapy assessment showed:

- Tightness of bilateral Achilles tendons with reduced ankle dorsiflexion (to plantargrade bilaterally)
- No decreased range of movement at hips, knees and ankle plantarflexion
- Hamstring stretch 70° (without foot stretch) bilaterally
- Signs of reduced balance
- Severe neuropathic pain
- Hypersensitivity of her feet.

Her consultant started her on gabapentin for the neuropathic pain and she was shown Achilles tendon and hamstring stretches and balance exercises. Sarah and her parents were encouraged to continue with these exercises 2–3 times daily. Sarah was reviewed regularly and showed progress in that she was able to maintain heel strike when walking and improved balance (she was having fewer episodes of falling at school).

Six months later a physiotherapy assessment was requested as Sarah's walking had deteriorated despite continuing with the regular exercises. On assessment she had no active dorsiflexion, was unable to heel-walk and unable to squat. Passively plantargrade could not be achieved bilaterally. She had a marked reduction in lower-limb power and was unable to stand with her heels on the floor. It was felt that this deterioration was due to vincristine chemotherapy, which can cause peripheral neurotoxicity. The proximal joint weakness could also have been due to a combination of steroids and vincristine. At this stage an immediate referral to orthotic services was made and Sarah was cast for ankle–foot orthoses (AFOs). The splints greatly helped and Sarah was able to function at the same level as her peers, was mobilizing well and achieving a good gait pattern. She and her parents were encouraged to continue with the exercise programme and contact physiotherapy services as required.

One year later (now 2 years since diagnosis), Sarah was re-referred to physiotherapy due to problems with splint-rubbing. This assessment revealed that she had in fact deteriorated. She had returned to toe-walking without the splints, had poor balance and marked loss of ankle range of movement but no neuropathic pain. After discussion with the orthotist it was felt that serial casting was appropriate to try to improve range of movement before recasting for AFOs. Sarah continued with serial casting for 3 weeks. She liked the casts and in fact felt more stable whilst wearing them and on removal was able to maintain heel strike on walking. She demonstrated a good gait pattern and improved balance. At this point she was recast for AFOs and encouraged to continue with the stretching programme.

Ten months later (now 9 months off completion of chemotherapy treatment) Sarah had started to toe-walk again, was only able to stand with knees hyperextended and hips flexed to maintain balance and could achieve plantargrade bilaterally. At this point she no longer wanted to wear splints or restart serial casting as she felt 'different' from her peers when at school. (She had started secondary school at this point.) It was felt the most appropriate course of action (to achieve optimum compliance) would be to recast for splints to wear at night and after school, continue with more regular stretches and maintain activity levels. Sarah was reviewed regularly and required regular reminders to continue with her stretching exercises and night splints. It was agreed with Sarah and her parents that if she deteriorated further splints would need to be worn when at school.

Eighteen months following completion of her chemotherapy Sarah's gait has improved slightly. She is mainly able to achieve heel strike, ankle range of movement has remained to plantigrade but she is continuing with night splints and stretches. At this stage she was advised to continue with the exercise regime and refer back to physiotherapy if mobility deteriorates.

CASE STUDY 20.3

Osteosarcoma

Jason had a history of generalized aches and pains in his legs for 6 months. In the previous month he had noticed swelling round his right lower thigh. A magnetic resonance imaging (MRI) scan was suggestive of a bone tumour; he was referred to the specialist orthopaedic hospital for further investigations. A chest computed tomography (CT) scan showed bilateral lung metastases, and a local biopsy was performed which confirmed a distal femoral osteosarcoma.

He returned to the local oncology centre, had a Hickman line inserted and commenced an initial 10-week (2 × 5-week cycles) course of chemotherapy. Initially Jason held his knee in flexion and was unable to extend it fully due to pain and marked swelling of his lower thigh. He also complained of back pain which was associated with his abnormal gait pattern. He was mobilized partially weight-bearing on crutches and commenced bilateral lower-limb exercises within the limits of discomfort. A wheelchair was provided for long distances. He was taught to get up and down stairs with crutches and the local social services occupational therapist visited the house to advise on any aids or adaptations which may be needed, such as temporary ramps, a commode, raised bed and bathing aids. The pain and swelling reduced over the next few weeks and Jason became progressively more mobile as his tumour shrank. He attended the physiotherapy gym at every inpatient admission for chemotherapy before he was attached to his intravenous lines. During this period he suffered from episodes of fever, loose stool and vomiting, and required unscheduled admissions for intravenous antibiotics.

He underwent excision of the tumour at the orthopaedic centre and replacement of the diseased bone by a tailor-made metallic endoprosthesis, which included a replacement knee joint.

Jason returned to his paediatric regional oncology centre 11 days postoperatively. He had an extensive scar from his upper thigh to below his patella. James was in pain and required analgesia before physiotherapy.

He was unable to straight-leg raise, had assisted/active knee flexion to 45° only and a flicker of quadriceps contraction. He was mobilizing as taught, partially weight-bearing on crutches by hyperextending his prosthetic knee replacement to provide stability on weight-bearing on the affected side. Jason found getting into and out of bed difficult and sitting with his leg dependent uncomfortable. Jason was given a continuous passive movement machine to improve his range of movement; he used this for up to 3 hours each day, alongside a programme of active exercises to regain strength and mobility. Two weeks later he had increased his active knee flexion to 90° but was still having difficulty with initiating quadriceps contraction.

Jason had previously been an active sportsman and was enthusiastic about trying hydrotherapy to encourage general activity and to assist quadriceps reactivation. After 1 month of surgery he mobilized with one stick and 2 weeks later he was walking short distances independently. He had his lung metastases removed surgically via thoracotomies and completed his courses of chemotherapy 4 months after surgery. He attended school parttime during this period and had a home tutor; Jason has decided to swim competitively next year.

REFERENCES

Almadrones L, Arcot R 1999 Patient guide to peripheral neuropathy. *Oncology Nurses Forum* 26: 1359–1360.

Berger B 1992 *Neurological Aspects of Paediatrics*. Boston: Butterworth Heineman.

Braith RW, Welsh MA, Mills RM et al 1998 Resistance exercise prevents glucosteriod induced myopathy in heart transplant patient. *Medicine and Science in Sport and Exercise* 30: 483–489.

Duffner PK, Horowitz ME, Krischer JP et al 1993 Post operative chemotherapy and delayed radiation in children less than 3 years of age with malignant brain tumours. *New England Journal of Medicine* 328: 1725–1731.

Estlin E 2005 *Central Nervous System Tumours of Childhood*. London: MacKeith Press.

Finlay JL, Boyett JM, Yates AJ et al 1995 Randomised phase III trial in children with high grade astrocytoma, comparing lomustine and prednisolone with eight drugs in one day regime. *Journal of Clinical Oncology* 13: 112–123.

Geyer R, Levy M, Berger MS et al 1991 Infants with medulloblastoma: a single institution review of survival. *Neurosurgery* 29: 707–710; discussion 710–711.

Gibson F, Evans M 1999 *Paediatric Oncology Acute Nursing Care*. London: Whurr.

Gillis TA, Donovan ES 2001 Rehabilitation following bone marrow transplantation. *Cancer* 92: 998–1007.

Grill J, LeDeley MC, Gamberelli D et al 2001 Postoperative chemotherapy without radiation for ependymoma in children under five years, a multi-centre trial of the French Society of Paediatric Oncology. *Journal of Clinical Oncology* 19: 1288–1296.

Harila-Saari A, Vainionpaa LK, Kovala TT et al 1998 Nerve lesions after therapy for childhood acute lymphoblastic leukaemia. *Cancer* 82: 200–207.

Hoelzer D, Gokbuget N, Ottoman O et al 2002 Acute lymphoblastic leukaemia. *Haematology* 1: 162–205.

Kirk E, Howard V, Scott C 1995 Description of posterior fossa syndrome in children after posterior fossa brain tumour surgery. *Journal of Paediatric Oncology Nursing* 12(4): 181–187.

MacArthur DC, Buxton N, Vloeberghs M et al 2001 Effectiveness of neuroendoscopic interventions in children with brain tumours. *Child's Nervous System* 17: 589–594.

Marchese VG, Chiarello LA, Lange BJ 2004 Effects of physical therapy intervention for children with acute lymphoblastic leukaemia. *Paediatric Blood Cancer* 42: 127–133.

Morland B, Whelan J 2004 *Paediatric Oncology,* 3rd edn. London: Arnold.

National Institute for Clinical Excellence (NICE) 2005 *Guidance on Cancer Services. Improving Outcomes in Children and Young People with Cancer.* London: NICE.

Pinkerton CR, Cushing P, Sepion B 1994 *Childhood Cancer Management – A Practical Handbook.* London: Chapman and Hall Medical.

Quasthoff S, Hartung HP 2002 Chemotherapy induced peripheral neuropathy. *Journal of Neurology* 249: 9–17.

Ryan J, Shaminski-Maher T 1995 Hydrocephalus and shunts in children with brain tumours. *Journal of Paediatric Oncology Nursing* 12(4): 223–239.

Shaminski-Maher T, Shields M 1995 Paediatric brain tumours: diagnosis and management. *Journal of Paediatric Oncology Nursing* 12: 188–198.

United Kingdom Children's Cancer Study Group (UK CCSG) 1999 *Incidence Rates of Childhood Cancer.* Leicester: UKCCSG.

Wisoff JH, Epstein FJ 1994 Management of hydrocephalus in children with medulloblastoma – prognosis factors for shunting. *Paediatric Neurosurgery* 20: 240–247.

Child and adolescent mental health

21 Child and adolescent mental health

Robyn M. Hudson

CHAPTER CONTENTS

INTRODUCTION

It can be perplexing to consider the role of the physiotherapist in the management of young people with mental health problems. These problems can be many and varied but are characterized by impairment in emotional and psychological well-being that subsequently affects the individual's ability to participate in daily tasks. When a young person is diagnosed as having a mental health problem, the implication is that the primary aetiology is psychological and thus requires a psychological treatment approach. However, physiotherapists working in this area manage very real physical problems such as poor cardiovascular fitness due to inactivity, weakness associated with disuse, odd and unusual gait patterns and provide advice and structure to support a return to premorbid functioning. They are valuable members of the multidisciplinary team assisting this population of young people toward recovery.

Illness in childhood and adolescence can have profound effects on education, socialization and identity development. Adolescence in particular is a time of identity formation and thus the reaction to illness can both affect self-development and in some cases influence the course of the illness. It has been noted by Muscari (1998) that: 'Many of these adolescents are not ready to surrender the disorder that has become their identity'. An awareness of this point is crucial to the successful treatment of young people with long-term ill health. It will not be possible to progress treatment in many cases unless the young person has made the appropriate psychological adjustment. It is essential that support is provided to the family to deal with issues arising from the young person's illness and to assist in changing unhelpful thoughts and behaviours within the family environment.

When children and adolescents experience prolonged periods in the health system, a return to normalcy can be challenging. It would seem necessary that clinicians move away from an impairment-focused assessment and treatment to one that focuses on activity and participation. As children and adolescents improve it is essential that thought is given to reintegration into the education system as well as ways to re-establish peer relations.

There are many illnesses that fall into the category of mental health; however only a few will be addressed in this chapter: anorexia nervosa (AN), chronic fatigue syndrome/myalgic encephalomyelitis (CFS/ME), conversion disorder and pervasive refusal syndrome (PRS). These patients may be seen in inpatient settings (acute ward, mental health unit, rehabilitation centre) or outpatient setting. Despite the number of environments and the differences between illnesses there are common themes in their management.

In order to assist recovery it is essential that a comprehensive, multidisciplinary team manage the young person. The members of the team will be influenced by the specific illness. For instance, dieticians have a large role in the management of AN. Where feasible, the team should reflect all stakeholders in health and education. All members must communicate with each other to ensure that consistent information is presented to the young person and family. It is also important to acknowledge that the young person and family are pivotal members of the team and without their cooperation it is not possible to progress.

It is key that any physiotherapy programme is patient goal-directed and reflects improved participation rather than a focus on symptom resolution. If the young person owns the program he or she will be more motivated to work with the team toward positive outcomes (Box 21.1).

ANOREXIA NERVOSA

AN ranks third among common chronic disorders in adolescents, surpassed only by asthma and obesity (Lucas et al

- Graded rehabilitation programme that addresses participation and focuses on ability
- Patient-oriented goals improve motivation and commitment to recovery
- Rapport and trust between therapist, family and young person are essential
- Clear, concise and consistent plan is identified
- Good communication between all professionals to ensure optimal management of a young person and understanding by the parents
- In the case of chronic fatigue syndrome/myalgic encephalomyelitis, pervasive refusal symptom and conversion disorder, there is a need to reduce the focus on symptoms

1991). It can be defined as the pursuit of thinness based on calorific restriction and increased calorific expenditure, which leads to an inability to maintain weight at or above what is considered to be within the normal (<85% of expected weight for age or a body mass index (BMI) <17.5 kg/m^2) (Thien et al 2000). It is widely agreed that the cause of AN is multifactorial in nature and studies have found links with depression, general anxiety disorders, a family history of AN and specific aspects of personality (Lilenfeld et al 1998, Strober et al 2000).

In the general population it is estimated that 19/100 000 females and 2/100 000 males suffer with AN (Pawluck & Gorey 1998). The highest rate is seen in adolescent girls, where the estimate is 7/1000 compared to 1/1000 for boys (Rastam et al 1989).

Medical management focuses on restoring appropriate weight and the reversal of the effects of a period of starvation such as amenorrhoea, osteoporosis, social isolation, depression and poor body image. Treatment strategies include inpatient admissions for intensive medical management, including refeeding, psychotherapy, antidepressants, behavioural therapy and selective serotonin reuptake inhibitors.

AN in the adolescent is characterized by bradycardia, reduced blood pressure, small heart size and a low resting cardiac output (Rowland et al 2003). AN also has a profound effect on the cardiovascular fitness of suffers. When challenged on treadmill or cycle exercise tests, maximal cardiac output ($V_{O_{2max}}$), blood pressure and heart rate responses are often lessened. It is thought that these changed responses to exercise testing are the result of alterations in the autonomic nervous system (Rowland et al 2003). Some suggest this is due to reduced activity in the sympathetic system whereas others suggest increased parasympathetic activity (Nudel et al 1984, St John Sutton

et al 1985, Kollai et al 1994, Petretta et al 1997). All of these factors not only influence the fitness of the individual but also the capacity to increase everyday participation as the patient recovers from the illness.

The use of exercise to improve fitness and thus activity and participation is controversial in the treatment of young people with AN. Exercise is considered by some authors to play a key role in the development of eating disorders and for others a way of maintaining the calorific expenditure and suppression of appetite (Davis et al 1997). It is not surprising then that there is a paucity of research into the use of exercise in this population.

Often young people are prevented from engaging in movement and exercise when being treated for AN. The risks of prolonged absence from exercise are well documented and can only compound effects of AN such as reduced bone mass, poor cardiovascular fitness, loss of muscle mass and an increased risk of atherosclerosis (Thien et al 2000). It is also thought that many young people with AN exercise covertly while engaged in treatment programmes. Thus policing by staff of this behaviour can lead to conflict between the young person and the treating team (Beaumont et al 1994, Thien et al 2000). So rather than enforce a restriction it may be of benefit to provide a supervised programme once the young person is medically stable and able to sustain a suitable weight.

Some researchers have had success with exercise programmes (Thien et al 2000). Table 21.1 outlines a programme that utilized stretching and strengthening. All patients participating in this programme commenced on level 1, remaining on each level for a complete week prior to progressing after team discussion. No differences were found between the exercise group and control for BMI or percentage body fat, and in fact for both groups there was an increase. Interestingly, the exercise group did indicate improvements on the quality-of-life measure beyond the control group. Another study demonstrated a greater increase in BMI for an aerobic exercise programme compared with the non-exercise group (Tokumura et al 2003). Despite limited research in the area, exercise is used by 71% of physiotherapists in the UK to treat AN (Mandy & Broadbridge 1998).

Therefore the benefits of exercise may be seen in improved compliance with the treatment programme but also as a counter to secondary effects of inactivity and AN, such as osteoporosis, poor strength, endurance and fitness. It may also teach the young person about healthy and sustainable ways to exercise, facilitating reintegration into regular activity patterns in the home environment.

It is also important to take into consideration the posture of young people with AN. The way we stand, sit and move communicates a lot about how we feel. Standard education of correct posture or the use of tape to provide feedback may be beneficial in addition to strengthening programmes (Beaumont et al 1994). It may also be useful to utilize relaxation techniques such as controlled breathing or guided imagery to assist the young person.

Table 21.1 Graded exercise protocol

Level	Description
1	Stretching exercises three times a week: sitting and lying <75% IBW or <19% BF
2	Stretching exercises three times a week: standing, sitting and lying 75% IBW or 19% BF
3a	Stretching exercise three times a week plus isometric exercise, one set three times per week for 3 weeks 80% IBW or 20% BF
3b	Stretching exercise three time a week plus isometric exercise, two sets three times per week plus low-impact cardiovascular exercise, twice per week after 3 weeks 80% IBW or 21% BF
4	Stretching exercise three times a week plus isometric exercise three times a week plus low-impact cardiovascular exercise three times a week 85% IBW or 21% BF
5	Stretching exercise three times a week plus resistive strengthening, one set three times a week plus low-impact cardiovascular exercise three times a week 90% IBW or 22.5% BF
6	Stretching exercise three times a week plus resistive strengthening, two sets three times a week plus low-impact cardiovascular exercise three times a week 95% IBW or 23% BF

Reproduced from Thien et al (2000) with permission from John Wiley.
IBW, ideal body weight; BF, body fat.

Communication between the team members and the young person must be clear and consistent. This is essential to ensure that the young person is aware of boundaries for engagement in exercise programmes but also to ensure trust.

The acute stages of management of AN require limits on activity and exercise in order to achieve a suitable weight. However, a supervised graded exercise programme will assist in reducing the secondary effects of starvation and inactivity, possibly improve compliance with treatment, reduce covert exercise and facilitate a return to normal activity.

CHRONIC FATIGUE SYNDROME

CFS/ME is defined as severe mental and physical fatigue that causes significant functional impairment of greater than 3–6 months with no medical explanation (Fukuda et al 1994, Viner et al 2004). The primary symptoms are listed in Box 21.2. Sometimes the term 'postviral fatigue' may also be used. However, this term is often used for those who have had fatigue and associated symptoms for

Box 21.2 Common symptoms of chronic fatigue syndrome/myalgic encephalomyelitis

- Constant fatigue
- Headache
- Poor concentration
- Reduced memory
- Muscle aches
- Joint pains
- Nausea
- Poor sleep quality
- Abdominal pain

a lesser amount of time, and for children who are under 10, for whom the diagnosis of CFS/ME can be made with less certainty. To date there is no identified cause for CFS/ME. Despite this, the prognosis for young people is positive. The majority are seen to improve within 2 years of attending a specialist centre and engaging in a rehabilitation programme (Joyce et al 1997, Viner et al 2004).

There are a number of different therapy options for young people diagnosed with CFS/ME. These include cognitive-behavioural therapy, family therapy, pacing and graded activity/exercise programmes or rehabilitation. Certainly there is support in the literature for the use of exercise programmes (Edmonds et al 2004).

The physiotherapist working with this population addresses the secondary effects of physical deconditioning as a result of inactivity, poor sleep patterns and reduced endurance and fitness. It can be helpful to address the notion of vicious and virtuous cycles with the young person and family in order to explain the role deconditioning can have on symptoms and equally the benefits of a rehabilitation programme (Figures 21.1 and 21.2).

The key to the management of young people with CFS/ME is to establish a baseline level of activity. This is considered to be the amount of activity that can be repeated each day with no exacerbation of symptoms. It is essential to ensure that the young person understands that this does not equate to a symptom-free day. The aim is to avoid the typical boom (high-activity day) and bust (low-activity day with exacerbation of symptoms) pattern. Some authors feel that frequent experience of this pattern can lead to avoidance of activity and a perception of activity being harmful (Nijs et al 2004, Gallagher et al 2005). The provision of a supervised, incremental programme assists in supporting the young person to break this cycle and to improve participation. The use of an activity diary can certainly assist in monitoring such activity behaviours and can be a useful outcome measure.

For young people with joint and muscle aches as a predominant feature of their presentation, a full assessment of their range of motion may be necessary to assess for benign joint hypermobility. The literature is mixed with regard to the coexistence of joint hypermobility and CFS/ME. Some suggest that a connective-tissue disorder may explain some symptoms in people with CFS/ME but others oppose this view (Barron et al 2002, van de Putte et al 2005). Regardless of the causal relationship, if hypermobility is noted, the necessary stabilizing and strengthening exercise should be provided.

Sleep is very often disturbed in adolescents with CFS/ME. They present with phasic changes or excessive amounts of time spent in bed. Consistently, rest does not alleviate the individual's fatigue and symptoms. Young people are therefore encouraged to establish a sleep routine and are advised on good sleep hygiene (Box 21.3).

Strength and fitness assessments play an important part in the assessment of the young person's abilities and also in the development of a graded activity programme. The literature has identified that patients with CFS/ME have reduced strength and fitness, thus supporting their inclusion in the management process (Fulcher & White 1997, 2000, van de Putte et al 2005). For assessments of strength and fitness to be meaningful outcome measures, it is essential that

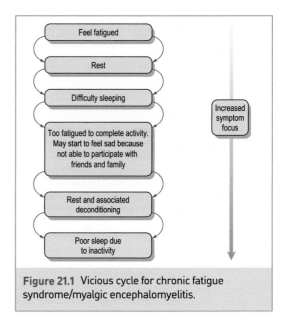

Figure 21.1 Vicious cycle for chronic fatigue syndrome/myalgic encephalomyelitis.

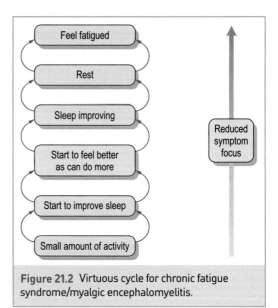

Figure 21.2 Virtuous cycle for chronic fatigue syndrome/myalgic encephalomyelitis.

they are functional measures and easily replicated in the clinical setting. Therefore, to assess strength, the number of stands completed from sitting in a minute can be a quick and efficient measure. Most commonly, submaximal exercise bike or treadmill tests are used (Fulcher & White 1998, Wallman et al 2004, Moss-Morris et al 2005). It is important when doing these tests that the young person feels that any effort is commendable and is encouraged to do the best possible. It is also essential to prepare the young person for possible secondary effects of exercise. Delayed-onset muscle soreness should be addressed so

Box 21.3 Components of good sleep hygiene

- Regular bed and get-up time. Set an alarm for getting up that is not within arm's reach. Try to get up immediately
- Quiet time prior to bed
- A dark room is good for sleeping but light is an important stimulus to waking
- Moderate temperature in bedroom
- Sleep in non-restrictive clothing
- Use guided imagery or relaxation techniques to settle to sleep
- No caffeinated drinks in the evening
- No television in bed
- No exercise prior to sleep
- Use the bed only for sleeping
- Be as active as possible during the day

that the young person does not interpret this as an exacerbation of symptoms, which would reinforce unhelpful thoughts about activity or exercise.

It has been suggested that exercise programmes may benefit patients with CFS/ME not only because they address deconditioning but also they may reduce symptom focus (Moss-Morris et al 2005). For this reason the rating of perceived exertion (RPE) scale can be a useful tool to measure change in cardiovascular fitness but also in perceived effort with the same amount of exercise (Borg 1970). Adults with CFS/ME have been found to terminate fitness testing at 91.5% of their age-predicted maximum compared with 97.5% for the sedentary controls and their RPE was also significantly higher for the activity output (Fulcher & White 2000).

Once the baseline of activity is set and a routine established, it is possible to start the increase in activity. The increment is negotiated with the young person and often relates to the goal. For instance, if the young person's goal is to attend full-time school by completion of the year, it may be that there is a small increase in the total number of lessons attended per week. Alternatively, if the goal focuses on attending a hike at the end of the year, it may be that the walking programme is increased by 1 minute each week. It is important to be imaginative when considering activities or exercises to be graded, to include activities that require mental and physical endurance and fitness. Also be practical in your expectations of the person's abilities. Ultimately, the value of the increment is not important, nor is the activity that is selected, as long as the young person slowly increases the amount of activity completed. Over the period of recovery young people may relapse and at this time it is important to provide encouragement, to re-establish the baseline and restart the process of rehabilitation as soon as possible.

Quantifying fatigue and the symptoms of CFS/ME is difficult. Visual analogue scales, the Chalder Fatigue Scale, Short Form 36 (SF-36, which is designed to measure health status across eight health concepts) and wellness scores have all been used as outcome measures in this population (Ware & Sherbourne 1992, Chalder et al 1993, Fulcher & White 1998, Viner et al 2004). Capturing this information will certainly assist the therapist in measuring improvement, together with monitoring cardiovascular fitness, strength and physical ability.

The use of a graded activity or exercise programme is well supported in the literature. It must encompass all activity in which the young person engages and be forward-thinking in terms of recovery.

CONVERSION DISORDER

Conversion disorder has many names, including hysterical paralysis, somatization disorder, functional disorder and psychosomatic presentation. All of these terms refer to a condition with symptoms and difficulties that appear neurological, or as the result of a physical condition that is not present despite a full medical investigation.

It is thought to occur more commonly in 10–15-year-olds and more often in girls than boys. The prevalence in the general population is estimated to be 15–20 per 100 000; however, when considering people who present to medical centres for investigations, the prevalence is much higher, at approximately 5–20% (Speed 1996). It is proposed that 82.5% of patients present with pseudoseizures, 7.5% with motor symptoms, 7.5% with sensory symptoms and 2.5% have a mixed presentation (Pehlivanturk & Unal 2002). In the majority of cases symptoms are the result of a minor trauma or injury. Factors have been identified that are thought to impair recovery, and include rigid personality trait, anxiety or depression; environmental factors such as domestic stress, feelings of parental rejection, unresolved grief and difficulties at school can all contribute (Leary 2003). It is also certain that recovery can be impeded and prolonged if the young person has an ally who champions the notion that the symptoms are organic (Leslie 1988). There are also positive prognostic factors such as recent onset of symptoms, a single symptom presentation and a good premorbid level of function (Pehlivanturk & Unal 2002).

It would seem from the literature that timely engagement in a graded activity programme can lead to a swift recovery in these young people (Calvert & Jureidini 2003). It is thought that a rehabilitation programme can legitimize a young person's symptoms and thus provide a dignified exit from the current predicament (Sullivan & Buchanan 1989). It is also believed that an inpatient stay may assist in breaking the negative behaviours that have become habitual in the home or school environment. This is especially important if the behaviour is being reinforced by overprotective or anxious families (Brazier & Venning 1997).

It is important that the multidisciplinary team communicates a consistent message to the family. The focus of communication is on the treatment of the problem rather than the cause. The symptom can be acknowledged, for instance if a pseudoseizure is witnessed, but is not the focus of the rehabilitation. Ordinarily, the young person will have had all differential diagnoses excluded so the team should feel confident with this approach. It may be helpful to provide a rationale for treatment using vicious and virtuous cycles, to shift focus from cause and symptom to improving function and ability (Brazier & Venning 1997). Parents and other family members are often quite keen to be involved and it may be helpful to set boundaries but designate particular tasks. If a specific strengthening or stretching programme seems appropriate, the family may be made responsible for this.

The initial physiotherapy assessment must ensure that there are no secondary changes associated with disuse. If muscle weakness or contracture is noted appropriate strategies should be instituted, such as positioning, stretching, strengthening and possibly hydrotherapy. It is also essential to ascertain any symptom patterns or discrepancy between assessment findings. For instance, is there a disparity between the strength assessment and gait disturbance? In the case of loss of balance, does the young person ever fall to the ground? Do pseudoseizures only occur in company and in an awake state? It may also be that short periods of remission may be seen, for instance when there is a need to get to the toilet quickly.

Goal-setting is of primary importance and all sessions need to focus on practice of tasks that link directly to the patient-identified goal. The young person must set the rate of progress in the programme. There should be no attempt to force the young person to do more than he or she feels able. As the young person is responsible for the goal and identifies strategies to achieve it, it is possible to encourage progress through the patient's own motivation to achieve these self-set goals (Calvert & Jureidini 2003). The goals must be clear and the steps to achieving this goal outlined. It is important to provide positive reinforcement for all achievements. For instance, having a star chart or graph that demonstrates progress can be good or functional improvements can be tied to privileges. Regardless, the focus is on the young person's ability and improvement.

Follow-up studies indicate that 85–97% of young people achieve complete recovery (Turgay 1990, Pehlivanturk & Unal 2002). So certainly, with a well-planned and executed rehabilitation programme, improvements should be swift and return to normal life ensured.

PERVASIVE REFUSAL SYNDROME

PRS is a severe and life-threatening disorder that was first described in 1991 and in 1997 specific diagnostic criteria were put forward (Lask et al 1991, Thompson & Nunn 1997). It is characterized by an active, conscious decision to refuse to eat, drink, talk, move or engage in any self-care with a determined resistance to engage in treatment. Although there is often no organic explanation for the presentation, it is crucial that all differential diagnoses are excluded: conversion disorder, AN, CFS/ME, depression, anxiety and somatoform disorder (Lask 2004). The number of patients reported in the literature is few. Despite this, an awareness of PRS is important, as it is possible that it may represent the extreme end of the spectrum of other disorders presented in this chapter.

It was originally thought that PRS was the result of sexual abuse; however, the consensus for the moment is a model of learned helplessness (Lask et al 1991, Thompson & Nunn 1997). The proponents of this model suggest that PRS is the result of events that are seen to be out of the young person's control, for instance, the death of someone close, frequent change of schools or even extreme conflict within the home. There have been no reported cases in the adult literature; the condition appears most often in girls aged between 8 and 15 years of age (Lask 2004).

Treatment for these young people is challenging and very long-term in nature. It is expected to take a year for the young person to recover (Lask 2004). The role of the physiotherapist initially is to minimize the effects of disuse. It may be necessary to institute a stretching routine or positioning using splints to maintain muscle range. In some cases hydrotherapy has also been utilized to provide an opportunity for movement (Nunn & Thompson 1996). It is essential that the young person has control over the physiotherapy management offered. This can be achieved by offering choice and suggesting what the future options may be.

A graded rehabilitation programme should be offered once the young person is ready. Any attempts to speed up the process are likely to lead to relapse. Refusal to engage in an activity or a decline in function will flag to the clinician that the young person is not ready for the next step. The graded rehabilitation programme is not dissimilar to those described earlier in this chapter. It is sufficient to say that all goals must be meaningful to the young person and to be of the patient's own choosing.

Young people with PRS require a team who are patient, understanding and supportive. They present a challenge to all who manage them.

CONCLUSION

For physiotherapists working in the realm of mental health there are significant rewards and challenges. Although a strong understanding of the physiotherapy problem is essential in each illness, it is also vital that there is an understanding of this problem within the context of the illness, the family, home and school environments.

CASE STUDY 21.1

Anorexia nervosa

Caitlyn presents as an outpatient, having recently been discharged from an inpatient stay. The multidisciplinary team feel that it is time to introduce an exercise programme for Caitlyn. It has also been noted that she frequently has neck and shoulder pain. She will continue to be monitored by the team for the next 12 months.

Key components to physiotherapy management

- Caitlyn's current level of fitness and strength are established to provide a strong objective measure of improvement
- It is essential that the physiotherapist is a member of the multidisciplinary team to ensure clear communication with Caitlyn and her family
- The team are open and clear about how her weight goals will affect the opportunities for progression

and participation of the exercise programme. A written contract is signed off by the therapist and Caitlyn. It is essential that the team and Caitlyn adhere to this agreement. It includes the physical goals identified by Caitlyn to ensure that, as the programme progresses to more mainstream activity, they are addressed and achieved

- As Caitlyn has only recently been discharged from hospital, it is important that she starts with a low-level stretch programme, to monitor the effect this has on her weight. An increase in frequency will be determined by achievement of her weight goals.

As Caitlyn also had shoulder and neck pain, once fully assessed it is appropriate to target the stretch programme to address this issue. Information is given about correct posture when using computers and completing other daily tasks.

CASE STUDY 21.2

Chronic fatigue syndrome

Matthew is a 14-year-old boy who has been referred to physiotherapy for the management of his chronic fatigue syndrome/myalgic encephalomyelitis (CFS/ME). He presents with a 36-month history of fatigue, headaches, tummy, muscle and joint pains. He arrives in a wheelchair, as he has found that when he walks for more than hour he becomes sore, especially in his legs and knees. Not long ago he spent most of his time in bed. He has not attended school full-time for 6 months. However, with his slight improvement he is now able to receive home tuition for 5 hours a week.

He goes to bed at 9 p.m., lies awake for a few hours and then sleeps on and off until 12 p.m. Often when he can't sleep he watches TV. Prior to becoming unwell, Matthew was very active – involved in many extracurricular activities such as cross-country running, karate and athletics. About once a week he feels really well. On these days he likes to meet his friends for some football in the park or to go for a bike ride with his family. He hopes to get better soon.

Key components to physiotherapy management

Length of illness: This can have many implications for recovery. It is likely that the family will have made many adjustments to accommodate the illness. This will need to be addressed alongside the physical issues.

Leg pains: This may be secondary to inactivity or a symptom of his CFS/ME.

- Assess calf muscle length
- If there is shortened muscle length, introduce stretching
- Assess joint range to investigate hypermobility
- If hypermobilily is evident, introduce stabilizing exercises.

Mobility: The use of a wheelchair can be useful to allow the family to participate in lengthy excursions outside the home. However, it is important to negotiate a graded withdrawal as Matthew improves.

School reintegration: Once home tuition is established, it may be timely to begin reintegration into school. Ideally, as attendance at school increases, the amount of home tuition decreases. It is best to start with afternoon lessons and to review the timetable fortnightly with gradual reintroduction on a lesson-by-lesson basis. The reintroduction of a lunch or break time is a way to re-engage with peers. It is essential that all stakeholders have input into the plan for reintegration.

Boom and bust pattern: Educate around the benefits of repeatable days and baseline activity. Suggest

continued

activity diary as a means of tracking this and also as a means of gauging improvement.

Sleep: Give sleep hygiene education (Box 21.3).

Age: Matthew is reaching a point in his development that suggests he can become more independent and responsible for treatment decisions. The use of contracts may facilitate increased ownership.

Encouragement: Focus on achievements: anticipate the good and bad days. Discuss strategies to manage this.

The rate of progress of the programme is set by Matthew. It is possible to grade any activity; it is only limited by Matthew's interests. Once the principles of the graded programme are understood, it may be possible to switch to e-mail or telephone contact to reduce the number of trips to the hospital, which can affect the young person's function for a number of days.

Example of initial contract for Matthew

Sleep: quiet time before bed: 9 p.m.

Lights out: 9.30 p.m.

Wake up: 8.30 a.m. using an alarm, Mum to come in at 8.45 a.m.

Out of bed: 9 a.m.

This includes weekends at the moment.

Activity: 5-minute walk at 10.30 a.m. and 3 p.m.

Unstack dishwasher every day

Cook dinner on Thursday nights – this includes talking to Mum about ingredients you need. So don't leave it until the last minute

Screen time: To be no more than 3 hours a day. This includes computer games, TV, internet access

School: Home tutor 2 p.m. Monday to Friday

Rests: half an hour at 11 a.m., and 3.30 p.m. after the walks. Remember this is quiet time, so no TV or computers.

Social: 10-minute phone call or e-mails to friends just to keep in touch each day. Also remember your social bank for the week is 2 hours – so make sure that you don't overspend at the start but spread it over the week.

CASE STUDY 21.3

Conversion disorder

Andrea has been in year 7 at her new school for almost a term now. During the last week of the holidays she had been complaining about a sore leg and then on the first Monday morning of term was unable to walk or even get out of bed. She just felt too sore. When she finally tried to walk she wobbled so badly that her Mum thought she might fall and hurt herself. Andrea stayed away from school for the first few days and since she was not showing any improvement, Mum took her to the general practitioner, who provided her with a wheelchair and sent her to the hospital. Andrea has been in hospital for the last week and has been diagnosed as having a conversion disorder. Her family is really worried about her.

Key components to physiotherapy management

- Ensure that all members of the team are communicating the same message to both Andrea and her family. It is essential that the team message is that rehabilitation is better than rest

- Establish goals that connect physical improvements to positive outcomes, such as going home, or entertainment, such as computer games. Place achievements on display for the whole team and family to admire. Star charts are useful. Delegating the task of completing the chart to Andrea will also improve engagement
- It is also essential that improvements in therapy are transferred to the ward environment. This can be achieved through demonstration on the ward and strong communication
- Providing a therapeutic environment that does not focus on the impairment or symptom provides a way to recover with no loss of face. Hydrotherapy may provide a way for Andrea to demonstrate improvement in her movement, an explanation for her recovery
- Engagement with a psychologist or similarly skilled individual to help Andrea and her family identify the trigger for the illness.

CASE STUDY 21.4

Pervasive refusal syndrome

Matilda is 13 years old. Over the last few weeks she has become less able to move, communicate or eat. She has been admitted to the ward with a diagnosis of pervasive refusal syndrome. She has had a nasogastric tube inserted. She has been wheelchair-dependent for 4 weeks and hasn't walked for 6 weeks. She communicates through grunting.

Initial physiotherapy management

- It is essential to engage with the young person. Matilda is likely to improve slowly and at her own pace. It is not possible to accelerate her improvement but it is essential to provide opportunities when she indicates it is time to improve and move forward
- Ensure that there is no contracture development. If contracture is noted, Matilda should be offered some choice in the management strategy and be given a full explanation of the pros and cons of each alternative, for instance a choice between a positioning programme or splinting.

Physiotherapy progression

- Once Matilda starts to move forward, it may be worth considering hydrotherapy. Establish goals that are achievable and meaningful for her. If Matilda does not feel in control of the pace and direction she is likely to relapse in her function. Always offer choice – for instance, crutches or a pick-up frame – but outline the implications of the choice. In this case crutches are easier to use in small places and provide a more normal gait pattern, although a pick-up frame may feel more stable
- It may be useful to work together with occupational therapy colleagues on transfers from the bed to wheelchair, and from wheelchair to toilet.

It is essential that Matilda is in control of the therapy pace and direction. This can be frustrating for staff and so it may be beneficial to have a debriefing or supervision environment to assist staff in the management of this type of patient.

REFERENCES

Barron D, Cohen BA, Geraghty MT et al 2002 Joint hypermobility is more common in children with chronic fatigue syndrome than in healthy controls. *Journal of Paediatrics* 141: 421–425.

Beaumont PJV, Arthur B, Russell JD et al 1994 Excessive physical activity in dieting disorder patients: proposals for a supervised exercise program. *International Journal of Eating Disorders* 15: 21–36.

Borg GA 1970 Perceived exertion rating as an indicator of somatic stress. *Scandinavian Journal of Rehabilitation Medicine* 2: 92–98.

Brazier DK, Venning HE 1997 Clinical practice review conversion disorders in adolescents: a practical approach to rehabilitation. *British Journal of Rheumatology* 36: 594–598.

Calvert P, Jureidini J 2003 Restrained rehabilitation: an approach to children and adolescents with unexplained sign and symptoms. *Archives of Disease in Childhood* 88: 399–402.

Chalder T, Berelowitz G, Pawlikowska T et al 1993 Development of a fatigue scale. *Journal of Psychosomatic Research* 37: 147–153.

Davis C, Katzman DK, Kaptein S et al 1997 The prevalence of high-level exercise in the eating disorders: etiological implications. *Comprehensive Psychiatry* 38: 321–326.

Edmonds M, McGuire H, Price J 2004 *Exercise Therapy for Chronic Fatigue Syndrome* [Cochrane review]. In: *Cochrane Database of Systematic Reviews*, issue 3.

Fukuda K, Straus SE, Hickie I et al 1994 International Chronic Fatigue Group. The chronic fatigue syndrome: a comprehensive approach to its definition and study. *Annals of Internal Medicine* 121: 953–959.

Fulcher KY, White PD 1997 Randomised controlled trial of graded exercise in patients with the chronic fatigue syndrome. *British Medical Journal* 314: 1647–1652.

Fulcher KY, White PD 1998 Chronic fatigue syndrome. A description of graded exercise treatment. *Physiotherapy* 84: 223–226.

Fulcher KY, White PD 2000 Strength and physiological response to exercise in patients with chronic fatigue syndrome. *Journal of Neurology, Neurosurgery and Psychiatry* 69: 302–307.

Gallagher AM, Coldrick AR, Hedge B et al 2005 Is the chronic fatigue syndrome an exercise phobia? A case control study. *Journal of Psychosomatic Research* 58: 367–373.

Joyce J, Hotopf M, Wessely S 1997 The prognosis of chronic fatigue and chronic fatigue syndrome: a systematic review. *Quarterly Journal of Medicine* 90: 223–233.

Kollai M, Bonyhay I, Jokkel G et al 1994 Cardiac vagal hyperactivity in adolescent anorexia nervosa. *European Heart Journal* 15: 1113–1138.

Lask B 2004 Pervasive refusal syndrome. *Advances in Psychiatric Treatment* 10: 153–159.

Lask B, Britten C, Krill L et al 1991 Children with pervasive refusal. *Archives of Disease in Childhood* 66: 866–869.

Leary PM 2003 Conversion disorder in childhood diagnoses: too late, investigated too much? *Journal of the Royal Society of Medicine* 96: 436–438.

Leslie SA 1988 Diagnosis and treatment of hysterical conversion reactions. *Archives of Disease in Childhood* 63: 506–511.

Lilenfeld LR, Kaye WH, Greno CG et al 1998 A controlled family study of anorexia nervosa and bulimia nervosa: psychiatric disorders in first-degree relatives and effects of proband comorbidity. *Archives of General Psychiatry* 55: 603–610.

Lucas AR, Beard CM, O'Fallon WM et al 1991 50 year trends in the incidence of anorexia nervosa in Rochester, Minn: a population base study. *American Journal of Psychiatry* 148: 917–922.

Mandy A, Broadbridge H 1998 The role of physiotherapy in anorexia nervosa management. *British Journal of Therapy and Rehabilitation* 5: 284–290.

Moss-Morris R, Sharon C, Tobin R et al 2005 A randomised controlled graded exercise trial for chronic fatigue syndrome: outcomes and mechanisms of change. *Journal of Health Psychology* 10: 245–259.

Muscari M 1998 Walking a thin line: managing care for adolescents with anorexia and bulimia. *American Journal of Maternal/Child Nursing* 23: 130–140.

Nijs J, Vanherberghen K, Duquet W et al 2004 Chronic fatigue syndrome: lack of association between pain-related fear of movement and exercise capacity and disability. *Physical Therapy* 84: 696–705.

Nudel DB, Gootman N, Nussbaum MP et al 1984 Altered exercise performance and abnormal sympathetic responses to exercise in patients with anorexia nervosa. *Journal of Paediatrics* 105: 34–37.

Nunn KP, Thompson SL 1996 The pervasive refusal syndrome: learned helplessness and hopelessness. *Clinical Child Psychology and Psychiatry* 1: 121–132.

Pawluck DE, Gorey KM 1998 Secular trends in the incidence of anorexia nervosa: integrative review of population-based studies. *International Journal of Eating Disorders* 23: 347–352.

Pehlivanturk B, Unal F 2002 Conversion disorder in children and adolescents. A 4-year follow-up study. *Journal of Psychosomatic Research* 52: 187–191.

Petretta M, Bonaduce D, Calfi L et al 1997 Heart rate variability as a measure of autonomic nervous system function in anorexia nervosa. *Clinical Cardiology* 20: 219–224.

Rastam M, Gillberg C, Garton M 1989 Anorexia nervosa in a Swedish urban region. A population based study. *British Journal of Psychiatry* 155: 642–646.

Rowland T, Koenings L, Miller N 2003 Myocardinal performance during maximal exercise in adolescents with anorexia nervosa. *Journal of Sports Medicine and Physical Fitness* 43: 202–208.

Speed J 1996 Behavioural management of conversion disorder: retrospective study. *Archives of Physical Medicine and Rehabilitation* 77: 147–154.

St John Sutton MG, Plappert T, Crosby L et al 1985 Effects of reduced left ventricular mass on chamber architecture, loda and function: a study of anorexia nervosa. *Circulation* 72: 991–1000.

Strober M, Freeman R, Lampert C et al 2000 Controlled family study of anorexia nervosa and bulimia nervosa: evidence of shared liability and transmission of partial syndromes. *American Journal of Psychiatry* 157: 393–401.

Sullivan M, Buchanan D 1989 The treatment of conversion disorder in a rehabilitation setting. *Canadian Journal of Rehabilitation* 2: 175–180.

Thien V, Thomas A, Markin D et al 2000 Pilot study of a graded exercise program for the treatment of anorexia nervosa. *International Journal of Eating Disorders* 28: 101–106.

Thompson SL, Nunn KP 1997 The pervasive refusal syndrome: the RAHC experience. *Clinical Child Psychology and Psychiatry* 2: 145–165.

Tokumura M, Yoshiba S, Tanaka T et al 2003 Prescribed exercise training improves exercise capacity of convalescent children and adolescents with anorexia nervosa. *European Journal of Pediatrics* 162: 430–431.

Turgay A 1990 Treatment outcome for children and adolescents with conversion disorder. *Canadian Journal of Psychiatry* 35: 585–589.

van de Putte EM, Uiterwaal CSPM, Bots ML et al 2005 Is chronic fatigue syndrome a connective tissue disorder? A cross sectional study in adolescents. *Paediatrics* 115: 415–422.

Viner RM, Gregorowski A, Wine C et al 2004 Outpatient rehabilitation treatment of chronic fatigue syndrome (CFS/ME). *Archives of Diseases in Childhood* 89: 615–619.

Wallman KE, Morton AR, Goodman C et al 2004 Randomised controlled trail of graded exercise in chronic fatigue syndrome. *Medical Journal of Australia* 180: 444–448.

Ware J, Sherbourne C 1992 The MOS 36-short form health survey (SF-36). *Medical Care* 30: 473–483.

Index